TEXTBOOK OF
SURGERY
Pocket Companion

SABISTON

TEXTBOOK OF

SURGERY

Pocket Companion

DAVID C. SABISTON, Jr., M.D.
James B. Duke Professor of Surgery
Chief of Staff
Duke University Medical Center
Durham, North Carolina

H. KIM LYERLY, M.D.
Assistant Professor of Surgery
and Immunology
Duke University Medical Center
Durham, North Carolina

W.B. SAUNDERS COMPANY
A Division of Harcourt Brace & Company
Philadelphia London Toronto Montreal Sydney Tokyo

W.B. SAUNDERS COMPANY
A Division of Harcourt Brace & Company

The Curtis Center
Independence Square West
Philadelphia, Pennsylvania 19106

TEXTBOOK OF SURGERY
POCKET COMPANION   ISBN 0–7216–8670–2

Printed in the United States of America.

Last digit is the print number: 9   8   7   6   5   4   3   2   1

CONTRIBUTORS

JOHN G. ADAMS, JR., M.D.
University of Missouri–Columbia School of Medicine

N. SCOTT ADZICK, M.D.
University of Pennsylvania School of Medicine

ROBERT W. ANDERSON, M.D.
Duke University Medical Center

PAUL S. AUERBACH, M.D., M.S.
Sterling Healthcare Group

ERLE H. AUSTIN III, M.D.
University of Louisville Medical School

WILLIAM H. BAKER, M.D.
Loyola University Chicago Stritch School of Medicine

CLYDE F. BARKER, M.D.
University of Pennsylvania School of Medicine

ROBERT H. BARTLETT, M.D.
University of Michigan School of Medicine

JAMES M. BECKER, M.D.
Boston University School of Medicine

FOLKERT O. BELZER, M.D. (deceased)
University of Wisconsin Medical School

MICHAEL E. BEREND, M.D.
Duke University Medical Center

JOHN J. BERGAN, M.D.
Loma Linda University Medical School

AMITAVA BISWAS, M.D.
Harvard Medical School

R. RANDAL BOLLINGER, M.D., PH.D.
Duke University Medical Center

R. MORTON BOLMAN III, M.D.
University of Minnesota

WILLIAM Z. BORER, M.D.
Thomas Jefferson University

JOHN BOSTWICK III, M.D.
Emory University School of Medicine

GENE D. BRANUM, M.D.
Emory University School of Medicine

KENNETH L. BRAYMAN, M.D., Ph.D.
University of Pennsylvania School of Medicine

ALYSON J. BREISCH, R.N., M.S.
Duke University School of Nursing

MURRAY F. BRENNAN, M.D.
Cornell University Medical College

GERT H. BRIEGER, M.D., Ph.D.
Johns Hopkins University School of Medicine

JOHN H. CALHOON, M.D.
University of Texas Health Science Center at San Antonio

JOHN L. CAMERON, M.D.
Johns Hopkins University School of Medicine

DAVID N. CAMPBELL, M.D.
University of Colorado Health Sciences Center

GRANT W. CARLSON, M.D.
Emory University School of Medicine

C. JAMES CARRICO, M.D.
University of Texas Southwestern Medical Center

JAMES CERILLI, M.D.
University of Rochester Medical Center

RAVI S. CHARI, M.D.
University of Toronto

WILLIAM G. CHEADLE, M.D.
University of Louisville School of Medicine

LAURENCE Y. CHEUNG, M.D.
University of Kansas School of Medicine

W. RANDOLPH CHITWOOD, Jr., M.D.
East Carolina University School of Medicine

BRYAN M. CLARY, M.D.
Duke University Medical Center

PIERRE A. CLAVIEN, M.D., Ph.D.
Duke University Medical Center

JOEL D. COOPER, M.D.
Washington University School of Medicine

JAMES L. COX, M.D.
Washington University School of Medicine

FRED A. CRAWFORD, JR., M.D.
Medical University of South Carolina

ROBERT D. CROOM III, M.D.
University of North Carolina School of Medicine

THOMAS A. D'AMICO, M.D.
Duke University Medical Center

MARK G. DAVIES, M.D., PH.D.
Duke University Medical Center

R. DUANE DAVIS, JR., M.D.
Duke University Medical Center

RICHARD H. DEAN, M.D.
Bowman Gray School of Medicine

HAILE T. DEBAS, M.D.
University of California, San Francisco

JEROME J. DeCOSSE, M.D., PH.D.
Cornell University Medical College

E. PATCHEN DELLINGER, M.D.
University of Washington School of Medicine

MARK E. DENTZ, M.D.
Duke University Medical Center

ARNOLD G. DIETHELM, M.D.
University of Alabama at Birmingham

GERARD M. DOHERTY, M.D.
Washington University

ROGER R. DOZOIS, M.D.
Mayo Medical School

ANDRÉ DURANCEAU, M.D.
University of Montreal

DAVID W. EASTER, M.D.
University of California, San Diego

JAMES M. EDWARDS, M.D.
Oregon Health Sciences University

JOSEPH R. ELBEERY, M.D.
East Carolina University School of Medicine

STEVE EUBANKS, M.D.
Duke University Medical Center

SAMIR M. FAKHRY, M.D.
University of North Carolina School of Medicine

JOHN A. FEAGIN, M.D.
Duke University Medical Center

AARON S. FINK, M.D.
Emory University School of Medicine

JOSEF E. FISCHER, M.D.
University of Cincinnati College of Medicine

ROBERT D. FITCH, M.D.
Duke University Medical Center

WILLIAM R. FLINN, M.D.
University of Maryland Medical School

M. WAYNE FLYE, M.D., Ph.D.
Washington University School of Medicine

THOMAS J. FOGARTY, M.D.
Stanford University School of Medicine

DOUGLAS L. FRAKER, M.D.
University of Pennsylvania School of Medicine

ALLAN H. FRIEDMAN, M.D.
Duke University Medical Center

DAVID FROMM, M.D.
Wayne State University

HERBERT E. FUCHS, M.D., Ph.D.
Duke University Medical Center

DAVID A. FULLERTON, M.D.
Northwestern University

STANLEY A. GALL, Jr., M.D.
St. John's Hospital

WILLIAM E. GARRETT, Jr., M.D., Ph.D.
Duke University Medical Center

WILLIAM A. GAY, JR., M.D.
Washington University School of Medicine

J. WILLIAM GAYNOR, M.D.
Children's Hospital of Philadelphia

COHAVA GELBER, PH.D.
Duke University Medical Center

ANNETINE C. GELIJNS, PH.D.
Columbia University College of Physicians and Surgeons

GREGORY S. GEORGIADE, M.D.
Duke University Medical Center

FARID GHARAGOZLOO, M.D.
Georgetown University School of Medicine

DONALD D. GLOWER, M.D.
Duke University Medical Center

J. LEONARD GOLDNER, M.D.
Duke University Medical Center

RICHARD D. GOLDNER, M.D.
Duke University Medical Center

CLEON W. GOODWIN, JR., M.D.
U.S. Army Institute of Surgical Research

JOHN GORECKI, M.D.
Duke University Medical Center

LAWRENCE J. GOTTLIEB, M.D.
University of Chicago School of Medicine

JOHN P. GRANT, M.D.
Duke University Medical Center

PAUL D. GREIG, M.D.
University of Toronto

KATHERINE P. GRICHNIK, M.D.
Duke University Medical Center

HERMES C. GRILLO, M.D.
Harvard Medical School

JAY L. GROSFELD, M.D.
Indiana University School of Medicine

FREDERICK L. GROVER, M.D.
University of Colorado Health Sciences Center

J. CAULIE GUNNELLS, Jr., M.D.
Duke University Medical Center

JEFFREY A. HAGEN, M.D.
University of Southern California, Los Angeles

PER-OTTO HAGEN, M.D.
Duke University Medical Center

CARL E. HAISCH, M.D.
East Carolina University School of Medicine

JOHN D. HAMILTON, M.D.
Duke University Medical Center

CHARLES B. HAMMOND, M.D.
Duke University Medical Center

WILLIAM T. HARDAKER, Jr., M.D.
Duke University Medical Center

ALDEN H. HARKEN, M.D.
University of Colorado

DAVID H. HARPOLE, Jr., M.D.
Duke University Medical Center

JOHN M. HARRELSON, M.D.
Duke University Medical Center

MARQUIS E. HART, M.D.
University of California, San Diego

JEFFREY S. HEINLE, M.D.
Boston Children's Hospital

JULIO HOCHBERG, M.D.
West Virginia University Health Sciences Center

WILLIAM L. HOLMAN, M.D.
University of Alabama at Birmingham

RICHARD A. HOPKINS, M.D.
Brown University School of Medicine

J. DIRK IGLEHART, M.D.
Duke University Medical Center

SUZANNE T. ILDSTAD, M.D.
University of Pittsburgh School of Medicine

ANTHONY L. IMBEMBO, M.D.
University of Maryland School of Medicine

GLYN G. JAMIESON, M.D.
University of Adelaide

MICHAEL E. JESSEN, M.D.
University of Texas Southwestern Medical Center at Dallas

OLGA JONASSON, M.D.
University of Illinois

R. SCOTT JONES, M.D.
University of Virginia School of Medicine

ROBERT H. JONES, M.D.
Duke University Medical Center

GREGORY J. JURKOVICH, M.D.
University of Washington

LARRY R. KAISER, M.D.
University of Pennsylvania School of Medicine

STEVEN S. KANG, M.D.
Loyola University Chicago Stritch School of Medicine

KEITH A. KELLY, M.D.
Mayo Medical School

ALLAN D. KIRK, M.D., PH.D.
University of Wisconsin Health Center

JAMES K. KIRKLIN, M.D.
University of Alabama at Birmingham

STUART J. KNECHTLE, M.D.
University of Wisconsin School of Medicine

THEODORE C. KOUTLAS, M.D.
East Carolina University School of Medicine

THOMAS J. KRIZEK, M.D.
University of South Florida

TERRY C. LAIRMORE, M.D.
Washington University School of Medicine

GREGORY J. LANDRY, M.D.
Oregon Health Sciences University

BERNARD LANGER, M.D.
University of Toronto

JEFFREY H. LAWSON, M.D., Ph.D.
Duke University Medical Center

ALAN T. LEFOR, M.D.
University of California, San Diego

GEORGE S. LEIGHT, Jr., M.D.
Duke University Medical Center

L. SCOTT LEVIN, M.D.
Duke University Medical Center

JONATHAN J. LEWIS, M.D., Ph.D.
Cornell University Medical College

R. ERIC LILLY, M.D.
Duke University Medical Center

JAMES E. LOWE, M.D.
Duke University Medical Center

H. KIM LYERLY, M.D.
Duke University Medical Center

GREG J. MACKAY, M.D.
The Nalle Clinic

RAYMOND G. MAKHOUL, M.D.
Medical College of Virginia

JOHN A. MANNICK, M.D.
Harvard Medical School

JAMES F. MARKMANN, M.D., Ph.D.
University of Pennsylvania School of Medicine

G. ROBERT MASON, M.D., Ph.D.
Loyola University Chicago Stritch School of Medicine

DOUGLAS J. MATHISEN, M.D.
Harvard Medical School

JAMES R. MAULT, M.D.
Duke University Medical Center

RICHARD L. McCANN, M.D.
Duke University Medical Center

DONALD E. McCOLLUM, M.D.
Duke University Medical Center

JOHN C. McDONALD, M.D.
Louisiana State University School of Medicine

DAVID C. McGIFFIN, M.D.
University of Alabama at Birmingham

ANTHONY A. MEYER, M.D., Ph.D.
University of North Carolina School of Medicine

WILLIAM C. MEYERS, M.D.
University of Massachusetts Medical Center

GREGORY L. MONETA, M.D.
Oregon Health Sciences University

FRANK G. MOODY, M.D.
University of Texas Medical School, Houston

A. R. MOOSSA, M.D.
University of California, San Diego

JON F. MORAN, M.D.
East Carolina University School of Medicine

ALAN J. MOSKOWITZ, M.D.
Columbia University College of Physicians and Surgeons

JOSEPH A. MOYLAN, M.D.
University of Miami School of Medicine

GORDON F. MURRAY, M.D.
West Virginia University Health Sciences Center

DAVID L. NAHRWOLD, M.D.
Northwestern University Medical School

ALI NAJI, M.D., Ph.D.
University of Pennsylvania School of Medicine

ELAINE E. NELSON, M.D.
Stanford Medical Center/Kaiser Permanente

JEFFREY A. NORTON, M.D.
Washington University School of Medicine

JAMES A. NUNLEY, M.D.
Duke University Medical Center

JOHN A. OLSON, JR., M.D., PH.D.
Washington University School of Medicine

SUSAN L. ORLOFF, M.D.
University of California, San Francisco

MARK B. ORRINGER, M.D.
University of Michigan Medical School

ALBERT D. PACIFICO, M.D.
University of Alabama at Birmingham

THEODORE N. PAPPAS, M.D.
Duke University Medical Center

DAVID F. PAULSON, M.D.
Duke University Medical Center

JOSE A. PEREZ, M.D.
Duke University Medical Center

WILLIAM S. PIERCE, M.D.
Pennsylvania State University College of Medicine

JEFFREY L. PLATT, M.D.
Duke University Medical Center

HIRAM C. POLK, JR., M.D.
University of Louisville School of Medicine

WALTER J. PORIES, M.D.
East Carolina University School of Medicine

JOHN M. PORTER, M.D.
Oregon Health Sciences University

BASIL A. PRUITT, JR., M.D.
University of Texas Health Science Center at San Antonio

SCOTT K. PRUITT, M.D., PH.D.
Duke University Medical Center

CEMIL M. PURUT, M.D.
Duke University Medical Center

MICHAEL F. REED, M.D.
Harvard Medical School

KEITH REEMTSMA, M.D., MED. SC.D.
Columbia University College of Physicians and Surgeons

J. G. REVES, M.D.
Duke University Medical Center

NORMAN M. RICH, M.D.
F. Edward Hebert School of Medicine,
Uniformed Services University of the Health Sciences

WILLIAM J. RICHARDSON, M.D.
Duke University Medical Center

LAYTON F. RIKKERS, M.D.
University of Wisconsin Clinical Science Center

MICHELLE L. ROBBIN, M.D.
University of Alabama at Birmingham

CARY N. ROBERTSON, M.D.
Duke University Medical Center

MICHAEL S. ROHR, M.D., PH.D.
Bowman Gray School of Medicine

ROLANDO ROLANDELLI, M.D.
Medical College of Pennsylvania and Hahnemann University

FRANCIS E. ROSATO, M.D.
Jefferson Medical College

ERIC A. ROSE, M.D.
Columbia University College of Physicians and Surgeons

JOEL J. ROSLYN, M.D.
Medical College of Pennsylvania and Hahnemann University

PABLO RUBINSTEIN, M.D.
New York Blood Center

DAVID C. SABISTON, JR., M.D.
Duke University Medical Center

JAMES D. ST. LOUIS, M.D.
Duke University Medical Center

PHILIP R. SCHAUER, M.D.
University of Pittsburgh

BRUCE D. SCHIRMER, M.D.
University of Virginia

STEVE J. SCHWAB, M.D.
Duke University Medical Center

STEWART M. SCOTT, M.D. (deceased)
Duke University Medical Center

SEAN P. SCULLY, M.D., Ph.D.
Duke University Medical Center

MARK W. SEBASTIAN, M.D.
Duke University Medical Center

H. F. SEIGLER, M.D.
Duke University Medical Center

GEORGE F. SHELDON, M.D.
University of North Carolina School of Medicine

G. TOM SHIRES, M.D.
Texas Tech University School of Medicine

G. TOM SHIRES III, M.D.
University of Texas Southwestern Medical Center at Dallas

JOSEPH B. SHRAGER, M.D.
Massachusetts General Hospital

KAREN S. SIBERT, M.D.
Duke University Medical Center

DONALD SILVER, M.D.
University of Missouri–Columbia School of Medicine

NORMAN A. SILVERMAN, M.D.
Case Western Reserve School of Medicine

RICHARD L. SIMMONS, M.D.
University of Pittsburgh School of Medicine

KEVIN M. SITTIG, M.D.
Louisiana State University School of Medicine

CRAIG L. SLINGLUFF, Jr., M.D.
University of Virginia School of Medicine

MILTON M. SLOCUM, M.D.
University of Missouri–Columbia School of Medicine

JAMES B. SNOW, Jr., M.D.
National Institutes of Health

HANS W. SOLLINGER, M.D., PH.D.
University of Wisconsin School of Medicine

JAMES H. SOUTHARD, PH.D.
University of Wisconsin Medical School

KEVIN P. SPEER, M.D.
Duke University Medical Center

THOMAS L. SPRAY, M.D.
University of Pennsylvania School of Medicine

ROBERT J. STANLEY, M.D.
University of Alabama at Birmingham

DELFORD L. STICKEL, M.D.
Duke University Medical Center

DAVID J. SUGARBAKER, M.D.
Harvard Medical School

BRUCE A. SULLENGER, PH.D.
Duke University Medical Center

R. SUDHIR SUNDARESAN, M.D.
Washington University School of Medicine

SCOTT J. SWANSON, M.D.
Harvard Medical School

TIMOTHY TAKARO, M.D.
Duke University Medical Center

JAMES L. TALBERT, M.D.
University of Florida College of Medicine

MARK TEDDER, M.D.
Duke University Medical Center

ANGUS W. THOMSON, PH.D., D.SC.
University of Pittsburgh School of Medicine

ROBERT D. TIEN, M.D., M.P.H.
Duke University Medical Center

DENNIS A. TURNER, M.D., M.A.
Duke University Medical Center

DOUGLAS TYLER, M.D.
Duke University Medical Center

ROSS M. UNGERLEIDER, M.D.
Duke University Medical Center

JAMES R. URBANIAK, M.D.
Duke University Medical Center

THOMAS PARKER VAIL, M.D.
Duke University Medical Center

PETER VAN TRIGT III, M.D.
Cardiovascular and Thoracic Surgeons of Greensboro

STEVEN N. VASLEF, M.D., Ph.D.
Duke University Medical Center

ROBERT B. WALLACE, M.D.
Georgetown University Medical Center

HENRY L. WALTERS III, M.D.
Wayne State University School of Medicine

JOHN L. WEINERTH, M.D.
Duke University Medical Center

SAMUEL A. WELLS, Jr., M.D.
Washington University School of Medicine

H. BROWNELL WHEELER, M.D.
University of Massachusetts Medical School

ANTHONY D. WHITTEMORE, M.D.
Harvard Medical School

ROBERT H. WILKINS, M.D.
Duke University Medical Center

DOUGLAS W. WILMORE, M.D.
Harvard Medical School

WALTER G. WOLFE, M.D.
Duke University Medical Center

BRUCE G. WOLFF, M.D.
Mayo Medical School

ROBERT J. WOOD, M.D.
Emory University School of Medicine

CHARLES J. YEO, M.D.
Johns Hopkins University School of Medicine

KARL A. ZUCKER, M.D.
University of New Mexico School of Medicine

PREFACE

The *Pocket Companion* is designed to provide an immediate source of key information on each surgical topic covered in the *Textbook of Surgery: The Biological Basis of Modern Surgical Practice*. It should be especially helpful in urgent situations, as the text fits conveniently into a coat pocket. It is particularly designed for medical students and residents as an immediate and readily available source of pertinent information. On numerous occasions, it is helpful to read a condensed version of a subject prior to a complete description, which can be read in a more leisurely manner. In all instances, the reader is referred to the 15th Edition for complete coverage of the topic, because the *Pocket Companion* represents the first step in the process.

Information included in the *Pocket Companion* is taken directly from the *Textbook of Surgery* and is prepared in a condensed form by the same authors. In each instance, the authors have been chosen because of their familiarity with and knowledge of the specific topic being addressed. Rapid strides in medicine continue, with increasing emphasis on its basic science aspects and its key role in the diagnosis and treatment of surgical disorders. In addition, several new chapters have been added and include:

Molecular Biology in Surgery by Drs. H. Kim Lyerly and Bruce A. Sullenger;

Clinical Outcomes in Surgery by Drs. Alan J. Moskowitz, Keith Reemtsma, Eric A. Rose, and Annetine C. Gelijns;

Laparoscopic Surgery by Drs. Steve Eubanks and Philip R. Schauer;

Plastic and Maxillofacial Surgery by Drs. Greg J. Mackay, Grant W. Carlson, Robert J. Wood, and John Bostwick III;

Surgical Management of Pulmonary Emphysema by Dr. James R. Mault;

Mesothelioma by Drs. David J. Sugarbaker, Michael F. Reed, and Scott J. Swanson.

The contributors to this edition have provided excellent summaries of their respective chapters in the *Textbook of Surgery*, and the editors are deeply appreciative of their fine efforts.

DAVID C. SABISTON, JR., M.D.
H. KIM LYERLY, M.D.

CONTENTS

1

THE DEVELOPMENT OF SURGERY:
Historical Aspects Important in the Origin and Development of Modern Surgical Science
Gert H. Brieger, M.D., Ph.D.

The history of disease is at least as old as the history of mankind. One can assume that surgical disease, or the surgical response to disease, is of similar antiquity. The basic forms of disease—tumors, infections, trauma, and congenital abnormalities—have existed unchanged. Today's surgeons obviously manage them in a different manner than did their colleagues of prehistoric times, yet some aspects of the surgeon's work are timeless.

By the thirteenth and fourteenth centuries, surgery was looked down on and avoided by physicians, who had received their education in the universities that were now arising all over Europe. Along with theology and law, medicine was usually one of the basic faculties. Surgeons, on the other hand, were often unlettered, lower-class men who were scorned in clerical circles. The surgeons were taught the ways of their craft by apprenticeship.

The barbers and surgeons of England had belonged to separate guilds since the fourteenth century. In 1540 a compromise as to the rights and duties of each was achieved, and a single company of barbers and surgeons was formed. Surgeons agreed to do no barbering, and the barbers restricted their surgery to dentistry. The union lasted 200 years. In 1745 it was dissolved, and the surgeons' company again existed independently, jealously guarding its prerogatives and protecting its interests. In 1800 George III chartered the Royal College of Surgeons of London, which by charter from Queen Victoria in 1843 became the Royal College of Surgeons of England.

Anatomic dissection began to be more common again at the end of the thirteenth century. With the first manual for dissection, written by Mondino de Luzzi in 1316, students had some guidance. The early dissections were still often confined to the bodies of animals and sometimes were really autopsies performed to ascertain the cause of death, especially if foul play were suspected. These dissections were usually the responsibility of the surgeon. Only by the middle of the fifteenth century did anatomic dissection become common enough that a special theater for it was built in Padua.

By the end of the fifteenth century and early in the sixteenth

---

See the corresponding chapter or part in the *Textbook of Surgery*, 15th edition, pp. 1–15, for a more detailed discussion of this topic, including a comprehensive list of references.

century, occasional illustrated medical works began to appear. Johannes de Ketham's *Fasiculus Medicinae* (Venice, 1491) and Berengario da Carpi's *Commentari . . . Super Anatomia Mundini . . .* are two of the best known. Others appeared, but the best and most lasting proved to be the *De Humani Corporis Fabrica* of Andreas Vesalius. The publication of the *Fabrica* in 1543 coincided with the publication of another great book in the history of science, the *De Revolutionibus Orbium Coelestium* of Nicolaus Copernicus.

The importance of Vesalius is that by his work and example he set forth a program. The famous frontispiece depicting him at the dissecting table, knife in hand, is itself programmatic. This young man, born in Louvain in 1514 and educated in Brussels and Paris, went to Padua to finish his medical studies. At the age of 23, upon receiving his degree, he was appointed professor of anatomy and surgery, an important academic combination for centuries to come.

There were numerous obstacles blocking the advance of surgery. Pain, infection, hemorrhage, and shock were four of the most difficult to overcome. As each was dealt with, the bounds of surgery enlarged. As the limits of surgery were extended, the field of the individual surgeons seems to have become more and more restricted.

Since the fundamental aim of all medical art and science has always been to alleviate human pain and suffering, the development of anesthesia for use during surgical operations ranks as one of the most dramatic discoveries in the annals of medicine. The use of alcohol, mandrake root, opium, and even bleeding or reduction of blood flow to the brain to reduce sensibility were known to the ancients in a crude sense, but the really effective use of general anesthesia can be dated very precisely to the 1840s. In 1842 a rural Georgia practitioner, Crawford W. Long, used ether in the removal of small skin tumors, but he did not report his results until 3 years after William Morton successfully etherized a patient for John Collins Warren on October 16, 1846, at the Massachusetts General Hospital. James Young Simpson of Edinburgh introduced chloroform in the next year, and a new age in surgery was born. Speed of operation would now no longer be the hallmark of the great surgeons.

Anesthesia found speedy acceptance. The same, unfortunately, cannot be said for the attempts to control infection. Wound healing in the days before Joseph Lister was a confused and depressing aspect of surgery. Wounding, either by accident or done by the surgeon, often was followed by what was called "irritative fever," usually lasting a few days and causing accumulation of pus in the wound.

In his earlier Edinburgh and Glasgow years, Lister investigated a number of problems closely related to surgery, such as inflammation, wound healing, and the role of blood coagulation in both. His approach to the problems of surgery was distinctly modern, in the sense that it was scientific and physiologic. Despite Lister's attempts to clean up his wards and to perform surgery as cleanly as possible, there was still an appalling rate of the common surgical complications of hospital gangrene, pyemia, and erysipelas among his patients.

In the years just before 1865, the French scientist Louis Pasteur slowly worked out what came to be a germ theory of disease. He clearly showed that fermentation and putrefaction, observed since ancient days, were caused by living, multiplying matter. He reasoned that pus formation, wound infection, and some fevers also must be caused by minute organisms from the environment.

Lister's first papers describing his method and its success appeared in 1867. In the following years, he changed the technical details of his method, added the steam-powered spray for the operating environment, and continued to fight for his idea in many publications. As the years went by, he was able to perform operations safely that previously no capable surgeon would have dared to attempt. The successful wiring of a fractured patella in 1877, which converted a closed fracture to an open one, brought much scorn on him, but patience, doggedness, and scrupulous attention to detail led eventually to complete success. Lister admitted in the 1880s that the spray was not necessary and indeed may have been harmful to operators and patients alike. He gracefully accepted the development of aseptic surgery by the Germans and acknowledged that it was but a step beyond his own work and a logical extension of it.

The acceptance of listerism was uneven and, in our retrospective view, seemingly quite slow. There were many reasons for this, most of them not tied to simple conservatism or resistance to change. Lister's method was complicated; the carbolic acid was an unpleasant nuisance and could actually be harmful; and the method was time-consuming and expensive and required assistance. Some surgeons and physicians believed the germ theory to be mere speculation; hence, the underlying theory or the rationale for Lister's technique also was slow to be accepted. Also, one must remember that many leading surgeons simply could not duplicate Lister's good results, hard as they might try. Theodor Billroth was one who tried the method, wanted to accept it, but found it somewhat frustrating. By the late 1870s he had adopted listerism fully, but not without much discouragement.

Among the many difficult technical problems faced by nineteenth-century surgeons was that of reconnecting the divided ends of hollow tubes, especially blood vessels and intestine. Just as cardiovascular surgery has captured both public and professional attention in the past two or three decades, 90 to 100 years ago abdominal surgery played the same role. The successful removal of an inflamed appendix before rupture, the Billroth operations for esophageal and gastric cancer causing obstruction, the improved hernia operations of Bassini and Halsted, and abdominal operations for such other reasons as diseases of the ovary all caused great excitement in the medical world of the late nineteenth century.

Much has been written in the last 100 years about the training of the surgeon, the proper qualifications, and what it means to be a surgeon. Between the simple apprenticeship or even the transfer of knowledge from father to son that held sway until the nineteenth century and the thorough grounding in pathology, research, and operative and postoperative management required of today's surgeon, much surgical history has passed.

The subject of surgical training in America invariably brings to mind the name of William S. Halsted, no doubt partly because of his famous address entitled, "The Training of the Surgeon," delivered at Yale in 1904. Halsted, who was born in New York City in 1852 and died in Baltimore 70 years later, made numerous important contributions to surgical technique and teaching.

Halsted developed improved methods for operating on hernias and cancer of the breast; he introduced the use of rubber gloves in surgery; and he constantly stressed the relationship of surgery to physiology. Careful handling of tissues and the minimization of blood loss were concepts he passed on to the many fine surgeons he trained over 30 years. Justifiable as has been his fame, Halsted was not solely responsible for establishing the surgical residency system as we know it. He himself would have been the first to note that the great German teachers of surgery, especially von Langenbeck and his pupils, including Billroth, were his models. Furthermore, Halsted's colleague, William Osler, deserves equal credit for instituting the system at Johns Hopkins.

Late twentieth-century surgery has become increasingly a part of human biology. It is not only skill with surgical tools that was for so long the hallmark of the leading surgeons but a knowledge of the body's physiologic processes and their control that has assumed equal, if not even greater, importance. Such knowledge has facilitated the development of techniques such as hypothermia, safer anesthesia, and the heart-lung machine. The great expansion of the surgeon's ability to play a role in an increasing number of afflictions has been materially influenced by the ability to regulate the body's fluids and electrolytes and especially by the advent of better means to control postoperative infections.

Perhaps nothing is more indicative of the great changes that have occurred, even in just the past 100 years, than the fact that surgery has moved from the theatricality and drama of the operating theater to the privacy and relative sterility of the operating room. No longer is the drama of the operation or the technical skill or virtuosity of the surgeon on center stage. In the old surgery it was the art that predominated. In the new surgery it is science. The focus has thus shifted increasingly from the operation itself to the results that now provide the drama.

2

MOLECULAR BIOLOGY IN SURGERY

H. Kim Lyerly, M.D., and Bruce A. Sullenger, Ph.D.

Deoxyribonucleic acid (DNA) consists of two strands of nucleotides wrapped around each other to form a complex double helix. The building blocks of each strand are deoxyribonucleotides, which consist of one of four bases—adenine (A), guanine (G), cytosine (C), and thymine (T)—a sugar-deoxyribose, and a covalently joined phosphate group. The double helical structure of DNA allows for the direct copying or replication of genetic instructions. This sequence of bases in a gene encodes the genetic instructions for the building of a specific peptide chain, and each amino acid is coded for by a specific set of three nonoverlapping nucleotide triplets known as *codons.*

A gene not only must include the instructions about the amino acid chain to be made but also must contain sequences that regulate the transcription of the gene to ensure that the protein product is made in its appropriate amounts, in the correct tissues, and at particular times during cellular development and differentiation. Almost all mammalian genes have flanking regulatory regions as well as sequences known as *introns* that interrupt their coding segments, called *exons.* Gene expression can be regulated at a number of points, including transcription, translation, and protein modification.

CELL GROWTH AND REGULATION

Signal transduction is defined as the conversion of an extracellular signal into the series of intracellular events that results in a cellular function. After the ligand binds to a specific cell surface receptor, the consequent conformational change, usually receptor dimerization, results in its activation. The receptor then associates with a coupler protein, usually a G protein, which, in turn, binds to an effector. Effectors catalyze the production of small molecules that act as second messengers in the cell and directly affect processes, such as the opening of a channel that, for example, results in the flow of ions. The net effect is a physiologic process, such as muscle contraction, secretion, or cell growth. Some processes are promptly evoked. Others, like cell division, require new protein synthesis, and the transcription factors involved in that process are also considered part of the signal transduction pathway.

The cyclins, proteins that increase or decrease at different stages of the cell cycle, regulate cyclin-dependent kinases,

---

See the corresponding chapter or part in the *Textbook of Surgery,* 15th edition, pp. 16–35, for a more detailed discussion of this topic, including a comprehensive list of references.

which in turn phosphorylate critical targets at specific points in the cell cycle. In addition to the cyclin control of cell division, another set of genes appears to regulate the cell cycle at a series of points that may serve to stop progression of the cell cycle if something has gone wrong.

THE HUMAN GENOME

It has been estimated that there may be somewhere between 50,000 and 200,000 important genes to be found and mapped. One of the most informative diseases includes the inherited hemoglobin disorders, of which examples exist that represent the broad spectrum of possible mutations including single-base changes or deletions and deletions of entire genes. Furthermore, mutations include insertions of new genetic material and inversions of stretches of DNA. Finally, in addition to mutations that directly affect the encoded protein product, mutations can occur that affect the regulatory regions of the gene that control the transcription and ultimately expression, as well as base substitutions that interfere with the processing or translation of messenger RNAs.

Thus there may already exist a reasonable idea of the repertoire of molecular abnormalities underlying single-gene disorders. Although the single-gene disorders have provided information regarding the nature of abnormalities that can occur and disrupt the expression of specific protein, when common disorders are considered, the potential for even more subtle changes within the context of complementary or confounding aberrations to have a profound influence on the function of cells is enormous. For this reason, the overwhelming complexity of more common disorders have not lent themselves to the molecular dissection portrayed in the less common single-gene disorders. In addition to the complexities involved in multiple-gene disorders evoked by the interaction of each of the genes involved, many of them have environmental factors that play a major role in their etiology.

CANCER GENETICS

The development of cancer is a complex and multistep process, originating in a phenotypically normal cell and culminating in the development of cells with deregulated growth characteristics and the ability to invade and metastasize. Cancer, even the nonhereditary forms, is considered a collection of polygenic disorders, since alterations in a number of genes have been shown to contribute to its origin and progression. In general, the genes that are altered in the development of cancer fall into three broad categories: oncogenes, the presence of which may cause cellular transformation; tumor suppressor genes, the absence of which may cause cellular transformation; and mutator genes. The genetic changes that are found in otherwise normal cells that lead to their transformation can be due to inherited defects, in which case a hereditary predisposition to cancer is found. In addition, genetic changes leading to cancer may be due to DNA rearrangements during the cell cycle, viral infection, exposure to mutagenic agents, or inherited defects in DNA replication or repair. These latter defects do not in themselves lead to transformation but may lead to an increase in the mutation rate in other genes directly responsible for the development of cancer. While understanding the mechanisms of proto-oncogene activation is important in understanding carcinogenesis, determining the normal function of proto-oncogenes has led to important insights into how cell division is turned on and off in the healthy organism. Some of the normal functions that have been widely found for the products of cellular proto-oncogenes involve signal transduction and cell division.

Although the presence of an oncogene can cause a cell to become transformed, the development of a cancer is a complex and multistep process in which a series of progressive changes culminates in deregulation of cell proliferation. The best characterized model of stepwise carcinogenesis is the colon, which has been studied extensively by Vogelstein and colleagues. Carcinogenesis in the colon is appreciated to evolve through a series of pathologically recognizable steps, from hyperplastic epithelium, to adenomatous polyps, to invasive carcinoma. The first histologically recognized step in neoplasia is a shift in the normal epithelium to continuous proliferation, leading to the formation of an adenomatous polyp. With time, certain adenomas grow and undergo pathologic changes in their morphology.

As mentioned, several genetic abnormalities occur commonly during the genesis of colorectal carcinoma, and the cumulative total of genetic abnormalities appears to be more important than the order of their appearance.

THE DIAGNOSIS AND TREATMENT OF DISEASE

Recombinant DNA and monoclonal antibody technology promise to revolutionize diagnostic medicine in the coming years. The earliest diagnostic uses of gene probes were for prenatal screening of fetal DNA and the detection of carrier states for genetic diseases. This new technology promises to revolutionize preventive genetics and offers the possibility of controlling many inherited diseases.

Gene probes, together with the use of polymerase chain reaction (PCR) technology, will have wide application in diagnostic pathology. Probes will become increasingly valuable for the rapid identification of malignant transformation. As demonstrated above in the case of colorectal cancer, the common adult solid tumors are associated with a number of activated proto-oncogenes and inactivated tumor suppressor genes. The practical applications of this knowledge are currently limited to a select number of cancers.

Medullary Thyroid Cancer (MTC) and the *RET* Proto-oncogene

The primary management goal in MEN 2 (multiple endocrine neoplasia Type 2) is to provide early treatment of affected presymptomatic individuals. Until recently, the most commonly used method of screening individuals within affected kindreds for the presence of MTC or premalignant C-cell hyperplasia was the measurement of plasma calcitonin levels following calcium and pentagastrin stimulation. In 1987, the gene for MEN 2A (and subsequently for MEN 2B and familial non-MEN medullary thyroid cancer [FMTC]) was localized by genetic linkage analysis to the centromeric region of chromosome 10. Recent studies have identified mutations in the *RET* proto-oncogene, which resides in the centromeric region of chromosome 10, in affected individuals in over 90% of kindreds with MEN 2A and MEN 2B and approximately 70% of those with FMTC. *RET* is a tyrosine kinase receptor expressed in normal human thyroid tissue, medullary thyroid carcinoma, and pheochromocytoma.

Individuals related to patients with MTC in whom a mutation in the *RET* proto-oncogene has been detected are all screened for the *RET* mutation. Asymptomatic family members who carry the *RET* mutation are then offered prophylactic thyroidectomy. Thyroidectomy in children identified to be carriers of the *RET* mutation is recommended at 5 years of age or at any time thereafter once the diagnosis is established.

Neuroblastoma and the N-*myc* Proto-oncogene

Neuroblastoma is a tumor of the autonomic nervous system and is the fourth most common pediatric malignancy. The clinical course of neuroblastoma can be unpredictable, with intrastage variability in response to similar treatments being especially common in advanced stages. N-*myc*, a proto-oncogene encoding a gene regulatory protein, has been demonstrated to be amplified within neuroblastoma cells. The number of copies of the N-*myc* gene in tissue present at different sites is similar to the number present in primary versus metastatic lesions. The number of copies is related to the clinical aggressiveness of the tumor and is a prognostic indicator independent of stage and age. N-*myc* amplification associated with any clinical stage or age places the patient at high risk for recurrence.

As mentioned above, the advent of recombinant DNA technology has allowed researchers to elucidate the genetic basis for an increasing number of inherited diseases. Gene therapy has been championed as a new and exciting approach for the treatment or prevention of such diseases. In its conception, gene therapy seemed quite simple: To treat a genetic deficiency, a functional copy of the defective gene was introduced into the cells of the deficient patient. The potential applications of gene therapy have grown to include the treatment of acquired diseases. Thus, broadly speaking, gene therapy can best be defined as the transfer of therapeutically useful genetic material to the cells of a patient.

3

CLINICAL OUTCOMES IN SURGERY

Alan J. Moskowitz, M.D., Keith Reemtsma, M.D.,
Eric A. Rose, M.D., and Annetine C. Gelijns, Ph.D.

Outcomes research can be defined as the set of research efforts that investigates the links between clinical interventions on the one hand and health and economic outcomes on the other. For example, outcome studies of coronary artery bypass grafting or abdominal aortic aneurysm repair might include an evaluation of the safety, efficacy, or cost-effectiveness of these procedures. In addition, outcomes research incorporates an analysis of which elements of care account for the outcomes achieved. An outcome analysis of abdominal aortic aneurysm repair might relate variables such as the previous experience of the surgeon, the use of special care units, or the type of graft used to predict the outcome of such surgery. These latter studies can provide important information about which providers and health care systems render better quality of care than others.

Over time, a wide variety of methods (including, among others, clinical trials, registries, and cohort studies) have evolved to assess patient outcomes. In addition, the endpoints have broadened to include not only survival and physiologic parameters but also quality of life, patient preferences, and cost-effectiveness. The following section reviews some of the strengths and weaknesses of current methods of evaluative research (see Table 1).

THE DESIGN OF CLINICAL STUDIES

Randomized, Controlled Clinical Trials

Generally speaking, clinical trials are any form of planned experiment that involve patients and are designed to elucidate the most appropriate treatment, management strategy, diagnostic test, or preventive measure for the future care of patients with a given medical condition or population at risk of developing a particular condition. Randomized, controlled trials, in general, employ techniques that help avoid biases that can distort the results of a study. These techniques, which are explored below, are comparative control groups that are concurrently treated, random assignment to treatment, uniformity of follow-up, and intention-to-treat-analysis.

COMPARATIVE CONTROL GROUPS. Randomized, controlled clinical trials are comparative: The experience of a control group of patients receiving standard therapy (or no

See the corresponding chapter or part in the *Textbook of Surgery,* 15th edition, pp. 36–54, for a more detailed discussion of this topic, including a comprehensive list of references.

TABLE 1. Current Methods of Evaluative Research

Method or Study Design	Description	Comments
Randomized clinical trial (RCT)	RCT is an experimental design for comparing treatments or management strategies for a clinical condition. To avert the introduction of confounding and measurement biases, the design calls for random assignment of patients to treatment groups, standardized approaches to delivering care and outcome evaluation, and when feasible, blinding of both patients and researchers. Further control for confounding is achieved at the analysis stage by comparing outcomes according to the original treatment assignments groups (i.e., by the intention-to-treat principle).	Although they are the strongest form of therapeutic evidence, RCTs can be time consuming, costly to conduct, and may have limited applicability, due to restrictive entry criteria and or unique venues of care.
Uncontrolled clinical trial (UCT)	UCT is an experimental design to assess the outcome of treatment or management in which only the experimental intervention is given; i.e., there are no comparative control patients.	The absence of a control population makes it difficult to sort out what part of the observed effect is actually related to the treatment and what might be attributed to spontaneous changes in disease activity or to the greater amount of follow-up care afforded patients in the experimental setting. However, when the natural history of the disease is well defined, varies little, and the measurement of outcome is irrefutable (e.g., death), this form of design can produce vary informative results.

Cohort study	Cohort study is a quasi-experimental investigative design in which a population of "similar" patients (a cohort) is followed prospectively, over time, to ascertain the risk and rate of developing clinical events of interest.	These studies are the next best thing to RCTs for evaluating prognosis and the effects of treatment. They are inefficient for studying rate associations and for studying diseases that have a long latency between exposure and manifestation of disease.
Case-control study	The case-control study is a quasi-experimental investigative design in which patients with and without a disease of interest are studied, retrospectively, to discern the association between prior exposure to a suspected risk factor and the development of disease.	This form of investigation is more efficient and less expensive than other study designs for evaluating uncommon clinical associations. Because of a greater susceptibility to bias, greater caution is required in interpreting results.
Case series or cross-sectional analysis	This is a survey of existing cases used to delineate the picture of a new disease or treatment complication by describing the prevalence of specific characteristics of the affected population.	Such studies can minimize the effects of selection bias, but they do not have a comparison group and therefore cannot put findings into context; they do not have a time dimension and therefore cannot provide direct evidence of the sequence of events that led to the disease or outcome; and they do not guard against biases in measurement or confounding.
Case reports or series of cases	These are detailed reports presenting one or more patients that manifest an unusual disease, disease presentation, or new or novel treatment approaches.	Such studies offer the weakest form of evidence. They do not have a defined population or comparison group and do not guard against measurement bias or confounding.

TABLE 1. Current Methods of Evaluative Research *Continued*

Method or Study Design	Description	Comments
Quantitative synthesis or meta-analysis	Meta-analysis is a group of techniques for critically reviewing and statistically combining the results of previously conducted research to give quantitative estimates of the weight of available evidence concerning the effects of treatments or risk of developing a particular disease or outcome.	A rigorous approach to conducting meta-analyses is necessary to avoid bias in the selection and interpretation of the articles included for study.
Decision analysis	Decision analysis is a formal analytic approach to making optimal choices. This form of mathematical modeling measures the likelihood and value of each potential outcome of a diagnostic or therapeutic choice and delineates the one yielding the highest benefit.	While such studies may offer insight into and reasoned solutions to clinical dilemmas, the simplifying assumptions made in modeling real problems can limit their clinical usefulness.
Cost-effectiveness (CE), cost-benefit (CB) analysis	These forms of economic analysis measure the health care resources consumed in delivering care in relation to the health benefits provided. CE studies are useful for determining how to allocate health care resources to yield maximum health benefits. CB studies determine whether there is a net dollar gain or loss from a health care expenditure.	Such studies are useful in guiding the delivery of health care when resources are limited. However, because cost data are difficult to obtain, a less desirable proxy is often used instead.

therapy when standard therapy does not exist) is compared with the experience of the experimental treatment group, also referred to as the *intervention group*. The control group gives the *expected rate* of the study outcome under the null hypothesis of no effect of the investigational intervention, while the intervention group gives the *observed rate* of this outcome under the investigational treatment.

For a controlled clinical trial to be a valid test of whether the intervention effect differs from the effect under the null hypothesis, both groups must have an equal probability of achieving the study outcome prior to administering the intervention; that is, they must be equally constituted in terms of their pretreatment likelihood of developing the outcome for study. To accomplish this, patients are randomly assigned to a treatment group.

INTENTION-TO-TREAT PRINCIPLE. Even though patients are assigned to a particular therapy at randomization, they do not always receive it. For a variety of reasons, patients may actually *cross over* from the experimental to control treatment group or vice versa. Factors that predict failure to receive therapy and cross overs almost invariably also predict the study outcome. Consequently, an analysis based on the treatment that the patient actually received (*as-treated analysis*) no longer compares randomly chosen groups that are equally likely to develop the outcome of interest. To ensure comparability between the study groups, the analysis should compare the groups that were composed at randomization, regardless of whether or not all patients received the assigned treatment. This analytic technique, which is referred to as *analysis by the intention-to-treat principle*, is the only valid method for testing the main hypothesis in a clinical trial. However, it may be supplemented by an *as-treated analysis* to support other endpoints, such as the analysis of complication rates.

CHRONOLOGIC BIAS. The concurrent comparison of control and experimentally treated patients is essential for avoiding chronologic bias. Chronologic bias can occur because diagnostic and therapeutic abilities change over time, and comparisons between control and intervention groups who are treated at different times, perhaps years apart, may reflect differences in an aspect of the care they received other than the effect of the intervention itself.

OBSERVATIONAL BIAS. Observational bias can occur whenever there are differences between how outcome observations are made in the control and experimental treatment groups. Observational biases can be prevented by (1) denying both the investigator and the patient knowledge of which treatment was received, that is, *double blinding*, (2) ensuring identical follow-up care for both groups of patients, and (3) documenting all outcome observations so that they can be verified by an independent, blinded observer.

Uncontrolled Clinical Trials

Trials are called *uncontrolled* if they do not contain a comparative control group and therefore describe the course of disease only in a single group of patients who have been exposed to a particular intervention (see Table 1). Such trials are problematic because the clinical courses of many diseases are fairly unpredictable: Spontaneous remissions in disease activity can occur that can be misinterpreted as a treatment effect. Moreover, patients in clinical trials may show improvement over what would be expected of standard care by virtue of the special attention that they receive and not because of the treatment itself. Such effects cannot be sorted out without a comparative control group.

When the outcome of interest is irrefutable (e.g., death) and the natural history is very well defined (e.g., uniformly fatal without treatment), uncontrolled trials can produce valid and highly informative results. Such is the case for congenital heart surgery, for instance, transposition of the great vessels, in which longitudinal studies of all patients treated at one center using a particular procedure have yielded important results.

Case Reports

Case reports, which are detailed presentations of a single patient or several patients, have a long tradition in medicine and have contributed greatly to its advancement (see Table 1). These reports are an important format for presenting the medical community with the description of an unusual disease, an unusual presentation of a disease, a new or novel procedure or treatment approach, or an unusual consequence of treatment. In the case of surgical innovation, for instance, lung volume reduction surgery, where, at the inception, major changes occur in technique, skill, and patient selection criteria, case reports serve as the major source of medical communication. In general, they often generate new hypotheses about disease frequency, risk, prognosis, and treatment.

What cannot be discerned from case reports are the frequencies of occurrence of the reported events. This limitation may unduly affect clinical behavior because the high visibility of the report may make the event seem more common than it really is. Furthermore, using this form of publication in a literature search to establish therapeutic efficacy is fraught with problems due to the proclivity of authors and journal editors to publish only successful cases.

In contrast to case reports, *case series* are prevalence surveys. They are used to delineate the picture of a rare disease or rare treatment complication by describing the prevalence of specific characteristics in the affected population. Because these studies do not report on the outcomes of patients followed over time, they do not provide prognostic information and therefore do not address issues of cause and effect. Also, without a comparison group, the within-group associations that are observed cannot be put into context.

Case-Control Studies

Case-control studies are a method for analyzing *nonexperimental* or *observational data* to discern the association between the exposure to a suspected risk factor and the development of disease (see Table 1). Patients who have a disease (cases) and a group of otherwise similar people who do not have the disease (controls) are selected, and investigators then look backward in time to determine the frequency of exposure to the suspected risk factor in the two groups. One can then calculate an estimate of the relative risk for developing disease related to the suspected risk factor, referred to as the *odds ratio*. In context of the case-control study, the odds ratio is just the odds of disease in exposed individuals relative to the odds of disease in nonexposed individuals.

Susceptibility to bias in case-control studies is related to two features of study design: (1) the groups to be compared are selected by the researcher and are not constituted naturally as in a cohort study (see below), and (2) the exposure to the suspected risk factor is measured after the disease has already occurred.

It is this vulnerability to bias that relegates such studies to hypothesis generation and hypothesis support rather than hypothesis confirmation. However, the efficiency of conducting case-control studies cannot be surpassed. Such studies are often the first piece of important evidence of disease association, which was the case with identifying maternal DES use as a risk factor for developing clear cell carcinoma of the vagina. With the rigorous attention to possible sources of bias, such studies can provide valid estimates of risk for rare clinical associations.

Cohort Studies

The epidemiologic concept of a *cohort* refers to a group of individuals who, at the time of their assembly, have characteristics in common, including not having yet experienced the outcome for study (see Table 1). Cohorts must be followed over time to study whether or not the outcome event of interest develops. Such studies are suitable for studying the risks of developing disease, prognosis following the development of disease, or response to treatment. While cohort studies are the next best thing to randomized, controlled trials for evaluating prognosis and the effects of treatment, they still are more susceptible to bias. Without the use of randomization, caution must be taken to avoid selection bias in the assembly of comparative cohorts.

Controlling for selection bias can be accomplished by (1) restriction, that is, limiting the range of characteristics of patients entered into the study, resulting in relatively homogeneous cohorts but risking the loss of generalizability; (2) matching, that is, for each patient in one cohort, selecting one or more patients with similar characteristics for the comparative cohort, which can be difficult to accomplish for more than a few characteristics; (3) stratification, that is, compare rates within subgroups with clinical characteristics that put them at the same risk of the outcome event, which can only be done for a few characteristics before statistical power is lost;

and (4) adjustment for difference in clinical characteristics between the cohorts. When differences between the cohorts are few, adjustment can be accomplished by standardizing the crude outcome rates between the cohorts so that equal weight is given to subgroups of similar risk. When differences are multiple, one can accomplish adjustment by using multivariable analysis. This method requires that the investigator construct a mathematical model (an equation) that relates the pertinent clinical characteristics of the patients to a prediction of the outcome event.

MEASURING CLINICAL END-POINTS

Clinical evaluative studies may include a spectrum of relevant end-points, ranging from physiologic and anatomic parameters to morbidity, mortality, health status, functional status, and quality of life. The notion of what constitutes valid end-points is in continual flux. Obviously, for interventions that aim to increase the survival and reduce the morbidity of a particular disease or condition, mortality and morbidity are the key end-points. The statistical methods for performing the requisite survival data analysis are a rigorous group of techniques that are well described in other texts. Many therapeutic interventions for today's chronic degenerative diseases, however, treat only symptoms. Thus improvement in functional status, health status, and quality of life are increasingly important end-points in clinical evaluation. Moreover, because chronic diseases often entail lifelong treatment, the health care resources consumed in achieving these health outcomes have become increasingly important considerations in the current economic environment. The remainder of this section is devoted to an overview of the techniques to assess quality of life, functional status, and economic cost of care.

Measuring Quality of Life and Patient Preferences

Overall quality of life is an all-inclusive concept that incorporates the ability of the individual to function physically, emotionally, and socially. For measuring the impact of medical interventions, however, a more limited definition is appropriate: *health-related quality of life* (HRQOL) includes those factors which immediately affect the health of the individual.

Instruments for measuring HRQOL fall into two broad categories: *generic* and *specific*. Generic measures assess general aspects of health-related quality of life that are applicable to a variety of populations and thus allow broad comparisons of the relative impact of disparate health care interventions. An example of this type of measure is the MOS 36-item Short-Form Health Survey. Specific instruments are geared to particular diseases or populations and focus on the functional limitations or disabilities produced by the disease of interest or are experienced by the populations of interest. By focusing on only important aspects of HRQOL that are relevant to the patients being studied, the measurement is more likely to be responsive to subtle changes in the function of those individuals over time.

Within these two broad categories of measurement there are two types of instruments: *health profiles* and *utility instruments*. Health profiles capture health status through questionnaires that ask about patient functional capabilities and symptomatology. These questionnaires are multidimensional constructs; that is, they are composed of questions that address each of the different concepts (dimensions or domains), that together, are thought to define health-related quality of life. In general, such concepts include physical functioning, mobility, cognitive functioning, self-care, emotional status, sensory function, and pain. Numeric scoring is accomplished by assigning points to the responses to each question and summing the scores for each concept or domain covered in the questionnaire. These scores have ordinal measurement properties with arbitrary magnitude. The more extreme values are better or worse than less extreme values (depending on the profile being used).

Utility measurements, which are also referred to as *preference-based measurements*, capture both the quality of life experienced by the patient and the strength of preference held for the health state relative to full health (assigned a score of 1) and death (assigned a score of 0). Scores less than zero, representing states worse than death, are possible. Utility scores are cardinal measures with interval scale properties and, accordingly, offer a greater ability to reason about the magnitude of scoring differences.

Quality-adjusted survival, measured in quality-adjusted life years (QALYs), is a complex outcome measure that captures features of both the survival and quality of life of the individuals being evaluated. Its calculation entails using quality adjustment factors to modify the measured survival for the quality of life experienced. Utility scores are commonly used as the quality adjustment factors. If, for example, an individual lives 70 years at full quality of life, he or she would have accumulated 70 quality-adjusted life years (70 years $\times$ 1.0 quality units). If, however, this patient's entire 70-year survival was at half of full quality, he or she would only have accumulated 35 quality-adjusted life years (70 years $\times$ 0.5 quality units). Having a single, unified outcome measure, such as a QALY, reflecting the multiple attributes of health believed to be germane to making therapeutic choices, facilitates the decision-making process considerably.

Assessing the Economic Impact of Clinical Care

The objective of an economic evaluation of a medical or surgical intervention is to measure the resources consumed (i.e., costs) in relation to the health benefits provided. An economic analysis can be undertaken from the following different perspectives: (1) society or the health care system, (2) third-party payers, (3) providers (including managed care organizations, hospitals, and clinicians), and (4) patients.

There are different methods of economic evaluation. Cost-benefit and cost-effective analyses both examine the costs as well as the benefits of alternative technologies. In a cost-benefit analysis, however, all costs and benefits are expressed in monetary terms. Expressing certain benefits, such as reductions in pain or increases in life expectancy, in dollar values is complex and requires a number of gross assumptions. Various techniques, such as the "human capital" approach or the "willingness to pay" method, have been employed, but they still have important limitations, and the results tend to be very controversial. Therefore, most economic evaluations today are cost-effectiveness analyses.

In a cost-effectiveness analysis, the health benefits are expressed in the most appropriate natural units, such as "cases successfully detected" or "years of life gained." In a so-called cost-utility analysis, which is a special form of cost-effectiveness analysis, the results are expressed as the cost per QALY gained.

Measuring health care costs is fraught with practical and conceptual difficulties. Although analyses have historically used the *charges* that providers bill as proxies for the cost of resources, charges may differ substantially from the resource costs of delivering care. This divergence may stem from cross-subsidization of less lucrative products and services by more profitable ones and cost-shifting to some patients and third-party payers from those who cannot pay all or part of their medical care bills. A less than perfect proxy for measuring costs is the *ratio-of-costs-to-charges* (RCC) method. With this method, charges billed are converted to actual hospital expenditures using a ratio of the actual costs to the charges billed; however, hospitals calculate RCCs only down to the department level. This means that the RCC loses accuracy when applied to individual patients who have undergone specific procedures, such as a lung transplantation. *Payments* relate to actual financial transactions but reflect differences in resource use only for services that are paid separately. *Resource costs,* the monetary value of actual resources used to deliver care, are the most desirable conceptually but usually require extensive data collection to obtain.

Different types of costs can be examined within an economic evaluation. Direct costs include those resource categories directly related to the technology being studied, such as personnel, medications, diagnostic testing, outpatient visits, costs of treatments required to manage side effects, or costs of treatments averted as a result of the health effects of a program. Direct costs also may include nonmedical costs, such as transportation of patients to and from the hospital, home health care services, or nursing home care. Indirect costs include earnings gained or lost by patients and the economic value of intangible costs such as pain, suffering, or quality of life; as mentioned, current methodology is limited in capturing such costs.

COMBINING THE RESULTS OF DIFFERENT STUDIES
Meta-analysis

Meta-analysis is a formal process for critically reviewing and statistically combining the results of previous research. When the definitive study of the effectiveness of a therapy is impractical or impossible to perform or is currently in progress and the decision to use this therapy must be made on the basis of existing studies that are perhaps multiple in number, smaller in sample size, and inconclusive, meta-analysis can help the decision-making process by giving quantitative estimates of the weight of available evidence.

This methodology can be used to analyze both randomized trials and epidemiologic data. The process of pooling existing studies can increase statistical power for measuring primary and secondary study end-points as well as increase the statistical power for subgroup analyses. It can help to resolve uncertainty when studies disagree and can answer questions that were not posed at the start of the individual studies. Moreover, it can improve estimates of therapeutic effect size or diagnostic accuracy.

FORMAL ANALYTIC METHODS FOR CLINICAL DECISION MAKING
Decision Analysis

When clinical trials are unavailable or unrepresentative of the patient at hand, clinicians are forced to make these decisions based on speculation from various pieces of evidence about the overall effect that a therapeutic option will have on the natural course of the patient's disease. The process of collating the various data sources and providing the appropriate weight for each datum can be a daunting task. *Decision analysis*, a formal analytic approach to making decisions under conditions of uncertainty, provides the structure for collating data from a variety of sources and helps project whether the benefits of the proposed intervention outweigh the risks. The process has been applied to decisions affecting the care of individual patients and groups, as well as to questions of health policy.

IMPACT OF THE OUTCOMES MOVEMENT ON THE PRACTICE OF SURGERY

In recent years, rigorous methods of clinical evaluation have increasingly supplanted subjective clinical experience in the assessment of new and existing surgical procedures. The dramatic restructuring of the U.S. health care system is reinforcing this trend.

In what ways can this type of research contribute to improving surgical practice? Obviously, these studies provide critical information to surgeons, as well as other physicians, about the effectiveness and cost-effectiveness of alternative surgical treatments. Presumably, this information should lead to more evidence-based use of existing surgical treatments and, more generally, the use of health care resources. In addition, outcomes studies may identify the elements of care that account for the outcomes achieved, also called *practice profiling*, thereby facilitating efforts by clinicians and hospitals to improve the outcomes of care in their institutions.

These profiles, and outcomes research in general, have use beyond self-assessment. First of all, they provide information on the risks and benefits of clinical interventions to prospective patients and the general public. This allows patients, in consultation with their physicians, to have a realistic look at the outcomes facing them, which facilitates making more informed choices based on willingness to accept risk. As such, outcomes research may contribute to a clinical decision-making process that better reflects patient preferences. Finally, outcomes research may provide important information to federal and state authorities, as well as to health care payers. In particular, it may assist in guiding licensure decisions, identification of centers of excellence for advanced tertiary care, and determination of appropriate benefit packages—all of these, in turn, will affect the quality and cost of care.

4

HOMEOSTASIS:
Bodily Changes in Trauma and Surgery
Douglas W. Wilmore, M.D.

Surgeons care for patients who experience sudden, rapid, and intense changes in normal physiology and metabolism. Such alterations occur following an elective operative procedure, but more dramatic perturbations arise following major accidental injury. Both these events interrupt normal fluid and electrolyte homeostasis, alter food intake, change tissue perfusion, and often disrupt vital organ function.

The human body responds to these stresses with dramatic resilience. Mechanisms are initiated to restore blood volume and redistribute blood flow to ensure perfusion of vital organs. Substrate is mobilized to provide a constant energy supply, and inflammatory responses are stimulated to initiate tissue repair and enhance host resistance. These biologic alterations that occur following injury and other stresses reflect a unique and indelible program that is genetically encoded in higher species. In strict Darwinian terms, these responses are the result of an evolutionary process that favors survival of the fittest in the struggle for existence. In teleologic terms, these responses have a purpose: to benefit the organism and aid recovery. Knowledge of homeostatic adjustments that occur in critically ill patients is essential for optimal patient care and necessary for rehabilitation and recovery from a life-threatening illness.

BODY COMPOSITION AND ITS RESPONSE TO SURGICAL STRESS

The body is composed of two major components: a non-aqueous and an aqueous phase. Body fat and extracellular solids such as bone make up the *anhydrous portion of the body*. The aqueous phase supports a heterogeneous mass of cells generally referred to as the *lean body mass*. These cells represent the functioning components of the body that actively exchange oxygen, glucose, and other metabolites.

These components of the body change with disease. For example, with congestive heart failure, total body water and exchangeable sodium increase. With starvation, skeletal muscle mass (a component of the lean body mass) decreases and adipose tissue is lost. Although body fat provides an excellent fuel source for the individual during stress, loss of lean body mass represents loss of body protein (i.e., nitrogen), and this is associated with loss of body structure and function. The erosion of body protein is not without consequences and, if

---

See the corresponding chapter or part in the *Textbook of Surgery*, 15th edition, pp. 55–67, for a more detailed discussion of this topic, including a comprehensive list of references.

moderately severe, delays wound healing, impairs immuno-logic responses to infection, and prolongs recovery.

HOMEOSTATIC RESPONSES TO SPECIFIC COMPONENTS OF INJURY

Clinical illness creates a variety of complex interacting ho-meostatic responses. The clinical features observed are the sum of changes known to occur following a single perturba-tion. These initiating factors include volume loss, underperfu-sion, simple starvation, tissue damage, and invasive infection. Each single alteration has been studied in detail, and it is well known that each perturbation stimulates a variety of hor-monal and chemical reactions that initiate the appropriate homeostatic adjustments. However, tissue damage and in-fection markedly accelerate catabolic responses, probably through the generation of cytokines. Although cytokines may function locally through paracrine and endocrine activities, they also may reach the bloodstream to exert systemic effects such as mediating fever, stimulating the elaboration of acute-phase proteins and leukocytes and causing the redistribution of trace elements (such as iron and zinc). In addition, cyto-kines such as interleukin-1 (IL-1) and tumor necrosis factor (TNF) may stimulate elaboration of pituitary hormones that also initiate and mediate metabolic responses.

RESPONSES FOLLOWING AN ELECTIVE OPERATION

The earliest response following a major operation is the stimulation of the pituitary-adrenal axis. Cortisol remains two to five times normal levels for approximately 24 hours after a major operation. In addition, urinary catecholamines are ele-vated for 24 to 48 hours after operation and then return to normal. Insulin is low and glucagon is elevated; this hormonal environment stimulates hepatic glycogenolysis and gluconeo-genesis. In addition, diminished food intake and elevated cortisol favor net skeletal muscle proteolysis. These amino acids are processed in the liver to urea, which is excreted in the urine. The operative stress also stimulates the secretion of aldosterone and antidiuretic hormone, which diminishes the excretion of free water. This retained fluid eventually returns to the circulation as the wound edema subsides, and diuresis commences 2 to 4 days following the operation.

RESPONSES FOLLOWING ACCIDENTAL INJURY

The events that occur following injury are generally graded responses: the more severe the injury, the greater the response. The events also change with time. Initially following injury there is a fall in metabolic functions and a decrease in core temperature, the *ebb* phase. With restoration of blood flow, the patient's metabolic rate rises, body temperature becomes elevated, and blood insulin levels are normalized.

These changes thus demonstrate the characteristic responses to injury, which include hypermetabolism (or increase in the resting metabolic rate), increased nitrogen loss, and accelerated gluconeogenesis. The hormonal environment favors accelerated breakdown of skeletal muscle protein, and this is reflected in the increased loss of nitrogen in the urine. Skeletal muscle amino acids, primarily alanine and glutamine, contribute their carbon skeletons to the synthesis of new glucose. In addition, glutamine buffers the acid load generated during this accelerated catabolism and also provides a specific fuel for rapidly growing cells, such as fibroblasts, enterocytes of the intestine, and stimulated macrophages and lymphocytes. The glucose is utilized by the injured tissue but is incompletely oxidized and generates lactate. The lactate is recycled to the liver and reconverted to glucose.

SUMMARY

Homeostatic adjustments constantly occur in surgical patients in an effort to maintain the *milieu intérieur* and ensure wound healing. Multiple factors, including diminished blood volume, tissue underperfusion, reduced food intake, extensive tissue damage, and invasive infection, initiate these responses via the neuroendocrine system. As a result of these physiologic adjustments, tissue perfusion is maintained, which supports the increased metabolic demands accompanying critical illness. Increased skeletal muscle proteolysis and accelerated gluconeogenesis are coupled responses that also occur; these biochemical alterations provide essential nutrients to support vital organ function and wound repair.

5

SHOCK:
Causes and Management of Circulatory Collapse

Robert W. Anderson, M.D., and
Steven N. Vaslef, M.D., Ph.D.

DEFINITION

Shock may be defined as a syndrome that occurs from inadequate perfusion of tissues. Alterations in cellular metabolism occur and lead to cellular dysfunction, elaboration of inflammatory mediators, and cellular injury. Current interpretations of shock view the syndrome as a continuum, ranging from subclinical deficits in perfusion to multiple organ dysfunction syndrome (MODS) or frank organ failure. The corollary of tissue hypoperfusion is tissue hypoxia, whereby oxygen demand exceeds oxygen supply.

CLASSIFICATION OF SHOCK

A classification system serves to delineate the various etiologies of shock and to provide a framework for establishing the diagnosis and instituting treatment. *Hypovolemic shock* occurs from hemorrhagic losses, such as occur with trauma, gastrointestinal bleeding, or ruptured aneurysms, or from plasma volume losses. Shock arising from plasma volume losses may be due to extravascular fluid sequestration, as might occur in pancreatitis, burns, and bowel obstruction, or it may arise from excessive gastrointestinal, renal, or insensible fluid losses. *Cardiogenic shock* occurs when the heart is unable to generate an adequate cardiac output to maintain tissue perfusion. Both intrinsic cardiac dysfunction and extrinsic etiologies of diminished cardiac output are incorporated in the category of cardiogenic shock. Intrinsic causes of cardiac dysfunction include myocardial infarction, cardiomyopathy, valvular heart disease, cardiac rhythm disturbances, and myocardial depression from drug toxicity or trauma. Extrinsic mechanisms of cardiogenic shock produce cardiac dysfunction by compressive or obstructive means. Tension pneumothorax, pericardial tamponade, and high levels of positive-pressure ventilation may all cause external compression of the heart that impedes diastolic filling and decreases cardiac output. Pulmonary embolism is an example of obstructive cardiogenic shock. *Neurogenic shock* may occur following spinal cord injury, severe head injury, or spinal anesthesia with failure of the sympathetic nervous system to maintain normal vascular tone. Arteriolar and venous vasodilation, with a reduction in peripheral vascular resistance and an increase in venous capacitance, is

See the corresponding chapter or part in the *Textbook of Surgery,* 15th edition, pp. 68–91, for a more detailed discussion of this topic, including a comprehensive list of references.

characteristic of neurogenic shock. *Vasogenic shock* is similar to neurogenic shock in that arteriolar and venous vasomotor tone is decreased; however, the mechanisms responsible for the development of these two entities are quite different. Whereas sympathetic denervation is implicated in the clinical syndrome of neurogenic shock, this mechanism is absent in vasogenic shock. Endogenous or exogenous vasoactive mediators are thought to play a major role in the development of vasogenic shock. Included in this category are shock associated with the systemic inflammatory response syndrome (SIRS), sepsis, anaphylaxis, adrenocortical insufficiency, and traumatic injuries.

PATIENT MONITORING

Expeditious restoration of perfusion and correction of the underlying pathology are the goals of resuscitation of patients in shock. Ongoing assessment of the patient's response to resuscitative efforts is essential to determine the efficacy of therapy. Most patients in moderate or severe shock, patients at high risk for developing postshock sequelae, or patients suspected of being incompletely resuscitated are optimally managed in a critical care setting.

Conventional monitoring techniques used to assess the adequacy of resuscitation in patients in shock have employed a number of modalities based on physical examination or laboratory data. Measures such as blood pressure, heart rate, central venous pressure, hematocrit, arterial blood gases, urine output, capillary refill, and skin turgor are rather insensitive in diagnosing shock or evaluating response to treatment because "abnormal" values reflect secondary effects of shock or tissue hypoxia. Thus endpoints such as adequate urine output or mean arterial pressure > 80 mm. Hg may not be appropriate or sensitive indicators of occult tissue hypoxia. Nevertheless, such measures are useful in guiding the initial resuscitation from shock.

In addition to the conventional parameters described above, there are some monitoring techniques, such as pulse oximetry, that are employed fairly routinely in the intensive care unit. Use of the flow-directed pulmonary artery catheter, in conjunction with an indwelling arterial cannula and blood gas analysis, can provide considerable hemodynamic and oxygen transport data that are extremely useful in directing therapy aimed at optimizing cardiac function and oxygen delivery. Cardiac output may be measured by the Swan-Ganz catheter utilizing the thermodilution technique. In addition to measuring left- and right-sided filling pressures and cardiac output, the pulmonary artery catheter also may provide some measures of oxygen balance.

Recent trends in critical care medicine have emphasized continuous on-line monitoring, which, when compared with intermittent monitoring, permits more information to be obtained in a more efficient manner. Previously undetected events may become unmasked; more prompt recognition of adverse events may be achieved; earlier therapeutic intervention may be accomplished; and the physiologic responses to various interventions may be assessed quickly with the use of continuous monitoring of mixed venous oxygen saturation ($S\bar{v}O_2$) or of cardiac output. A number of methods have been developed that allow the continuous measurement of cardiac output, including thoracic electrical bioimpedance, "continuous" thermodilution using a modified pulmonary artery catheter, a combination of oximetry and on-line metabolic gas analysis, and Doppler methods.

Other methods that have been used to assess the adequacy of resuscitation from shock include measurement of serum lactate concentration, measurement of the lactate-to-pyruvate ratio, and gastrointestinal tonometry.

PATHOPHYSIOLOGY OF SHOCK

Consequences of tissue hypoperfusion may include tissue hypoxia, anaerobic metabolism, acidosis, elaboration of inflammatory mediators, circulatory redistribution with early involvement of the splanchnic circulation, cellular injury, septic complications, and MODS.

Impaired tissue hypoperfusion leads to decreased oxygen delivery relative to oxygen needs. In the resting state, $\dot{D}O_2$ and $\dot{V}O_2$ are well matched, resulting in a $\dot{D}O_2$ that normally exceeds $\dot{V}O_2$ by three- to fourfold. This corresponds to an oxygen extraction ratio (O_2ER) of 0.25 to 0.33. Under conditions of either increased energy expenditure or decreased $\dot{D}O_2$, the normal $\dot{D}O_2$–$\dot{V}O_2$ relationship is disrupted. The physiologic response to restore homeostasis under such conditions is to increase O_2ER in order to supply the basal O_2 requirements and preserve aerobic metabolism. The increased O_2ER may become clinically apparent by a fall in $S\bar{v}O_2$. As long as the tissues are able to extract enough O_2 to maintain aerobic metabolism, $\dot{V}O_2$ remains constant and independent of $\dot{D}O_2$. If, on the other hand, further increases in O_2ER are inadequate to maintain tissue oxygenation, a critical O_2ER is reached, above which $\dot{V}O_2$ becomes dependent on $\dot{D}O_2$, and anaerobic metabolism supervenes.

When oxygen delivery is insufficient to meet cellular oxygen demands, anaerobic glycolysis occurs. As cellular oxygen supply diminishes, lactate production increases and pyruvate concentration diminishes. Thus increases in the blood lactate concentration and the blood lactate-to-pyruvate (L/P) ratio have been observed under conditions of anaerobic metabolism.

The homeostatic response to hypoperfusion and hypoxia is to preserve oxygen delivery to the heart and brain by selectively, but inhomogeneously, diverting blood flow from other tissues, particularly the skin, subcutaneous tissues, and gastrointestinal tract. The splanchnic circulation appears to be especially vulnerable to this redistribution of blood flow.

Gut dysfunction may be a manifestation of the *effect* of shock, but it also may be an important *cause* of the perpetuation of various shock syndromes. The pathogenesis of gut injury involves at least two different mechanisms: those related to hypoxia and those related to reperfusion injury once blood flow is reestablished. Hypoxic injury causes mucosal ischemia, which leads to the disruption of the normal epithelial cell barrier. Reperfusion occurs with the accumulation of toxic oxidants, which may lead to cellular injury. As a consequence of intestinal mucosal injury, gut permeability may increase, allowing enteric flora or bacterial toxins to *translocate* across the gut wall and invade the host via lymphatic or portal venous routes.

MEDIATORS OF SHOCK AND SEPSIS

Shock, like sepsis, induces a complicated cascade of physiologic events that is brought about through the action of a number of inflammatory and neuroendocrine mediators. The mediators of the inflammatory response include a large and growing cadre of molecules with important but incompletely defined roles in the development, progression, and perpetuation of the various shock syndromes. Depending on the severity of the injury or insult, the systemic inflammatory response may be self-limited or may escalate to the point of multiple organ dysfunction. In addition to having direct effects on target cells, many of these inflammatory mediators potentiate the actions of one another to produce an amplified host response. Some of the mediators with key roles in shock and/or sepsis include *endotoxin, complement fragments C3a and C5a, kinins, eicosanoids* (prostaglandins, thromboxanes, and leukotrienes), *nitric oxide, cytokines* (interleukins, tumor necrosis factor, colony-stimulating factors, and interferons), *platelet-activating factor,* and *oxidants.*

In response to injury, stress, or infection, there is an increase in the circulating levels of catabolic, or stress, hormones. Release of catechols produces tachycardia, increased inotropy, and peripheral vasoconstriction, as well as increased metabolic rate, increased glycogenolysis, increased gluconeogenesis, and inhibition of insulin secretion by the pancreas. Release of adrenocorticotropic hormone stimulates cortisol output, the effects of which include proteolysis, lipolysis, and gluconeogenesis. Glucagon release also contributes to gluconeogenesis and glucose intolerance. The renin-angiotensin system may be activated due to adrenergic vasoconstriction in the kidneys. The resultant release of angiotensin II leads to further vasoconstriction, which may exacerbate ischemia and shock. Aldosterone and vasopressin are also released, leading to salt and water retention.

DIAGNOSIS AND MANAGEMENT OF SHOCK: GENERAL APPROACH

The ultimate goals in the management of shock are to restore perfusion and adequate oxygen delivery to tissue. No matter what the etiology of shock, the basic algorithm to restore hemodynamic stability and tissue perfusion is the same in the initial evaluation. Many patients will likely need a pulmonary artery catheter placed in order to optimize cardiac output and oxygen delivery. Reasonable initial resuscitation goals include (1) maintaining pulmonary capillary wedge pressure (PCWP) between 15 and 18 mm. Hg, (2) achieving a mean arterial pressure between 60 and 80 mm. Hg, (3) maintaining $S\bar{v}O_2 > 65\%$ to 70%, and (4) achieving delivery-independent oxygen consumption. In order to reach these goals, patients may require the use of pharmacologic agents to improve cardiac inotropy (dobutamine, dopamine, epinephrine), decrease afterload (nitroglycerin, nitroprusside), or increase mean arterial pressure (agents with alpha-adrenergic effects, such as norepinephrine, moderate doses of epinephrine, and phenylephrine). Measures also should be instituted to treat the inciting cause of shock, eliminate infectious or inflammatory foci with appropriate surgical intervention and antibiotics, and provide early nutritional support.

SPECIFIC SHOCK SYNDROMES

HYPOVOLEMIC SHOCK. Hypovolemia accounts for the most commonly encountered shock syndrome in surgical patients. Hypovolemic shock occurs when a loss of body fluids is sufficient to cause intravascular volume depletion and when compensatory mechanisms fail to restore normal tissue perfusion.

Clinical signs and symptoms of hypovolemic shock depend on the severity of the intravascular volume deficit. A loss of 15% or less of the circulating blood volume is generally well tolerated by most patients without any hemodynamic signs of shock. The first sign of hypovolemic shock may be a decrease in the pulse pressure (difference between systolic and diastolic pressures) due to an increase in catecholamine levels. As the circulating blood volume is reduced even further, tachycardia and hypotension may become evident. Concomitantly, urine output falls, normal skin turgor is lost, and mental status changes occur.

Blood tests are infrequently helpful in situations of acute volume losses because of the fluid shifts that occur, but they may be helpful in detecting less acute, occult fluid losses. Hemoconcentration may occur, as evidenced by an increase in hemoglobin concentration, hematocrit, and the BUN/creatinine ratio. Hypernatremia may be observed after excessive free water losses, as with insensible losses due to a large burn wound. If the clinical picture of hypovolemic shock is unclear, it is helpful to place a central venous line or, preferably, a pulmonary artery catheter for hemodynamic monitoring. The characteristic hemodynamic profile of hypovolemic shock reflects low filling pressures, decreased cardiac output, decreased $S\bar{v}O_2$, and increased systemic vascular resistance.

Initial management of hypovolemic shock includes an assessment of the patient's airway and a determination of the adequacy of ventilation and oxygenation. Essentially all patients with severe shock and circulatory collapse will require tracheal intubation and mechanical ventilation. Direct pressure on bleeding external wounds may be applied to control obvious hemorrhage. Two large-bore intravenous lines should be established, and an initial fluid bolus should be administered. Ordinarily, isotonic electrolyte solutions, such as Ringer's lactate solution, are infused in the initial stages of resuscitation. If hypotension persists after a 2-liter fluid challenge, ongoing volume losses are likely, and blood transfusion must be considered if the clinical situation is compatible with hemorrhagic shock. Fully crossmatched blood is preferred, but type-specific or type O packed red blood cells may be necessary in life-threatening hemorrhage. Controversy exists regarding the use of colloid solutions, hypertonic saline solutions, or a combination of these solutions in the treatment of hypovolemic shock.

CARDIOGENIC SHOCK. Cardiogenic shock occurs when the heart fails to generate an adequate cardiac output to maintain tissue perfusion. This type of shock, whether due to intrinsic or extrinsic causes, may be regarded as pump failure. The patient may appear anxious, tachycardic, and tachypneic, with cool, clammy, mottled skin and oliguria. In addition, there may be signs of increased preload, such as distended neck veins, and the presence of an S_3 heart sound, pulmonary rales, and peripheral edema. Prior history of cardiovascular disease may be useful in establishing the diagnosis.

Laboratory data, particularly arterial blood gases, serum electrolytes, and cardiac enzymes, may be useful in the diagnosis and management of cardiogenic shock. A chest radiograph and electrocardiogram should be done in all cases of suspected cardiogenic shock in order to identify acute, as well as chronic, disease. An echocardiogram can provide valuable information about cardiac function, as well as about any structural abnormalities of the heart. If pulmonary embolism is considered, a ventilation-perfusion scan or pulmonary angiogram should be obtained.

Invasive monitoring using a pulmonary artery catheter is frequently required to optimize cardiac function and oxygen delivery in cases of cardiogenic shock. Typical hemodynamic findings in cardiogenic shock include a low cardiac output (<2.2 liters/min./sq. m.), an elevated systemic vascular resistance, and elevated filling pressures.

The diagnosis of compressive cardiogenic shock must be entertained in any patient with a history of trauma who presents with hypotension. Patients with *tension pneumothorax* may present with profound hypotension, absence of breath sounds on the affected side, hyperresonance to percussion on the affected side, distended neck veins, and a trachea deviated to the opposite side. Immediate treatment by decompression of the pleural space may be lifesaving and should be carried out without obtaining a confirmatory chest radiograph. *Pericardial tamponade* may be seen following trauma, particularly after penetrating wounds to the heart, but also may be seen with pericardial effusions due to renal failure or malignant processes. The findings of Beck's triad, consisting of hypotension, distended neck veins, and muffled heart sounds, and of pulsus paradoxus may be helpful in diagnosing pericardial tamponade. Echocardiography is very sensitive in detecting pericardial effusions. Patients in shock due to pericardial tamponade may respond initially to the administration of intrave-

nous fluids to increase preload. Pericardiocentesis should be
performed in patients suspected of having a pericardial effusion who fail to respond or transiently respond to initial measures.

Principles of management of intrinsic cardiogenic shock,
like other forms of shock, are to optimize cardiovascular function, improve oxygen delivery, and restore tissue perfusion.
To achieve these goals, manipulation of preload, afterload,
and cardiac contractility is necessary, as is optimization of
the myocardial oxygen supply-to-demand ratio. Supplemental
oxygen should be administered and mechanical ventilation
instituted, if indicated. Initial hemodynamic interventions
should be aimed at correcting arrhythmias and optimizing
preload. Most patients in cardiogenic shock have higher than
normal filling pressures, with the PCWP > 15 mm. Hg. Patients with a noncompliant left ventricle, however, may require high filling pressures, with the PCWP in the range of 18
to 20 mm. Hg. A reasonable initial goal is to manipulate the
preload until PCWP is between 15 and 18 mm. Hg. This may
be accomplished with fluid administration to increase preload
or with diuretics or venodilators to decrease preload.

The sympathomimetic inotropic agents commonly used include dopamine, dobutamine, and epinephrine. The choice of
which agent to use depends on the patient's hemodynamic
parameters. When both afterload reduction and inotropic support are desirable, dobutamine is frequently the drug of
choice. Vasodilators, such as nitroprusside or nitroglycerin,
may be useful in patients with evidence of elevated filling
pressures, low cardiac output, elevated systemic vascular resistance, and normal or raised blood pressure. If pharmacologic manipulations of preload, afterload, and contractility fail
to improve cardiac function, use of the intra-aortic balloon
pump may be considered to provide diastolic augmentation
and to reduce left ventricular afterload.

NEUROGENIC SHOCK. Neurogenic shock occurs when
sympathetic denervation produces an impairment in vasomotor tone. Loss of vasomotor tone in both the arteriolar and
venous systems leads to a decrease in systemic vascular resistance, a large increase in venous capacitance, a decrease in
venous return to the heart, and a decrease in cardiac output.
Hypotension and bradycardia, along with warm, dry extremities, are included in the classic description of neurogenic
shock, but tachycardia is frequently observed. The mainstay
of treatment of neurogenic shock is to improve cardiac filling
by intravenous volume administration. Placement of the patient in the Trendelenburg position may assist in increasing
venous return to the heart. The use of alpha-adrenergic agonist agents such as phenylephrine is rarely indicated if restoration of an effective intravascular volume has been carried out.

ANAPHYLACTIC AND ANAPHYLACTOID SHOCK.
Anaphylaxis is an allergic response mediated by IgE antibody.
Anaphylactoid reactions are not immunologically mediated.
The symptoms of both anaphylactic and anaphylactoid reactions are similar and are due to the activation and release of
inflammatory mediators, which lead to vasodilatation, increased capillary permeability, bronchospasm, airway edema,

and circulatory collapse. Initial management consists of ensuring an adequate airway, providing oxygen and intravenous fluids, and administering epinephrine. Bronchospasm may further be treated by inhaled nebulized solutions of metaproterenol or albuterol. Secondary therapy may include the use of aminophylline, corticosteroids, and antihistamines.

HYPOADRENAL SHOCK. Shock due to adrenocortical insufficiency should be considered in patients who have a history of glucocorticoid therapy or in patients with no previous history of adrenocortical insufficiency who develop severe shock refractory to volume and pressor resuscitation. Hypoglycemia in a hypotensive patient may suggest the diagnosis, which may be supported by the findings of hyponatremia and hyperkalemia. The diagnosis should be established by performance of the rapid adrenocorticotropic hormone stimulation test, but institution of steroid therapy should not be delayed in unstable patients while waiting for the laboratory results.

SHOCK ASSOCIATED WITH SIRS, SEPSIS, AND MULTIPLE ORGAN DYSFUNCTION SYNDROME. Multiple organ failure is the most common cause of death in intensive care units. Noninfectious insults, such as trauma, pancreatitis, burns, and massive transfusions, may produce a MODS that is clinically indistinguishable from that due to culture-proven infectious causes. There is a clinically recognizable pathophysiologic progression from SIRS to sepsis to shock and, ultimately, to MODS.

Patients in shock associated with sepsis or SIRS frequently have fever, tachycardia, hypotension, oliguria, and altered mental status. The hemodynamic profile may vary. In the early stages, a hyperdynamic profile exists, manifested by elevated cardiac index and a decreased systemic vascular resistance. The intravascular volume is expanded and vasodilatation occurs in peripheral arterial and venous capacitance vessels, while the splanchnic circulation may remain underperfused. Hypermetabolism is typically seen, reflected by increases in resting energy expenditure, gluconeogenesis, catabolism, and oxygen consumption. In contrast, during the late, or preterminal, stage of shock associated with sepsis or SIRS, a hypodynamic response is sometimes seen. The hypodynamic response is indicative of a decompensated circulatory state.

Patients in septic shock, by definition, have positive microbial cultures. In adults, septic shock is associated most frequently with pneumonia, gastrointestinal perforation, biliary tract infection, urinary tract infection, burn wounds, and line sepsis from indwelling intravascular catheters.

The number of organs involved in MODS is a prognostic indicator of mortality, as is the existence of particular combinations of dysfunctional organs (e.g., liver and lung). Pulmonary dysfunction appears at an early stage of MODS. The acute lung injury in MODS reflects the pathophysiologic pulmonary manifestations of a systemic inflammatory process. The adult respiratory distress syndrome (ARDS) is characterized by ventilation-perfusion abnormalities, noncardiogenic pulmonary edema, decreased functional residual capacity, refractory hypoxemia, diffuse infiltrates on chest radiographs,

and decreased lung compliance. Treatment is largely supportive, including the use of mechanical ventilation. The mortality
rate for ARDS exceeds 50%.

Gastrointestinal dysfunction in MODS may include gastritis
or ulcerations, ileus, pancreatitis, acalculous cholecystitis, malabsorption, and mucosal atrophy. Breakdown of the gut mucosal barrier predisposes to the translocation of bacteria or toxins
that can perpetuate the inflammatory process.

The liver appears to play a pivotal role in the progression
and outcome of MODS. The vital metabolic functions of the
liver, as well as the host defense functions of the Kupffer cells,
are key processes, which, when perturbed, contribute to the
high morbidity and mortality associated with MODS when
severe hepatic dysfunction exists.

Renal dysfunction in MODS may arise as the result of
tissue hypoperfusion or direct tissue damage by activated
inflammatory cells and their mediators. Vasoconstrictive
mechanisms, redistribution of blood flow, and inadequate perfusion pressure may all contribute to renal dysfunction.

Pre-existing cardiovascular disease predisposes the patient
to more severe cardiac dysfunction during the course of
MODS. A myocardial depressant factor, possibly tumor necrosis factor, may exist.

The best treatment for shock associated with sepsis or SIRS
is preventing the progression to MODS. As with other forms
of shock, aggressive resuscitation to establish optimal levels
of oxygen delivery and oxygen consumption should be the
goal. Several studies have demonstrated that increased survival may be seen in patients who can generate a hyperdynamic response early in the course of sepsis or SIRS. Thus
attempts to improve oxygen delivery and oxygen consumption in order to achieve delivery-independent oxygen consumption seem warranted, at least in the early stages of SIRS
or sepsis. Such therapy has not proven to be of benefit when
MODS is fully developed.

Oxygen delivery can be optimized by using a rational combination of volume expansion, provision of red blood cell
mass, and appropriate use of pharmacologic agents. Beta agonists, vasodilators, and occasionally, alpha agonists, may improve cardiac contractility, decrease afterload, and increase
mean arterial or perfusion pressure, respectively. Patients with
shock due to sepsis or SIRS have a high mortality as the
syndrome progresses to MODS.

Patients with sepsis or presumed sepsis should be treated
with appropriate antibiotics, surgical débridement, and drainage when indicated. Reduction of "second hits" should be
achieved through meticulous care to lines and catheters and
by early nutritional support, preferably via the enteral route.

Therapies for shock due to sepsis or SIRS and/or MODS
have been directed primarily at supporting organ function.
New approaches are being evaluated that aim to modulate
the stress response by blocking the activation or action of key
mediators or by enhancing immune function. Results from
recent human clinical trials evaluating antimediator therapies
have not demonstrated clear outcome benefits.

6

FLUID AND ELECTROLYTE MANAGEMENT OF THE SURGICAL PATIENT

G. Tom Shires III, M.D., and G. Tom Shires, M.D.

Fluid and electrolyte management is an integral part of the care of surgical patients, and it may be a critical factor in certain patients. Many diseases and injuries, as well as operative trauma, have a great impact on the physiology of body fluids and electrolytes, far greater than the changes associated with a simple lack of alimentation. Therefore, a thorough understanding of the metabolism of salt, water, and other electrolytes and of certain metabolic responses is essential to the care of surgical patients.

ANATOMY OF BODY FLUID COMPARTMENTS

Total Body Water

Water constitutes between 50% and 70% of total body weight. Using deuterium oxide or tritiated water for measurement of total body water (TBW), the average normal value is 60% of body weight for young adult males and 50% for young adult females. The water of the body is divided into three functional compartments. The fluid within the body's diverse cell population, *intracellular water*, represents between 30% and 40% of the body weight. The *extracellular water* represents approximately 20% of the body weight and is divided between the *intravascular fluid*, or plasma (5% of body weight), and the *interstitial fluid*, or extravascular, extracellular fluid (15% of body weight).

CLASSIFICATION OF BODY FLUID CHANGES

The disorders in fluid balance may be classified in three general categories: disturbances of volume, concentration, and composition. Of primary importance is the concept that although these disturbances are interrelated, each is a separate entity.

If an isotonic salt solution is added to or lost from the body fluids, only the *volume* of the extracellular fluid is changed. The acute loss of an isotonic extracellular solution, such as intestinal juice, is followed by a significant decrease in the

---

See the corresponding chapter or part in the *Textbook of Surgery*, 15th edition, pp. 92–111, for a more detailed discussion of this topic, including a comprehensive list of references.

extracellular fluid volume and little, if any, change in the intracellular fluid volume. Fluid will not be transferred from the intracellular space to refill the depleted extracellular space as long as the osmolality remains the same in the two compartments.

If water alone is added to or lost from the extracellular fluid, the *concentration* of osmotically active particles will change. Sodium ions account for most of the osmotically active particles in the extracellular fluid and generally reflect the tonicity of other body fluid compartments. If the extracellular fluid is depleted of sodium, water will pass into the intracellular space until osmolality is again equal in the two compartments.

The concentration of most other ions within the extracellular fluid compartment can be altered without significant change in the total number of osmotically active particles, thus producing only a *compositional* change. For instance, a rise of the serum potassium concentration from 4 to 8 mEq. per liter would have a significant effect on the myocardium, but it would not significantly change the effective osmotic pressure of the extracellular fluid compartment. Normally functioning kidneys minimize these changes considerably, particularly if the addition or loss of solute or water is gradual.

An internal loss of extracellular fluid into a nonfunctional space, such as the sequestration of isotonic fluid in a burn, peritonitis, ascites, or muscle trauma, is termed a *distributional* change. This transfer or functional loss of extracellular fluid internally may be extracellular (e.g., as in peritonitis) or intracellular (e.g., as in hemorrhagic shock). In any event, all distributional shifts or losses contract the *functional* extracellular fluid space.

Volume Changes

An excess or deficit of extracellular fluid (ECF) volume must be diagnosed by clinical examination of the patient. Direct measurement of the ECF volume using sodium bromide or radioactive sodium sulfate is feasible in a research setting but is of limited use clinically because of the complexity of the tests. Several laboratory tests, however, indirectly reflect changes in ECF volume. The blood urea nitrogen (BUN) rises with an ECF deficit of sufficient magnitude to reduce glomerular filtration.

VOLUME DEFICIT. Extracellular fluid volume deficit is by far the most common fluid disorder in the surgical patient. The loss of fluid is not water alone, but water and electrolytes in approximately the same proportion as that in which they exist in normal ECF. The most common disorders leading to an ECF volume deficit include losses of gastrointestinal fluids due to vomiting, nasogastric suction, diarrhea, and fistula drainage. Other common causes include sequestration of fluid in soft tissue injuries and infections, intra-abdominal and retroperitoneal inflammatory processes, peritonitis, intestinal obstruction, and burns.

VOLUME EXCESS. Extracellular fluid volume excess is generally iatrogenic or secondary to renal insufficiency. Both the plasma and the interstitial fluid volumes are increased. In a healthy young adult, the signs are generally those of circulatory overload, manifested primarily in the pulmonary circulation, and of excessive fluid in other tissues. In an elderly patient, for instance, congestive heart failure with pulmonary edema may develop rather quickly with a moderate volume excess.

Concentration Changes

The serum sodium level is used to estimate total body fluid osmolality. Because the extracellular and intracellular fluid compartments are separated by a membrane that is freely permeable only to water, osmolality is approximately the same in the two spaces. Any change in the number of particles (osmolality) in one compartment will initiate an appropriate transfer of water between the two spaces. Therefore, even though the sodium ion is largely confined to the extracellular compartment, its level reflects total body fluid osmolality. Hyponatremia and hypernatremia can be diagnosed by clinical manifestations, but discernible signs and symptoms are not generally present until the changes are severe. Changes in concentration should be noted early by appropriate laboratory tests and corrected promptly.

Composition Changes

Compositional abnormalities of importance include changes in acid-base balance and concentration changes of potassium, calcium, and magnesium.

The four types of acid-base disturbances are respiratory alkalosis or acidosis and metabolic alkalosis or acidosis. Use of the CO_2 content and knowledge of the patient's disease may allow an accurate diagnosis in the uncomplicated case. However, use of the CO_2 content alone is generally inadequate as an index of acid-base balance. In the acute phase, respiratory acidosis or alkalosis may exist without any change in the CO_2 content; determinations of the pH and P_{CO_2} from a freshly drawn arterial blood sample are necessary for diagnosis.

Unfortunately, more complex acid-base disturbances are encountered frequently. Combinations of respiratory and metabolic changes occur and may represent compensation for the initial acid-base disturbance or may indicate two or more coexisting primary disorders (e.g., a *primary* respiratory acidosis complicated by a *primary* metabolic acidosis or alkalosis).

POTASSIUM ABNORMALITIES. Ninety-eight per cent of the potassium in the body is located in the intracellular compartment at a concentration of approximately 150 mEq. per liter, and it is the major cation of intracellular water. Although the total extracellular potassium in a 70-kg. male would approximate only 63 mEq. (4.5 mEq. per liter $\times$ 14 liters), this small amount is critical to cardiac and neuromuscular function.

HYPERKALEMIA. The signs of significant hyperkalemia are limited to the cardiovascular and gastrointestinal systems.

The gastrointestinal symptoms include nausea, vomiting, intermittent intestinal colic, and diarrhea. The cardiovascular signs are apparent on the electrocardiogram initially, with high peaked T waves, widened QRS complex, and depressed ST segments. Disappearance of T waves, heart block, and diastolic cardiac arrest may develop with increasing levels of potassium. Treatment of hyperkalemia consists of immediate measures to reduce the serum potassium level, withholding of exogenously administered potassium, and correction of the underlying cause when possible.

HYPOKALEMIA. A more common problem in the surgical patient is hypokalemia, which may occur as a result of excessive renal excretion, movement of potassium into cells, prolonged administration of potassium-free parenteral fluids with continued obligatory renal loss of potassium (>20 mEq./day), parenteral nutrition with inadequate potassium replacement, and loss of gastrointestinal secretions.

The treatment of hypokalemia involves, first, prevention of this state. In the replacement of gastrointestinal fluids, it is safe to replace the upper limits of loss, since an excess is readily handled by the patient with normal renal function. No more than 40 mEq. should be added to 1 liter of intravenous fluid, and the rate of administration should not exceed 20 mEq. per hour unless the electrocardiogram is being monitored.

NORMAL EXCHANGE OF FLUID AND ELECTROLYTES

Knowledge of the basic principles governing both the internal and the external exchanges of water and salt is mandatory for care of the patient undergoing major operative surgery. The stable internal fluid environment, which is maintained by the kidneys, brain, lungs, skin, and gastrointestinal tract, may be compromised by severe surgical stress or direct damage to any of these organs.

WATER EXCHANGE. The normal individual consumes an average of 2000 to 2500 ml. of water per day; approximately 1500 ml. of water is taken by mouth, and the rest is extracted from solid food, either from the contents of food or as the product of oxidation. The daily water losses include 250 ml. in stools, 800 to 1500 ml. as urine, and approximately 600 to 900 ml. as insensible loss through the skin and the lungs. A patient deprived of all external access to water must still excrete a minimum of 500 to 800 ml. of urine per day in order to excrete the products of catabolism, in addition to the mandatory insensible loss through the skin and lungs.

SALT GAIN AND LOSSES. In a normal individual, the daily salt intake varies between 50 and 90 mEq. (3 to 5 gm.) as sodium chloride. Balance is maintained primarily by the kidneys, which excrete the excess salt. Under conditions of reduced intake or extrarenal losses, normal kidneys can reduce sodium excretion to less than 1 mEq. per day within 24 hours after restriction. For practical considerations, then, normal losses may be relatively free of salt in the healthy individual with normal renal function.

Gastrointestinal losses are usually isotonic, although there is considerable variation in their compositions. These should be replaced by isotonic salt solutions. It is also important to reiterate that distributional or sequestration losses of extracellular fluid at any point in the operative or postoperative course also represent isotonic losses of salt and water.

FLUID AND ELECTROLYTE THERAPY

Parenteral Solutions

A good available isotonic salt solution for replacing gastrointestinal losses and ECF volume deficits, in the absence of gross abnormalities of concentration and composition, is lactated Ringer's solution. This solution is *physiologic* and contains 130 mEq. of sodium balanced by 109 mEq. of chloride and 28 mEq. of lactate. Lactate is used instead of bicarbonate, since the former is more stable in intravenous fluids during storage. The lactate is readily converted to bicarbonate by the liver following infusion. Concern about the ability of the liver to metabolize lactate is unwarranted even when infusing large quantities of lactated Ringer's solution to patients in hemorrhagic shock. This fluid has minimal effects on normal body fluid composition and pH even when infused in large quantities. Other balanced salt solutions are available, some with sodium acetate or bicarbonate instead of lactate; all are considered interchangeable.

Isotonic sodium chloride contains 154 mEq. of sodium and 154 mEq. of chloride per liter. The high concentration of chloride above the normal serum concentration of 103 mEq. per liter imposes on the kidneys an appreciable load of excess chloride that cannot be excreted rapidly. Thus a dilutional acidosis may develop. This solution is ideal, however, for the initial correction of an ECF volume deficit in the presence of hyponatremia, hypochloremia, and metabolic alkalosis.

A frequent choice for maintenance fluid in the postoperative period, 0.45% sodium chloride in 5% dextrose solution, provides free water for insensible losses and some sodium for renal adjustment of serum concentration. With added potassium, this is a reasonable solution to use for maintenance requirements in an uncomplicated patient requiring only a short period of parenteral fluids.

CORRECTION OF VOLUME CHANGES. Changes in the volume of ECF are the most frequent and important abnormalities encountered in the surgical patient. Depletion of the ECF compartment without changes in concentration or composition is a common problem. The diagnosis of volume changes is made almost entirely on clinical grounds. The signs that are present in an individual patient depend not only on the relative or absolute quantity of ECF that has been lost but also on the rapidity with which it is lost and the presence or absence of signs of associated disease.

Volume deficit in the surgical patient may result from external loss of fluids or from an internal redistribution of ECF into nonfunctional compartments. Often it involves a combination of the two, but the internal redistribution is frequently overlooked.

Fluid replacement should be started and changed according to the response of the patient noted on frequent clinical observation. Reliance on a formula or single clinical sign to determine adequacy of resuscitation is unwise. Rather, reversal of the signs of the volume deficit, combined with stabilization of the blood pressure and pulse, and an hourly urine volume of 30 to 50 ml. are used as general guidelines. An adequate hourly urine output, although usually a reliable monitor for volume replacement, may be totally misleading, however. For example, the excessive administration of glucose may cause osmotic diuresis. Additionally, the rapid administration of salt solutions may transiently expand the intravascular volume, increase the glomerular filtration rate, and create an immediate outpouring of urine, although the total ECF space remains quite depleted.

The choice of a proper fluid for replacement depends on the existence of concomitant concentration or compositional abnormalities. With pure ECF volume loss or when only minimal concentration or compositional abnormalities are present, the use of a balanced salt solution is desirable.

RATE OF FLUID ADMINISTRATION. This varies considerably, depending on the severity and type of fluid disturbance, the presence of continuing losses, and the cardiac status. In general, the most severe volume deficits may be replaced safely initially with isotonic solutions at a rate of 1000 ml. per hour, reducing the rate as the fluid status improves. Constant observation by a physician is mandatory when administration exceeds 1000 ml. per hour. At these rates, however, a significant portion may be lost as urinary output owing to a transient overexpansion of the plasma volume.

In elderly patients, associated cardiovascular disorders do not preclude correction of existing volume deficits, but they do require slower, more careful correction with appropriate monitoring, including the central venous or pulmonary artery and wedge pressures.

7

PRINCIPLES OF PREOPERATIVE PREPARATION OF THE SURGICAL PATIENT

Hiram C. Polk, Jr., M.D., and William G. Cheadle, M.D.

The modern preparation of the patient for operation characterizes the emergence of all the surgical disciplines from art to science.

ASSESSMENT OF OPERATIVE RISK

Calculation of operative risk is a major component of the relative rewards and risks of treatment for a specific illness. The overt nature of the surgical method magnifies the significance of adverse results and permits a clear understanding of this expression in the therapeutic ratio—that is, the relative harm (risk) and the relative good (benefit) that are *likely* to follow a specific operation for a specific illness in a specific patient. The *natural history* of a given illness must be known to evaluate such potential benefit. The capacity for sound clinical *judgment* is the ultimate characteristic of the mature physician.

PERSONAL RELATIONSHIPS

When an operation is being considered, a genuine bond of communication and personal responsibility must be established between the surgeon and the patient. The patient's confidence is based on real understanding, allowing him or her to participate, when appropriate, in judgments affecting risks, future lifestyle, and the postoperative recovery. The *specific permission* for conduct of an operative procedure is a focal point of medical, legal, and sociologic discussion. Local custom and recent legal practice often determine which of these is most appropriate.

GENERAL PREPARATION OF THE PATIENT

Psychologic Preparation

A frank but optimistic discussion of the possibilities ahead is valuable to the patient undergoing a major surgical procedure. The preoperative steps, as well as drainage devices and various forms of intubation, should be enumerated, justified, and explained in detail. The surgeon must not equivocate in

---

See the corresponding chapter or part in the *Textbook of Surgery,* 15th edition, pp. 112–117, for a more detailed discussion of this topic, including a comprehensive list of references.

discussing possible disfiguring operations. When an illness is apt to have a clinically significant course beyond the duration of the early posthospital follow-up, it is usually very reassuring for the surgeon to explain his or her continuing commitment to the patient.

Physiologic Preparation

BLOOD VOLUME CONSIDERATIONS. Numerous chronic disease processes are associated with anemia. The key issue is tissue oxygen delivery (O_2), which can be enhanced by increased cardiac output, hemoglobin concentration, or O_2 extraction. Transfusion to achieve a hemoglobin of 10 gm. per 100 ml. allows adequate O_2 delivery given normal tissue blood flow.

OTHER FLUID DEFICITS. Plasma and extracellular fluid deficits are significant in both volume and concentration. Special problems are presented when the volume deficiencies are pre-existing or concealed. *Pre-existing* losses may represent vomitus and/or diarrhea occurring before hospitalization. *Concealed* or "third space" losses, in which blood, plasma, or extracellular fluid is extravasated, are often associated with fractures, major burns, and peritonitis. Hourly determinations of urinary output, hemoglobin concentration, appearance of the mucous membranes, and skin turgor can reveal problems. Isotonic losses of sodium, chloride, and potassium may produce profound volume deficiencies, which must be replenished with similar isotonic solution (e.g., lactated Ringer's solution).

TIMING AND PARAMETERS. Urgency of the operation is the major determinant in the time available for correction of fluid and electrolyte balance. Not all volume and concentrational deficits need to be corrected before operation is undertaken. In general, the longer a patient has been ill, the more time one can take to correct the deficiencies. In other words, the patient has adjusted physiologically to the deficiency induced by the illness. One must be certain that the rapid replenishment of such deficits does not impose a risk greater than the illness itself.

Nutrition

Nutritional replenishment and supplementation have become common (and expensive) worldwide surgical practices; these pertain only to elective procedures in terms of preoperative preparation. A recent Veterans Administration cooperative study showed that severely malnourished patients benefit from prolonged preoperative nutritional supplementation.

Prevention of Infection

During preoperative evaluation, the patient should be protected from any patient with extramural or hospital-acquired infections. The proposed operative site should be cleansed with an appropriate antiseptic agent on several occasions before operation, and shaving should be done either as close to the time of operation as is feasible or not at all, with substitution of either clipping or depilatory agents where removal of hair is desired. Antibiotic prophylaxis is highly effective when used just before, during, and immediately after an operation. However, one must always balance the risk of an adverse effect of an antibiotic with its potential benefit. The agent selected should have sustained antibiotic activity in the surgical wound itself.

SPECIFIC ORGANS AND SYSTEMS

CARDIOVASCULAR. The capacity of the patient to increase cardiac output in response to intra- and postoperative challenges is perhaps the most fundamental determinant of survival following complex operations. Goldman determined important risk factors that predict fatal or life-threatening complications of cardiac origin after *noncardiac* operations, which include congestive heart failure, acute myocardial infarction, and unstable angina operations. Preoperative pulmonary wedge pressure monitoring with and without challenge has identified some patients with prohibitive cardiac risk and has allowed others to be improved prior to operation.

RESPIRATORY. Postoperative complications include atelectasis, pneumonia, and embolism. Preoperative teaching, evaluation, pulmonary physiotherapy, and antibiotics may reduce such risk. Patients at increased risk for thromboembolism include those with a clear history or clinical signs of prior thrombosis or embolism, those likely to have prolonged operations or perineal operations requiring the use of stirrups, and those with certain reconstructive operations on the hip. The clinician may then employ a number of methods for reducing the risk of thromboembolism, including pneumatic compression stockings, exercises, early ambulation, and variable degrees of anticoagulation.

RENAL. With appropriate perioperative hydration, renal complications of major surgical endeavors have become relatively uncommon. With the screening procedures of blood urea nitrogen determination, creatinine determination, and urinalysis, one may proceed to an operation and subsequent fluid therapy reasonably confident that the patient will tolerate judiciously managed fluid loads with ease. The most common cause of oliguria on surgical services continues to be *hypo*volemia rather than incipient renal failure.

HEPATIC. The signs and symptoms of significant liver impairment are detectable on standard examinations. Only lifesaving procedures should be attempted in Child's C patients, and an attempt at conversion to Child's A or B by prolonged nutritional support and diuretics substantially reduces operative risk.

NEUROLOGIC. Maintaining cerebral function via appropriate oxygenation and circulation is vitally important to the anesthesiologist and the surgeon. Of special concern is the prevalence of occult cerebrovascular disease in the elderly, who constitute a major proportion of patients requiring surgical attention.

SPECIAL PROBLEMS

Pulmonary aspiration is a dreaded surgical complication, the treatment of which remains inadequate, whereas prevention is simple. In almost no circumstances should general anesthesia be induced without specific attention to evacuation of the patient's stomach, ascertained in any questionable case by the surgeon. Mechanical preparation of the colon is wise prior to any operation in the abdomen.

8

BLOOD TRANSFUSIONS AND DISORDERS OF SURGICAL BLEEDING

Samir M. Fakhry, M.D., and George F. Sheldon, M.D.

PREPARATION AND USE OF BLOOD COMPONENTS

The ability to replace blood loss is an important prerequisite in modern surgical practice. Approximately 60% of all blood products given to patients are transfused at or near the time of surgery. Component therapy is the accepted standard for optimal management of the blood supply. Blood is collected and separated into its individual components to optimize therapeutic potency: packed red blood cells (RBCs), plasma, platelets, cryoprecipitate, and proteins. Blood is withdrawn from the donor and mixed with citrate solution to prevent coagulation by binding calcium (e.g., citrate phosphate dextrose, CPD). Storage and refrigeration of RBCs result in a "storage lesion" including altered hemoglobin affinity for oxygen, decrease in pH, changes in RBC deformability, hemolysis, and an increase in concentration of potassium, phosphate, and ammonia. Transfusion of refrigerated blood contributes to the development of hypothermia. Many of these changes are reversed after transfusion or result in different metabolic patterns than predicted. Cookbook-type formulas for infusion of fresh-frozen plasma (FFP), platelets, calcium, bicarbonate, and so on for a set number of units of RBCs are contraindicated and may result in added risk to the patient. Therapy should be based on demonstrated deficiencies and the clinical condition of the patient. The following are guidelines for transfusion but cannot substitute for the judgment of an experienced clinician.

RED BLOOD CELLS

Packed RBCs can be stored in CPDA-1 (citrate-phosphate-dextrose-adenine) for 35 days at 1 to 6° C, but platelets degenerate under these conditions. Levels of factors V and VIII decrease significantly, but other factors remain unchanged. The decision to transfuse and the amount to transfuse depend on the clinical situation. The use of a hematocrit of 30% (or a hemoglobin of 10 gm. per 100 ml.) as a "transfusion trigger" is no longer acceptable without considering the clinical situation. Compensatory mechanisms maintain oxygen delivery when hemoglobin or hematocrit fall, including increased cardiac

---

See the corresponding chapter or part in the *Textbook of Surgery,* 15th edition, pp. 118–136, for a more detailed discussion of this topic, including a comprehensive list of references.

output, increased extraction ratio, increase in 2,3-DPG concentrations in the RBC, rightward shift of the oxyhemoglobin curve, and volume expansion. Healthy patients tolerate acute anemia to hemoglobin levels of 7 gm. per 100 ml. or less provided they have a normal intravascular volume and high arterial oxygen saturation. Patients with significant cardiopulmonary disease should receive RBC transfusion whenever clinically indicated to prevent cardiac ischemia. A stable, asymptomatic patient generally should not receive packed RBCs solely for a hematocrit below 30%. Each unit of packed RBCs usually raises the hematocrit approximately 2% to 3% in a 70-kg. person, although this varies.

PLATELETS

Platelet transfusions are indicated for patients suffering from or at significant risk of bleeding due to thrombocytopenia and/or platelet dysfunction. Single, random-donor units of platelets are prepared from single donors; patients receive 6 to 10 units per transfusion. Multiple-unit, single-donor platelets are harvested from one donor by apheresis to yield as many platelets as 6 to 10 single, random-donor units. Multiple-unit, single-donor platelets can be obtained by apheresis from donors who are selected by human lymphocyte antigen (HLA) type to yield HLA-matched platelets. Following platelet transfusion in the adult, the platelet count obtained at 1 hour should rise at least 5000 platelets per μl. per unit of platelets transfused. Patients may experience a lesser response, especially after repeated transfusions and the development of alloimmunization or because of fever, sepsis, splenomegaly, drug effects, or uremia. When alloimmunization is the cause of the poor response, single-donor or HLA-matched units may provide an adequate response. Platelets should not be transfused prophylactically without either microvascular bleeding, a low platelet count in a patient undergoing a surgical procedure, or a platelet count that has recently fallen below 10,000 per μl. Patients receiving massive transfusion should not automatically receive prophylactic platelets in the absence of microvascular bleeding. In such patients, hypothermia plays an important role in depressed platelet function, and platelet transfusion is generally ineffective.

FRESH-FROZEN PLASMA

Fresh-frozen plasma (FFP) is used to replace clotting factors in patients with coagulopathy as a result of liver dysfunction, congenital absence of clotting factor, or transfusion of factor-deficient blood products. A unit of FFP contains near-normal levels of all clotting factors and will increase factor levels by about 3%. Adequate clotting is usually achieved with factor levels above 30%; higher levels are advisable in patients undergoing operative or invasive procedures. Low factor levels or abnormal prothrombin time (PT) or activated partial thromboplastin time (aPTT) in a patient with clinical bleeding will identify patients needing FFP. FFP should not be used routinely by preset formula after RBC transfusion (e.g., 2 units of FFP for every 5 units of packed RBCs) or "prophylactically" after cardiac bypass or other procedures. FFP should not be used as a volume expander.

CRYOPRECIPITATE

Cryoprecipitate is useful in the treatment of factor deficiency (hemophilia A), von Willebrand's disease, and hypofibrinogenemia and may aid in the treatment of uremic bleeding. Each 5- to 15-ml. unit contains 80 units of factor VIII and about 200 mg. of fibrinogen. Cryoprecipitate is usually administered as a transfusion of 10 single units and provides a smaller volume load than FFP.

RISKS OF BLOOD TRANSFUSION

Transfusion of blood products can result in serious complications, including death. Blood products should be considered potentially dangerous "drugs." Although most transfusion reactions are minor febrile responses, transfusion of incompatible RBCs related to clerical error is potentially fatal. The transmission of HIV and viral hepatitis remains the major infectious risk of transfusion. The risk of transmission of HIV is estimated at 1 in 220,000 per unit. With the recent introduction of donor screening for surrogate markers for non-A, non-B hepatitis and for antibodies to hepatitis C virus, the risk of posttransfusion hepatitis has been reduced to less than 1% per patient. Blood components contain viable lymphocytes capable of mounting a graft-versus-host response in immunocompromised recipients. Transfusion may modify the recipient's immune response, as has been demonstrated with renal transplantation, and may increase reccurrence rates of solid tumors when administered at the time of surgical resection.

EVALUATION OF PATIENTS WITH DISORDERS OF HEMOSTASIS OR COAGULATION

An accurate history and examination offer the most valuable sources of information regarding the risk of perioperative bleeding. This includes a history of a bleeding tendency, significant hemorrhage with invasive procedures or a family history of such problems, easy bruisability, frequent mucosal bleeding, high menstrual flow in females, and hepatic, renal, metabolic, or endocrine disorders. The intake of medications should be elicited, especially aspirin and nonsteroidal anti-inflammatory drugs (NSAIDs). Excessive bruising, joint deformities, petechia or ecchymosis, hepatosplenomegaly, excessive mobility of joints, and increased skin elasticity suggest disorders associated with excessive perioperative bleeding. For most patients undergoing minor surgery not involving extensive dissection, laboratory testing is unlikely to provide additional information over a properly performed history and physical examination. Routine preoperative laboratory screening is useful in patients undergoing major surgery involving body cavities, significant dissection, or creation of raw surfaces and in patients with an abnormal history or examination. Patients with infection, sepsis, malnutrition, organ failure, and other major systemic disorders also warrant preoperative screening. Commonly recommended tests include the prothrombin time (PT), the activated partial thromboplastin time (aPTT), a complete blood count with platelet count, and in some patients a bleeding time (BT). If suspicion of a specific factor deficiency exists (e.g., a family history of hemophilia), then specific factor assays should be obtained.

DISORDERS OF HEMOSTASIS OR COAGULATION

Hemostasis is the physiologic cessation of bleeding. When blood vessel injury occurs, tissue factor (TF) and collagen are exposed. Platelets aggregate and adhere, forming a platelet "plug." Vasoconstriction also occurs to decrease blood flow. Initiation of the coagulation cascade occurs by interaction of TF with circulating factor VII. Prothrombin is converted to thrombin, which converts fibrinogen to fibrin. The fibrin monomers and entrapped platelets form a hemostatic thrombus. Stabilization of the fibrin clot occurs by cross-linking of fibrin monomers under the effect of factor XIII. Organized clot formation and arrest of bleeding result. Local blood flow, vasodilatory influences, and regulatory feedback mechanisms limit extension of the thrombus systemically. Fibrinolysis with dissolution of the fibrin thrombus then begins. Hemostatic and coagulation mechanisms allow the prompt repair of a local injury in the microcirculation without progression to a systemic reaction. Acquired coagulation defects are more common than congenital defects and include the following:

VITAMIN K DEFICIENCY. Bleeding results from depletion of the vitamin K–dependent clotting factors, factors II, VII, IX, and X, protein C, and protein S. Intramuscular or subcutaneous vitamin K may be given in doses of 10 to 25 mg. per day for 3 days to replete body stores.

ANTICOAGULANT DRUGS. Including coumadin and heparin. Treatment of bleeding caused by coumadin consists of either vitamin K or FFP for life-threatening bleeding. Heparin can be neutralized with intravenous protamine sulfate: 100 units of heparin equals 1 mg. of protamine.

HEPATIC FAILURE. Associated with varying degrees of coagulopathy. In patients with severe liver dysfunction, large volumes of FFP may be required to normalize factor levels. Up to 2 units of FFP may be needed every 2 hours in patients with complete liver failure.

RENAL FAILURE. Renal disease and uremia cause a reversible bleeding disorder largely related to platelet dysfunction. DDAVP, 0.3 μg. per kg. IV, results in a decrease in BT and increased factor VIII activity. Cryoprecipitate is also helpful in normalizing prolonged BTs.

HYPOTHERMIA. A common, underdiagnosed cause of altered coagulation, especially with massive transfusion.

DISSEMINATED INTRAVASCULAR COAGULATION (DIC). A systemic thrombohemorrhagic disorder associated with well-defined clinical situations and laboratory evidence of procoagulant activation, fibrinolytic activation, and inhibitor consumption as well as biochemical evidence of end-organ damage or failure.

Among the more common congenital disorders are the following:

VON WILLEBRAND'S DISEASE. Quantitative or qualitative defects of von Willebrand's factor, important in platelet function and as a plasma carrier of factor VIII. DDAVP and cryoprecipitate are effective therapies.

HEMOPHILIA. Deficiency of factor VIII (hemophilia A or classic hemophilia) or factor IX (hemophilia B or Christmas disease). DDAVP may temporarily raise factor VIII levels in patients with mild hemophilia A. FFP may be used to replace factors VIII and IX, but the volumes required in severe hemophilia are large and not practical. Cryoprecipitate is a good source of factor VIII but is rarely used when specific factor VIII concentrates are available. Two types of concentrates are available for treatment of hemophilia A: plasma-based and recombinant preparations. In general, 1 unit per kg. of factor VIII will raise levels by 2%. For treatment of hemophilia B, the traditional therapy is prothrombin complex concentrate, which contains not only factor IX but all the vitamin K–dependent clotting factors. High-purity factor IX concentrate is now available.

9

METABOLISM IN SURGICAL PATIENTS:
Protein, Carbohydrate, and Fat Utilization by Oral and Parenteral Routes
Josef E. Fischer, M.D.

Over the past several years, the process of nutritional support has changed so that the enteral route has become preferred. It was assumed previously that the enteral route would not work in the critically ill, but with attention to detail in striving to use this route, the enteral route has become the preferred methodology, with total parenteral nutrition (TPN) serving only when the enteral route is not feasible.

REQUIREMENTS

The minimal protein requirements for a nonseptic patient at rest are 55 mg. of nitrogen per kg. of body weight. For parenteral nutritional support, the "safe" value is considerably higher: 1.75 to 2.0 gm. of protein equivalent per kg. per 24 hours. This is likely higher in sepsis. The conversion factor between nitrogen and protein is 1 gm. of nitrogen to 6.25 gm. of mixed protein. The caloric requirement is approximately 35 cal. per kg. per 24 hours, with a calorie/nitrogen ratio of 1 gm. of nitrogen per 150 cal. In sepsis or trauma, the ratio is slightly lower, at 1:100. In resting starvation, approximately 75% of calories are derived from fat, which is fortunate indeed because the viscera, such as liver and kidney, derive most of their energy from fat. Carbohydrate provides approximately 10%, and protein, much of which is converted to carbohydrate, provides approximately 15%. The basal energy requirements can be determined by either metabolic cart or by the Harris-Benedict equation (basal energy expenditure = 66.5 + 13.7 W + 5.0 H − 6.8 A [male]; 655.1 + 9.56 W + 1.85 H − 4.68 A [female], where W = weight in kg.; H = height in cm.; and A = age in years), with an activity adjustment for both. In trauma or sepsis, the contribution of protein increases, since the amount of carbohydrate derived from protein increases so that protein constitutes approximately 20% of the caloric load. Resting energy requirements are increased 10% to 20% in trauma, probably up to 50% in sepsis, and in burns, since major burns represent the most severe metabolic insult, up to 100%. A major portion of this increase in the metabolic requirement of burns can be avoided by early (within 3 hours)

See the corresponding chapter or part in the *Textbook of Surgery*, 15th edition, pp. 137–175, for a more detailed discussion of this topic, including a comprehensive list of references.

enteral feeding. This presumably is secondary to the decrease in translocation of gut bacteria or their products across the gut and the release of cortisone, which this engenders.

During nutritional support, lipids make up anywhere between 20% and 50% of the caloric supply. It is probably not efficacious in most situations to use more than 50% of lipid because of the specific dynamic action of carbohydrate, although the requirement is considerably less.

GROUPS AT RISK

It has become possible recently to identify the group at risk from malnutrition. It should be stressed that this is not individual. One cannot pick out the individual who will be at increased risk, but 60% of a group that is identified as being malnourished will have an immunologic deficiency that will contribute to sepsis and a worse outcome. The characteristics of this group are (1) weight loss of greater than 10% and probably 15% of body weight over the most recent 3 to 4 months, (2) serum albumin in the hydrated resting state of less than 3 gm. per 100 ml., (3) confirmatory information including a serum transferrin of less than 220 mg. per 100 ml., and (4) anergy to injected skin antigens. Others have proposed that functional measurements such as hand dynamometry are equally efficacious. Global nutritional assessment also has been used with good results.

SHORT-TERM SUPPLEMENTATION

Once these individuals are identified, short-term nutritional supplementation has now been shown to reverse the undesirable effects of malnutrition. Most of these studies have been carried out with TPN, and it is not clear what the duration of nutritional supplementation should be, but it is probably in the range of 5 to 7 days. When preoperative TPN is used, at least as used in patients who are mildly or moderately malnourished, the incidence of nosocomial infections and the undesirable side effects more than make up for any beneficial effect of nutritional supplementation.

ROUTE OF NUTRITIONAL SUPPORT

Enteral nutrition is preferred for several reasons. First, the normal ingress of the nutrients is through the gut. Material supplied through the gut enters the portal circulation and is first delivered to the liver, where its normal role of continual uptake, processing, and storage with release upon hormonal-neural stimulation takes place. It may be that the liver requires most of the calories to pass through it in order to maintain its integrity. Enteral nutrition can be provided through the stomach or through the small intestine. Most authorities prefer to have a tube passed into the small intestine to decrease the risk of aspiration. Gastric motility may change suddenly in sepsis, and the patient may aspirate; this is less likely to happen if the tube is in the small bowel. Most of the advantages of the gut have been ascribed to improvements in the gut mucosal barrier, and while this may play a role in burns and in hemorrhagic shock, there is little evidence to suggest that this plays a major role elsewhere. Increased hepatic protein synthesis may be another mechanism by which this may be achieved.

Parenteral nutrition may be carried out peripherally using a relatively small amount of dextrose and a relatively large amount of lipid. It is difficult to maintain nitrogen equilibrium in patients for a prolonged period of time, so the central approach is used. The role of lipid has changed; initially lipid was used for essential fatty acids, but it is now utilized for a significant amount of calories. Calories given as 25% lipid will result in optimal visceral protein synthesis.

INDICATIONS

Indications may be divided into four categories: (1) primary therapy (value established), (2) primary therapy (efficacy not shown), (3) supportive therapy (efficacy shown), and (4) controversial.

Primary Therapy, Value Established

1. Enterocutaneous fistulas.
2. Short-bowel syndrome.
3. Renal failure. The use of essential amino acids and hypertonic dextrose results in improved survival and a shorter duration of renal failure.
4. Burns. Enteral nutrition has improved efficacy, decreased catabolic drive, and improved survival.
5. Hepatic failure. Improvement in encephalopathy and, in some studies, decreased mortality. When combined with operation in patients with cirrhosis of the liver, preoperative TPN with a branched-chain amino acid–enriched mixture results in fewer complications.
6. Weight loss prior to major surgery. Five to seven days of TPN is required. Data are lacking with respect to enteral nutrition. In patients with neoplastic disease, efficacy has only been shown in neoplasms of the upper gastrointestinal tract.
7. Trauma. Early feeding via the gut has been shown to result in fewer complications and fewer infections.

Primary Therapy, Efficacy Not Shown

1. Inflammatory bowel disease. Remission can be induced by either enteral or parenteral nutrition but is transient.
2. Anorexia nervosa, in patients who refuse to eat and whose thought processes have been compromised by weight loss.

Supportive Therapy, Efficacy Shown

1. Acute radiation and chemotherapy toxicity. Some investigators propose that the addition of glutamine helps in regen-

eration of the gut mucosa. It should be pointed out that glutamine is a fuel for tumors.

2. Patients on respirators for prolonged periods.

3. Patients with large upper wounds such as decubitus ulcers.

Controversial

1. Sepsis. High branched-chain amino acid mixtures (45%, generally high in leucine) may be slightly more efficacious in severely ill septic patients and in patients with bone marrow transplants, for example.

2. Cancer. There is little question that in some experimental studies, tumor growth is accelerated by the use of TPN. This area is still controversial, and its resolution probably awaits the determination of solutions that may lack certain nutrients required by tumors.

3. Nutritional pharmacology. Over the past several years, nutritional pharmacology, which is the use of naturally occurring nutrients as drugs, has become more important. The following are prominent in this area: glutamine as a preferred gut fuel — efficacy has yet to be shown; arginine — supranormal amounts of arginine may be useful in improving host resistance (it should be remembered that arginine is a precursor of nitric oxide); fish oil, with the change in the precursors of prostaglandins to the omega-3 fatty acids; and nucleotides. An enteral diet utilizing nutritional pharmacology of most of these materials has been shown to decrease length of stay and, if complications occur, decreased mortality from such complications.

COMPLICATIONS

Enteral Nutrition

1. Aspiration due to changing gut motility in sepsis and inappropriate technique are most common.

2. Diarrhea from hyperosmolality into the small bowel without sufficient free water. This may result in perforation and pneumatosis intestinalis.

3. Misplacement of the tube into the main stem bronchus, resulting in fatal aspiration.

Parenteral Nutrition

1. Technical misadventures in the placement of the needle in a crowded thoracic inlet, including, most commonly, pneumothorax (6%), laceration of vein or artery, and so on.

2. Metabolic complications. Mostly related to glucose but may include hypophosphatemia and hypokalemia.

3. Sepsis. May be bacterial in origin, usually relating to poor technique in caring for the catheter, and fungal sepsis, of which the port of entry is probably through the gastrointestinal tract.

10

SURGICAL ASPECTS OF DIABETES MELLITUS

Olga Jonasson, M.D.

Diabetes mellitus is a disorder of carbohydrate metabolism causing hyperglycemia. The consequences of diabetes derive from elevated levels of blood glucose and a deficiency in insulin. The major aim of therapy is consistent normoglycemia through diet, oral hypoglycemic agents, and exogenous insulin. Insulin is normally produced in the beta cells of pancreatic islets as proinsulin and a connecting peptide (C peptide). When it is necessary to measure insulin production in patients receiving exogenous insulin, it is advisable to measure the C peptide molecule.

Diabetics have fasting blood glucose levels greater than 140 mg. per 100 ml. on at least two occasions. Measurement of glycosylated hemoglobin (HgAl$_c$) indicates mean blood glucose levels over time. *Patients with hyperglycemia from any cause must be treated appropriately with insulin to normalize their blood glucose levels during any acute illness, stress, or operation.*

About 20% of diabetic patients have insulin-dependent diabetes mellitus (IDDM) and have little or no endogenous insulin production. They are prone to ketosis and iatrogenic hypoglycemia. Most diabetics have non–insulin-dependent diabetes mellitus (NIDDM); are older, obese, and hypertensive; and often have advanced accelerated atherosclerosis and heart disease. Hyperglycemia can be delayed or prevented in these patients through diet and lifestyle changes, emphasizing exercise and cessation of smoking. Sulfonylureas or biguanides may be used to stimulate insulin secretion. Exogenous insulin is given if oral drugs fail to normalize blood glucose levels and during any time of stress, such as infection or a surgical procedure. Patients with diabetes secondary to pancreatic insufficiency or disease are "brittle," in that the important counterregulatory hormones such as glucagon are also absent. They are especially prone to the development of hypoglycemia.

COMPLICATIONS

Metabolic Complications

The immediate effect of hyperglycemia is glucosuria and osmotic diuresis. Absence of insulin causes breakdown of fatty acids into ketoacids as fuel for the brain, and the excess ketone bodies appear in the plasma and urine. If this is uncorrected, diabetic ketoacidosis (DKA) occurs, with extreme hyperglycemia, dehydration, ketosis, and acidosis. Leukocytosis

---

See the corresponding chapter or part in the *Textbook of Surgery*, 15th edition, pp. 176–185, for a more detailed discussion of this topic, including a comprehensive list of references.

and abdominal pain due to delayed gastric emptying are often present. The inciting cause for this catastrophic metabolic cascade is often found to be sepsis or stress. Patients with NIDDM usually do not become ketoacidotic but may develop even more serious hyperglycemia associated with coma (nonketotic hyperosmolar hyperglycemia).

Hyperglycemia is directly related to the susceptibility of diabetics to infections. The most common site of infection in diabetics is the urinary tract. Necrotizing cellulitis and fasciitis can occur especially in the perineal region of male diabetics who have recently had urethral catheterization (Fournier's gangrene). This polymicrobial infection with aerobic and anaerobic organisms must be treated with prompt, aggressive surgical débridement, colostomy, and systemic antibiotics.

Neuropathy and the Diabetic Foot

A peripheral neuropathy develops in diabetic patients with long-standing diabetes. Peripheral neuropathy of the feet and distal lower extremity causes loss of protective sensation in the foot. Minor trauma may develop into a serious necrotizing infection with tissue loss. Aggressive débridement and antibiotic administration are necessary.

Autonomic Neuropathy

Gastroparesis with delayed gastric emptying and gastric dilatation may cause hypoglycemia in patients receiving insulin. Bethanechol, metoclopramide, and erythromycin may increase gastric motility, but surgical procedures have been ineffective. Intractable diarrhea and steatorrhea and esophageal dysmotility also may occur. Esophagoscopy should be performed in diabetic patients with dysphagia because *Candida* infection of the esophagus is commonly found. Treatment with fluconazole is indicated. Hypotonicity and failure to empty occur in the urinary bladder and contribute to the high rate of urinary tract infections in diabetics. This may be treated successfully initially by educating the patients in double-voiding techniques and in self-clean intermittent catheterization. Diabetic patients should be evaluated preoperatively for the presence of cardiac neuropathy by measuring the electrocardiogram R-R interval during a Valsalva maneuver or measuring orthostatic changes in pulse rate and blood pressure.

Diabetic renal disease develops in patients with diabetes for at least 15 years. Because of the pre-existing hyperfiltration in poorly controlled diabetic patients and their chronic osmotic diuresis and dehydration, they are highly susceptible to the nephrotoxic effects of iodinated radiologic contrast agents. Diabetic patients who are scheduled for angiography, CT scanning, or even oral cholecystography must be prepared by correction of pre-existing dehydration with infusion of 0.45% saline for 12 hours before and 12 hours following administration of the contrast agent. Angiotensin-converting enzyme inhibitors (ACE inhibitors) delay or halt progression of early diabetic nephropathy.

Atherosclerosis and
Coronary Artery Disease

The strong likelihood of significant coronary artery occlusive disease must be considered when undertaking surgical treatment of any diabetic patient. It is unwise to perform any but the most simple procedures on a diabetic patient in an outpatient setting.

In the diabetic patient with lower leg ischemia, septic foci must be dealt with by aggressive débridement and local amputations. Only when the infection is controlled should surgical reconstruction be considered. Sepsis, not ischemia, is the greatest cause of major amputation.

MANAGEMENT

The basic goal of management of diabetes is the consistent maintenance of a normal blood glucose. Patients with NIDDM can respond well to diet and exercise alone. Patients with IDDM and many patients with secondary diabetes require insulin. Iatrogenic hypoglycemia, a common occurrence in insulin-treated patients, should be treated by oral carbohydrates, but an unconscious patient requires an IV bolus of 20 ml. of 50% glucose, repeated as necessary, and an IV infusion of 5% or 10% dextrose until the blood glucose is above 100 mg. per 100 ml. and the patient is conscious.

Diabetic patients require insulin infusions during illness and operative stress. Fluid and electrolyte imbalance, blood pressure abnormalities, infection, and diminished wound healing are the risks of hyperglycemia in the surgical patient, and they are more serious than the risks of hypoglycemia during insulin treatment in a well-monitored surgical patient.

Diabetic patients with severe hyperglycemia may have abdominal pain and rigidity mimicking an acute abdomen. It is important to keep in mind that the precipitating cause for the development of DKA or the nonketotic hyperosmolar syndrome might be an acute abdominal condition. The treatment of severe hyperglycemia must precede any operative intervention. It is most important to treat the acidosis and dehydration; correction of the blood glucose follows. Resuscitation should take place in a monitored setting, such as the intensive care unit. Patients with changes in mental status likely require endotracheal intubation; a nasogastric tube must be placed because all severely hyperglycemic patients have gastric stasis.

Transplantation of vascularized whole pancreas has become a relatively safe procedure. Arterial blood supply is established by an end-to-side anastomosis to the iliac artery, and venous drainage is to the iliac vein; a small portion of duodenum surrounding the pancreatic duct opening is anastomosed to the urinary bladder. Recent graft survival rates reach 75% in most centers, and patient survival rates exceed 90%. Patients with a successful pancreas transplant report improvement in quality of life and feelings of well-being.

11

ANESTHESIA AND POSTOPERATIVE ANALGESIA

Mark E. Dentz, M.D., Katherine P. Grichnik, M.D.,
Karen S. Sibert, M.D., and J.G. Reves, M.D.

THE ROLE OF THE ANESTHESIOLOGIST IN THE CARE OF THE SURGICAL PATIENT

The anesthesiologist, like the surgeon, has a critical role in caring for the patient coming for a surgical procedure. This care extends from the preoperative to the operative and into the postoperative periods. Adjunctive care of hospitalized patients is also an important part of an anesthesiologist's job. This includes care of patients during procedures outside the operating suite, care of patients for radiologic procedures, hyperbaric medicine, and care of the patient with chronic pain. Further, the skills of the anesthesiologist are often required in the management of patients who suffer cardiopulmonary arrests.

PREOPERATIVE ASSESSMENT AND ANESTHETIC RISK

The challenge for the anesthesiologist is to function as the patient's internist in the perioperative period as well as to provide anesthesia safely during the surgical procedure. During the preoperative interview with the patient, the anesthesiologist attempts to obtain all pertinent information that gives him or her a complete portrait of the patient's physical health status, level of anxiety, and specific risk factors for complications from anesthesia. Physical examination focuses on the airway, heart, and lungs, looking for any previously unrecognized disease and for any factors that could present difficulties with airway management and intubation. The planned surgical procedure is the major determining factor in assessing an individual patient's risk for perioperative complications and in deciding which anesthetic technique—local anesthesia alone or with sedation, regional anesthesia, or general anesthesia—will be most appropriate. While it certainly is difficult to separate out the risks of anesthesia from those of operation, most studies have suggested that approximately 1 death per 10,000 anesthetics is totally attributable to anesthesia.

MONITORING

Monitoring of a patient's physiologic functions during the procedure is one of the primary responsibilities of the anesthe-

---

See the corresponding chapter or part in the *Textbook of Surgery*, 15th edition, pp. 186–206, for a more detailed discussion of this topic, including a comprehensive list of references.

siologist. The standards for basic intraoperative monitoring as stated by the American Society of Anesthesiologists require that the patient's ventilation, circulation, oxygenation, and temperature be evaluated continually during all anesthetics. This is accomplished with a variety of monitors, including precordial and esophageal stethoscopes, intermittent blood pressure monitors, continuous electrocardiography, pulse oximetry, and temperature probes. Also, depending on the type of surgical procedure and the physical status of the patient, specialized monitors may be required to assess specific organ systems.

ANESTHESIA TECHNIQUES

The induction of anesthesia, in general, falls into two categories: general and regional anesthesia. *General anesthesia* involves inducing a state of unconsciousness with analgesia, amnesia, and immobility. This goal can be accomplished with a combination of intravenous and inhalational medications. Further, usually some degree of control of a patient's airway is part of the introduction of a general anesthetic. Mask ventilation is usually accomplished with positive-pressure ventilation as necessary. Depending on the surgical procedure and the patient's comorbid disease, the anesthesiologist may choose to continue mask ventilation (spontaneous or controlled), place a laryngeal mask airway, or intubate the patient with a cuffed or uncuffed endotracheal tube.

Anesthesia is maintained with intravenous drug delivery (bolus or infusion) and/or inhalational drug delivery through the ventilating circuit. The maintenance period of anesthesia is characterized by adjusting the level of anesthesia to the surgical stimulus, monitoring vital bodily functions, treating abnormalities of hemodynamics or other organ function, and ensuring a quiet surgical field.

At the end of the operation, the disposition of the patient is determined in conjunction with the surgeon. If the patient is to be transferred to an intensive care unit (ICU), the anesthesiologist may elect not to allow the patient to emerge from anesthesia and may take the patient to the ICU anesthetized with ventilation controlled. However, if the patient is to be transferred to the postanesthesia care unit (PACU) in anticipation of going home or to a ward bed, the anesthesiologist usually allows the patient to emerge from anesthesia.

Regional anesthesia is often divided into major conduction anesthesia and major nerve block. *Major conduction anesthesia* includes epidural and spinal anesthesia. Epidural and spinal anesthesia share the goal of interruption of afferent neural impulses by deposition of drugs close to the spinal cord. Epidural anesthesia is most often accomplished by epidural space cannulation and subsequent infusion of local anesthetic agents and/or opioids. Spinal anesthesia involves the placement of anesthetic drugs into the subarachnoid space via puncture of the dura mater. The benefits of major conduction anesthesia are multifold. Patients can have control over their own respiratory function; patients receive less medication to achieve anesthesia; and postoperative analgesia is enhanced.

Further, there may be beneficial effects on respiratory function, cardiac function, release of stress hormones, coagulation and blood loss.

Major nerve blockade is also a form of regional anesthesia. Some of the most utilized blocks are the brachial plexus blocks for arm and shoulder procedures, cervical plexus blocks for neck and carotid procedures, femoral-sciatic nerve blocks for upper and lower leg procedures, three-in-one nerve (femoral, obturator, and lateral femoral cutaneous nerves) blocks for upper leg procedures, popliteal fossa nerve blocks for lower leg procedures, and ankle blocks for foot procedures. Further, paravertebral blocks may be used to perform certain upper abdominal and thoracic procedures, and retrobulbar blocks are used for eye procedures.

POSTANESTHESIA CARE UNIT

The postoperative period is one of multiple physiologic and pharmacologic changes. This time period includes complex pharmacology surrounding emergence and reversal of anesthesia, as well as physiologic changes related to surgical trauma. Intensive care for a period of time in the PACU is therefore critical to successful surgical outcomes. The patient's vital signs, hemodynamics, and recovery are monitored closely, and initial postoperative orders from the primary care team are carried out as the patient is prepared for eventual transfer to a ward bed. Airway management is exceedingly important as patients are being readied for transfer to a ward bed with less monitoring capabilities.

ACUTE PAIN MANAGEMENT

The alleviation of acute pain has made major progress over the course of the last decade. Much attention has been focused on the concept of preemptive analgesia utilizing opioids, nonsteroidal anti-inflammatory agents, and regional analgesia. Preventing and alleviating pain may be associated with both reduced morbidity and mortality.

Intravenous Patient-Controlled Analgesia (PCA)

PCA is a device that allows patients to give themselves pain medication in a highly controlled fashion. After analgesia has been established with a loading dose of opioid, patients give themselves small doses of opioids to maintain their level of analgesia (Table 1). Advantages of PCA are immediate medication delivery, rapid onset of analgesia, and patient control over pain medication. Potential disadvantages with PCA are less contact with the nursing staff and patient fears that they could inadvertently administer an overdose or possibly become addicted to the opioid. Patients should not be able to give themselves too much; therefore, lockout intervals and safe maximum doses are built into the program.

TABLE 1. Doses of Opioids and Settings for
Patient-Controlled Analgesia

Drug	Dose (μg./kg.)	Lockout Interval (minutes)	Loading Dose (μg./kg.)
Morphine	20–30	8–12	50–100
Meperidine	200–250	8–12	500–750
Fentanyl	20–40	5–8	0.5–1
Hydromorphone	2–4	6–10	20–40
Sufentanil	0.01–0.02	5–8	0.1–0.2

Epidural Analgesia

Epidural analgesia using opioids and local anesthetics has been used extensively in the management of acute postoperative pain. Epidurally administered opioids diffuse to the spinal cord through multiple routes to act presynaptically and postsynaptically at specific receptors (mu, delta, and kappa). Epidural opioid analgesia does not affect other sensory modalities or motor functions.

Local anesthetics act to inhibit nerve impulses (including pain impulses) by inhibition of sodium channels along nerve fibers. Local anesthetics affect multiple sensory modalities, including pain, sensation, and motor function. The degree of loss of sensory or motor function depends on the local anesthetic and the concentration of local anesthetic used.

Epidural analgesia can relieve pain in a segmental fashion, resulting in localized analgesia with less systemic effects than intravenous analgesia. Epidural analgesia may be effected with opioids (Table 2), local anesthetics, or a combination of the two.

Advantages of epidural analgesia include excellent pain relief, decreased sedation with more rapid recovery to preoperative levels of consciousness, and earlier mobilization after operation with increased ability to cooperate with respiratory therapy and physical therapy. This may lead to a decreased incidence of pulmonary complications and venous thrombosis. Further, epidural analgesia also may improve graft flow in patients following vascular procedures through mild sympathetic blockade. Earlier return of bowel function, decreased stress response, shorter hospitalizations, and decreased morbidity have all been associated with epidural analgesia.

TABLE 2. Commonly Used Epidural Opioids

Drug	Bolus Dose (mg./kg.)	Infusion Concentration (mg./ml.)	Infusion Rates (ml./hr.)
Fentanyl	0.001–0.002	0.0025–0.01	4–10
Morphine	0.03–0.10	0.1–0.2	1–5
Meperidine	0.35–0.7	1–2.5	4–10
Hydromorphone	0.01–0.02	0.05–0.1	1–5

Transdermal Opioids

Transdermal fentanyl patches have been approved for use in patients with cancer-induced pain. Many studies have already been performed exploring the role of transdermal fentanyl in the management of postoperative pain. Transdermal fentanyl may obviate the need for a functioning gastrointestinal tract or an intravenous or epidural catheter.

These patches provide the predicted amount of medication in the range of *25 to 100 µg. per hour.* Since the skin is not uniform, the rate of transfer will vary with the site on which the patch is placed as well as the gender, age, skin, blood flow, sweat gland activity, temperature, and pH of the skin.

Nonsteroidal Anti-Inflammatory Drugs

Nonsteroidal anti-inflammatory analgesics (NSAIDs) may be used in the management of postoperative pain both as a sole agent or in combination with other analgesics. The use of NSAIDs may reduce the requirements for opioids. NSAIDs all have the ability to produce antipyretic, analgesic, and anti-inflammatory effects, but the relative proportions vary with the different agents.

Multiple forms of NSAIDs have been used, including oral, rectal, intramuscular, and intravenous. One of the most commonly used agents is ketorolac tromethamine, an NSAID that is approved by the Food and Drug Administration for intravenous, intramuscular, and oral administration. This agent is an effective analgesic with a paucity of side effects. As with all NSAIDs, there is potential for enhanced surgical or gastrointestinal bleeding, renal dysfunction, and platelet dysfunction.

SUMMARY

The art and science of anesthetic practice have existed as a unique medical specialty for a relatively short period of time. The focus of the anesthesiologist has changed from merely providing amnesia, analgesia, and muscle relaxation for surgery to aggressive management of surgical stress, prior coexisting diseases, and hemodynamic parameters as part of an anesthetic. This requires an extensive knowledge of pharmacology, physiology, anatomy, and pathology integrated with knowledge about the actions and effects of anesthetic agents and techniques. Further, the anesthesiologist's role in care of the patient has extended beyond the borders of the operating room to the critical care unit, on pain management teams, as part of respiratory care teams, and as part of emergency response teams. The mutually dependent relationship of surgeons and anesthesiologists is unique to medicine, where two specialists work side by side at the same time, each with respective duties, but both ensuring optimal patient care through communication, cooperation, and competence.

12

WOUND HEALING:
Biologic and Clinical Features
N. Scott Adzick, M.D.

Wound healing occurs with a sequential cascade of overlapping processes leading to restoration of tissue integrity. *Primary intention* healing occurs in closed wounds, which are wounds in which the edges are approximated, for example, a skin incision closed with sutures. *Secondary intention* healing occurs when the wound edges are not apposed, for example, an open punch skin biopsy wound. *Contraction* occurs with open wounds and enhances closure by pulling normal tissue over the defect. Contraction is distinct from *contracture*, which is the loss of tissue mobility due to a shrinking scar. Both open and closed wounds heal with the same basic repair processes.

The amount of tissue injury and degree of contamination influence the speed and quality of healing. Small, clean closed wounds heal quickly with little scar formation, whereas large, open, dirty wounds heal slowly with significant scar. Recent insights into the basic molecular events involved in tissue repair promise to facilitate clinical wound healing.

REPAIR PROCESSES

The overlapping processes of wound repair are conceptually defined as inflammation, epithelialization, granulation, and fibroplasia.

Inflammation

After tissue injury, vessels immediately constrict, and then platelets aggregate and degranulate. Thromboplastic tissue products are exposed. The coagulation and complement cascades are initiated. The coagulation mechanisms activate prothrombin to thrombin, which converts fibrinogen to fibrin; fibrin is then polymerized into stable clot. As thrombus is formed, hemostasis in the wound is achieved. After the transient vasoconstriction, local small vessels dilate secondary to the effects of kinin, complement components, and prostaglandins. An efflux of white blood cells (first neutrophils, later monocytes) and plasma proteins enters the wound site. The early neutrophil infiltrate scavenges cellular debris, dirt, and bacteria. Activated complement fragments attract neutrophils and help kill bacteria. Monocytes infiltrate later at the wound site and differentiate into macrophages that are crucial in the orchestration of tissue repair. Macrophages not only continue

See the corresponding chapter or part in the *Textbook of Surgery,* 15th edition, pp. 207–220, for a more detailed discussion of this topic, including a comprehensive list of references.

to consume tissue and bacterial debris but also secrete multiple growth factors. These peptide growth factors activate and attract local endothelial cells, fibroblasts, and epithelial cells to begin their respective repair functions. Depletion of monocytes and macrophages causes a severe alteration in wound healing with poor débridement, delayed fibroblast proliferation, and inadequate angiogenesis.

Granulation

Granulation tissue is characterized by its beefy-red appearance, which is a consequence of endothelial cell division and migration to form a rich bed of new capillary networks (angiogenesis) at the wound site. Fibroblasts migrate into the wound using the newly deposited fibrin and fibronectin matrix as a scaffold. Fibroblasts proliferate and synthesize new extracellular matrix. Thus the directed growth of vascular endothelial cells occurs simultaneously with fibroplasia during granulation tissue formation, stimulated by platelet and activated macrophage products. Granulation is most prominent in wounds healing by secondary intention.

The initial wound matrix is provisional and is composed of fibrin and the glycosaminoglycan (GAG) hyaluronic acid. Because of its large water or hydration shell, hyaluronic acid provides a matrix that enhances cell migration. Adhesion glycoproteins, including fibronectin, laminin, and tenascin, are present throughout the early matrix and facilitate cell attachment and migration. Integrin receptors on cell surfaces bind to the matrix GAGs and glycoproteins. As fibroblasts enter and populate the wound, they use hyaluronidase to digest the provisional hyaluronic acid–rich matrix, and larger, sulfated GAGs are deposited. Concomitantly, collagens are deposited by fibroblasts onto a fibronectin and GAG scaffold in a disorganized array. Collagen Types I and III are the major fibrillar collagens comprising skin extracellular matrix. Type III collagen is initially predominant in wounds compared with normal skin, but as the wound matures, Type I collagen is deposited in increasing amounts. The majority of collagen is Type I in both wounds and normal skin.

Epithelialization

Within hours after injury, morphologic changes in keratinocytes at the wound margin are evident. In skin wounds, the epidermis thickens, and marginal basal cells enlarge and migrate over the wound defect. Once a cell begins migrating, it does not divide until epidermal continuity is restored. Fixed basal cells in a zone near the cut edge of the wound continue to divide, and their daughter cells flatten and migrate over the wound matrix as a sheet. Cell adhesion glycoproteins, tenascin and fibronectin, provide a "railroad track" to facilitate epithelial cell migration over the wound matrix. Keratinocytes lay down laminin and Type IV collagen as part of their basement membrane. The keratinocytes then become columnar and divide as the layering of the epidermis is established, thus re-forming a barrier to further contamination and moisture loss.

Fibroplasia

Ultimately, the outcome of mammalian wound healing is scar formation. Disorganized collagen deposition plays a prominent role in scar. As the collagenous matrix forms, densely packed fibers fill the wound site. The balance of collagen synthesis and degradation favors collagen deposition. The wound remodels slowly over months to form a mature scar. The initially dense capillary network and fibroblast infiltrate regress until relatively few capillaries and fibroblasts remain. Wounds become stronger with time. Wound tensile strength increases rapidly from 1 to 6 weeks after wounding. Thereafter, tensile strength increases at a slower pace and has been documented to increase up to 1 year after wounding in animal studies. However, the tensile strength of wounded skin at best only reaches approximately 80% that of unwounded skin. The final result of repair is scar, which is brittle and less elastic than normal skin and does not contain any skin appendages such as hair follicles or sweat glands.

GROWTH FACTORS: REGULATORS OF REPAIR

Growth factors play a prominent role in the regulation of wound healing. These polypeptides are released by a variety of activated cells at the wound site. They act in either a paracrine or autocrine manner to stimulate or inhibit protein synthesis by cells in the wound. They also chemoattract new cells to the wound. Myriad growth factors are present in wounds, and many have overlapping functions.

Platelet-derived growth factor (PDGF) is released from platelet alpha granules immediately after injury. PDGF attracts neutrophils, macrophages, and fibroblasts to the wound and serves as a powerful mitogen. Macrophages, endothelial cells, and fibroblasts also synthesize and secrete PDGF. PDGF stimulates fibroblasts to synthesize new extracellular matrix, predominantly noncollagenous components such as GAGs and adhesion proteins. PDGF also increases the amount of fibroblast-secreted collagenase, indicating a role for this cytokine in tissue remodeling.

Transforming growth factor-beta (TGF-β) directly stimulates collagen synthesis and decreases extracellular matrix degradation by fibroblasts. It is released from platelets and macrophages at the wound. In addition, TGF-β is released from fibroblasts and acts in an autocrine manner to further stimulate its own synthesis and secretion. TGF-β also chemoattracts fibroblasts and macrophages to the wound. Through these mechanisms, TGF-β can augment fibrosis at the wound site.

Angiogenesis is stimulated by acidic and basic fibroblast growth factors (aFGF and bFGF, respectively). Both endothelial cells and macrophages produce aFGF and bFGF. These growth factors are bound by heparin and the GAG heparan sulfate in the extracellular matrix. Basement membrane serves as a storage depot for bFGF, which is released when the heparin components of the basement membrane are degraded. The FGFs stimulate endothelial cells to divide and form new capillaries. They also chemoattract endothelial cells and fibroblasts.

Epithelialization is directly stimulated by at least two growth factors: epidermal growth factor (EGF) and keratinocyte growth factor (KGF). EGF is released by keratinocytes to act in an autocrine manner, whereas KGF is released by fibroblasts to act in a paracrine manner to stimulate keratinocyte division and differentiation.

Multiple other growth factors affect wound repair. For example, insulin-like growth factor-1 (IGF-1) stimulates collagen synthesis by fibroblasts, and IGF-1 functions synergistically with PDGF and bFGF to facilitate fibroblast proliferation. Interferon-gamma has been shown to downregulate collagen synthesis. The various interleukins mediate inflammatory cell functions at the wound site.

Surgeons may soon have the ability to enhance repair by adding or deleting growth factors from healing wounds. Addition of growth factors has augmented repair in animal models of impaired wound healing conditions such as diabetes, chronic steroid use, or chemotherapy.

CLINICAL FACTORS THAT AFFECT WOUND HEALING

Nutrition

The precise calorie requirements for optimal wound healing have not been defined. Protein depletion impairs wound healing if recent weight loss exceeds 15% to 25% of body weight. Wound dehiscence risk is increased in hypoalbuminemic patients, signifying the detrimental effect of chronic malnutrition on repair.

Vitamin C (ascorbic acid) deficiency causes scurvy. Vitamin C is necessary for hydroxylation of proline and lysine residues. In patients with this deficiency, normal amounts of fibroblasts are present in the wound, but they produce an inadequate amount of collagen. Without hydroxyproline, newly synthesized collagen is not transported out of cells. Without hydroxylysine, collagen fibrils are not cross-linked.

Vitamin A (retinoic acid) requirements increase during injury. Severely injured patients require supplemental vitamin A to maintain normal serum levels. Vitamin A also partially reverses the impaired healing in chronically steroid-treated patients. Vitamin B_6 (pyridoxine) deficiency impairs collagen cross-linking. Vitamin B_1 (thiamine) and vitamin B_{12} (riboflavin) deficiencies cause syndromes associated with poor wound repair. Trace metal deficiencies such as zinc and copper have been implicated in poor wound repair because these divalent cations are cofactors in many important enzymatic reactions. Zinc deficiency is associated with poor epithelialization and chronic, nonhealing wounds.

Oxygen, Anemia, and Perfusion

Wounds require adequate oxygen delivery to heal well. Ischemic wounds heal poorly and have a much greater risk of infection. Conversely, increased oxygen delivery at the wound improves wound healing. Anemia in the normovolemic patient is not detrimental to wound repair as long as the hematocrit is greater than 15%, because oxygen content in blood does not affect wound collagen synthesis. Tissue proliferation is the ultimate determinant of wound oxygenation and nutrition. To optimize wound repair, those factors leading to wound ischemia should be prevented. Sutures should not be placed too tightly. The patient should be kept warm, pain should be well controlled to prevent vasoconstriction, and hypovolemia should be treated.

Diabetes Mellitus and Obesity

Wound healing is impaired in diabetic patients by unknown mechanisms. Healing is enhanced if glucose levels are well controlled. Obese patients with diabetes have impaired wound healing independent of glucose control and insulin therapy. Poor wound perfusion and necrotic adipose debris probably contribute to impaired healing in both diabetic and nondiabetic obese patients.

Corticosteroids, Chemotherapy, and Radiation Therapy

Pharmacologic steroid use impairs healing, especially when given in the first 3 days after wounding. Steroids reduce wound inflammation, collagen synthesis, and contraction. Both radiation and chemotherapeutic agents have their greatest effects on dividing cells. The division of endothelial cells, fibroblasts, and keratinocytes is impaired in irradiated tissue, which slows wound healing. Irradiated tissue usually has some degree of residual endothelial cell injury and endarteritis that causes atrophy, fibrosis, and poor tissue repair. Chemotherapeutic agents are not administered until at least 5 to 7 days postoperatively to prevent impairment of the initial healing events.

Infection

Wound contamination by bacteria causes clinical wound infection and delays healing if more than 10^5 organisms per mg. of tissue are present. Infected wounds are erythematous and tender and commonly have drainage. The patient may be febrile. Immediate wound opening with suture removal and débridement is essential. Administration of antibiotics treats surrounding cellulitis.

FETAL WOUND HEALING

Unlike the adult, the fetus heals skin wounds with regenerative-type repair, not with scar formation. The epidermis and dermis are restored to a normal architecture in which the collagen matrix pattern in the wound is reticular and unchanged from unwounded dermis. The wound hair follicle and sweat gland patterns are normal. In contrast, adult tissue injury due to several diseases processes causes scar and fibrosis. Examples include pulmonary fibrosis, hepatic fibrosis, keloids, intraperitoneal adhesions, and burn wound contractures. An understanding of the biology of scarless fetal wound repair may help surgeons develop therapeutic strategies to avert scar and fibrosis.

13

BURNS:
Including Cold, Chemical, and Electrical Injuries

Basil A. Pruitt, Jr., M.D., Cleon W. Goodwin, Jr., M.D.,
and Scott K. Pruitt, M.D., Ph.D.

BURN INJURY

An estimated 1.4 to 2 million persons are burned each year, with over 5000 burn-related deaths reported in 1991. While the majority of burn injuries are of limited extent and can be cared for on an outpatient basis, approximately 270 patients per million population per year require hospital care. Within this group, a smaller subset, 82 per million population per year, is classified as having major burn injury. Criteria for major burn injury include (1) second- and third-degree burns involving more than 20% of the body surface area (BSA) in patients under 10 or over 50 years of age; (2) second- and third-degree burns of more than 20% BSA in other age groups; (3) significant burns of the face, hands, feet, genitalia, perineum, or skin overlying major joints; (4) full-thickness burns that involve more than 5% BSA in patients of any age; (5) significant electrical injury, including lightning injury; (6) significant chemical injury; (7) lesser burns associated with inhalation injury, concomitant mechanical trauma, or significant pre-existing medical disorders; and (8) burn injury in patients who will require special social, emotional, or long-term rehabilitative support, including cases of suspected or actual child abuse and neglect. Patients meeting these criteria should be treated at a center specializing in burn care.

INITIAL CARE OF BURN PATIENTS

At the scene of the injury, the patient should be removed from the heat source, and burning clothing should be extinguished. Chemical-soaked clothing should be removed, and chemical agents should be diluted with copious lavage. In addition, 100% oxygen should be administered to any patient suspected of having inhaled significant amounts of carbon monoxide, and an endotracheal tube should be inserted in patients with severe inhalation injury. In the Emergency Department, intravenous fluid resuscitation should be initiated (see below); a medical history should be obtained; a rapid but complete physical examination should be performed; blood should be drawn for laboratory analysis; and the patient should be weighed.

See the corresponding chapter or part in the *Textbook of Surgery,* 15th edition, pp. 221–252, for a more detailed discussion of this topic, including a comprehensive list of references.

The depth of the burn injury should then be estimated. First-degree burns are red in color, with a dry or moderately blistered surface, and are painful. Second-degree burns are pink or mottled red in color, with bullae or a moist weeping surface, and are painful. Third-degree, or full-thickness, burns are pearly white, charred, translucent, or parchmentlike in color, with a surface notable for dryness and thrombosis of superficial vessels. These burns are insensate. Next, the extent of the burn should be estimated using either the Rule of Nines or a burn diagram. Based on the total BSA of second- and third-degree burns and the patient's weight, fluid needs can then be estimated for adequate resuscitation (see below).

PATHOPHYSIOLOGY OF THERMAL INJURY

A number of physiologic derangements occur following thermal injury. The initial drop in cardiac output seen early after burn injury can be reversed by adequate volume resuscitation. Following resuscitation, a hypermetabolic state ensues with supranormal cardiac output. Alterations in the coagulation system include early depression of platelet and fibrinogen levels, with normalization and subsequent supranormal levels following resuscitation. Gastrointestinal manifestations include ileus, with return of motility by the third to fifth postburn day, and perhaps alterations in mucosal permeability. The multiple defects in host immunologic responsiveness observed following burn injury may play a critical role in the development of infectious complications in burn patients.

FLUID RESUSCITATION

Fluid resuscitation should be started as soon as possible in all patients with burns of 15% or more BSA. For fluid administration, a large-bore peripheral IV catheter should be inserted, preferably through unburned skin. Fluid requirements are then calculated based on the patient's weight and extent of burn. Using one such formula, the modified Brooke formula, 2.0 ml. per kg. per percent BSA burn of lactated Ringer's solution is administered in the first 24 hours postburn, with one-half this requirement being administered over the first 8 hours and the remainder being infused over the next 16 hours. Colloid-containing fluids are unnecessary during this time period. Patients who may characteristically require greater than estimated volumes of fluid include those with electrical injury, those with inhalation injury, those with delayed resuscitation, and those who are burned while intoxicated with ethanol. During the second 24 hours postburn, colloid-containing fluids are used to replace any persistent plasma volume deficits. Additional electrolyte-free fluid such as 5% dextrose in water is infused in a volume sufficient to maintain urinary output and replace insensible losses.

The volume of fluid actually infused is governed by the patient's response. The amount of fluid administered should be sufficient to maintain vital signs and an hourly urine output of 30 to 50 ml. in adults and 1 ml. per kg. in children weighing less than 30 kg. Thus insertion of a urinary catheter is essential. Invasive monitoring should be reserved for patients who do not respond to resuscitation as anticipated.

INHALATION INJURY

Inhalation injury, a chemical tracheobronchitis and acute pneumonitis due to irritative products of incomplete combustion, is frequently present in patients admitted to burn centers and exerts its greatest mortality-enhancing effect in patients in whom anticipated mortality is from 40% to 75%. Inhalation injury should be suspected in any patient burned in a closed space or during a period of impaired mentation due to inebriation, drug overdose, or head trauma. Signs suggestive of inhalation injury include head and neck burns, singed nasal vibrissae, brassy cough, hoarseness and wheezing, bronchorrhea, and unexplained hypoxemia. The production of carbonaceous sputum is a specific sign of inhalation injury, but carbon-stained bronchial secretions may be cleared from the airway prior to examination of the patient.

With respect to diagnostic tests, a chest roentgenogram is notoriously insensitive in detecting even severe inhalation injury. Occasionally, pulmonary function testing and xenon-133 ventilation-perfusion pulmonary scintiphotography aid in the diagnosis of inhalation injury. Fiberoptic bronchoscopy is useful in the diagnosis of inhalation injury and, when an endotracheal tube is placed over the bronchoscope prior to the examination, allows immediate artificial airway placement under direct vision.

BURN WOUND CARE

Attention should be directed to the burn wound only after resuscitation has been initiated and hemodynamic and respiratory stability has been established. The burn wound should first be cleansed with a surgical detergent, and all loose nonviable tissue should be gently débrided. A topical antimicrobial agent should then be applied. Three topical agents, all of which are in clinical use, are mafenide acetate (Sulfamylon) burn cream, silver sulfadiazine (Silvadine) burn cream, and 0.5% silver nitrate soaks. While all three agents have specific advantages and disadvantages, they each effectively control invasive burn wound infection and burn wound sepsis.

Excision of the burned tissue in full-thickness and most deep partial-thickness burns should be carried out as soon as possible after resuscitation is complete. Excision procedures should be limited to 20% of total BSA or 2 hours operative time, and the wound produced by excision must be closed by autografting or by the application of a biologic dressing or skin substitute.

The goal of burn wound care is the timely, definitive closure of the wound. Wounds ready for split-thickness skin grafting are those which have been excised or those treated by nonexcisional methods, which are characterized by absence of residual nonviable tissue and pooled secretions; firm, red, finely granular granulation tissue; a surface bacterial count of less that 10^5 organisms per sq. cm. of wound surface; and absence of beta-hemolytic streptococci. Adherence and vascularization of allografted skin to a wound also indicate readiness for definitive split-thickness autografting. For wound closure in patients with limited donor sites, research directed at improving the usefulness of cultured epithelial sheets is actively under way.

Prior to definitive wound closure with autografted skin, the burn wound may be covered with a biologic dressing. Viable cutaneous allografted skin is the biologic dressing of choice because it prevents wound desiccation, promotes maturation of granulation tissue, limits bacterial proliferation in the burn wound, prevents exudative protein and red cell loss, decreases wound pain, thereby facilitating movement in involved joints, diminishes evaporative water loss from the burn, thus decreasing heat loss, and serves to protect tendons, vessels, and nerves. Lyophilized skin also may be used. Cutaneous xenografts are readily available but are less effective as physiologic dressings and allow survival of greater numbers of subgraft bacteria. In addition, amnion has been used as a biologic dressing. Finally, a number of synthetic membranes have been proposed as skin substitutes, with several collagen-based bilaminate membranes showing clinical effectiveness.

ELECTRICAL INJURY

Tissue damage caused by electrical current is most severe at the contact sites but also may involve underlying tissues and organs along the route of the current. Thus seemingly small areas of cutaneous burn may overlie extensive areas of devitalized tissue and may lead to severe underestimation of fluid resuscitation requirements. In addition, edema formation in the injured tissues beneath the investing fascia may compromise blood flow and require fasciotomy.

Electrical injury may also cause a variety of other adverse pathophysiologic sequelae. Neurologic changes, including peripheral neuropathy and spinal cord deficits, may occur. Fractures may be caused by tetanic contractions of muscles during the injury or by associated trauma. An increased incidence of cholelithiasis also has been reported to occur within 2 years of electrical injury. Patients sustaining electrical injury to the head and neck frequently develop cataracts. Cardiopulmonary arrest commonly occurs following lightning injury and should be treated by prompt initiation of cardiopulmonary resuscitation.

CHEMICAL INJURIES

The severity of a chemical burn is related to the concentration of the chemical agent, the amount of agent in contact with the tissue, and the duration of the contact. Thus all contaminated clothing must be removed promptly, and immediate copious water lavage should be initiated to dilute the agent and reduce the heat content of injured tissues. Irrigation of the wound should be carried out for at least 30 minutes. Chemical injuries of the eye may require irrigation for up to 72 hours.

Several agents require more specific therapy. Hydrofluoric acid injury should be irrigated initially with benzalkonium chloride solution, or calcium gluconate gel should be applied. After initial water lavage, phenol burns should be lavaged with a lipophilic solvent such as polyethylene glycol to remove residual phenol. White phosphorus injuries, most of which result from ignition of military munitions, should be irrigated with saline and covered with a moistened dressing to prevent ignition of the phosphorus particles prior to their removal.

METABOLIC ALTERATIONS AND NUTRITIONAL SUPPORT

The metabolic response following burn injury increases in magnitude in proportion to burn extent, and these changes appear to be mediated by increases in catacholamine (principally norepinephrine) production and excretion. Postburn hypermetabolism is manifested by increased oxygen consumption, elevated cardiac output and minute ventilation, increased core temperature, wasting of lean body mass, and increased urinary nitrogen excretion. Blood flow to the burn wound is markedly exaggerated in relationship to total body blood flow, and this enhanced need appears to drive the hypermetabolic response to burn injury.

Nutritional needs in the burn patient can be measured by indirect calorimetry, predicted by use of any of several formulas or estimated (for adults with burns of over 70% BSA) as being 2000 to 2200 cal. and 12 to 18 gm. of nitrogen per sq. m. of BSA per day. Since most patients will not be able to meet these nutritional requirements by spontaneous oral intake, nutritional support may be necessary. In patients with a functional gastrointestinal tract, the enteral route is preferred, but parenteral nutritional support may be necessary in some patients.

COMPLICATIONS IN BURN PATIENTS

Despite the application of topical antimicrobial agents, bacteria in the burn wound may escape control and invade underlying tissue. To identify invasive burn wound infection as early as possible, it is mandatory that the entire burn wound be examined each day. Conversion of an area of partial-thickness burn to full-thickness necrosis and the appearance of focal areas of black or dark hemorrhagic discoloration are the most common changes indicative of burn wound infection.

Histologic examination of a burn wound biopsy is the most rapid and the only reliable means of making the differentiation between microbial colonization of nonviable tissue, which is present in all burn wounds, and the presence of microorganisms in unburned, viable tissue that is characteristic of invasive burn wound infection. Surface cultures of the wound have no role in making this diagnosis. Histologic confirmation of invasive infection requires an immediate therapeutic response, with change of the topical agent to mafenide acetate and initiation of systemic antibiotic therapy, followed by excision of the infected tissue.

While the incidence of bacterial wound infections has decreased, the incidence of nonbacterial wound infections has increased. *Candida* species commonly colonize the wound without invasion, and therapy is required only if tissue invasion occurs. *Aspergillus* species and the *Phycomycetes* are more aggressive burn wound invaders that are most often seen late in the hospital course. Phycomycetic infections are characterized by rapidly expanding soft tissue ischemic necrosis with a peripheral rim of subcutaneous edema and frequent hematogenous dissemination to remote tissues. If treatment with topical antifungal agents and systemic amphotericin-B and prompt wide excision fail to control the infection in an involved limb, amputation may be necessary.

As the incidence of fatal burn wound infection has decreased, infections in other sites have increased as principal causes of death in burn patients. Bronchopneumonia, due to airborne bacteria, is most commonly caused by *Staphylococcus aureus* and gram-negative opportunistic bacteria and commonly occurs early in the postburn period. Hematogenous pneumonia, due to microorganisms arising from a remote septic site, is less common and occurs late in the postburn course. Suppurative thrombophlebitis, which can occur in any previously cannulated vein, is a possible septic source that should not be overlooked. Other infectious complications include acute endocarditis and suppurative sinusitis.

Gastrointestinal complications of the burn patient are the same as those of other critically ill patients and include ulcerations, acalculous cholecystitis, and pancreatitis. Acute ulceration of the stomach and duodenum (Curling's ulcer) is effectively controlled by prophylactic antacids or pharmacologic H_2 histamine receptor blockade.

COLD INJURY

The injury produced by exposure to cold depends on the coldness of the temperature, the duration and time course of exposure, and the environmental conditions that can influence the effects of low temperature. Frostbite results in the actual freezing of tissue and produces damage by tissue ice crystallization, cellular dehydration, and microvascular occlusion. The vascular system is particularly susceptible to freeze injury and appears to be the primary target organ of frostbite, with endothelium being most sensitive.

Frostbite is classified into four levels of severity based on appearance after thawing, with fourth-degree frostbite resulting in full-thickness necrosis of skin extending into underlying muscle and bone. Determination of tissue viability is all but impossible during the first several weeks following injury and often can be made only after the gangrenous tissue has demarcated or sloughed.

Treatment of frostbite begins with removal of wet and constricting clothing, followed by wrapping of the patient in warm blankets and oral administration of hot fluids. Rapid rewarming of the frozen part is the single most effective therapeutic maneuver for preserving potentially viable tissue and is accomplished by placing the part in water at 40° C. After rewarming has been achieved, wound care consists of daily cleansing with a surgical detergent/disinfectant solution. Early débridement increases tissue loss and should be avoided unless supervening infection develops.

Nonfreezing cold injuries include trench foot, immersion foot, and pernio or chilblain. Treatment of these conditions is supportive and consists of rapid rewarming and meticulous local care. Prolonged exposure to cold also may lead to total body hypothermia, the hallmark of which is a core (rectal) temperature below 34° C. Prompt initiation of rewarming is the most important intervention.

14

PRINCIPLES OF OPERATIVE SURGERY:
Antisepsis, Technique,
Sutures, and Drains

Julio Hochberg, M.D., and Gordon F. Murray, M.D.

ANTISEPSIS AND ASEPSIS

Antisepsis is the use of antimicrobial chemicals on human tissue, whereas *disinfection* employs these agents on inanimate objects. Hygienic hand washing, preoperative preparation of the patient's skin, gloving and sterile draping during operations, isolation precautions, autoclaving of instruments, and proper waste disposal are all examples of the aseptic technique.

Aseptic Procedures

THE OPERATING ROOM. The operating room (OR) should provide an environment that is as free of bacterial contamination as possible. Appropriate ventilation rapidly clears bacteria from the air. However, organisms recovered from air often are not those which cause wound infection. The most important source of contamination is the patient, and the secondary source is the OR team.

THE PATIENT. Infections that develop from operations classified as clean-contaminated, contaminated, or dirty are caused primarily by bacteria already present in the operative field. Preparation of the patient's skin before an incision is one of the most important methods of decreasing infection in clean operations.

Intact skin can withstand very strong disinfecting agents, whereas cells of a fresh surgical wound are very susceptible to further damage. In heavily contaminated wounds, high-pressure irrigation can decrease the number of bacteria.

Age, obesity, diabetes, cirrhosis, uremia, and connective tissue disorders, as well as hereditary or induced immunodeficiency states, have all been associated with increased infection rates.

THE OR TEAM. The OR team should scrub 3 to 5 minutes with an antiseptic before each operation. Agents such as iodophors or chlorhexidine combined with a detergent have proved effective. During the operation, a face mask should cover the mouth and nose. Gloves perform a dual function: They protect the patient from the hands of the surgeon and protect the surgeon from potentially contaminated blood. A

See corresponding chapter or part in the *Textbook of Surgery,* 15th edition, pp. 253–263, for a more detailed discussion of this topic, including a comprehensive list of references.

sterile gown prevents the transmission of bacteria to the patient. The primary function of the sterile drapes is to define and preserve the sterile field during the operation.

SURGICAL TECHNIQUE

INCISIONS. An incision should be planned properly as to shape, direction, and size. In general, incisions are made along the normal skin lines. In reoperations, every attempt should be made to use the original incision. Skin incisions should be made with the stainless steel surgical scalpel. Incision of the skin should be perpendicular to the epidermal surface. Skin margins should be handled gently to minimize necrosis that may promote infection or delay healing.

DISSECTION. The least amount of trauma will be accomplished by dissecting natural tissue planes. The surgeon's index finger will readily dissect many lightly adherent normal tissue planes. A blunt-tipped scissors is excellent for opening tissue planes that are too dense for finger or sponge dissection.

DÉBRIDEMENT. The most important single factor in the management of the contaminated wound is the débridement. It removes tissue heavily contaminated by bacteria or foreign bodies and protects the patient from the threat of invasive infection.

HEMOSTASIS. The objectives of hemostasis are to minimize blood loss during and after an operation and to prevent hematoma. It is also imperative to maintain a clear, bloodless field during incision and dissection. Hemostasis of large vessels is obtained by ligatures, suture ligatures, or metal clips.

WOUND CLOSURE. Wounds containing less than 10^5 bacterial organisms per gram of tissue will nearly always heal primarily following closure. When the wound is contaminated by exceedingly large numbers of organisms, primary closure probably should be delayed. Closure of dead space by sutures potentiates the development of infection. When wounds involve vital structures that may be destroyed by exposure, flaps must be transposed immediately. Newly developed skin-stretching devices can now be used in difficult skin closures.

SUTURING. Simple interrupted sutures coapt the wound edges and correct any intervening gaps or discrepancies in height. Subcuticular sutures are an excellent choice when good cosmetic results are desired. Running cuticular suture is an easy and rapid method of skin closure and is readily removed postoperatively. Vertical mattress sutures are intended to gain both a secure grasp of tissue and a good approximation of the skin margins.

DRESSING. During the early postoperative period (48 hours), the fresh incision should be protected by dressings until epithelialization is completed. Draining and infected wounds require dressings that can absorb exudate and remove necrotic tissue remnants after surgical débridement. When skin loss is extensive, biologic dressings are helpful in achieving wound coverage and protection against bacterial invasion and evaporative loss. When the site of any injury is immobilized, lymphatic flow is reduced, thereby minimizing the spread of the wound microflora.

SUTURE REMOVAL. The proper timing for suture removal is determined by the amount of tension on the wound edges, concurrent chemotherapy, exogenous steroid administration, the presence of sepsis, and cosmetic considerations. Percutaneous sutures may create a sinus tract, and a typical railroad track appearance can be the final result.

PROPHYLACTIC ANTIBIOTICS. Previous studies indicating that "a load of antibiotics should be on board" before operation apparently were not correct. Considerable experience has shown that antibiotics can be started intravenously when the need for antibiotic therapy appears during the surgical procedure, with just as good results as if prophylactic antibiotics were started before the procedure.

ELECTROCAUTERY. A unipolar electrosurgical unit is used both for surgical dissection and for hemostasis. The cutting cautery may significantly save operative time and diminish the blood loss during massive excisional operation. A bipolar cautery is more precise and confines the damage to the tissues between the tips of the cauterizing forceps. It is indicated to control bleeders in microvascular and microneural operations.

ARGON BEAM COAGULATOR. The argon beam coagulator (ABC) allows unipolar coagulation in a nontouch technique. The bolus of argon gas blows any oxygen away from the impact site, reducing smoke production, which is advantageous in laparoscopies.

SURGICAL LASER. This is a new, multi-purpose tool that can cut, coagulate, and vaporize tissues, weld, and selectively destroy pigmented pathologic tissues. Surgeons can now employ energy from light as a scalpel. Forward penetration of the laser beam is least with the argon laser, intermediate with the CO_2 laser, and deepest with the neodymium:yttrium-aluminum-garnet (Nd:YAG) laser.

CUSA KNIFE. The Cavitron ultrasonic surgical aspirator (CUSA) functions as an acoustic vibrator and selectively fragments and aspirates tissue of high water and low collagen content, that is, tumors, sparing other tissues such as blood vessels and nerves. The main advantages of the CUSA over the laser are, first, the rapidity with which it can debulk large volumes of tumor and, second, the fact that it does not produce char as it resects.

SUTURES AND NEEDLES

SELECTION OF SUTURE MATERIAL. The choice of suture for a particular procedure should be based logically on the known physical and biologic characteristics of the suture material and the healing properties of the sutured tissues. Adequate suture tensile strength is required for wound closure, but the finest suture that will hold the tissues together safely should be used. All sutures should be avoided in dirty, contaminated, or infected wounds whenever possible.

Absorbable Sutures

CATGUT. Catgut is made from the intestines of cattle or sheep. The absorption rate of plain catgut is about 10 days.

Chromic catgut has been treated with a chromium salt to retard its absorption to 20 days. Plain catgut usually will evoke a greater inflammatory reaction than chromic catgut.

POLYGLYCOLIC ACID. Polyglycolic acid (Dexon) is a braided synthetic suture material. Total reabsorption by hydrolysis occurs 60 to 90 days postoperatively. Dexon is useful in muscle, fascia, capsule, tendon, and subcuticular skin closure.

POLYGLYCONATE. Polyglyconate (Maxon), a monofilament suture, has the best *in vitro* knot security and tensile strength when compared with other synthetic absorbable sutures.

POLYGLACTIC ACID. Polyglactic acid (Vicryl) is a braided synthetic suture. The tensile strength is very high (second to that of Dexon), and it is completely absorbed in 60 days. It is extremely useful as a completely buried suture to approximate wound edges.

POLYDIOXANONE. Polydioxanone (PDS) is a monofilament synthetic suture with a long duration of absorbability and an extremely high tensile strength. This low-reactive suture can maintain its integrity in the presence of bacterial infection.

Nonabsorbable Sutures

SILK. Silk is a protein filament obtained from the silkworm larva. The suture has good tensile strength, is easy to handle, and has excellent knot characteristics.

POLYESTER. Constructed of polyester fibers (Dacron), these braided sutures have superior strength and durability. The uncoated suture (Mersilene) tends to cut slightly when pulled through tissue; thus Teflon (Tevdek), silicone (Ti-Cron), and polybutilate (Ethibond) have all been employed in its manufacture.

NYLON. Nylon is available in both monofilament and multifilament forms. It is very strong and smooth, but extra care must be taken when tying to prevent knot slippage. Its smooth monofilament composition ensures facile passage through tissue and minimal reaction. Nylon sutures are the most commonly used sutures in cutaneous surgery.

POLYPROPYLENE. A monofilament suture material, Prolene provides smooth passage through tissues and minimal tissue reaction. Easy removability renders it an ideal suture for a running intradermal stitch.

STAINLESS STEEL. Wire is the strongest and least reactive suture. However, its handling characteristics are very poor. Wire is used mainly in surgery of ligaments, tendons, and bones.

Selection of Needles and Needle Holders

Needle selection is determined by the type of tissue to be sutured, the tissue's accessibility, and the diameter of the suture material. The traumatic needle holder has rounded jaw edges to avoid structural damage to either monofilament suture or needles.

Staples

Stapling is faster than a traditional hand-sewn effort, reducing operation and anesthesia time, tissue trauma, blood loss. Contemporary devices include a great variety of skin and internal stapling instruments.

Skin Tapes

Skin tapes are pervious to sweat, maintain the integrity of the epidermis, lessen the likelihood of wound infection, and prevent suture marks. In children, selection of skin tapes avoids the ordeal of suture placement and removal.

Surgical Adhesives

Autologous fibrin glue is a biologic adhesive consisting of fibrinogen, factor XIII, fibronectin, thrombin, apoprotinin, and calcium chloride. It is effective in stabilizing esophagogastric, small-intestinal, and nerve anastomoses. The autologous fibrin glue is prepared from single-donor human plasma, eliminating the danger of multidonor pools.

DRAINS

For either prophylactic or therapeutic indications, the surgeon should select the form of drainage, either passive or active, that is best suited for the purpose intended. The drain must be appropriate to the demands of the viscosity or the volume of the expected drainage. In general, prophylactic drainage may be best accomplished by the use of closed wound suction drainage. As the volume or complexity of drainage increases and therapeutic drainage is indicated, passive and sump drains are more efficacious. Four types of drains are used primarily: Penrose drain, closed suction drain, sump drain, and the closed suction Penrose drain. Percutaneous catheter drainage represents a new method that is proving to be exceedingly valuable.

15

SURGICAL INFECTIONS

I

Surgical Infections and Choice of Antibiotics

E. Patchen Dellinger, M.D.

The modern surgeon has the responsibility to understand infections and must realize that knowledge of many aspects of microbiology, immunology, and pharmacology is essential to complement surgical skills. Basic understanding of how the body defends itself against infection is essential to a rational application of surgical and other therapeutic principles in the control of infection.

CAUSES OF WOUND INFECTION

Infections of surgical wounds occur whenever the combination of microbial numbers and virulence in the wound is sufficiently large to overcome the local host defense mechanisms and establish progressive growth. Careful studies of the bacterial flora of surgical wounds taken at the time of closure have shown that one or more types of organisms can be cultured from most wounds. Even so, overt infection is unusual unless surgical principles have been violated or large numbers of organisms have been introduced into the wound.

PREVENTION OF WOUND INFECTION

Preventing infectious complications is more practical than treating them. Fortunately, strict adherence to the principles of wound care can prevent the vast majority of infectious complications in surgical practice. Whenever possible, all cutaneous infections should be controlled or cleared before an elective operation. A distant-site infection at the time of an elective clean operation doubles the postoperative infection rate. When the operative area is shaved the night before the procedure, the injury of shaving itself promotes bacterial growth. This practice increases the infection rate about 100% when compared with removing the hair by clippers at the time of the procedure or not removing it at all. As many as 90% of the members of an operative team puncture or tear their gloves during a long operation. The safest practice is to wear two pairs of gloves, with one pair a half size larger than

---

See the corresponding chapter or part in the *Textbook of Surgery,* 15th edition, pp. 264–280, for a more detailed discussion of this topic, including a comprehensive list of references.

usual beneath the standard-size pair. This practice reduces the risk of getting the patient's blood onto the surgeon's hands, but it is equally effective in keeping the surgeon's bacteria out of the patient's wound.

Importance of Surgical Technique

Gentle care of the tissues to minimize local damage is extremely important in preventing wound infection. All devitalized tissues and foreign bodies should be removed from traumatic wounds. Foreign bodies left in a wound decrease the minimal infective dose of a bacterial inoculum 10,000-fold or more. Not only must all contaminated foreign bodies be removed from grossly contaminated wounds, but one should try to avoid introducing new foreign bodies such as prostheses, grafts, and suture materials. Monofilament suture is preferable to multifilament in contaminated wounds. Hematomas, seromas, or dead spaces favor bacterial localization and growth and prevent the delivery of phagocytic cells to such foci. In a large potential dead space in an operative wound that is potentially contaminated, the best way to prevent fluid collection and infection is to use a closed-suction drain. However, because a foreign body in a wound increases the risk of infection, the benefit of fluid removal and obliteration of dead space must be balanced against the effect of the foreign body. Open drainage of wounds with Penrose-type drains increases the degree of contamination and the incidence of infection.

In heavily contaminated wounds, delayed primary closure minimizes serious infection. With this technique, the subcutaneous tissues and skin are left open and "packed" loosely with gauze after fascial closure. The number of phagocytic cells at the wound edges progressively increases, peaking about 5 days after the injury. Capillary budding is intense at this time, and closure usually can be accomplished successfully even when there is heavy bacterial contamination, since phagocytic cells can be delivered to the site in large numbers. The number of organisms required to initiate an infection in a surgical incision progressively rises as the interval of healing increases, up to the fifth postoperative day.

Social Considerations

Traditionally, surgeons have monitored and recorded the incidence of postoperative surgical-site infections. Accurate and continued surveillance of the incidence of wound infection with feedback to the surgeon reduces the incidence of wound infection by about 50%. Infection rates should be determined at 30 days postoperatively rather than at discharge because more than half the infections occur after discharge. However, with the surgical load in most hospitals and modern low infection rates, it is not possible to see a statistically significant difference in infection rates over intervals shorter than several months. However, each infection should be discussed in the surgical complications meeting and should be categorized as apparently avoidable or apparently unavoidable. If the review reveals that any of the known adjunctive measures to reduce wound infection risk were omitted, then it is an apparently avoidable infection. The goal of surveillance and quality assurance should be to achieve zero avoidable infections.

Reducing the Bacterial Load by Prophylactic Chemotherapy

The decision to use prophylactic antibiotic therapy must be based on the evidence for possible benefit against the evidence for possible adverse effects. Indiscriminate or blind use of antibiotics should be discouraged because it may elicit antibiotic-resistant strains of organisms or serious hypersensitivity reactions. Prolonged use of prophylactic antibiotics also may mask the signs and symptoms of established infections, making diagnosis more difficult.

Prophylactic systemic antibiotics are not indicated during straightforward, clean operations with no obvious bacterial contamination or insertion of a foreign body. When the incidence of wound infections is less than 1%, the potential for reducing this low infection rate does not justify the expense and side effects of antibiotics. Prophylactic antibiotic therapy is no substitute for careful surgical technique using established surgical principles, and its indiscriminate or general use is not in the best interest of the patient. Antibiotic agents can be used effectively only as adjuvants to adequate surgical procedure.

Clinical situations in which prophylactic systemic antibiotic therapy usually helps almost always involve a brief period of contamination by organisms that can be predicted with reasonable accuracy. These antibiotics reduce infection with clinical benefit in the following circumstances: (1) high-risk gastroduodenal procedures, including operations for gastric cancer, ulcer, obstruction, or bleeding, or when effective suppression of gastric acid has been accomplished, or in operations for morbid obesity; (2) high-risk biliary procedures, including operations in patients over 60 years old, those for acute inflammation, common duct stones, or jaundice, and in patients with prior biliary tract operations or endoscopic biliary manipulation; (3) resection and anastomosis of the colon or small intestine (see below); (4) cardiac procedures through a median sternotomy; (5) vascular procedures for the lower extremities or abdominal aorta; (6) amputation of an extremity with impaired blood supply, particularly with a current or recent ischemic ulcer; (7) vaginal or abdominal hysterectomy; (8) primary cesarean section; (9) operations entering the oropharyngeal cavity in continuity with neck dissections; (10) craniotomy; (11) the implantation of any permanent prosthetic material; (12) known gross bacterial contamination in any wound; and (13) accidental wounds with heavy contamination and tissue damage. In such instances, the antibiotic should be given by the intravenous route as soon as possible after injury. The two best-studied situations are penetrating abdominal injuries and open fractures.

Oral nonabsorbable antibiotics to suppress both aerobic and

anaerobic intestinal bacteria before scheduled surgical procedures of the colon also have been successful in controlled trials. Neomycin plus erythromycin given only on the day before operation, 19, 18, and 9 hours before the procedure, is the most well-established combination. Thorough mechanical cleansing of the intestinal tract is a critically important component of the oral regimen. Several reports demonstrate a reduced infection rate with the combination of oral nonabsorbable and intravenous antibiotics, and this is currently the most common practice among colorectal surgeons in the United States.

Prophylactic antibiotics are more effective when started preoperatively and when therapeutic blood levels are maintained throughout the operative period. Antibiotics started after bacterial contamination are less effective, and it is completely without value to start prophylactic antibiotics after wound closure. For elective procedures, the first dose of prophylactic antibiotics should be given intravenously when anesthesia is induced. A single dose, depending on the drug used and length of operation, is often sufficient. For prolonged operations, the prophylactic agent should be repeated at intervals of 1 to 2 half-lives for the drug being used. It is almost never indicated to give prophylactic antibiotic coverage for more than 12 hours for a planned operation.

The most important determinant in choosing a prophylactic antibiotic is whether or not the planned procedure is expected to involve obligate colonic anaerobic bacteria (*Bacteroides* species). For operations on the colon or distal ileum or during appendectomy, an agent effective against *Bacteroides* species such as cefotetan must be used. If anaerobic flora are not expected, then cefazolin is the prophylactic drug of choice. For patients allergic to cephalosporins or when methicillin-resistant *Staphylococcus aureus* is common, vancomycin can be used. If an intestinal procedure is planned, then an agent active against gram-negative rods such as aztreonam or an aminoglycoside and an agent with activity against anaerobes such as clindamycin or metronidazole also must be used. Prophylactic antibiotics are generally ineffective in clinical situations in which continuing contamination is apt to occur.

NATURE, DIAGNOSIS, AND TREATMENT OF SURGICAL INFECTIONS

Surgical infections are distinguished from medical infections by the presence of an anatomic or mechanical problem that must be resolved by operation or other invasive procedure to cure the infection. Such procedures include, but are not limited to, incising and draining an abscess, opening an infected wound, removing an infected foreign body, repairing or diverting a bowel leak, or draining an intra-abdominal abscess with a percutaneous catheter. Antibiotic treatment of a surgical infection without this mechanical solution does not resolve the infection. The most important aspect of the initial approach to a surgical infection is the recognition that operative intervention is required.

SOFT TISSUE INFECTIONS. The most obvious example of a surgical infection is an abscess that does not resolve without drainage. An abscess may be mistaken for cellulitis when it is located deeply beneath overlying tissue layers and it cannot be readily detected by physical examination. Superficial abscesses on the trunk and head and neck are most commonly caused by *S. aureus*, often combined with streptococci. Abscesses in the axillae often have a prominent gram-negative component. Abscesses below the waist, especially on the perineum, frequently harbor a mixed aerobic and anaerobic gram-negative flora. Necrotizing soft tissue infections, both clostridial and nonclostridial, are less common than subcutaneous abscesses and cellulitis but much more serious conditions whose severity may be unrecognized initially. These infections are marked by the absence of clear local boundaries or palpable limits. This lack accounts both for their severity and for the frequent delay in recognizing their surgical nature. These infections are marked by a layer of necrotic tissue, which is not walled off by a surrounding inflammatory reaction and thus does not present a clear boundary. In addition, the visible degree of involvement is substantially less than that of the underlying tissues. A clostridial infection involves underlying muscle and is termed *clostridial myonecrosis* or *gas gangrene*. Most nonclostridial and some clostridial necrotizing infections spread in the subcutaneous fascia, between the skin and the deep muscular fascia. These infections have been described under a variety of labels but are most commonly called *necrotizing fasciitis*. Rapid progression of a soft tissue infection, a marked hemodynamic response to infection, or the failure to respond to conventional nonoperative therapy may be the earliest signs of a necrotizing soft tissue infection. An apparent cellulitis with ecchymoses, bullae, any dermal gangrene, extensive edema, or crepitus suggests an underlying necrotizing infection and mandates operative exploration to confirm the diagnosis and provide definitive treatment. Operative treatment requires excision of involved tissues for clostridial myonecrosis. Nonclostridial infections often can be managed by wide incision and débridement and do not usually require amputation.

INTRA-ABDOMINAL AND RETROPERITONEAL INFECTIONS. Most serious intra-abdominal infections require surgical intervention for resolution. Use of antibiotics for fever and abdominal pain before diagnosis may obscure subsequent findings and delay diagnosis and certainly delays definitive operative management. If too ill to receive antibiotics, the patient is also too ill to avoid operative intervention with definitive diagnosis and treatment. Mortality from serious intra-abdominal or retroperitoneal infection remains high (5% to 50%), and morbidity is substantial.

Regardless of the initial antibiotic choice and operative procedure, there is a significant chance that a change in antibiotics may be required and that reoperation may be necessary. Outcome is improved by early diagnosis and treatment. The risk of death and of complications increases with increased age, pre-existing serious underlying diseases, and malnutrition. Initial treatment for intra-abdominal infection consists of cardiorespiratory support, antibiotic therapy, and operative intervention. Since most intra-abdominal infections yield three to five different aerobic and anaerobic pathogens, specific, targeted antibiotic therapy is not possible at first, and the initial choice must be empirical, designed to cover a range of possible organisms. For infections acquired in the community with a small likelihood of resistant gram-negative rods and for a patient who is not severely ill, empirical therapy can be initiated with cefoxitin, cefotetan, ticarcillin/clavulanate, or ampicillin/sulbactam. For a more severely ill patient or a patient who has been in the hospital or has recently been treated with antibiotics, more comprehensive treatment is needed, using imipenem, piperacillin/tazobactam, or a combination of a third-generation cephalosporin or ciprofloxacin combined with either clindamycin or metronidazole.

CT scans precisely localize intra-abdominal abscesses, permitting selected abscesses to be drained percutaneously under radiologic or ultrasound guidance. If the abscess is single and has a straight path to the abdominal wall that does not transgress bowel, it is amenable to percutaneous drainage. If percutaneous drainage is not successful, an open operation may be required. Most pancreatic "abscesses," which are more often diffusely infected, necrotic, peripancreatic retroperitoneal tissue, require transabdominal operation and débridement. A pelvic abscess may be amenable to transrectal or transvaginal drainage.

POSTOPERATIVE FEVER. Approximately 2% of all primary laparotomies are followed by an unscheduled operation for intra-abdominal infection, and about half of all serious intra-abdominal infections are postoperative. Wound infections are more common but less serious. However, most febrile postoperative patients are not infected, and indeed, a significant proportion of infected patients may not be febrile, depending on the definition of "fever." Fever in the first 3 days following operation most likely has a noninfectious etiology. However, when the fever begins 5 or more days postoperatively, the incidence of wound infections exceeds the incidence of undiagnosed fevers. Neither the prolongation of perioperative prophylactic antibiotics nor the initiation of empirical therapeutic antibiotics is indicated without a presumptive clinical diagnosis and a plan for operative intervention when indicated. The two important infectious causes of fever likely in the first 36 hours after a laparotomy are an injury to bowel with intraperitoneal leak or an invasive soft tissue infection beginning in the wound and caused either by beta-hemolytic streptococci or clostridia. The diagnosis is made by examination of the patient and inspection of the wound and Gram stain of wound fluid.

GENERAL PRINCIPLES. Whichever antibiotics are employed, the goal of therapy is to achieve adequate levels at the site of infection. Each patient should be evaluated frequently to assess response to treatment. If improvement has not occurred within 2 to 3 days, one should be concerned about the reasons why the patient is failing to improve. Likely answers include (1) the initial operative procedure was inadequate, (2) the initial procedure was adequate but a complication has occurred, (3) a superinfection has developed at a new site, (4) the drug choice is correct but given in an insufficient amount, or (5) another or a different drug is needed. The choice of antibiotics is not the most common cause for failure unless the original choice was clearly inappropriate, such as failing to provide coverage for anaerobes in an intra-abdominal infection. For most surgical infections, there is not a specific duration of antibiotics known to be ideal. After 3 to 5 days, the local responses of new capillary formation and inflammatory infiltrate provide a competent local defense for fresh wounds. For deep-seated or poorly localized infections, longer treatment may be needed. A good guideline is to continue antibiotics until the patient shows an obvious clinical improvement based on clinical examination and has had a normal temperature for 48 hours or more. Signs of improvement include improved mental status, return of bowel function, and spontaneous diuresis.

Antibiotic-associated colitis due to *Clostridium difficile* is a significant superinfection that can occur in hospitalized patients with mild to serious illness. Diagnosis is by endoscopy, stool assay for the characteristic toxin, and stool culture to recover *C. difficile*. Treatment is supportive with fluid and electrolytes, withdrawal of the offending antibiotic, if possible, and oral metronidazole to treat the superinfection. Vancomycin should be reserved for metronidazole failures. In rare instances when an overwhelming colitis does not respond to medical management, emergency colectomy may be required.

II

Surgical Aspects of Acquired Immunodeficiency Syndrome

Douglas Tyler, M.D., and H. Kim Lyerly, M.D.

The acquired immunodeficiency syndrome (AIDS) is characterized by profound defects in cellular immunity leading to opportunistic infections and unusual neoplasms. AIDS was first recognized in 1981 and is caused by a human retrovirus termed *human immunodeficiency virus Type 1* (HIV-1). HIV-1 has a unique tropism for the CD4 molecule found on T-helper/inducer cells and monocytes-macrophages. Following infection of such cells, intracellular replication of HIV-1 leads to the production of infectious progeny and to the destruction or dysfunction of the infected cell. It is the quantitative or

See the corresponding chapter or part in the *Textbook of Surgery*, 15th edition, pp. 280–286, for a more detailed discussion of this topic, including a comprehensive list of references.

qualitative deficiency in T-helper/inducer lymphocytes that produces the immune defects in AIDS, because these cells control the proliferation of natural killer cells and cytotoxic T cells.

Acute infection with HIV-1 may cause a mononucleosis-like syndrome, but after the acute infection, a variable asymptomatic period may occur that may last for as long as 7 to 10 years. This asymptomatic period may be followed by a period of symptomatic disease consisting of constitutional signs including weight loss, fever and night sweats, or infections that do not meet the criteria for the complete syndrome of AIDS. These features comprise the AIDS-related complex. Other manifestations of progressive HIV-1 infection include immune thrombocytopenia and neurologic disease. AIDS represents the most severe manifestation of infection with HIV-1; most, if not all, of those infected develop AIDS with a mean period of 8 years. AIDS is characterized by a progressive lymphopenia, predominantly of T-helper/inducer cells, that is clinically manifested by susceptibility to life-threatening opportunistic infections and malignancies. Such infections and/or neoplasms are typically recurrent, and life expectancy is estimated to be 1 to 2 years without specific anti-HIV-1 therapy but has increased with improved management of opportunistic infections.

Zidovudine (AZT) is a thymidine analogue that acts as a chain terminator for the reverse transcriptase–driven elongation of HIV-1 DNA. The use of AZT has lead to an improvement in the quality and length of life for patients with AIDS and has been demonstrated to decrease the number and severity of opportunistic infections in these patients. There is currently no curative therapy for AIDS. The standard method of testing for HIV-1 infection is by the identification of anti-HIV-1–specific antibodies. After infection, such antibodies are usually present within 6 to 8 weeks and can be detected by using an enzyme-linked immunoabsorbent assay or Western blot analysis. After infection with HIV-1, a number of individuals may remain seronegative for weeks to years. Confirmation of infection in these individuals relies on the direct detection of HIV-1 by viral culture, the demonstration of HIV-1–specific proteins in body fluids, or the detection of HIV-1–specific nucleic acid sequences in cellular material.

EPIDEMIOLOGY

Risk groups for the development of AIDS include homosexual or bisexual males, intravenous drug abusers, hemophiliacs receiving factor VIII concentrates, recipients of blood or blood products, heterosexual partners of infected individuals, and children of a parent with AIDS or at risk for AIDS. Transmission of HIV-1 is through sexual contact with infected partners, direct exposure to contaminated blood or blood products, and perinatal transmission from infected mothers to their offspring.

OCCUPATIONAL RISK OF HEALTH CARE WORKERS

HIV-1 can be transmitted to health care workers through occupational exposure; however, it is difficult to assess the magnitude of risk for such exposure. Combined data from 10 prospective studies indicate that the risk for HIV-1 transmission from a single parenteral exposure is 0.37%. There is no evidence at present of HIV-1 transmission following a single mucous membrane exposure. Occupational exposure is minimized by implementation of universal blood.

TRANSFUSION-ASSOCIATED AIDS

Transmission of HIV-1 has been documented after transfusion of whole blood, packed red blood cells, fresh-frozen plasma, cryoprecipitate, and platelets (single-donor blood products). Blood products derived from pooled plasma also can transmit HIV-1. Transmission of HIV-1 by transfusion has become rare since the introduction of voluntary deferral of donors at risk for HIV-1 infection and the routine testing of all donations. The estimated risk of acquiring HIV-1 ranges from 1 in 36,000 to 1 in 10,000 per unit of blood transfused. The current risk of HIV-1 infection from organ transplantation is unknown but is thought to be comparable with the risk from blood transfusion.

CLINICAL FEATURES

Most of the morbidity observed in AIDS patients is related to overwhelming infections. Clinical syndromes that occur frequently include diffuse pneumonia, fever, diarrhea, central nervous system disorders, generalized lymphadenopathy, and esophagitis. Although infectious complications are a prominent feature in AIDS, unusual neoplasms are also encountered in large number. These include Kaposi's sarcoma (KS) and non-Hodgkin's lymphoma. KS encountered in AIDS patients is characterized by the sudden onset and often widespread appearance of lesions involving not only skin but oral mucosa, lymph nodes, and visceral organs. The average survival of patients is 18 months; however, visceral involvement implies a poor prognosis. Small, localized lesions may be treated by electrodesiccation and curettage or by surgical excision, and KS tumors generally are responsive to local radiation; however, it has not been demonstrated that local or systemic therapy for KS alters the ultimate course of the disease.

Most AIDS-related lymphomas are B-cell tumors of high-grade pathologic type, and as many as 63% may present with Stage IV disease. The therapy of choice for AIDS-related lymphomas is unknown because multiagent chemotherapy may worsen the patient's immune dysfunction and susceptibility to infection. Median survival of patients with AIDS-related lymphoma is less than 1 year but has improved. The incidence of non-Hodgkin's lymphoma appears to be increasing, especially in those treated with AZT.

SURGICAL CONSIDERATIONS IN HIV-1–INFECTED INDIVIDUALS

HIV-1–infected individuals not only are susceptible to standard medical problems and surgical disorders but also may tolerate surgical interventions differently from nonimmunosuppressed individuals as well as be susceptible to a variety of unique conditions that frequently require surgical intervention.

EVALUATION BY ORGAN SYSTEM

ESOPHAGUS. Diffuse esophagitis secondary to *Candida albicans* (most frequently), herpes simplex virus, or cytomegalovirus (CMV) is the most common lesion observed. Empirical therapy with ketoconazole (*Candida*) or acyclovir (herpesvirus) may be successful; however, endoscopy and biopsy may be required to differentiate these lesions. Esophageal ulceration, thought to be secondary to an as yet undefined virus, may occur. KS lesions of the esophagus may bleed or rarely cause pharyngeal obstruction and thus require excision.

STOMACH AND DUODENUM. Commonly encountered lesions include KS, non-Hodgkin's lymphoma, and CMV infections. KS lesions are usually asymptomatic but are the most common cause of upper gastrointestinal bleeding in HIV-1–infected individuals and can occasionally cause gastric outlet obstruction. Surgical excision is required if radiotherapy, chemotherapy, or immunotherapy fails to control the tumor. Non-Hodgkin's lymphoma may cause hemorrhage, obstruction, or perforation. Surgical excision is preferable to chemotherapy initially because intestinal perforation secondary to extensive tumor lysis after chemotherapy may occur. CMV infections of the stomach and duodenum cause ulceration, which may perforate and require surgical intervention. Despite operation, morbidity and mortality following perforation secondary to CMV are high.

LIVER. The majority of HIV-1–related opportunistic infections and the neoplastic complications of HIV-1 infection, KS and non-Hodgkin's lymphoma, may affect the liver, but operative intervention is rarely required for therapy. Liver biopsy is occasionally indicated, and liver abscesses occasionally may require surgical intervention for drainage. Constitutional symptoms and abnormal liver function tests are indicative of liver involvement. Most patients with AIDS have serologic evidence of previous hepatitis B infection. Other types of viral hepatitis are also common.

GALLBLADDER AND BILIARY TRACT. Numerous cases of acute acalculous cholecystitis have been documented in HIV-1–infected individuals. Inciting organisms include *Cryptosporidium* and CMV (most commonly), *Campylobacter*, and *Candida*. Diagnosis is by ultrasonography, and cholecystectomy is the treatment of choice. This operation is usually well tolerated in asymptomatic HIV-1–infected individuals but has a high morbidity and mortality in patients with AIDS.

Papillary stenosis and sclerosing cholangitis are observed

with surprising frequency in HIV-1–infected individuals. Cryptosporidiosis and CMV infection are the likely causes. Extrinsic compression of the bile ducts secondary to KS lesions, lymphadenopathy, or lymphoma should be excluded by ultrasonography and/or CT scanning. Papillary stenosis can be relieved by endoscopic sphincterotomy; sclerosing cholangitis, by balloon dilation and stenting. Surgical intervention may be required for relief of extrinsic compression or when endoscopic sphincterotomy fails.

INTESTINE. HIV-1–related neoplastic lesions affecting the intestine include non-Hodgkin's lymphoma and KS. Lymphomas are usually symptomatic, presenting with signs of pain, fever, night sweats, weight loss, jaundice, ascites, obstruction, bleeding, and/or perforation. Diagnosis is by CT scan. Surgical intervention is frequently indicated and is advised before chemotherapy for the prevention of intestinal perforation secondary to postchemotherapy tumor lysis. Intestinal KS lesions are present in 40% to 50% of patients with cutaneous KS lesions but are usually asymptomatic. Lesions causing bleeding or obstruction may require surgical excision.

CMV infection may cause intestinal perforation, necessitating surgical exploration and segmental bowel resection. Morbidity and mortality after such a procedure remain high (40%) because of the lack of appropriate systemic antiviral therapy. Several organisms can cause an inflammatory response in the terminal ileum that mimics regional enteritis or appendicitis, leading to surgical exploration. These include *Yersinia, Campylobacter, Shigella, Salmonella,* and *Mycobacterium avium-intracellulare.*

APPENDIX. Whereas appendicitis occurs in HIV-1–infected individuals via the same mechanisms through which it occurs in seronegative individuals, appendiceal obstruction also may follow AIDS-related neoplasms such as KS and lymphoma. Appendicitis is often more difficult to diagnose in patients with AIDS, since they frequently have chronic abdominal complaints.

COLON. Lesions affecting the colon in HIV-1–infected individuals are predominantly infectious in nature. CMV infection can lead to perforation requiring surgical intervention. A number of bacterial and parasitic organisms can cause a severe colitis, which usually persists with abdominal pain and diarrhea.

ANUS AND RECTUM. Anorectal complaints are common in HIV-1–infected individuals, especially homosexuals and AIDS patients. Symptoms include pain, discharge, incontinence, bleeding, mass, and/or tenesmus. Such symptoms may be caused by a wide variety of viral, bacterial, fungal, protozoal, and helminthic infections; lesions such as anal fissures, fistulas, and perirectal abscess or tumors such as KS, lymphoma, or squamous cell carcinoma are common. The frequency of these lesions in AIDS patients appears to increase their risk of developing anal and rectal carcinoma. Treatment of the various anorectal lesions should be as conservative as possible because patients appear to heal poorly after attempted surgical therapy.

EVALUATION BY CLINICAL SIGNS OR SYMPTOMS

ABDOMINAL PAIN. Abdominal pain affecting HIV-1–infected patients is seen more commonly in late-stage disease (AIDS), and its occurrence appears associated with reduced patient survival. There appear to be four general syndromes of abdominal pain: (1) epigastric pain with or without esophageal symptoms, (2) right upper quadrant pain with or without jaundice, (3) right iliac fossa pain, and (4) diffuse abdominal pain.

Epigastric pain is usually secondary to esophagitis but also can be caused by gastritis, duodenitis, gastric malignancy, or non–HIV-1–related processes such as peptic ulcer disease. Endoscopy is the diagnostic test of choice. Right upper quadrant pain is usually secondary to either acute cholecystitis, hepatitis, or papillary stenosis/sclerosing cholangitis. Initial evaluation involves ultrasound. A HIDA scan can confirm the diagnosis of acute cholecystitis; ERCP should be performed if the patient is jaundiced or has dilated bile ducts. Right iliac fossa pain should be worked up with ultrasound and/or laparoscopy to rule out appendicitis. Diffuse abdominal pain is usually secondary to an infectious process in the colon. Colonoscopy is usually more informative than CT scans. Surgery is rarely required unless bleeding, obstruction, or perforation is present.

THROMBOCYTOPENIA. The etiology of thrombocytopenia in HIV-1 infection is unclear but appears related to antibodies against HIV-1 that crossreact with certain platelet antigens. Major bleeding episodes are rare. AZT can increase platelet counts in 70% of patients. Splenectomy is reserved for patients who do not respond to AZT.

GASTROINTESTINAL BLEEDING. Gastrointestinal bleeding is an unusual occurrence in HIV-1–infected individuals. Most lesions causing gastrointestinal bleeding are directly related to HIV-1 infection. Such lesions include KS and non-Hodgkin's lymphoma. Because these lesions are frequently treatable, gastrointestinal bleeding should be treated aggressively in HIV-1–infected individuals who are not terminally ill.

LYMPHADENOPATHY. Generalized lymphadenopathy is a relatively common finding in patients with HIV-1 infection. The recognition of HIV-1 as the etiologic agent in AIDS and the development of accurate serologic tests for antibodies to HIV-1 have rendered routine diagnostic lymph node biopsy unnecessary. Selective use of lymph node biopsy may assist in the diagnosis of a specific infection, lymphoma, or disease process and thus alter the clinical management of the patient.

OTHER CONSIDERATIONS

POSTOPERATIVE COURSE. Postoperative morbidity and mortality in HIV-1–infected individuals appear to be related to the patient's underlying immunocompetence and the nature of the underlying illness requiring surgery. Asymptomatic HIV-1–infected individuals undergoing elective surgical procedures have no more problems with wound healing and postoperative infection than do the normal population. There is a debate regarding the healing ability of patients with AIDS after elective procedures. Surgical intervention in this patient population, however, has been reported to occasionally exacerbate underlying HIV-1 infection. Extremely high morbidity and mortality are reported following emergent surgery in AIDS patients.

16

BITES AND STINGS

Elaine E. Nelson, M.D., and Paul S. Auerbach, M.D., M.S.

SNAKEBITES

TOXICOLOGY. Most medically significant bites are from snakes belonging to either the Crotalidae (pit viper) or the Elapidae (coral snake) families. Envenomation increases vascular permeability, damages erythrocytes and muscle cells, and causes tissue necrosis. Deleterious effects on the cardiovascular, pulmonary, renal, hematologic, and neurologic systems can occur.

CLINICAL MANIFESTATIONS. Approximately 20% of bites by pit vipers do not cause envenomation. These appear as puncture wounds associated with minimal pain. Inoculation with venom produces burning pain within minutes, followed by edema and erythema. Ecchymoses, hemorrhagic bullae, and lymphangitis can develop. Patients typically complain of weakness, nausea, vomiting, perioral paresthesias, metallic taste, and fasciculations. Pulmonary edema, hypotension, renal failure, and disseminated intravascular coagulation can occur. Coral snakes produce primarily a neurotoxic venom with minimal local complaints only.

MANAGEMENT. Cryotherapy, incision and suction, tourniquets, and electric shock therapy are no longer recommended. If the patient remains asymptomatic 6 hours after a pit viper bite or 24 hours after a coral snake bite, it is unlikely that envenomation occurred. The wound should be cleansed thoroughly, débrided, splinted, and soaked in Burow's solution. Fasciotomies should be performed if compartment pressures are over 30 mm Hg. Tetanus status should be current. A broad-spectrum antibiotic is recommended.

ANTIVENIN THERAPY. Antivenin is the primary treatment modality for systemic envenomation. The use of antivenin for minor envenomation is controversial. Significant hypersensitivity reactions to antivenin can occur. Therefore, skin testing should be performed before it is administered. Between 5 and 20 vials of antivenin are administered, depending on the severity of the envenomation. A separate antivenin is available for coral snakes.

MAMMALIAN BITES

TREATMENT. Patients attacked by animals are at risk for blunt and penetrating trauma. X-rays should be obtained to diagnose fractures, joint and skull penetration, and foreign bodies. Tetanus prophylaxis is necessary. The wound should be meticulously débrided and irrigated.

See the corresponding chapter or part in the *Textbook of Surgery*, 15th edition, pp. 287–295, for a more detailed discussion of this topic, including a comprehensive list of references.

Primary closure of selected bites produces the best outcome for the patient without increasing the risk of infection. This is especially true for head and neck wounds, where aesthetic results are important. Healing of face wounds by secondary intention produces unacceptable scars. The primary goal for repairing bite wounds to the hand is to maximize functional outcome. Healing by secondary intention is recommended for most hand bites, especially with the clenched-fist injury. Tendon and nerve injuries should be managed by delayed repair. The method of repair used for bite wounds to other body parts depends on the risk factors associated with the particular injury. Primary closure should be avoided in high-risk bites such as puncture wounds, bites to the hand, and bites in immunocompromised patients.

MICROBIOLOGY. Infections are usually polymicrobial, with *Staphylococcus* and *Streptococcus* species and anaerobes present. *Pasteurella multocida* is the primary organism responsible for infections in cat bites, and *Eikenella corrodens* has been isolated from human bites. Prophylactic antibiotics are recommended for patients with high-risk bites. Cat bites can be treated with penicillin and dicloxacillin. Recommended antibiotics for bites from other animals include dicloxacillin or cephalexin. Human bites can be treated with a second- or third-generation cephalosporin or a combination of dicloxacillin and ampicillin. Cefuroxime or amoxicillin/clavulanic acid is acceptable for all bites. The decision to administer rabies prophylaxis depends on the animal species and the nature of the event. The local health department can help determine the risk of rabies in patients suffering from animal bites or scratches.

ARTHROPOD BITES

BLACK WIDOW SPIDERS. The black widow spider produces a neurotoxic venom with minimal local properties. Envenomation causes muscle spasms and adrenergic stimulation. Other symptoms include fasciculations, vomiting, headache, paresthesias, fatigue, and salivation.

Mild envenomation is managed with local wound care, including cleansing, applying ice, and administering tetanus prophylaxis. Narcotics and benzodiazepines can relieve muscular pain. Significant envenomation might benefit from antivenin therapy. Antivenin is recommended for pregnant women, children under 16 years of age, individuals over 60 years of age, and patients with severe reactions such as hypertension, respiratory distress, and seizures. Skin testing is necessary. The initial recommended antivenin dose is 1 vial, repeated as necessary.

BROWN RECLUSE SPIDERS. Venom from brown recluse spiders produces local hemolysis, coagulation, and platelet aggregation and causes initial blister development. These conditions can progress to vasoconstriction and ultimately tissue necrosis. Systemic features are uncommon but can include headache, vomiting, fever, arthralgias, coagulopathy, and a maculopapular rash.

The bite site should be elevated and an ice compress applied. Antibiotics should be administered and tetanus status made current. Brown recluse bites that do not develop necrosis within 72 hours usually heal well and require no additional therapy. More severe lesions may benefit from dapsone administration. Early surgery and steroid administration are controversial. Severe cases might require eventual wide excision and split-thickness skin grafting.

HYMENOPTERA. Most arthropod envenomations are by bees, wasps, and ants. Histamine and serotonin are responsible for local reactions and pain, and peptides and enzymes are responsible for the allergic reactions. A sting in a nonallergic individual produces immediate pain followed by a wheal reaction. Large local reactions present as erythematous, painful, and pruritic areas. Anaphylaxis develops in 0.3% to 3% of the general population and consists of mild urticaria and angioedema to cardiorespiratory arrest.

The stinger should be removed and the bite site cleansed. Ice therapy, lidocaine, or a vinegar-and-salt solution can alleviate pain. Antihistamines can decrease pruritus. Persons with severe local reactions may be given prednisone. Mild anaphylaxis is treated with subcutaneous epinephrine and intravenous antihistamines. Severe cases may require intravenous fluids, vasopressors, bronchodilators, and endotracheal intubation. All persons with previous severe systemic allergic reactions to Hymenoptera stings and adults with isolated dermal reactions might benefit from venom immunotherapy.

MARINE TRAUMA AND ENVENOMATION

GENERAL MANAGEMENT. Injuries from marine organisms can range from mild local complaints to systemic collapse from major trauma or severe envenomation. Initial management includes stabilizing the patient and administering antivenin (available for box jellyfish, sea snakes, and stonefish) followed by local wound care. Tetanus status should be updated. Radiographs should be obtained to diagnose foreign bodies and fractures.

WOUND CARE. Wounds should be irrigated with normal saline and débrided. Primary closure should be avoided in distal extremity wounds, punctures, and crush injuries. Patients with large abrasions, lacerations, puncture wounds, or hand injuries and immunocompromised patients should receive prophylactic antibiotics. Third-generation cephalosporins, ciprofloxacin, trimethoprim/sulfamethoxazole, or doxycycline provide adequate coverage for the gram-positive and gram-negative microorganisms found in water, including *Vibrio* species.

NONVENOMOUS AQUATIC ANIMALS. These include sharks, eels, alligators, crocodiles, barracudas, sea lions, and needlefish. Injuries range from major trauma to minor bites and puncture wounds. The patient should be treated as a trauma victim, with special attention paid to wound management and antibiotic coverage.

ENVENOMATION. Fire coral, hydroids, Portuguese man-of-war, jellyfish, sea nettles, and sea anemones belong to the phylum Coelenterata. These organisms carry venomous stinging cells called *nematocysts*. Mild envenomation causes skin irritation. Severe envenomation presents with fever, vomiting, malaise, hypotension, and rare cardiorespiratory arrest. Therapy consists of detoxification of nematocysts by applying dilute acetic acid (vinegar—critical with box jellyfish), baking soda, or isopropyl alcohol. The remaining nematocysts are removed by using a razor and shaving cream. Systemic steroids are administered to manage postenvenomation inflammation. Prophylactic antibiotics are usually unnecessary.

Stingrays attack by thrusting spines into a victim, producing puncture wounds and lacerations with contiguous necrosis. Systemic complaints include weakness, nausea, diarrhea, headache, muscle cramps, and rare seizure or cardiorespiratory arrest. The wound should be irrigated, soaked in nonscalding (45° C) hot water, débrided, and left opened. Residual spines can be located with radiographic studies or MRI scans. Injuries from stonefish, scorpionfish, and lionfish are treated similarly; antivenin is available for stonefish envenomation. Sea urchin spines may need to be removed in the operating room with surgical magnification.

17

TRAUMA:
Management of Acute Injuries
Gregory J. Jurkovich, M.D., and C. James Carrico, M.D.

The crucial role of the trauma surgeon mandates a working knowledge of prevention, prehospital care, emergency room care, and rehabilitation in addition to the direction and provision of acute surgical care. This chapter will focus on the acute management of specific injuries. The important issues in trauma care systems are discussed in the main text.

INITIAL RESUSCITATION OF THE ACUTELY INJURED PATIENT

Initial care of the injured patient necessitates two assumptions. The first is that the patient may have more than one injury; the second is that the obvious injury is not necessarily the most important one. The key to initial care is an approach predicated on prioritizing injuries by their life-threatening potential. The priorities of initial trauma care are often referred to as the ABCs of trauma resuscitation.

AIRWAY. The crucial first step in the management of the injured patient is securing an adequate airway. In the majority of severely injured patients, this involves endotracheal intubation. The potential for cervical spine injury always should be considered, and injudicious movement of the neck in the process of *endotracheal* intubation must be avoided. *Nasotracheal* intubation is an option in the spontaneously breathing patient without midface injury. In rare patients, a surgical airway (tracheostomy) may be required.

BREATHING. When an adequate airway is secured, ventilation must be ensured. The three most common reasons for ineffective ventilation following successful placement of an airway are malposition of the endotracheal tube, pneumothorax, and hemothorax. There is generally time to perform a chest radiograph before invasive therapeutic procedures. However, with a high suspicion of tension pneumothorax in the patient with profound hemodynamic instability, urgent needle catheter decompression before chest radiography can be both diagnostic and therapeutic.

CIRCULATION. Control of obvious hemorrhage, placement of an intravenous line, and fluid resuscitation are next and each of high priority. Intravenous cannulas are usually placed percutaneously in the arm or groin. They should be large bore, and a minimum of two should be placed. Lines should not be inserted distal to extremity wounds with potential vascular injury. Alternative access sites are the saphenous

---

See the corresponding chapter or part in the *Textbook of Surgery,* 15th edition, pp. 296–339, for a more detailed discussion of this topic, including a comprehensive list of references.

cutdown route or intraosseous infusion in children under the age of 6 years. With the exception of the use of the large (8-French) introducer catheter, subclavian venipuncture is not a rapid route for fluid administration and is best reserved for monitoring response to fluid therapy. Fluid resuscitation begins with a 1000-ml. bolus of lactated Ringer's solution for an adult or 20 ml. per kg. for a child.

DISABILITY/NEUROLOGIC ASSESSMENT. At this juncture, a brief examination to determine the severity of neurologic injury is indicated. This includes calculation of the Glasgow Coma Scale, which is a method of both following the evolution of neurologic disability and prognosticating future recovery.

EXPOSURE FOR COMPLETE EXAMINATION. The next step is to completely, but expeditiously, re-examine the patient for diagnosis of other injuries. Appropriate laboratory and radiologic tests are obtained. Additional lines, catheters (nasogastric, Foley), and monitoring devices are now placed as needed. A priority treatment plan based on these initial findings should be established.

The management of *specific* injuries follows. It is organized to reflect, in general, the probability that these specific injuries will impact negatively on airway, breathing, and circulation. Thus thoracic and abdominal injuries are first, followed by the head and central nervous system, the neck, the face, and finally the extremities.

MANAGEMENT OF SPECIFIC INJURIES

Thoracic Injuries

A quarter of civilian trauma deaths are caused by thoracic trauma, and two thirds of these deaths occur after the patient reaches the hospital. Despite this high mortality, only 10% to 15% of thoracic injuries require a thoracotomy. The simple lifesaving maneuvers of airway control and tube thoracostomy effectively treat the majority of chest trauma victims. The treatment of specific thoracic injuries is outlined below.

CHEST WALL AND LUNGS

RIB FRACTURES. Rib fractures are the most common thoracic injury. With simple fractures, pain on inspiration is the principal symptom. Localized pain, tenderness, and occasionally crepitus confirm the diagnosis. A chest film should be obtained for exclusion of other intrathoracic injuries and not necessarily for identification of the rib fracture. Narcotics, intercostal nerve blocks, and muscle relaxants are usually adequate treatment. For more severe injuries, hospital admission for pain relief, cough assistance, and endotracheal suction may be necessary for several days, particularly in elderly patients. Rib belts and adhesive taping, although formerly popular, should be avoided because the resultant limitation in motion increases the incidence of retained secretions and atelectasis. Fracture of the upper ribs (1–3), clavicle, or scapula implies significant trauma, and associated major vascular injury must be suspected, although angiography may be employed selectively.

FLAIL CHEST. With segmental fractures of multiple ribs, chest wall instability may be so severe as to limit the effectiveness of spontaneous respirations. This is known as *flail chest*. Endotracheal intubation and mechanical ventilation may be required. Tachypnea, hypoxia, and hypercarbia are indications for intubation and mechanical ventilation.

PULMONARY CONTUSION. Respiratory difficulty in patients with flail chest injury is invariably aggravated by an underlying pulmonary contusion, although pulmonary contusion also can appear without any evidence of rib fracture, particularly in children. Fluid and blood from ruptured vessels enter the alveoli, interstitial spaces, and bronchi and produce localized airway obstruction. Pulmonary compliance decreases, and ventilation becomes more difficult. Positive end-expiratory pressure ventilation may be helpful in restoring functional residual capacity and reducing intrapulmonary shunts. Excessive fluid administration should be avoided.

PNEUMOTHORAX. Pneumothorax is the accumulation of air in the potential space between the visceral and parietal pleura following either a full-thickness violation of the chest wall or laceration of the visceral pleura. Accumulation of air in this space under pressure is known as a *tension pneumothorax*. Sufficient accumulation of air in this space collapses the lung and shifts the mediastinum into the contralateral thorax, causing hypoxia and a diminished venous return to the heart. Prompt venting of a tension pneumothorax can be lifesaving, and virtually all traumatic pneumothoraces should be treated with a tube thoracostomy to water-seal drainage. An *open pneumothorax* is a defect in the chest wall that provides a direct communication between the pleural space and the environment. A large wound provides an alternative air pathway of less resistance than the normal tracheobronchial tree. Inability to generate negative intrathoracic pressure causes lung collapse and marked paroxysmal shifting of the mediastinum with each respiratory effort. Diagnosis is usually apparent, since each inspiration draws air into the interpleural space, causing the characteristic "sucking chest wound." Treatment consists of prompt closure of the defect with a sterile dressing followed by venting of the chest with either a flutter valve or chest tube for treatment of the possible resultant tension pneumothorax.

HEMOTHORAX. Hemothorax occurs in some degree in almost every patient with a diagnosable chest injury. Although an upright chest film can reveal an intrathoracic accumulation of as little as 200 ml. of blood, a supine film may miss collections of up to 1 liter. Since the lung itself is a low-pressure system, spontaneous hemostasis occurs for all but central hilar injuries or injury to the intercostal or internal mammary arteries. Tube thoracostomy with a 32- to 36-French chest tube placed in the sixth or seventh intercostal space at the midaxillary line should be promptly performed. When massive hemothorax is present, preparation for collection of the blood for autotransfusion should be made before tube insertion.

In 85% of patients, tube thoracostomy is the only treatment required. However, an initial thoracic blood loss greater than 1500 ml. (30% blood volume) or an ongoing loss of 250 ml. (5% blood volume) for 3 consecutive hours is generally an indication for exploratory thoracotomy. This is only a guideline, however, and the clinical situation and overall condition of the patient should be the most influential factors.

TRACHEAL AND BRONCHIAL INJURIES. Tracheal and bronchial injuries are unusual but may be caused by blunt or penetrating trauma. Presenting signs are generally dramatic, with significant hemoptysis, hemopneumothorax, subcutaneous crepitance, and respiratory distress; mediastinal and deep cervical emphysema; or pneumothorax with a massive air leak. Emergency treatment usually consists of inserting the endotracheal tube (via endoscopic control) beyond the injury to facilitate ventilation and prevent aspiration of blood. Tube thoracostomy is required for hemo- or pneumothorax. Primary surgical repair is generally indicated.

HEART AND AORTA

MYOCARDIAL CONTUSION. A direct blow to the sternum with subsequent cardiac bruising is known as a *myocardial contusion*. The cardiac injury may vary from superficial epicardial petechiae to transmural damage. Dysrhythmia is the most common presenting finding, although right ventricular dysfunction and decreased cardiac output may occur. The major difficulty in treatment is early recognition. Although cardiac CPK isoenzymes are widely employed, they have not been shown to be adequately sensitive or specific diagnostic tests. Electrocardiograms may show nonspecific ST-T wave changes or dysrhythmias. Cardiac monitoring for 24 hours is indicated if electrocardiographic abnormalities are present or if a major contusion is suspected. Echocardiography is helpful in diagnosing ventricular dysfunction and in detecting blood in the pericardium. The management of myocardial contusion is supportive.

CARDIAC TAMPONADE. Most frequently caused by penetrating thoracic injuries, cardiac tamponade is occasionally observed in blunt thoracic trauma from superior vena caval or atrial rupture, coronary artery laceration, or descending dissection of an aortic tear. Accumulation of as little as 150 ml. of blood in the pericardial sac may significantly impair diastolic filling. Beck's classic triad of distended neck veins, muffled heart sounds, and hypotension is present in only one-third of patients with tamponade. Pulsus paradoxus is even less frequently discernible. Pericardiocentesis can be both diagnostic and temporarily therapeutic. However, approximately 15% of pericardiocenteses yield false-negative results because of a clotted hemopericardium. Therefore, echocardiography before open pericardiotomy is advisable if it can be obtained promptly. If the patient is *in extremis*, emergency thoracotomy with pericardiotomy and cardiac repair should be performed.

AORTA. Rupture of the thoracic aorta is the most lethal injury following blunt chest trauma. The exact mechanism of injury is not fully understood, but it is thought that the descending portion of the aortic arch undergoes flexion or torsion, disrupting the aortic wall at the ligamentum arteriosum immediately distal to the left subclavian artery. Most patients with aortic rupture die immediately from exsanguination, but in approximately 20% the periaortic tissue temporarily contains the hematoma. Survival depends on prompt diagnosis and treatment. A suggestive mechanism of injury and a widening of the mediastinal shadow should prompt angiography, even though only 20% to 43% of patients with a widened mediastinum have aortic injury. Other radiographic signs suggestive of aortic injury include loss of the contour of the aortic knob, shift of the trachea and the nasogastric tube to the right, apical capping, and left hemothorax.

DIAPHRAGM AND ESOPHAGUS

Penetrating lacerations of the diaphragm outnumber blunt ruptures at least four to one. Both may produce herniation through the diaphragm, and both require repair, even small stab wounds. With isolated diaphragm injuries, diagnosis may be difficult. The initial chest film may be normal in 30% of patients with right-sided diaphragmatic rupture. Herniation of the viscera may not occur immediately, and the patient may present months or years later with incarceration of abdominal contents in the hernia. Fortunately, the diagnosis is often made incidentally at the time of laparotomy, since most patients have concomitant intra-abdominal injuries.

Blunt injury to the esophagus is rare, and penetrating injuries are rarely isolated. The most common symptom of esophageal perforation is extreme chest pain with the slow evolution of fever several hours later. Regurgitation of blood, hoarseness, dysphagia, or respiratory distress also may be present. Suspicious radiographic findings are mediastinal air and widening, presence of a foreign body, pleural effusion, or hydropneumothorax. All gunshot wounds traversing the mediastinum should be evaluated for possible esophageal injury. Both endoscopy and esophagography have reported sensitivities that vary from 50% to 90% and should be considered complementary studies. Esophageal injury requires immediate débridement, suture closure, and drainage. Delays of 12 to 24 hours may preclude primary repair and mandate proximal diversion and distal feeding access.

Abdomen: Mechanisms and Diagnosis of Injury

In the awake, alert, responsive patient with *isolated* abdominal injury, the physical examination and history are quite accurate in predicting the presence of significant visceral injury. However, in the patient with altered level of consciousness or multiple injuries, an impaired ability to recognize abdominal pain makes diagnosis more difficult. The overall sensitivity (95%), specificity (98% to 99%), and accuracy (97%) of diagnostic peritoneal lavage make this technique the mainstay for diagnosis of intraperitoneal injury in the multiple-injury trauma patient. Computed tomography (CT) is useful in assessing the abdomen of the *hemodynamically stable* patient and is particularly useful in assessing the retroperitoneum, an anatomic area of injury for which diagnostic peritoneal lavage is not helpful. Peitzman and colleagues have listed five indications for abdominal CT scans in *hemodynamically stable* trauma victims: (1) an equivocal abdominal examination, (2) closed head injury, (3) spinal cord injury, (4) hematuria, and (5) patients with pelvic fractures and significant bleeding.

The diagnosis of intraperitoneal injury in penetrating abdominal trauma remains controversial. In general, gunshot wounds require laparotomy; stab wounds can be more selectively managed. It should be emphasized that if there is any doubt regarding the potential for intra-abdominal injury, exploratory laparotomy remains the best method of evaluation and treatment.

Abdomen: Intraperitoneal Injuries

SPLEEN

The spleen is the most commonly injured intra-abdominal organ. Splenectomy is no longer the only management option for splenic injuries. Trauma surgeons also must consider splenic repair or nonoperative management as viable options in select patients, with recognition of the rare but highly lethal syndrome of overwhelming postsplenectomy sepsis (see main text). Splenorrhaphy (repair) can be considered for injuries to all areas of the spleen except the central hilar area. Although the reported success rate of splenic repair varies, most large trauma centers report splenic salvage rates to be between 40% and 60% of all splenic injuries. In patients with multiple intra-abdominal injuries or extensive peritoneal contamination from visceral perforation, it is good surgical judgment to weigh the benefits of splenic salvage against the safer and more expedient course of splenectomy. In addition, splenic salvage is probably not warranted if only 50% or less of the splenic substance is to be preserved.

The safety and effectiveness of nonoperative management of selected pediatric patients with isolated splenic injuries are acceptable, but similar management in adults is controversial. The unknown incidence of delayed splenic rupture and the incidence of associated injuries are reasons often given for avoiding nonoperative management. An additional factor considered in determining the risk of nonoperative management versus splenorrhaphy or splenectomy is the risk of blood transfusion.

LIVER

The liver is the second most commonly injured organ following blunt trauma and is the most commonly injured abdominal organ following penetrating trauma. Over 50% of all liver injuries are nonbleeding at the time of initial exploration, and an additional 20% can be managed by direct suture ligation, cautery, or hemostatic agents. The remaining severe liver injuries can be difficult to manage and are responsible for the high overall liver injury mortality of 11% and morbidity of 22%.

With deeper lacerations, bleeding may be so significant initially as to prevent adequate exposure. Direct compression and inflow occlusion (Pringle maneuver) are effective maneuvers for providing exposure and allowing direct ligation of vessels and biliary radicals. Although the exact length of warm ischemia time tolerated by the human liver is not known, inflow occlusion for at least 20 minutes, and perhaps up to 1 hour, appears to be well tolerated. Liver lacerations should not be sutured closed. This predisposes to liver abscesses and hemobilia. Closed-suction drainage should be provided in all cases.

Selective ligation of the right or left hepatic artery is necessary in less than 1% of all liver injuries; injudicious hepatic artery ligation may cause liver infarction. The proper hepatic artery must never be ligated. Resection of hepatic parenchyma is also unusual following liver injuries. In one large review consisting of over 1300 liver trauma patients, hepatic resectional débridement was performed in only 36 patients (2.6%), hepatotomy and vessel ligation in 50 patients (3.7%), and segmentectomy in 18 patients (1.3%). Formal hepatic lobectomy was performed in only 12 patients (0.9%). Today, packing of the site of bleeding is often successful, followed by later removal of the pack. Packing controls the hemorrhage, and associated injuries, coagulopathy, and hemodynamic status make attempts at direct repair unwise.

If inflow occlusion is unsuccessful, it is presumed that the patient has a retrohepatic inferior vena cava injury, hepatic vein injury, or juxtacaval intraparenchymal hepatic vein injury. In this rare circumstance, atrial-caval shunting may be considered. The liver injury is tightly packed, extended exposure is obtained, and both hepatic vascular inflow and outflow are controlled. Despite this technique, mortality for retrohepatic caval and intraparenchymal hepatic vein injuries exceeds 50%.

STOMACH

Most full-thickness gastric injury is due to penetrating trauma. Gastric rupture secondary to blunt trauma is rare, but vigorous ventilation with an endotracheal tube misplaced in the esophagus can cause iatrogenic gastric rupture in the trauma patient. If there is any reason to suspect a gastric injury, the gastrocolic omentum must be opened widely so that the entire posterior surface of the stomach may be inspected completely. If there is any blood in the gastrohepatic ligament, the lesser curvature of the stomach must be examined closely. Most gastric injuries can be treated simply with débridement and closure in layers.

SMALL INTESTINE

The incidence of small bowel injury approaches 50% for all penetrating abdominal injuries and ranges from 5% to 15% following blunt abdominal trauma. During any laparotomy for trauma, the entire small bowel should be examined meticulously. Abdominal wall entrance and exit wounds cannot be used to predict the likely site of a small bowel injury. Each tear, as it is encountered, should be controlled in order to prevent further leakage and contamination. Simple lacerations of the small bowel are generally sutured with a single layer of interrupted nonabsorbable Lembert sutures after removal of any devitalized tissue. Where damage to the bowel wall is extensive, or where multiple tears are situated fairly close to one another, resection of the involved segment rather than repair of the individual perforations is preferred.

COLON AND RECTUM

Because of a concern for anastomotic breakdown following primary repair, it has long been thought that the safest way of managing most colon injuries is by colostomy. This concept has dominated modern management of colon wounds and can be traced to the surgical experience of World War II, when colostomy was credited with reducing mortality from colonic injury to 37%, down from World War I mortality of 60% for colon injuries treated by primary repair. However, the need for uniform colostomy in civilian colon trauma has been challenged, the premise being that unlike war injuries, most civilian colon wounds are due to low-velocity handguns or stab wounds. As a consequence, many trauma surgeons maintain that more than half of all civilian colon injuries can be treated by primary repair instead of exteriorization or colostomy.

Primary repair is generally applicable only to the stable patient without a history of hypotension, minimal soilage or contamination, intact colon blood supply and minimal colon tissue loss, and few or no associated injuries. In addition, most surgeons treat the various anatomic components of the colon with some unique distinction. There is a general trend to repair *right* colon injuries and *stab* wounds or *low-velocity* gunshot wounds primarily. More significant penetrating injuries and most blunt injuries to the right colon are managed by right colectomy; primary reconstruction via ileotransverse colostomy may be performed in a stable patient in whom there is an isolated injury with no evidence of shock or gross fecal contamination. Otherwise, a right colectomy is accompanied by the creation of an ileostomy and mucous fistula. The same guiding principles for primary repair of minor wounds can be followed for the left colon, although resection with primary anastomosis is generally not recommended owing to the different vascularity, fecal consistency, and bacterial contamination. More extensive left colon injuries are treated by resection with proximal end colostomy and distal mucous fistula or Hartmann's pouch. Stab wounds and low-velocity gunshot wounds of the transverse colon also can be considered for primary repair or exteriorized as loop colostomies.

RECTUM. Primary closure is *not* used *without colostomy* if the wound is full thickness and occurs above the dentate line. Presacral drains and rectal stump washout are employed. For wounds below the dentate line, débridement, repair, and drainage without colon diversion are appropriate.

Abdomen: Retroperitoneal Injuries

DUODENUM

Whereas the diagnosis of penetrating duodenal injuries is generally made during laparotomy immediately following injury, the insidious nature of many blunt duodenal injuries makes the initial diagnosis difficult. This delay may be lethal. One report documents a fourfold increase in mortality (11% versus 40%) if the diagnosis was delayed longer than 24 hours.

Early diagnosis requires a high index of suspicion in patients with appropriate injury mechanisms. Serum amylase determination should be obtained initially and, if elevated, repeated at 6-hour intervals. An early suspicion of retroperitoneal duodenal rupture is best confirmed (or excluded) by a Gastrografin upper gastrointestinal series or abdominal CT scan with oral and intravenous contrast enhancement. Diagnostic peritoneal lavage is unreliable in detecting duodenal injuries, but approximately 40% of patients with duodenal injury have associated intra-abdominal injuries that cause a positive diagnostic peritoneal lavage and subsequent surgical exploration.

Most (80% to 85%) duodenal wounds can be safely repaired primarily. Approximately 15% to 20% require more complex procedures. Protection of a tenuous duodenal repair may be aided by lateral tube duodenostomy or duodenal drainage via a retrograde jejunostomy or by complete diversion of gastric contents away from the duodenum either by a Berne duodenal "diverticulization" (antrectomy and Billroth II gastrojejunostomy) or by "exclusion" of the pylorus and duodenal diversion via a loop gastrojejunostomy.

Duodenal hematomas usually do not require operative intervention. The initial diagnostic Gastrografin examination (CT or upper gastrointestinal study) should be followed by barium to provide greater detail needed to detect the "coiled spring" or "stacked coin" sign. Continuous nasogastric suction should be employed and total parenteral nutrition begun. The patient should be re-evaluated with upper gastrointestinal contrast studies at 5- to 7-day intervals. Operative exploration and evacuation of the hematoma may be considered if resolution has not occurred after 2 weeks of conservative therapy.

PANCREAS

Combined morbidity and mortality of approximately 50% emphasizes the significance of pancreatic injuries. Associated injuries are common because the pancreas is surrounded by major abdominal organs and blood vessels. Concomitant vascular injuries are responsible for half of all pancreatic trauma deaths and nearly all the immediate deaths. Infection is responsible for the majority of the late deaths. The key determinant of long-term outcome is the presence or absence of pancreatic duct injury, since this determines the likelihood of postoperative complications. The implication of these observations is that the first priority in managing pancreatic trauma should be control of hemorrhage and repair of intestinal injuries to limit bacterial contamination. A diligent search for potential pancreatic duct injury should follow.

Preoperative evaluation of patients with penetrating abdominal wounds and possible pancreatic injury is relatively straightforward, since abdominal exploration is generally warranted. The evaluation of patients with blunt injury is more complex. Serum amylase determination has limited sensitivity or specificity for pancreatic injury. In one report, the serum amylase level was elevated in only 16% of patients with penetrating pancreatic injuries and in only 61% of those with blunt pancreatic trauma. Isoamylase differentiation does not increase the test's accuracy. Nonetheless, an elevated serum or peritoneal lavage effluent amylase level raises concern about pancreatic injury and mandates further evaluation by either CT scan or surgical exploration.

At operation, the majority (95%) of pancreatic injuries can be diagnosed by careful inspection following adequate exposure. The remaining 5% of injuries may require more elaborate investigative techniques for diagnosis of ductal injury, such as contrast studies through the biliary tree, ampulla, or tail of the pancreas when there is major concern about the integrity of the main pancreatic duct. The routine performance of intraoperative pancreatography when proximal duct injury is strongly suspected decreased the postoperative morbidity rate from 55% to 15% in the authors' institution.

The principles of managing pancreatic injuries are to control hemorrhage, débride devitalized tissue, provide adequate external drainage of injuries or resections, and preserve as much functional pancreatic tissue as possible. The difficult decisions in managing pancreatic trauma involve patients with parenchymal disruption and major duct injury. In general, distal pancreatic duct injuries are treated by resectional débridement. Proximal duct injuries are treated by a combination of wide drainage, resection, or enteric drainage. A more detailed discussion of the management of pancreatic injuries is provided in the main text.

MAJOR ABDOMINAL VESSELS

The mortality from abdominal vascular trauma ranges from 15% to 80%, highest for aortic wounds, followed by superior mesenteric vessels and iliac vessels, and lowest for vena caval wounds, although suprarenal wounds can be very difficult to repair. One third of abdominal vascular trauma patients present to the emergency room in shock. Rapid control of the injury is therefore the primary management goal, and since most injuries are due to penetrating wounds, immediate triage to the operating room is simplified and must be expedited.

Operative control of major vessel hemorrhage can be chal-

lenging. If active hemorrhage is encountered, it must be controlled immediately, initially by packing. Any retroperitoneal
hematoma should suggest the possibility of associated vascular injury. Specific approaches to individual intra-abdominal
vessels depend on the location of the surrounding hematoma.

Midline suprarenal hemorrhage is perhaps the most difficult
to control, since the aorta, celiac axis, mesenteric vessels, or
vena cava may be responsible. In addition, with the usual
penetrating wound, associated gastric, duodenal, or pancreatic
injuries are likely. Proximal aortic control may be attempted
via direct aortic compression through either the gastrohepatic
ligament or a left anterolateral thoracotomy. Rotation of the
descending colon, spleen, pancreas, and left kidney to the
midline allows complete exposure of the aorta from the hiatus
to the aortic bifurcation. The left diaphragmatic crux may be
divided to provide even more proximal exposure. Suprarenal
vena caval injuries are approached with an extended Kocher
maneuver and retraction of the liver superiorly. Retrohepatic
vena caval injuries (see Liver) are extremely difficult to control
and are generally lethal.

Midline infrarenal hematomas usually can be approached directly through the retroperitoneum or the base of the mesentery, and direct control with vascular clamps can be accomplished. The maneuvers utilized are similar to those used in
the approach to abdominal aortic aneurysms.

Lateral hematomas may be due to renal parenchymal or vascular injury. Preoperative evaluation with "one-shot" intravenous pyelography is often helpful. Following blunt trauma, if
the kidney is well perfused and the hematoma small and
nonexpanding with no urine leak, no further exploration is
required (see Urinary Tract). In penetrating trauma, however,
all lateral hematomas should be explored and the path of
injury meticulously followed. Renal vascular control should
be obtained first before opening Gerota's fascia. This step,
while often unnecessary, appears to decrease the incidence of
nephrectomy.

The approach to *pelvic hematomas* again depends on the
mechanism of injury. A retroperitoneal pelvic hematoma following blunt trauma should *not* be explored (see Pelvic
Injuries). Pelvic bone fixation and angiography with embolization have a role in managing these injuries. Penetrating pelvic
wounds, however, require exploration of the projectile or stab
pathway. Injuries to the common or external iliac artery
should be repaired, if at all possible. In contrast, injuries to
the internal iliac artery can be ligated with impunity, even if
they occur bilaterally.

URINARY TRACT

There is no degree of hematuria that is diagnostic of major
urinary tract injury, and the absence of hematuria does not
exclude significant injury. Therefore, a key principle to be
applied in diagnosing urologic trauma is to suspect injury by
assessing the mechanism and forces involved. Signs of a lower
urinary tract injury include blood at the urinary meatus, a
"high riding" or misplaced prostate that cannot be palpated

on rectal examination, urinary retention, bladder distention, or the desire to void but an inability to empty the bladder. In the presence of these signs, a retrograde urethrogram is indicated before attempts at inserting a Foley catheter. The presence of pelvic crush injury also suggests the need to obtain a retrograde cystourethrogram for evaluation of bladder or urethral injury, even in the absence of blood at the meatus.

Specific signs of upper urologic tract injury include either gross or microscopic hematuria. If upper urinary tract injury is suspected, the initial evaluation depends in part on the patient's associated injuries and hemodynamic stability. If the patient requires emergent surgical therapy for associated injuries, a limited "one-shot" intravenous pyelogram may be obtained in the emergency room or on the operating room table by the rapid intravenous injections of 60 ml. of high-density contrast medium followed by a flat-plate radiograph of the abdomen and pelvis in 1 to 5 minutes. This study generally identifies the presence or absence of functioning kidneys but is an extremely limited study that may falsely fail to identify a renal outline in the presence of shock. In the hemodynamically stable patient, either intravenous pyelography or CT with intravenous contrast is an effective method of evaluating the urinary tract, although CT scans provide more detailed information about both the urologic injury and the potential associated intra-abdominal and retroperitoneal injuries. The degree of renal parenchymal injury identified on CT scans is also useful in classifying the injury and defining management plan. Demonstration by either CT scan or intravenous pyelography of the apparent presence of a solitary kidney or a lack of function of a segment of the kidney is an indication for immediate arteriography.

Pelvic Injuries

Pelvic fractures are the third most common injury sustained in motor vehicle accidents. The majority require straightforward skeletal management, but approximately 20% are complex crush injuries and open pelvic fractures with mortality in excess of 50%.

Examination begins by administering the anteroposterior and lateral compression for assessment of instability and pain. A rectal and vaginal examination must be performed to assess blood, fragments, mucosal lacerations, and prostate location in the male. Blood at the urethral meatus requires retrograde urethrocystography before insertion of a Foley catheter. The initial radiographic examination should include an anteroposterior plain film of the pelvis. More select views, including CT, may be indicated as time and the patient's condition allow but must not take precedence over the search for associated injuries.

The management objectives in a patient with a pelvic fracture are control of hemorrhage, skeletal fixation, and treatment of associated injuries. Massive blood loss (up to 20 units) can occur into the retroperitoneal space from arterial or venous injuries or the fracture line itself. Extensive collateralization, difficult exposure, and release of the tamponade effect of the posterior peritoneum make surgical exploration of pelvic hematomas generally frustrating and fruitless. Application of the pneumatic antishock garment may be beneficial as a temporizing agent, pending either immediate skeletal fixation or angiographic evaluation and embolization. If pelvic hematoma-related blood requirements exceed 4 to 6 units, either angiographic intervention or emergent skeletal fixation may be indicated. There currently exist no comparative data for determining which method or approach is superior, nor are there exact indications for their use.

Approximately 25% of pelvic fracture victims have associated intra-abdominal injury. Diagnostic peritoneal lavage should be performed in the supraumbilical location, since false-positive rates range from 16% to 50% if it is performed in the standard infraumbilical location. A grossly positive peritoneal lavage is generally an indication for immediate exploratory celiotomy. Computed tomography is an alternative diagnostic modality in the hemodynamically stable patient.

Central Nervous System Injuries

CRANIUM AND BRAIN

The two guiding principles of initial care are (1) *assessment of injury severity* and (2) *protection of the brain from further injury* until definitive diagnosis and therapy can be achieved. The treatment plan depends on identifying the two fundamental head injuries: focal or diffuse. Focal injuries consist of mass lesions that cause neurologic dysfunction, largely by brain compression, and often require surgical evacuation. Diffuse brain injuries are equally frequent and cause prolonged coma without intracranial masses. These do not require surgical therapy but can be as devastating as focal injuries.

ASSESSMENT OF INJURY SEVERITY. The severity of brain injury can be estimated in less than 1 minute by evaluating three factors: *level of consciousness, pupillary function,* and *lateralized weakness* of the extremities.

Level of consciousness is best assessed by the Glasgow Coma Scale (GCS), a system that evaluates eye opening, best motor response, and verbal response. *Pupillary function* is assessed by the size, equality, and response to bright light. Whether or not there has been ocular injury, any pupillary asymmetry greater than 1 mm. must be attributed to intracranial injury unless proved otherwise. With few exceptions, the largest pupil is on the side of the mass lesion. The *lateralized extremity weakness* is detected by testing motor power in patients able to cooperate or by observing symmetry of movement in response to painful stimulus. As the severity of injury increases, lateralized weakness is more difficult to recognize, and small differences may be important.

The presence of any of the following criteria suggests serious injury: (1) a GCS score of less than 10, (2) a decrease in the GCS score by 3 or more regardless of the initial GCS score,

(3) pupillary inequality greater than 1 mm. regardless of the GCS score, (4) lateralized extremity weakness regardless of the GCS score, (5) markedly depressed skull fractures, and (6) open cranial wounds with brain exposed.

PROTECTION FROM FURTHER INSULT. Delivering adequate oxygen to the brain is the primary goal in preventing further injury. Arterial oxygen content must be optimized. This often involves intubation, oxygen supplementation, and mechanical ventilation. If urgent intubation is required, paralytic agents, pharyngeal anesthesia, and barbiturate induction limit the massive elevation of intracranial pressure (ICP) that may occur. Brain injury *per se rarely* causes hypotension during the early period following trauma, but the brain is extremely susceptible to hypoxia and inadequate perfusion. Cerebral perfusion pressure (MAP − ICP) greater than 40 mm. Hg must be maintained by appropriate fluid and blood replacement while volume overload is avoided.

Even after relatively short periods of ischemia, the brain may respond to reperfusion in a pathologic manner with prompt and severe brain swelling and marked increases in ICP. Elevated ICP can best be managed in the early phases of injury by controlled hyperventilation to PCO_2 values in the low-mid 20s. Decreasing brain water with diuretics or hyperosmotic agents also may be helpful.

DEFINITIVE CARE. Definitive care begins with a definitive diagnosis, which is established exclusively by computed tomography. Cranial CT has a high priority in the evaluation of a patient with an altered level of consciousness or lateralizing neurologic signs. It should be performed as soon as cardio-respiratory stability has been achieved and a lateral cervical spine roentgenogram demonstrates no fracture or dislocation. Seriously injured patients who are intubated should receive neuromuscular blockage during the study. A good-quality CT scan identifies focal mass lesions and allows the diagnosis of diffuse brain injury. *Focal injuries* with significant mass effect require surgical evacuation; patients with these injuries go directly to the operating room.

Patients with *diffuse brain injury* are managed in the intensive care unit. Monitoring devices for ICP are placed for on-line management of intracranial hypertension in both groups. Principal treatment efforts are directed toward controlling intracranial hypertension, providing adequate cerebral oxygenation, and preventing infectious complications of prolonged coma. Although both barbiturates and glucocorticoids have been advocated in the management of severe head injury, recent clinical evidence does not support their use.

VERTEBRAE AND SPINAL CORD

All patients with blunt trauma must be treated initially as if they have a spinal cord injury. Proper care of the potentially unstable spine begins at the scene of injury with proper immobilization of the head, neck, and spine on a backboard and continues until the spine has been proved stable. Careful follow-up examinations must be made during a traumatized patient's hospitalization if there are complaints of pain in the back or neck; if weakness, numbness, or loss of control of extremities or sphincters develops; or if only screening radiographs were obtained during admission evaluation.

The history and physical examination should specifically assess the presence of any spinal column pain or transient neurologic abnormalities. If a neurologic deficit is present, the examination focuses on defining the neurologic level of injury and on determining whether there is sparing of some spinal cord function across this level. A patient with a complete spinal cord injury has no distal motor or sensory function. Most incomplete spinal cord injuries exhibit mixed motor and sensory sparing rather than a classic pattern of partial injury. Sacral sparing may be the only evidence that paralysis may not be complete. The natural history of incomplete cord injuries is improvement. If deterioration is observed, emergency diagnostic and surgical treatment may be warranted. Since changes in the neurologic examination are so crucial, it is essential that neurologic function be recorded accurately in the prehospital and emergency room notes to allow later comparison.

Good-quality roentgenograms are essential and must be accomplished before moving the neck of all blunt trauma patients, particularly those who are unconscious, obtunded, or complaining of neck pain. The initial screening view is a cross-table lateral of the supine patient. Formal anteroposterior, lateral, and odontoid views should be obtained before the cervical spine is "cleared," but flexion and extension radiograms are rarely indicated and only if the patient is conscious and cooperative. Computed tomography and magnetic resonance imaging have a role in defining in greater detail the spinal cord and bony column injury in the hemodynamically stable patient.

Neck Injuries

The neck is classically divided into anatomic triangles. Penetrating wounds that enter through the anterior triangle or sternocleidomastoid muscle have a high likelihood of significant vascular, airway, or esophageal injury. In contrast, wounds to the posterior triangle rarely involve the esophagus, airway, or major vascular structures, although, if they are directed inferiorly, intrathoracic injury can occur. The other major anatomic landmark in the neck is the platysma muscle. Wounds that fail to penetrate the platysma are considered superficial and do not warrant extensive evaluation. Wounds that penetrate the platysma mandate hospital admission and either immediate operative exploration or further diagnostic evaluation.

The anterior neck is further divided into three zones defined by horizontal planes. Zone I injuries (low neck) have the highest mortality because of the risk of major vascular and intrathoracic injury. Zone II injuries (midneck) are the most common but have the lowest mortality. Significant injury is generally apparent, and exposure of vital structures is readily accomplished. Zone III wounds (high neck) risk injury to the distal carotid artery, salivary glands, and pharynx. Operative exposure can be particularly difficult.

Nearly all patients with platysma-penetrating wounds and clinical signs of vascular, airway, or esophageal injury (shock, hemorrhage, expanding hematoma, hemoptysis, hematemesis, subcutaneous emphysema, others) require prompt operative exploration. Patients with "clinically silent" platysma-penetrating wounds should at least be admitted to the hospital. At Harborview Medical Center in Seattle, the authors continue to explore the majority of neck wounds that penetrate the platysma. More specifically, injuries to the base of the skull and thoracic outlet (Zone III and Zone I) require angiography before, and occasionally in lieu of, exploration. Injuries to the midneck (Zone II) are generally managed by exploration without prior invasive diagnostic studies.

The signs of neck injury following blunt trauma can be subtle, but the consequences of an overlooked injury can be devastating. A neurologic deficit unexplained by head CT findings in a patient with blunt neck trauma mandates four-vessel angiography. Hoarseness, dysphagia, hemoptysis, or hematemesis in such victims portends airway and/or esophageal injury. Patency of the airway must be ensured. Panendoscopy and esophagography should be employed liberally. Computed tomography can be extremely helpful in delineating laryngeal injuries.

Maxillofacial Injuries

While preserving sight and speech and minimizing deformity are important goals, they occupy a relatively low priority in the care of the multiply injured patient. Rather, it is a fact that maxillofacial trauma is frequently associated with upper airway compromise and difficult hemorrhage that mandate attention in the initial resuscitation of the trauma victim. Definitive airway control can be difficult in the presence of facial injuries, and the physician always must be prepared and equipped to perform emergency tracheostomy.

Severe hemorrhage in conjunction with a facial fracture can be a particularly vexing problem. Hemorrhage typically occurs from the nasal or oral cavity and usually can be controlled by fracture reduction combined with anterior and posterior nasopharyngeal packing. Substantial hemorrhage in a patient with severe midface fractures that is not controlled by these techniques should arouse suspicion of laceration of one or both internal maxillary arteries or basilar skull fracture with internal carotid artery involvement. If these maneuvers fail to control hemorrhage, immediate angiographic evaluation and embolization are indicated and generally preferred over operative attempts at external carotid artery or selective branch ligation.

The initial examination of the patient includes palpation of all external facial features, evaluation of ocular muscle activity, and visual acuity examination. A gloved hand should be used to intraorally assess maxillary stability, dentition, and the mandibular contour. However, the diagnosis of maxillofacial trauma has been revolutionized by CT. The accuracy of CT scanning is unsurpassed when compared with plain radiographs or tomography, particularly in the evaluation of certain soft tissue injuries and injuries to the paranasal sinuses, orbits, and mandibular condylar heads. This information can be extremely useful to the surgeon in directing a treatment plan. The management of specific maxillofacial injuries is discussed in greater detail in the main text.

Extremity and Peripheral Vascular Injuries

The management of most musculoskeletal injuries is discussed in other sections of this text. The following section highlights three key areas of trauma care involving the extremities: early fracture stabilization, soft tissue injury, and vascular trauma.

EARLY FRACTURE STABILIZATION

Hemorrhage due to massive disruption or transection of major blood vessels constitutes the only situation in which extremity injuries are immediately life-threatening. However, multiple long bone fractures have been recognized recently to have a strikingly adverse impact on survival following injury. Although specific treatment of fractures is not addressed in this chapter, the crucial role of early fracture fixation in the care of the multiply injured victim cannot be overlooked. Early fixation of long bone fractures decreases the incidence of adult respiratory distress syndrome, fat embolization syndrome, and subsequent development of sepsis and multiple organ failure. The exact mechanism of this beneficial effect remains unknown but appears to be related to the *early* fracture stabilization with subsequent diminished inflammatory response and an ability to rapidly mobilize the patient and begin early feedings. Early discharge of the patient from the intensive care unit undoubtedly has additive beneficial effects.

SOFT TISSUE INJURIES

The principles of management of soft tissue injuries are débridement of devitalized tissue, restoration of adequate blood supply, and adequate coverage of vital structures including nerves, blood vessels, tendons, and other soft tissues subject to desiccation. All lacerations and penetrating injuries of the extremities should be cleansed and meticulously débrided. No maneuver contributes as much to the prevention of tetanus or gas gangrene infection as *complete débridement of all devitalized tissue*. Patients with tetanus-prone wounds should be evaluated for immunization status and treated accordingly (see main text). Re-exploration under anesthesia generally should be planned within the next 24 hours, particularly if there is any question regarding the viability of residual tissues. Rapidly spreading cellulitis, crepitus, erythema, and unexplained pain in an extremity are indications for immediate surgical exploration and débridement.

Restoration of blood supply to an injured extremity receives high priority, since as little as a few hours of ischemia may cause tissue necrosis and subsequent amputation. The classic signs of vascular compromise include *pain, pallor,* and *pulselessness,* although more subtle findings such as delayed capillary refill and venous congestion are signs of vascular compromise that jeopardize healing of soft tissue wounds and invite secondary infection.

Adequate soft tissue coverage of exposed vital structures is essential for preventing desiccation, secondary infection, and vascular suture disruption. Although primary closure of native soft tissue is ideal, this is often impossible owing to the presence of contaminated or ischemic tissue, infection, or large-area soft tissue defects. Early closure with auto-, allo-, or xenografts of skin can provide temporary coverage pending more elaborate soft tissue reconstructive maneuvers such as free muscle flaps or combined muscle and skin rotational flaps.

PERIPHERAL VASCULAR INJURIES

Penetration, perforation, transection, and lateral lacerations are the usual forms of injury among patients with penetrating wounds, whereas fracture of the intima with obstruction and thrombosis is the usual type of arterial injury following blunt trauma. Both mechanisms also may induce significant arterial spasm in the vicinity of the injury that diminishes extremity blood flow, but which will improve spontaneously. Because of the possibility of hidden lacerations or the delayed development of aneurysm or arteriovenous fistulas, injuries *near* all major blood vessels should be explored thoroughly or otherwise evaluated. Whereas some authors have advocated only observation of wounds in proximity to blood vessels without major signs of vascular injury, these very reports contain case studies of delayed diagnoses and overlooked injuries. Although this particular issue remains controversial, current consensus favors angiographic or noninvasive (Doppler ultrasonography) evaluation for wounds in proximity to major vessels.

Preoperative angiography is generally helpful in order to plan the operative approach and ascertain the extent of damage, especially if blunt trauma or multiple vascular injuries are involved. It is of less benefit in penetrating trauma with obvious vascular injury. An unstable patient should not undergo angiography. Spontaneous cessation of bleeding is often only temporary, and the sudden recurrence of severe hemorrhage is likely.

Vascular injuries are often associated with long bone fractures in the distal part of the leg. In particular, fracture dislocation at the level of the knee is often associated with combined popliteal artery and vein injury, and arteriography should be routinely considered with a "free floating" or posterior knee dislocation. Popliteal vascular trauma is particularly devastating, causing amputation more often than any other arterial injury. Complex combined vascular and orthopedic injuries demand coordination of operative approach and often require temporary vascular conduits while bony repair is performed.

The principles of operative treatment of vascular injuries of the extremity are identical to those described elsewhere for elective vascular repair. However, fasciotomy is used perhaps more often in the trauma setting and is usually necessary when there are combined popliteal artery and vein injuries, when the patient has extensive bony and muscular injury, or following prolonged shock or several hours of extremity ischemia time. Current techniques allow routine and frequent measurements of compartment pressures and accurately indicate those patients who require fasciotomy. The authors favor a double-incision, four-compartment fasciotomy with full incision of the skin.

Whether venous injuries are best treated by repair or by ligation is still controversial. Data compiled by the Vietnam Vascular Registry revealed a significant reduction in the morbid sequelae of lower extremity venous injuries treated by repair instead of ligation, especially when associated arterial injuries were present. Civilian trauma experience supports this observation, and most trauma surgeons perform simple venorrhaphy repair of major (unpaired) venous lacerations in the stable patient. However, the incidence of post-repair thrombosis following more complex repairs is high, and the extra time required may be ill-advised in the multiply injured or unstable patient. If ligation is performed, prolonged postoperative elevation and elastic extremity wrapping reduce edema and decrease late morbidity.

18

SURGICAL COMPLICATIONS

A. R. Moossa, M.D., Marquis E. Hart, M.D.,
and David W. Easter, M.D.

Any deviation from normal recovery and return to regular function is a postoperative complication. Some complications may be unavoidable; others are preventable by careful preoperative anticipation and advice (cessation of smoking, correction of obesity, respiratory exercise, meticulous surgical technique intraoperatively, and early correction of abnormalities postoperatively).

POSTOPERATIVE FEVER AND INFECTION

Fever is a common response to an operation observed in nearly half of patients following major procedures. No infection is found in 80%, and pyrexia resolves spontaneously within a few days. A careful clinical examination is essential initially with attention to the timing and pattern of the fever.

INFECTIOUS CAUSES OF PYREXIA. Most infections follow intraoperative contamination at the operative site via airways during general anesthesia or from cannulas and catheters. Hospital-acquired pathogens are often involved and are difficult to treat because of antibiotic resistance. Local factors predisposing to infection include ischemia, devitalized and necrotic tissues, hematoma formation, and the presence of foreign bodies. These provide an ideal environment for bacteria by protecting them from host defenses. Systemic factors include neonates, the elderly, diabetes mellitus, hepatic disease, disseminated malignancy, malnutrition, obesity, and drugs (i.e., steroids, alcohol, chemotherapeutic agents). Clinical manifestations include signs of a local inflammatory response (heat, pain, redness, mass). Systemic manifestations are chills, rigors, and elevated core body temperature. Fever beginning within 24 hours suggests atelectasis and urinary tract or wound infections. Abscesses usually become evident in the second week, with recurrent spiking pyrexia. Intravenous and urinary catheters should be examined. Pulmonary infections are common, since atelectasis often follows general anesthesia, aspiration, or the use of contaminated ventilation equipment. Patients who smoke and those with nasogastric tubes are more at risk. Urinary tract infections are associated with indwelling catheters, bladder outflow obstruction, and anorectal operations. Cellulitis and phlebitis, lymphangitis, and regional lymphadenopathy may be seen with infected venous cannulas. Central line sepsis is more occult and requires cultures of blood or the catheter tip.

See the corresponding chapter or part in the *Textbook of Surgery,* 15th edition, pp. 341–359, for a more detailed discussion of this topic, including a comprehensive list of references.

NONINFECTIOUS PYREXIA. Postoperative fever may be a manifestation of disseminated malignancy, reaction to drugs or blood transfusion, formation of a hematoma, or inflammation around an intravenous catheter after administration of irritant fluids or drugs. Deep venous thrombosis may manifest as mild pyrexia after the fifth day. Acute pancreatitis after upper abdominal surgery, especially in mild cases, may not be evident from the amylase or lipase levels, and a computed tomographic scan may be required for diagnosis. Supportive care is usually adequate. Some conditions may be precipitated by surgical stress. Thyroid storm and pheochromocytoma are life-threatening. Beta blockade and antithyroid therapy have to be instituted in the former, and both alpha and beta blockade along with nitroprusside for control of hypertension and catecholamine release are needed in the latter. Malignant hyperthermia manifests with fever, tachycardia, rigidity, skin mottling, and cyanosis in the susceptible individual shortly after induction of anesthesia, and is treated with dantrolene, bicarbonate, insulin, and active cooling of the patient; mortality is 30%.

MISCELLANEOUS CAUSES

Thrombophlebitis. Usually a noninfective, inflammatory reaction at the site of the intravenous cannula, thrombophlebitis is a common cause of fever after the third postoperative day. Occasionally, bacterial infection with suppurative phlebitis ensues, which requires excision of the vein.

Postoperative Parotitis. This complication is observed in the elderly and debilitated. Malignancy, dehydration, and poor oral hygiene are predisposing factors. The infection is usually staphylococcal and occurs within 2 weeks of operation. The parotid gland is swollen and tender, and a drop of pus may be seen at the intraoral opening of Stensen's duct. Cultures should be obtained and the appropriate antibiotic instituted. Incision and drainage may become necessary, care being taken to avoid facial nerve damage.

WOUND COMPLICATIONS

HEMATOMA. The formation of hematoma is due to the collection of blood in the wound, usually owing to imperfect hemostasis. Aspirin and low-dose heparin may increase risk slightly. Patients on anticoagulants or with coagulopathy have a higher risk. Hypotension at operation and hypertension postoperatively may contribute to wound hematoma formation. On examination, a fluctuant, discolored swelling in the wound is found. Small hematomas may resorb, but they increase the incidence of wound infection. Larger hematomas should be evacuated and any bleeding vessel ligated with wound closure. Neck hematomas are dangerous because they may expand rapidly and compress the trachea.

SEROMA. Seroma is a collection of fluid other than blood or pus. This usually follows liquefaction necrosis of fat or interruption of lymphatics (i.e., mastectomy, nodal dissection, groin operations). Treatment is aspiration and compression.

WOUND INFECTION. A collection of pus in the wound

signifies infection. It may be primary or secondary to a hematoma or seroma. Treatment is incision and drainage. Skin sutures or staples must be removed along with any necrotic tissue. Irrigation, packing, and covering have the same efficacy provided free drainage is achieved.

WOUND FAILURE. A partial or total disruption of any or all layers of the wound indicates wound failure. It may be early (wound dehiscence) or late (incisional hernia). Chest wounds rarely dehisce; if they do, it is usually following median sternotomy. Laparotomy wounds have a 1% incidence of "burst abdomen" with a 20% mortality; it is largely preventable by secure mechanical closure of the wound. Infection is a major local factor. Predisposing systemic factors include sepsis, uremia, malnutrition, diabetes, liver failure, and corticosteroid therapy. Serosanguineous fluid discharge from the wound is a pathognomonic sign. Sudden evisceration following an episode of coughing or retching may be the presentation. Management begins with reassurance, analgesia, covering the wound with moist sterile towels, and surgical repair under general anesthesia with nonabsorbable, interrupted, nonreactive sutures employing healthy tissues and deep bites.

RESPIRATORY COMPLICATIONS

ATELECTASIS. Atelectasis is the most common complication following general anesthesia. It denotes loss of patency and collapse of small airways and alveoli. Stasis in the airways with accumulation of secretions predisposes to infection, especially at the lung bases. Clinical signs include rales, diminished breath sounds, and bronchial breathing accompanied by rapid pulse and fever with radiologic evidence of consolidation due to associated pneumonia. Cessation of smoking, avoidance of prolonged anesthesia, and physiotherapy in the bronchitic patient are important preventive measures. Postoperatively, management is rigorous physiotherapy, postural drainage, suction (via endotracheal tube, mini-tracheostomy, bronchoscopy), nebulized bronchodilators, mucolytic agents, and antibiotics as deemed necessary. Assisted mechanical ventilation may be required. Analgesia is important.

ASPIRATION PNEUMONITIS. Aspiration of the sterile acid contents of the stomach produces a chemical burn of the airway. The presence of food particles adds insult by encouraging an intense inflammatory reaction as well as blockage of distal airways by larger particles. Clinically the patient is dyspneic and cyanosed soon after the aspiration, with chest radiographs revealing interstitial pulmonary edema. Arterial blood gases show hypoxemia and hypercarbia. Rapid deterioration to respiratory failure may occur.

ASPIRATION PNEUMONIA. The oropharynx contains bacteria, primarily anaerobes. Aspiration of the contents of the oropharynx is a common cause of pneumonia. Aspiration pneumonia may progress to pulmonary abscess, which is characterized by foul-smelling sputum and a fluid level in a cavity on chest film.

PULMONARY EDEMA. Pulmonary edema presents as orthopnea, hypoxia, and elevated jugular venous pulse. Confirmation is by clinical examination and chest film. Treatment is by upright positioning of the patient, oxygen administration, and restriction of intravenous fluids. An electrocardiogram is important for outlining any cardiac causes (infarction, arrhythmias). Drugs include diuretics, digoxin, and morphine. Mechanical ventilation and phlebotomy may be indicated.

IMMEDIATE POSTOPERATIVE RESPIRATORY DEPRESSION. This usually is due to narcotic agents and/or muscle relaxants used in anesthesia. It should be recognized and treated accordingly. Other conditions that may present similarly are aspiration, laryngeal edema, massive atelectasis, pneumothorax, and hypothermia. These may be exacerbated by mechanical ventilation and thus should be excluded.

ACUTE RESPIRATORY FAILURE. Respiratory failure is the inability to maintain adequate gas exchange in the lungs. In practical terms, it is PaO_2 less than 60 mm. Hg or $PaCO_2$ more than 60 mm. Hg (in the absence of metabolic alkalosis) on breathing room air. It may have an insidious onset with increasing respiratory rate and effort. Management is geared toward increasing oxygenation and reducing the work of breathing. It includes intermittent mandatory ventilation, which provides ventilatory support; positive end-expiratory pressure for reinflating the collapsed alveoli; or a combination of both. Continuous positive airway pressure may be an alternative to positive end-expiratory pressure in patients who require intervention for hypoxemia without hypercarbia or ventilatory insufficiency.

SHOCK

Acute circulatory failure, commonly termed *shock*, is a well-known surgical complication. Hypotension is the usual presenting feature of all types of shock. Occasionally, low blood pressure could be due to vasovagal reflex or orthostatic changes. Shock can be classified into three categories according to the etiology: (1) hypovolemic, (2) cardiogenic, and (3) septic. Hypovolemic shock is due to a fall in circulating blood volume and is the most frequent cause of postoperative shock. Cardiogenic shock is usually secondary to myocardial ischemia or infarction, arrhythmias, cardiac tamponade, pulmonary embolism, adrenal insufficiency, myocardial depression (as in sepsis), and fluid overload especially in the elderly with pre-existing myocardial disease. Septic shock occurs when infection from gram-negative or gram-positive organisms or a fungus produces septicemia. Clinically, this may present as either warm shock or cold shock. The final common pathway in shock is inadequate tissue perfusion for meeting metabolic demands. Any form of shock must be recognized and treated early before irreversible multiorgan damage ensues.

RENAL FAILURE

Acute renal failure must be considered in any patient with oliguria after an operation. When the hourly urinary output is less than 0.5 ml. per kg. per hour (35 ml. per hour for a 70-kg. man), renal failure is secondary to prerenal, renal, or postrenal causes. Prerenal failure implies an inadequate renal blood flow and usually is a direct result of diminished circulating blood volume. Acute parenchymal renal failure is caused by obstruction of the urinary tract and usually presents as anuria. It is important to exclude bladder outflow obstruction in such patients. Proper assessment of the patient and identification of the cause of renal failure are mandatory in management. An intravenous fluid challenge is usually helpful in evaluating the etiologic factor. Patients at risk may require a central venous or pulmonary artery catheter prior to administration of intravenous fluids. If urinary output remains low but blood volume is normal, an intravenous infusion of mannitol 25 gm., furosemide 25 mg. over 20 minutes, or a low-dose infusion of dopamine (2 to 5 mg. per kg. per min.) may be considered. The use of diuretics is controversial.

Lack of response to the measures outlined suggests acute or postrenal failure. At this stage, the possibility of postrenal failure must be excluded especially in patients following operations involving a retroperitoneal or pelvic dissection. This usually involves an imaging procedure such as intravenous pyelography, cystoscopic retrograde pyelography or technetium-labeled diethylene tetramine pentaacetic acid (DTPA) scan. When renal failure is established, an acute renal failure regimen is instituted. This involves close attention to fluid balance, hemofiltration or dialysis, or peritoneal dialysis.

DEEP VEIN THROMBOSIS AND PULMONARY EMBOLISM

Thrombosis of lower limb and pelvic veins is an important cause of morbidity, both because of its frequency and because of the potentially fatal consequences related to pulmonary embolism.

Clinically, the classic features of deep vein thrombosis are calf swelling, tenderness, elevated temperature, and a positive Homans' sign. These may be absent, and the first manifestation may be a fatal pulmonary embolus. The risk factors include obesity, old age, oral contraception, malignancy, trauma, immobility, and certain specific surgical procedures involving the prostate, hip joint, and pelvis. Venography is the standard among diagnostic investigations, others being Doppler ultrasonography, ^{125}I-fibrinogen studies, and plethysmography. Prophylactic measures directed to prevention of deep vein thrombosis and pulmonary embolism may be divided into mechanical devices that prevent venous pooling and stasis and drugs that inhibit blood coagulation. Pneumatic calf compression is the only mechanical measure with proven efficacy. The use of various pharmacologic agents remains controversial. The most studied and frequently used method is a subcutaneous heparin regimen of 5000 units preoperatively and every 12 hours thereafter until the patient is mobile. It is doubtful whether these measures reduce the incidence of pulmonary embolism.

ALIMENTARY TRACT DYSFUNCTION

In the postoperative period, the normal propulsive activity of the gastrointestinal tract is temporarily depressed. The term *paralytic ileus* is a misnomer because small bowel motility rapidly returns.

Complications involving the alimentary tract include acute gastric dilation, gastroduodenal mucosal hemorrhage, intestinal obstruction, fecal impaction, colitis, anastomotic leak, and dysfunctions of the hepatobiliary-pancreatic system. Patients with acute dilation of the stomach usually present with severe pain and dyspnea, although sometimes it is insidious in nature. Treatment consists of gastric decompression with a nasogastric tube and fluid replacement. Gastroduodenal mucosal hemorrhage is a well-recognized complication in severely ill and septic postoperative patients. Histamine-receptor antagonists are recommended both as a prophylactic measure and for definitive therapy. Under extreme situations, an operation may be required. Intestinal obstruction may be the result of paralytic ileus or mechanical obstruction. Acute colonic pseudo-obstruction is a localized form of paralytic ileus affecting the large bowel. Mechanical obstruction is most often caused by postoperative adhesions or an internal hernia. The initial treatment is conservative, but if the obstruction persists or increasing abdominal signs develop, laparotomy should be performed. Fecal impaction is treated with laxatives and enema; occasionally, manual evacuation under general anesthesia is necessary. Postoperative diarrhea is occasionally due to *Shigella, Salmonella*, or *Campylobacter*. Patients treated with antibiotics are at risk of bacterial overgrowth with resistant staphylococci and occasionally a more serious condition termed pseudomembranous colitis. This is associated with *Clostridium difficile*, an anaerobic bacterium that releases a toxin.

Anastomotic leakage is usually a technical complication. The successful outcome of an anastomosis depends on many factors including good blood supply, impermeable mechanical apposition of serosa to serosa, avoidance of tension on the anastomotic line, and avoidance of gross contamination. Colonic anastomoses are more prone to leak. Pericolic abscess and enterocutaneous fistula may follow a leak. More seriously, a diffuse peritonitis may result, and it requires rapid resuscitation with intravenous fluids and nasogastric aspiration followed by laparotomy.

The incidence of hepatobiliary complications is greatest after operations on the liver, biliary tract, and pancreas, but they may occur after any operation involving general anesthesia. Anesthetic agents, particularly halothane, have been implicated as a cause of potentially fatal postoperative hepatitis, especially after re-exposure to the same agent. Extrahepatic obstruction is caused by direct surgical injury to the bile ducts, retained common bile duct stones, tumors, or pancreatitis.

NEUROLOGIC AND PSYCHOLOGICAL COMPLICATIONS

Operations on the brain or spinal cord and spinal or epidural anesthesia are associated with occasional focal lesions.

Septic emboli may cause a brain abscess. Peripheral nerves may be damaged during operative procedures. Stroke occurs in 1% to 3% of patients after carotid endarterectomy or other reconstructive operations on the extracranial portion of the carotid system. Cerebral injuries are capable of producing convulsions. Epilepsy or metabolic derangements also may cause convulsions in the postoperative period.

Anxiety and fear are normal in patients who undergo surgical procedures. Confusion is common in the elderly, and sleep deprivation, which is especially common in patients in intensive care units, may cause disorientation and hallucinations. Patients requiring a stoma, mastectomy, or amputation may perceive an alteration in body image. Postoperative psychosis occurs in approximately 0.2% of cases but is much higher following open heart surgery. Postoperative delirium could be due to factors such as drug dependency, dementia, brain lesions, or metabolic abnormalities including uremia and hepatic insufficiency.

19

ACUTE RENAL FAILURE IN SURGICAL PATIENTS:
Prevention and Treatment

R. Randal Bollinger, MD., Ph.D.,
and Steve J. Schwab, M.D.

Acute renal failure (ARF) is a potentially lethal complication
in the surgical patient. Despite recent advances in dialysis and
intensive care support, almost half the patients who develop
ARF in the postoperative period die. The severity of the
trauma, the magnitude of the surgical procedure, the gravity
of underlying medical conditions that predispose to ARF, and
the high incidence of sepsis all contribute to multiorgan failure
with high mortality. Prompt and effective treatment of each
component of the multifaceted etiology of ARF can prevent
the syndrome and offers the surgical patient the best likelihood of survival.

Acute renal failure is defined as an abrupt decline in renal
function sufficient to cause retention of nitrogenous waste.
This definition of ARF does not depend on the urinary output
of the patient. The emphasis is on the quality of the urine
rather than on the quantity, since nonoliguric forms of ARF
occur quite frequently. Whether or not oliguria is present, a
progressive rise in blood urea nitrogen and serum creatinine
concentration in the posttrauma or postoperative period
should suggest ARF.

CLASSIFICATION

When renal failure occurs abruptly, *acute* renal failure is
present. When the azotemia develops gradually over many
weeks or months, the renal failure is termed *chronic*. If a
patient in renal failure presents with asymptomatic azotemia,
the differentiation of acute from chronic disease may be difficult. Several aspects of the history and radiologic examination,
particularly the presence of small, "end-stage" kidneys, provide the correct classification of the patient's disease. Renal
failure is termed *oliguric* if less than 400 ml. of urine is produced in 24 hours. Patients with *nonoliguric* renal failure produce large volumes of isosthenuric urine but are unable to
clear nitrogenous wastes.

Acute renal failure is conveniently classified according to
its cause as prerenal, renal, or postrenal. Each of these may
present in either the oliguric or nonoliguric form, and all
are associated with a rising blood urea nitrogen and serum
creatinine. The difficult problem posed by surgical patients is
to distinguish a normal kidney that is attempting to correct
an abnormal internal environment (prerenal failure) from a

See the corresponding chapter or part in the *Textbook of Surgery*, 15th
edition, pp. 360–381, for a more detailed discussion of this topic,
including a comprehensive list of references.

kidney that is no longer able to maintain the internal environment (renal failure).

Acute renal failure is initiated most commonly by a critical underperfusion of the kidneys with consequent intense arteriolar vasoconstriction with resulting ischemic tubular injury. In other circumstances, direct tubular cell damage is sustained from a toxin such as aminoglycoside or amphotericin. Myoglobin or hemoglobin pigment may cause direct tubular injury with intratubular obstruction when proteins coagulate. Iodinated contrast material and nonsteroidal anti-inflammatory drugs may be cellular toxins but are also powerful mediators of intrarenal vasoconstriction. When tubular damage is sustained, a number of factors converge to maintain the renal failure. These include backleak of filtrate across disrupted tubular barriers, intraluminal obstruction from cell swelling and sloughing, persistent vasoconstriction that serves to perpetuate cellular ischemia, and changes in glomerular capillary membrane permeability. Even in apparently intact renal tubular cells, the intracellular metabolism that supports the transport functions of the cell is severely disturbed from hypoxia, free oxygen radical accumulation, and high levels of free ionized cytoplasmic calcium. The result is failure in the homeostatic maintenance of the extracellular fluid and failure to excrete accumulating toxic metabolic wastes. Biochemical alterations in acute renal failure include retention of nitrogenous wastes, metabolic acidosis, hyperkalemia, hyponatremia, hyperphosphatemia, hypocalcemia, and hypermagnesemia.

CONDITIONS THAT PREDISPOSE TO ACUTE RENAL FAILURE

ARF is a frequent complication of surgical procedures. The most common cause of ARF is acute tubular necrosis. Of the approximately 30 patients annually per million population who require dialysis for ARF, 20 patients have acute tubular necrosis, three quarters of these as a complication of surgical procedures. Many factors cause this high incidence of ARF in the postoperative period. An important factor is the severity of any underlying diseases, both medical conditions existing in the patient before operation and the trauma or illness that necessitated the surgical procedure. Exposure to anesthetic agents and incompatible blood transfusion, both possible causes of ARF, are high-risk factors for the surgical patient. The most important factor, however, is hypovolemia from preoperative fluid restriction, surgical fluid loss, surgical blood loss, and gastric tube drainage of fluids. The already ischemic kidney in the hypovolemic patient may be easily injured by nephrotoxic antibiotics and other drugs. The combination of toxic and ischemic damage to tubular epithelium is the direct cause of postoperative ARF.

PREVENTION OF ACUTE RENAL FAILURE

Any postrenal problem that is allowed to persist may cause acute tubular necrosis. Postoperative and posttrauma patients with a sudden onset of anuria should be considered to have mechanical obstruction of the ureters or lower urinary tract until this possibility has been excluded. Operative or traumatic injury of the urinary tract in the retroperitoneal or pelvic areas is suspected whenever absolute anuria develops, since total anuria is rarely seen in the intrinsic renal and prerenal forms of ARF. The diagnosis can be established by cytoscopy, retrograde catheterization of the ureters, and radiologic techniques, including ultrasonography, intravenous pyelography, and computed tomographic scan of the abdomen. The cystogram and urethrogram demonstrate traumatic rupture of the bladder and disruption of the urethra, respectively. These causes of postrenal ARF should be suspected in cases of pelvic fracture, particularly if the rectal examination reveals displacement of the prostate gland.

Prerenal causes of ARF are prevented by optimizing volume status, cardiac function, and blood pressure while avoiding nephrotoxins and infections. Extracellular volume can be estimated by physical examination in many cases. When it cannot be judged accurately, central venous pressure or pulmonary capillary wedge pressure must be measured. An important means of evaluating the volume status in oliguric patients is by fluid challenge. The intravascular volume is increased by infusing crystalloid or colloid until the wedge pressure is raised to 15 to 18 cm. H_2O. A brisk diuresis suggests a prerenal cause for the oliguria. If oliguria persists, an intrinsic renal problem is suspected.

The mean arterial blood pressure must be restored to normal levels and vasoconstriction reversed for maintenance of the glomerular filtration rate above 60 ml. per minute and avoidance of activation of the renin-angiotensin system. In patients who are oliguric after hypotension, the blood pressure should be monitored by means of an intra-arterial cannula. Blood pressure should be restored to a mean pressure of 80 mm. Hg and maintained at that level by adequate volume replacement. The extracellular volume replacement is adequate if urinary output is 40 ml. or more per hour and the central venous pressure is normal.

Treatment with a loop diuretic such as furosemide or an osmotic agent such as mannitol may reverse early ARF by flushing the tubules and reducing their oxygen consumption. This treatment may convert oliguric renal failure to the nonoliguric form, but it does not alter the course of acute tubular necrosis. High-output renal failure is easier to manage clinically and may have a better prognosis for survival. Although loop diuretics are effective agents for increasing urinary flow in postoperative and posttrauma patients, they should not be used until the extracellular fluid volume has been restored to normal. Furosemide may convert homeostatic oliguria to ARF by inducing a large urine loss in a patient who is already volume depleted and whose oliguria is a normal response to the physiologic condition. To guard against the indiscriminate and dangerous use of loop diuretics, measurement of central venous or left atrial pressure should be made before administration of loop diuretics to an oliguric patient. When the extracellular fluid volume is proved normal, up to 200 mg. of furosemide or 12.5 gm. of mannitol may be given intravenously as a bolus, or continuous furosemide infusion may be used. Alternatively, 5 μg. per kg. per minute of dopamine, a nonpressor dose, may be administered to increase renal blood flow directly. If these measures fail to reverse the acute oliguria, further diuretic therapy is not helpful, and dialysis should be instituted as metabolic abnormalities or uremic symptoms develop. In cases of hemorrhagic or septic shock, diuretic therapy may be given as part of the resuscitation. If the pulmonary capillary wedge pressure is normal or low, mannitol is an appropriate agent. If the wedge pressure is high, furosemide is a better choice. Dopamine should be part of either regimen, but diuretic therapy is no substitute for adequate volume replacement. In fact, even dopamine given alone can dehydrate critically ill patients.

DIAGNOSIS OF ACUTE RENAL FAILURE

A systematic approach to the patient with oliguria and a rising creatinine concentration is of great importance. The physician must first consider prerenal and postrenal causes of the deteriorating renal function before concluding that intrinsic renal tubular damage has occurred. When the distinction between prerenal failure and ischemic tubular necrosis is unclear, the patient's response to careful volume expansion and optimization of cardiac performance is assessed. It is essential to consider the possibility that volume contraction, compromised cardiac output, or some toxic insult is superimposed on pre-existing chronic renal insufficiency. The most important diagnostic test may be volume restitution and improving the cardiac performance. Critically ill patients with multiple clinical problems and recent tissue injury suggest not only acute ischemic tubular necrosis but the concomitant presence of prerenal and postrenal compromises. ARF in the postoperative setting is commonly associated with combinations of volume depletion, third-spacing body fluids, heart failure, and intrinsic tubular injury from ischemia and toxins and perhaps even an element of urinary tract obstruction. Failure to systematically consider each of these possible causes for a decline in renal function delays specific effective therapy and jeopardizes renal recovery.

Evaluation should begin with a careful *clinical assessment,* including consideration of the clinical context, review of the clinical course, and physical examination with attention to blood pressure, heart rate, orthostatic changes, and serial changes in body weight. Detailed examination of intake and output is essential. Fluid intake should match fluid losses both in quantity and in quality.

Laboratory studies should include urinalysis, urine and plasma osmolality, urea, creatinine, and sodium. These values may be used to calculate urine diagnostic indices that are helpful in the differential diagnosis of acute renal failure. For example, the fractional excretion of sodium (FE_{Na}) may be calculated using the simultaneous urinary and plasma spot levels of sodium and creatinine as follows: $\%FE_{Na} = UN_{Na}/P_{Na}$ divided by $U_{Creat}/P_{Creat} \times 100\%$. In prerenal azotemia the FE_{Na} is less than 1% of filtered load, whereas established tubular injury is associated with FE_{Na} values above 3%. Each of these *diagnostic indices* is useful and should be employed routinely; together they can provide highly accurate diagnostic information. However, each test has proven exceptions and should not be interpreted rigidly. For example, radiocontrast-induced ATN is often associated with FE_{Na} values below 1%. Efforts should be directed toward improving circulatory hemodynamics, treating infection, relieving obstruction, and removing nephrotoxins. Following the clinical course while making these improvements may prove to be the most important diagnostic maneuver.

Sophisticated *radiographic studies* may be necessary when the diagnosis remains unclear. Radiologic techniques detect hydronephrosis, impairments in renal blood flow, unusual size, shape, or location of the kidney, and abnormalities of the collecting system. Plain films show renal size and radiopaque stones. Ultrasonography demonstrates obstruction, morphologic changes, and stones. Radionuclide scans document perfusion, function, and urinary extravasation. Intravenous pyelography demonstrates the level of an obstruction. Computed tomographic scanning defines location, size, and morphologic change of the kidney and disease in adjacent organs. Arteriography is useful in patients with suspected arterial lesions.

Biopsy is reserved for those cases of ARF in which the diagnosis of acute tubular necrosis appears doubtful and one or more intrinsic renal etiologic factors may be present, such as acute glomerular nephritis, acute interstitial nephritis, or acute vasculitis. When postrenal and prerenal causes of ARF have been excluded in a surgical patient, the majority have acute tubular necrosis, so renal biopsy has a *very* limited role in management. An exception is the renal transplant patient with ARF, in whom biopsy differentiates acute rejection from acute tubular necrosis, drug toxicity, and recurrent primary disease. Percutaneous needle biopsy of the native kidney has some risk (e.g., a 9% complication rate in one series) and should be performed only for clear indications such as prolonged renal failure beyond 3 weeks. It is contraindicated in the presence of bleeding diathesis or uncontrolled hypertension.

MANAGEMENT OF THE PATIENT WITH ESTABLISHED ACUTE RENAL FAILURE

When oliguria and/or a rise in blood urea nitrogen and creatinine supervenes in the postoperative patient, the clinician should be alert to the possibility of evolving ARF. Attention should be directed toward seeking and excluding specific reversible causes of the apparent deterioration of renal function. When the reversible factors have been corrected and the urinary indices have established tubular injury, a program of therapy should be undertaken immediately.

HYPERKALEMIA. Early attention must be given to fluid and electrolyte status of the patient with ARF, particularly hyperkalemia, which is the most serious electrolyte abnormality. The threat of hyperkalemia is cardiac arrest. The severity of hyperkalemia can be judged by the electrocardiographic changes, which include peaked T waves, prolongation of PR intervals, loss of P waves, and widening of the QRS complex. These changes indicate diminished cardiac excitability and imminent cardiac standstill. When significant electrocardiographic changes are apparent, emergent therapy is indicated.

First, a calcium infusion with 1 or 2 ampules of 10% calcium gluconate should be given over 5 to 15 minutes for stabilizing the cardiac membranes and reversing the toxic effects of hyperkalemia. This membrane-stabilizing action of calcium is immediate in onset but is relatively short-lived. It is often lifesaving, but other therapy must be instituted to actually lower the serum potassium and remove the excess potassium from the body. These therapies include the intravenous administration of concentrated glucose, insulin, and sodium bicarbonate.

Glucose and insulin therapy is best administered as a 10% glucose solution with 20 to 30 units of regular insulin per liter. The rate of intravenous administration should be titrated according to serial serum potassium values but may be administered as rapidly as 500 ml. per hour. Glucose-insulin therapy may be initiated with a bolus of 50 to 100 ml. of 50% glucose plus 10 units of regular insulin intravenously, followed by the drip infusion. The action of glucose and insulin begins within 10 minutes and persists for as long as the drip is continued. Sodium bicarbonate is either administered as a bolus over 5 to 10 minutes or diluted in 5% to 10% glucose in water and infused slowly. Potassium levels may be decreased transiently by administering bicarbonate, glucose, and insulin simultaneously (e.g., 45 mEq. $NaHCO_3$ in 1000 ml. of $D_{10}W$ with 20 units of regular insulin). Both forms of therapy lower the serum potassium by driving potassium into cells rather than removing it from the body. Ultimately, therefore, enteral administration of cation-exchange resins such as sodium polystyrene sulfonate (Kayexalate) or dialytic therapy must be employed to remove the potassium from the body. Each therapy has its limitations. With glucose-insulin infusion, water overload with progressive hyponatremia is a concern, and with large amounts of sodium bicarbonate, volume overload, pulmonary congestion, and hypernatremia are problems. Cation-exchange resins are most effective if they are administered orally with sorbitol. The presence of an ileus or intestinal injury precludes this mode of administration, and one must then rely on the less effective but still useful rectal route of administration. Precipitous reduction in serum potassium via hemodialysis can be associated with complex ventricular arrhythmias, particularly if other electrolyte disturbances coexist. Continuous electrocardiographic monitoring is mandatory.

FLUID VOLUME. Careful monitoring of fluid intake and output along with daily weights can prevent volume overload in the patient with ARF. If the patient is oliguric, excessive salt and water input cause hypertension and pulmonary edema. The clinician should restrict fluid intake to match actual fluid losses plus 500 to 700 ml. per day of insensible loss and 200 ml. per day per degree of fever. It is important that frequent regular quantitation of all fluid losses be performed because nasogastric drainage, wound drainage, stool losses, or urinary flow vary from hour to hour. It is best that standing orders for a fixed amount of fluid per day not be written because fluid administration must match fluctuating losses and determine necessary administration of blood products, antibiotics, nutrition, and so on. Volume overload in the oliguric patient can be treated with phlebotomy or some mode of dialysis.

HYPONATREMIA. Evolution of hyponatremia indicates

that free water intake is exceeding free water elimination. Severe hyponatremia is often a contributing factor to the encephalopathy and propensity to convulsions that complicate ARF when administered intravenous fluid is excessive and hypotonic. When hyponatremia evolves, free water restriction must be prescribed. If the serum sodium concentration falls below 120 mEq. per liter, convulsions are imminent. Dialysis is the only maneuver that can correct hyponatremia in this situation; administration of hypertonic sodium chloride in the oliguric patient who is usually already fluid overloaded is to be avoided. Hyponatremia is best managed by an awareness of how it might evolve and preventing it.

METABOLIC ACIDOSIS. Metabolic acidosis often accompanies acute renal failure, especially in association with major surgical therapy, traumatic injury, or sepsis. In the hypercatabolic patient, acid production is substantially increased, and the markedly reduced renal function allows no means for excretion of the accumulating acid or the regeneration of consumed bicarbonate. Harmful effects from the progressive metabolic acidosis include nausea, vomiting, and cerebral dysfunction, as well as cardiac depression, insulin resistance, impaired cellular metabolism, and hyperkalemia. Metabolic acidosis is treated with oral administration of Shohl's solution, intravenous or oral sodium bicarbonate, or dialysis. Enough alkali must be administered not only to repair the already existing acidosis but also to maintain arterial pH and bicarbonate reserves at a level that will match the daily endogenous acid production from catabolism. In the average resting adult, daily acid production is approximately 1 mEq. per kg. per day. Therefore, 70 to 100 mEq. of alkali would suffice to maintain acid-base balance. However, in the hypercatabolic patient with tissue injury, recent surgical therapy, or sepsis, endogenous acid production can be two to three times this amount, which must be matched by alkali administration. Such large amounts of sodium bicarbonate expand extracellular volume, may precipitate pulmonary edema, and are often associated with hypernatremia. If large amounts of sodium bicarbonate are required to maintain arterial pH, dialytic therapy must be initiated.

HYPOCALCEMIA AND HYPERPHOSPHATEMIA. Hypocalcemia and hyperphosphatemia occur most commonly in the patient who has experienced tissue necrosis from crush injury or burn. When the serum phosphate exceeds 6 mg. per 100 ml., magnesium-free phosphate-binding antacids should be prescribed to minimize elevations in the calcium-phosphate product and attenuate soft tissue deposition of calcium-phosphate crystals. Ionized calcium in acute renal failure is usually near normal owing to acidosis, uremia, and hypoalbuminemia. Infusion of calcium is therefore unnecessary unless carpopedal spasm or tetany develops. If phosphate is not lowered, infusion of calcium produces soft tissue precipitation of calcium phosphate. Ultimately, dialysis may be required to control phosphate and calcium balance.

USE OF DIALYSIS

Dialysis should be initiated when there is life-threatening hyperkalemia, severe acidosis, volume overload, uremic encephalopathy, or uremic pericarditis. Dialysis is best initiated prophylactically before the occurrence of any of these life-threatening complications of ARF rather than as an urgent procedure. The goals of dialysis are to (1) remove uremic nitrogenous metabolites and ameliorate the uremic state, (2) correct metabolic acidosis, (3) remove excess fluid, (4) normalize serum electrolyte concentrations, (5) improve platelet and leukocyte function, and (6) permit effective hyperalimentation. There are currently three forms of renal replacement therapy for use in patients suffering from ARF. Hemodialysis, peritoneal dialysis, and hemofiltration are each available in a series of modifications. Each mode of therapy has its own advantages and disadvantages. Consultation with a nephrologist for selecting and initiating renal replacement therapy is usually the best course of action.

MANAGEMENT OF LATE COMPLICATIONS

The major factor that determines patient survival in ARF is the nature and severity of associated illnesses. The evolution of complications during the course of renal failure dramatically affects patient prognosis. More than 50% of patients who die in the setting of ARF do so because of sepsis and pulmonary infections. Respiratory and cardiac failure represent another 25%, and severe bleeding is responsible for 10% to 15% of patient deaths. Malnutrition is a frequent concomitant and probably a primary permissive factor. When the postoperative patient with ARF is stabilized with regard to acute fluid and electrolyte complications and intensity of uremia is being controlled by an individualized dialysis prescription, attention must be directed toward preventing and managing these late complications.

PROGNOSIS

Untreated ARF in surgical patients rapidly causes death from fluid overload or hyperkalemia. When early resuscitation efforts are successful, infection, which causes 50% to 80% of deaths, becomes the overwhelming concern. In patients who have severe, multisystem trauma, ruptured abdominal aortic aneurysms, major surgical procedures for advanced cancer, abdominal catastrophes, or cardiovascular circulatory failure in addition to their ARF, mortality greater than 50% is reported in nearly every series. With early, aggressive, repeated dialysis for prevention of the metabolic derangements associated with ARF and successful management of the late complications of bleeding, sepsis, and drug intoxication, most patients recover renal function after postoperative ARF. A spectrum of outcomes was observed among survivors of acute tubular necrosis: 30% to 40% of patients had normal renal function, 40% to 50% had complete clinical recovery but persistent defects in glomerular or tubular function, 10% required medical management, and the remaining 10% to 20% required dialysis. Even during the recovery phase, prevention by avoidance of insults that might reinjure the recovering kidneys is much easier, most cost effective, and more successful than is treatment of ARF.

20

TRANSPLANTATION

I

Historical Aspects
R. Randal Bollinger, M.D., Ph.D.,
and Delford L. Stickel, M.D.

ANCIENT ACCOUNTS OF TRANSPLANTATION

Transplantation, the removal or partial detachment of a part of the body and its implantation to the body of the same or a different individual, has fascinated mankind for centuries. Legends of transplantation are recorded in the early written histories of both Eastern and Western cultures. Homer in his *Iliad* describes the monstrous Chimaera, a remarkable creature of transplanted animal parts created by the gods. This mythical hybrid animal had parts of a goat, a lion, and a serpent. All three of its heads breathed fire. The term *chimera* is now used in transplantation to describe individuals who possess hybrid characteristics such as the circulating cells of both donor and recipient after bone marrow transplantation. The Christian legend of Cosmas and Damian describes transplantation of a black leg to the amputation stump of a white parishioner as one of the miraculous feats of these two medical martyrs. Tragically, in 1492 two boys were bled to death in a vain attempt to save the life of Pope Innocent VIII by means of transfusion of young blood. Ancient Hindu surgeons described methods for repairing defects of the nose and ears about 700 B.C., and a Chinese document written about 300 B.C. contained a legendary account of organ transplantation.

A new Western tradition of transplantation surgery arose during the Renaissance in Bologna. The sixteenth century anatomist and surgeon Tagliacozzi developed his technique for reconstructing the nose by use of a flap of skin from the inner aspect of the upper arm. He carved the flap of skin in the shape of the patient's nose and then sutured it to the forehead and inner surface of the cheek, leaving a slender attachment to the arm for maintaining blood supply until circulation was re-established from the face. Following this painful procedure, the patient had to sit upright with the arm alongside the face and the head turned toward the arm for the next 3 weeks of healing, at which time the attachment to the arm was severed. The technique is still in use, known as the *tagliacotian flap* or the *Italian method.*

See the corresponding chapter or part in the *Textbook of Surgery*, 15th edition, pp. 382–389, for a more detailed discussion of this topic, including a comprehensive list of references.

EARLY EXPERIMENTS IN TRANSPLANTATION

The Scottish surgeon John Hunter (1728–1793) is rightfully known as the father of experimental surgery because of his pioneering research. Several of his experimental procedures involved transplantation, including autografting a cock's claw to its comb and xenografting a human tooth to the comb of a cock. A number of connective tissue transplant procedures including skin and cornea were performed successfully for the first time during the eighteenth and nineteenth centuries.

The first well-documented report of successful free auto-grafts of skin was in 1804 by Baronio, who experimented with sheep, although free autografts of human skin may have been used successfully centuries before. In 1822, Bunger reported successful use of a free full-thickness human skin autograft for repair of a nasal defect. In 1870, Reverdin reported that small grafts of epidermis on a granulating surface increased in size and grew out to coalesce with adjacent grafts. In 1886, Thiersch in Germany described the resurfacing of wounds with large sheets of split-thickness skin. Such grafts are still sometimes termed *Thiersch's grafts*, although essentially the same procedure was reported 14 years earlier by Ollier in France.

Corneal xenografts attempted early in the nineteenth century were unsuccessful. A corneal allograft between two gazelles was reported by Bigger in 1835, but the necessity of using a cornea from the same species was not recognized until 1872 to 1880, when successful corneal allografts were reported in animals and in man. Refinements of operative techniques, methods of preservation of grafts, and systems of graft procurement were subsequently developed. During the period 1925 to 1945, corneal transplantation emerged as a widespread and accepted therapeutic practice.

TRANSPLANTATION IN THE TWENTIETH CENTURY

The first long-functioning renal transplant was reported by Ullmann in March 1902. He transplanted kidneys in dogs with use of magnesium tube stents and ligatures for making the vascular anastomoses. That same year, the French surgeon Alexis Carrel reported his new technique of suturing blood vessels together by use of triangulation and fine silk suture material. His revolutionary technique was rapidly applied to the problems of organ transplantation. Between 1902 and 1912, Carrel and Guthrie of Chicago performed a large series of animal transplantation experiments, including the transfer of blood vessels, kidneys, hearts, spleens, ovaries, thyroids, extremities, and even the head and neck. In 1905, in his preliminary communication entitled "The Transplantation of Organs," Carrel stated, "This operation consists of extirpating an organ with its vessels, of putting it in another region, and of uniting its vessels to a neighboring artery and vein. If the organ is replaced in the same animal from which it was removed the operation is called an *autotransplantation*. If it is placed in another animal of the same species, it is called a *homotransplantation*, while if it is placed into an animal of a different species, the operation is called a *heterotransplantation*. The correct modern terminology is *syngeneic, allogeneic,* and *xenogeneic* transplantation, as shown in Table 1. Depending on the site of implantation, grafts are termed *orthotopic* if surrounded by the same type of tissues or located in the same part of the body after transplantation. Otherwise, they are termed *heterotopic*.

PROBLEM OF REJECTION. Although the immunity theory of graft rejection was postulated by several authors during the first decade of the century, the theory was questioned largely because there was no direct evidence that circulating antibody—the traditional hallmark of immunity—was involved in the rejection process. Cellular immunity, histocompatibility antigens, and immunologic tolerance were important discoveries in the understanding of transplant rejection.

In 1914, Murphy reported lymphocytic infiltrates in host tissues surrounding rejecting transplanted tumors, and by 1954, certain forms of immunity were observed to be transferable to an unimmunized subject by lymphoid cells and not by serum, a phenomenon designated *adoptively acquired immunity.* Jensen observed that a second graft did not survive as long as the first when a mouse received two grafts of a tumor separated by an interval of several days, and he suggested that immunity was responsible for the difference. This *second-set phenomenon* was observed in human skin graft recipients by Holman while treating burn patients at the Johns Hopkins Hospital in the 1920s. In 1932, Shinoyi in Japan described the specificity of the second-set phenomenon. Gibson and Medawar, working in England in 1943, reported similar observations with burn patients, and use of the term *second-set* dates to this report. Medawar demonstrated the immunologic specificity of the phenomenon, which was observed uniformly only when the same donor was used for both the first and the second sets of grafts. Medawar also contrasted the histologic characteristics of first- and second-set rejections. First-set rejection was predominantly a cellular event, whereas both cellular and humoral mechanisms were involved in the rejection of the second-set of grafts.

HISTOCOMPATIBILITY ANTIGENS. When immunity, both cellular and humoral, had been established as the cause

TABLE 1. Transplantation Terminology

Recent Nomenclature	Old Nomenclature	Relationship of Donor and Recipient of Graft
Syngeneic (isogeneic) graft	Autograft	Same individual
	Isograft	Same species and genetically identical
Allogeneic graft	Homograft	Same species but not genetically identical
Xenogeneic graft	Heterograft	Different species

of graft rejection, study was focused on the antigens that both stimulated graft rejection and were the targets of the ensuing immune response. The antigens responsible for graft rejection and the genetic control of these antigens were extensively studied in the mouse by Jensen, Little, Gorer, and Snell. The serologic identification of human transplantation antigens began in 1952 when Dausset discovered a leukocyte antigen responsible for transfusion reactions. In 1958 Payne found that antileukocyte antibodies were frequent in the sera of multiparous women, thus establishing a rich source of reagents for tissue typing. The new system of tissue matching was first used for selection of appropriate donors and recipients by Hamburger of Paris. In 1964, Payne reported the first clear evidence that these leukocyte antigens segregated in families as a genetic system. Terasaki in 1964 introduced the sensitive and specific microlymphocytotoxicity test. Definition of the HLA system, the major histocompatibility gene complex of man, was the result of a series of international workshops begun in 1964 by Amos. A major advance that same year was the discovery that lymphocytes from potential donors and recipients, when mixed together in tissue culture, undergo a vigorous proliferative response. This reaction, termed a *mixed lymphocyte culture*, became, along with microlymphocytotoxicity, a major method for histocompatibility testing.

IMMUNOLOGIC TOLERANCE. Chimerism was found to occur naturally in dizygotic cattle twins by Owen in 1945. He reported that each of such twins carry two different types of erythrocytes, and he postulated that the marrow of each individual had become populated by cells of both *in utero* when the circulation of the two placentas was mixed. Owen successfully exchanged skin grafts between the cattle twins, and in 1955 Simonson reported that kidneys as well as skin could be readily transplanted between them. In 1953, Billingham, Brent, and Medawar reported their experiments on "actively acquired tolerance of foreign cells" with use of inbred strains of mice of various ages. It became clear that the barrier between self and non-self could be overcome if the exposure to alloantigens occurred in the neonatal period. Grafts established on the fetus survived permanently, and the host was tolerant to other grafts from the donor strain; grafts performed more than a day or two after birth were rejected, and the rejection of subsequent grafts from the donor strain was accelerated. Animals rendered tolerant prenatally or neonatally were normal except for being chimeras and for being specifically nonreactive to antigens of the donor. Many subsequent studies have been directed toward the objective of inducing tolerance in the adult by methods that would be applicable to therapeutic transplantation in man. Since an effective method of producing acquired tolerance to transplantation antigens in adult animals and humans has not yet been discovered, the progress of transplantation has depended on the development of methods of immunosuppression.

IMMUNOSUPPRESSION. Total-body irradiation was used extensively for preventing rejection of grafts in experimental animals before it was used in the first successful human allografts from living, related donors in Paris and in Boston.

TABLE 2. The Era of Organ Replacement

Organ	First Experimental Animal Success	First Extended Human Survival
Kidney	1902 Ullman	1954 Murray
Heart	1905 Carrel and Guthrie	1967 Barnard
Pancreas	1922 Banting and Best	1966 Lillehei
Liver	1955 Welch	1967 Starzl

Although one allograft lived for 25 years, radiation therapy as an immunosuppressive agent was judged "too blunt, nonspecific and unpredictable." Schwartz and Dameshek reported in 1959 that the capacity of rabbits to form antibody was blocked by 6-mercaptopurine, which Calne and Zukoski used successfully in canine renal transplants. Hitchings and associates developed an imidazole derivative termed *azathioprine* in 1961 that could be administered conveniently and safely in an oral form. Murray, Hume, and Starzl reported clinical successes with azathioprine that same year, thus initiating the modern era of transplantation. With the advent of chemical immunosuppression, the brief but exciting history of clinical transplantation began. For the first time, several vascularized organs were transplanted with regular success, as shown in Table 2.

II

The Immunology of Transplant Antigens

Jeffrey L. Platt, M.D.,
and Pablo Rubinstein, M.D.

The first organ transplants were performed at the beginning of the twentieth century by Floresco, Carrel, and Ullmann. Transplants between different individuals, *allografts,* were observed to function for days, sometimes weeks, but ultimately to fail; transplants that were put back into the donor from which they originated, *autografts,* were observed to function indefinitely. The contributions of these experimental surgeons comprised landmarks in vascular surgery because they demonstrated for the first time that a kidney or potentially any organ removed from its natural environment and reimplanted surgically would function, if only temporarily. Those early

---

See the corresponding chapter or part in the *Textbook of Surgery,* 15th edition, pp. 389–399, for a more detailed discussion of this topic, including a comprehensive list of references.

experiments were the first demonstration of the fundamental principles of transplantation—that autografts are always successful, whereas allografts in a randomly bred population of donors and recipients are always rejected, and that rejection proceeds more rapidly than conventional immune responses. This chapter considers briefly the immunologic basis for rejection of allografts and the mechanisms that make this immune response so rapid and intense.

HISTOCOMPATIBILITY. *Histocompatibility* is the ability of a tissue or an organ to survive after grafting. In the broadest sense, it reflects various immune and nonimmune factors that allow a graft to survive in a foreign environment. With the discovery that the fate of allografts is governed by the immune reaction of the recipient against genetically determined cell surface structures in the donated organ, the term has referred more narrowly to the genetic determinants of graft rejection.

The concept that there is a genetic trait associated with histocompatibility can be traced to the work of C. O. Jensen, a Danish biologist. In 1903, Jensen discovered that tumors arising in an inbred strain of mouse could be maintained by transplanting pieces of the tumor tissue between members of that strain; however, if the tumor was transplanted into a mouse of a different strain, it would grow for a period of days and then regress and disappear. If the tumor was transplanted into a mouse in which the tumor had regressed previously, it would disappear almost immediately. The fate of tumor transplants in inbred mice was pursued further by C. Little and E. E. Tyzzer, who showed with the outcome of tumors transplanted into crosses between inbred and randomly bred mice that acceptance and growth of a tumor transplant depended on the joint presence of many genes. Ultimately, Little was able to conclude that resistance to tumor grafts reflects inheritance of a number of independently segregating, co-dominant genes, each existing as multiple alleles, and that the inheritance of the genes by the tumor (not the recipient) follows classic mendelian rules. Little also suggested that the regression of tumor grafts and the fate of normal tissue grafts might be governed by the same processes. These observations provide the basis for current concepts of the genetics of transplantation.

Little's work was continued by George D. Snell, who used inbred mice to examine in great detail the role of histocompatibility, or *H*, genes in tumor transplantation, characterizing the "strength" of different H genes as a specific feature of the gene. That the mechanism of failure of tumor allotransplants is immunologic was proposed on general grounds by many investigators, including Jensen, but a formal demonstration was first provided in the 1930s by Peter Gorer based on the observations that the outcome of tumor grafts could be predicted based on expression of an antigen in the tumor that was not expressed in the recipient and that graft recipients develop antibodies against the transplantation antigens of the donor. Further resolution was achieved by Gorer and Snell, who, together with the mouse geneticist Lyman, showed that transplantation antigens were inherited at a locus, which Snell called *H-2*. The strong histocompatibility locus was later found to be a complex of genes called the *major histocompatibility complex*, or *MHC*. J. Dausset discovered that patients who had received multiple transfusions of blood and were thus subject to transfusion reactions contained in their serum antibodies specific for leukocyte alloantigens, ultimately called *human leukocyte antigens* (HLA), and these antigens were analogous to the murine H-2 antigens. Although these antibodies could define some markers of the MHC, they were not in most cases the mediators of allograft rejection, for the transfer of immune serum was found to have no detrimental impact on the fate of free tissue grafts such as the skin. Rather, Mitchison demonstrated on the basis of cell transfer experiments that it is the lymphoid cells, later called *T lymphocytes* because of their origin in the thymus, which are responsible for causing the rejection of primary allografts (in sensitized subjects, antibodies can cause graft injury and rejection as discussed in Chapter 20–VI). How T lymphocytes recognize an allograft, the relationship between recognition and the inheritance of MHC antigens, and how the lymphocytes become recruited so rapidly to cause rejection of the graft in a period of days became central questions in transplant immunology.

HISTOCOMPATIBILITY AND THE PHYSIOLOGY OF CELLULAR IMMUNE RESPONSES

The immune response to a foreign antigen consists of two phases: recognition of the foreign antigen and the action of those lymphocytes or other cells called into the reaction by activated lymphocytes on the foreign antigen or organism that expresses it. The immune response to allogeneic tissues and organs is unique in that it is nearly universal in its occurrence and it is very rapid and powerful. The physiologic role of histocompatibility antigens accounts for these properties. The following sections consider how MHC molecules contribute to the development of immune responses, focusing on cellular immune responses, because these are the primary cause of allograft rejection.

IMMUNE RECOGNITION. T cells recognize foreign antigens via cell-surface glycoproteins called the *T-cell antigen receptor* (TcR). The TcR is a heterodimer consisting of α and β chains each approximately 40 to 45 kd which in structure resemble immunoglobulin. Unlike immunoglobulins, the TcR does not bind to "free" antigens but rather only binds to antigens that are associated with MHC Class I or Class II molecules. Cells bearing TcR that recognize MHC Class I express the CD8 molecule, and cells bearing TcR that recognize MHC Class II express the CD4 molecule. The first step in the recognition of foreign antigen by T cells and thus in the development of an immune response is *antigen presentation*. In this process, antigens become associated with MHC molecules and are expressed on the cell surface in such a way that the antigen can be recognized by a T cell.

MHC CLASS II MOLECULES. MHC Class II molecules

are heterodimers consisting of a 32-kd α chain and 28-kd β chain expressed mainly by specialized antigen-presenting cells such as macrophages and dendritic cells. In humans, endothelial cells also express MHC Class II molecules. The structural organization of MHC Class II molecules includes four extracellular domains, a transmembrane region, and a cytoplasmic "tail." The tertiary structure of MHC Class II antigens provides a pocket or antigen-binding cleft between the two polypeptide chains. Foreign proteins taken up by antigen-presenting cells are cleaved by proteases to yield peptides of varying length and amino acid composition. Peptides of 12 to 24 amino acids and having certain amino acids at critical points become firmly bound to the pocket in exchange for the *Class II invariant-chain peptide* (CLIP) that occupies the antigen-binding cleft, stabilizing the complex and preventing premature binding of endogenous peptides to the Class II molecule. Certain MHC peptides are preferentially taken up by the MHC Class II peptide-binding cleft. The propensity of MHC Class II antigens to be associated with MHC peptides is an important factor contributing to the strength of alloimmune responses.

Expression of foreign peptides in association with MHC Class II molecules provides a target for T cells bearing TcR that recognize polymorphic α_1 and β_1 domains of the Class II molecules plus the peptide. Whether the presentation of antigen in this way leads to activation of the T cell depends on the probability that an antigen-presenting cell bearing a given peptide will encounter a T cell able to recognize the particular peptide-MHC complex, the density of those particular peptide-MHC complexes on the surface of the antigen-presenting cell, and the state of activation of the antigen-presenting cell. However, under ordinary conditions, the probability is very low that a given peptide expressed in association with MHC Class II on an antigen-presenting cell will encounter a T cell specific for that peptide so expressed. For many foreign antigens, the frequency of responder cells is 10^{-4} to 10^{-5}, and for some specificities, only 10 or fewer T cells exist. However, inflammation involves several mechanisms that favor activation of T cells. Local trauma, infection, inflammation, and the like activate antigen-presenting cells, which in turn increases phagocytosis, antigen processing, and synthesis of MHC Class II molecules. If these changes occur in concert, antigen-presenting cells express higher concentrations of MHC molecules bearing foreign peptides.

MHC CLASS I MOLECULES. MHC Class I molecules consist of a 45-kd α chain and β_2-microglobulin, a 12-kd glycoprotein that is not encoded by the MHC complex. The functional organization of Class I, like that of Class II, includes four extracellular domains, a transmembrane region, and a cytoplasmic "tail." The Class I molecule is configured so as to make a groove that harbors an antigenic peptide, so the correct folding of the Class I MHC proteins depends on the presence of peptides simultaneously with the α chain and β_2-microglobulin. The peptide and polymorphic regions of the α_1 and α_2 domains bind to the T-cell receptor. A nonpolymorphic region of the α_3 domain binds to CD8.

The types of peptides that bind to MHC Class I molecules and the mechanism by which such peptides are taken up distinguish MHC Class I from Class II molecules. The peptides presented by Class I are generated from antigenic molecules present in the cytosol because of synthesis in the cell itself. Peptide transporters carry the peptides (8 to 11 amino acids) into the endoplasmic reticulum, where the Class I assembly takes place. The major transporter of peptides destined to be associated with MHC Class I molecules is a protein called *TAP* (transporter associated with antigen processing). TAP mediates the transport of small peptides into the lumen of the endoplasmic reticulum. TAP's ability to attach to a given peptide determines in part the immunogenicity of the peptide. These features of the MHC Class I–T-cell system allow recognition of molecules synthesized in the nucleus or cytoplasm of the cells but not the potentially vast array of foreign proteins taken up by phagocytosis.

T-CELL ACTIVATION. The second series of events in the development of immune responses leads to the activation of T lymphocytes. This process generally requires the delivery to a resting T cell of two types of signals, one provided by stimulation of the TcR by MHC-antigen complexes and one provided by accessory or "co-stimulatory" signals. Signals generated by the binding of TcR to MHC-peptide complexes are generated by CD3 molecules that consist of combinations of δ (25 kd), ε (20 kd), γ (20 kd), and ζ (16 kd) chains that are noncovalently associated with TcR chains. CD3 chains anchor protein tyrosine kinases, which, following stimulation of the TcR, initiate a cascade of signals. The cytoplasmic domains of the CD4 and CD8 cells are associated with protein tyrosine kinase, which contribute signals as well.

Stimulation of the TcR activates protein tyrosine kinases on CD3 and co-receptor molecules, which phosphorylate various T-cell proteins. One consequence of this process is activation of phospholipase C, which catalyses the metabolism of inositol phosphates. The products of these phosphates serve as second messengers, causing an increase in intracellular Ca^{2+} and activation of protein kinase C. These interactions in turn contribute to transcriptional activation of key T-cell genes such as interleukin-2. Second or co-stimulatory signals contributing to the activation of T cells may be generated when a T-cell surface glycoprotein, CD28, interacts with the corresponding ligands B7-1 or B7-2 expressed by antigen-presenting cells. Other T-cell surface molecules and cytokines also may deliver this second signal to T cells. Stimulation of the TcR alone, without the coordinate stimulation of co-stimulatory receptors, fails to induce T-cell activation and ultimately renders the T cell resistant to appropriate stimulation for a period of time. This resistance to stimulation, commonly called *anergy*, is an important mechanism for preventing inadvertent activation of T cells or activation by autoantigens.

MHC RESTRICTION AND THE T-CELL REPERTOIRE. Cellular immune responses are governed by two central "rules." One is that foreign antigens are only recognized in association with MHC molecules. The second is that antigens normally part of the T-cell host, regardless of their ability to be incorporated into MHC, do not elicit cellular responses when complexed with MHC molecules, that is, tolerance. MHC restriction and tolerance are brought about in part by the processes involved in the development of the T-cell repertoire in the thymus.

THE IMMUNE RESPONSE TO ALLOANTIGENS AND ALLOGENEIC CELLS

The structural characteristics of transplantation antigens and the way in which they are presented account for the extraordinary *immunogenicity* of allografts. The immunogenicity of transplantation antigens reflects in part their polymorphism; that is, the amino acid sequences of these proteins differ among individuals in the population. Immunogenicity also reflects which of the structural features of MHC Class I and Class II facilitate incorporation into the peptide-binding cleft of MHC molecules.

A very important factor contributing to the strength of alloimmune responses is that MHC antigens on allogeneic cells can be recognized "directly" on the allogeneic cell on which allogeneic MHC plus allogeneic peptide resemble self MHC plus foreign peptide. The mechanism explains the very high (10%) proportion of T cells able to recognize an allogeneic cell in comparison with the 1 in 10,000 to 1 in 100,000 that ordinarily recognize a foreign peptide presented by self MHC. Not only can a very large proportion of T cells recognize MHC antigens on allogeneic cells, but a very significant fraction of potential responding cells are activated by exposure to allogeneic antigen-presenting cells.

THE HUMAN MHC: HLA

The HLA system is composed of a large number of genes homologous with MHC genes of other species. HLA is located in chromosome 6. The Class I region encodes more than 15 genes, including the classic transplant genes A, B, and C, as well as HLA-E, F, and G and four pseudogenes, H, J, K, and L.

The Class II region contains more than 25 genes, including the loci for the α and β chains of the Class II "professional" transplantation antigens DR, DQ, and DP. The region also includes two α genes, DMA and DNA, and two β genes, DMB and DOB, genes for the low-molecular-weight proteins (LMPS) LMP2 and LMP3 and for the transporter molecules TAP1 and TAP2.

The Class III region, lying between Class II and Class I, contains more than 30 genes, among which are the genes encoding the complement components factor B, C2, and both C4 molecules, both tumor necrosis factor genes α and β, and the heat-shock proteins Hsp 1H and Hsp 70-2.

The polymorphism of HLA molecules reflects the existence of multiple alleles at one locus. Discerning alleles depends not only on the presence of such alleles but also on having methods to disclose their differences. Serologic methods are the mainstay of Class I and Class II typing. In addition, cellular typing techniques and typing at the DNA level, including RFLPs, specific hybridization of amplified (by PCR) polymorphic regions, and even the determination of their nucleotide sequence, are often used. In addition to the techniques applied to MHC typing, prospective graft recipients are usually tested via a "crossmatch" for antibodies against the donor that might cause injury in the period immediately following transplantation.

The importance of HLA typing on the outcome of transplants has been a central question in transplantation for many years. In clinical studies in which graft recipients are treated with immunosuppressive agents, the survival of renal allografts between HLA-matched siblings is approximately 90% at 1 year, compared with approximately 80% for HLA-mismatched siblings. However, HLA typing is generally not conducted before cardiac or liver allotransplants are performed (because there is not sufficient time); yet the results of these transplants are better than the results of kidney transplants, for which HLA typing is routinely performed. Matching for HLA-A, -B, and -DR does appear to have a small but significant impact on survival of cardiac allografts.

III

Mechanisms and Characteristics of Allograft Rejection

Jeffrey L. Platt, M.D.,
and Pablo Rubinstein, M.D.

THE IMMUNOLOGIC BASIS OF ALLOGRAFT REJECTION AND TOLERANCE

The beginning of modern transplantation biology can be traced to the work of Peter Medawar, a biologist, and Thomas Gibson, a surgeon, in the early 1940s. Medawar and Gibson carried out a classic experiment in which a series of skin grafts were placed on a patient with extensive burns. Some of the grafts were taken from the patient's own uninvolved skin, that is, autografts, and some were from another individual, that is, allografts. All the skin grafts healed, but within 15 to 23 days, the allografts had degenerated and contained an abundant mononuclear cell infiltrate, while the autografts showed no evidence of damage. A second series of allografts placed on the patient 15 days after the first were destroyed within a week; a second series of autografts healed normally.

See the corresponding chapter or part in the *Textbook of Surgery,* 15th edition, pp. 400–408, for a more detailed discussion of this topic, including a comprehensive list of references.

Medawar concluded that the hastened deterioration of the second set of allografts compared with the first set was caused by an immune reaction of the recipient against the graft, and on the basis of these and subsequent studies, he deduced some of the basic principles of alloimmune responses. First, the reaction against tissue allografts engenders immunologic "memory," since the "second set" response can be observed long after a first graft is destroyed. Second, the response is donor-specific, since recipients sensitized to one donor reject that donor's skin very rapidly but simultaneously accord a "first set" reaction to a graft from a third-party donor. Third, alloimmunity is systemic, since the placement of a graft in one location sensitizes the recipient against a graft placed in another location.

In the meantime, Ray Owen, a geneticist, discovered the concept of immunologic tolerance based on the discovery that twin cattle may have two kinds of erythrocytes, some bearing the blood group antigens of autologous hematopoietic cells and others the blood group of the fraternal twin. This observation showed that the discrimination between self and nonself, long a dogma of immunology and particularly of transplantation, was "learned" or acquired, not merely inherited.

The first clues about the immunologic mechanisms of graft rejection derived from the study of delayed-type hypersensitivity. Nearly all immune responses were thought to be mediated by antibodies, the one exception being delayed-type hypersensitivity (DTH). The immunologic mechanism underlying the DTH reaction was first revealed by Landsteiner and Chase, who demonstrated in 1942 that contact sensitivity is transferable by cells and not by serum. A potential relationship between DTH and the allograft reaction was elucidated in 1954 by Mitchison, who showed that lymph node and spleen cells but not serum harvested from allograft recipients could "adoptively" transfer immunologic resistance to allografts, thus providing compelling evidence of a cellular immune basis for allograft rejection.

As the era of clinical renal transplantation was ushered in by the clinical application of immunosuppressive therapy in the early 1960s, new types of rejection were seen. Hyperacute rejection and acute vascular rejection were seen in primarily vascularized grafts such as kidney or heart transplants. Others, such as chronic rejection, could only been seen if the more vigorous types of rejection were averted by immunosuppressive therapy.

ACUTE CELLULAR REJECTION

An organ or tissue transplanted between unrelated individuals is usually destroyed by acute cellular rejection within 7 to 14 days unless the recipient receives immunosuppressive therapy. Even if the recipient of an allograft is treated with immunosuppressive agents, acute cellular rejection is observed in about 50% of cases, usually within 6 months of transplantation, but sometimes after a year or longer. In some cases, cellular rejection proceeds more rapidly and aggressively than expected. Such responses may be observed in recipients who have been presensitized to donor antigens and thus have a more rapid cellular or humoral immune response upon re-exposure to those antigens.

Acute cellular rejection is characterized by histologic changes consisting of interstitial edema, capillary damage, and dense cellular infiltrates consisting mainly of lymphocytes and macrophages. Acute cellular rejection is a manifestation of a cellular immune response of the recipient directed against the donor. The events leading to acute cellular rejection include sensitization leading to activation of alloreactive T cells, trafficking of lymphocytes from the site of activation to the graft, and graft injury caused by immunologic effector mechanisms.

Sensitization is thought to be initiated when donor cells enter the lymphatics or the circulation and are carried to the local lymph nodes or to the spleen. In the case of organ transplants, sensitization may occur in the graft itself. Regardless of the location, the recipient's T cells brought into contact with antigen-presenting cells of the donor (or antigen-presenting cells of the recipient carrying donor peptides) become activated. After the recipient's immune response is triggered, the recipient's T cells and mononuclear cells migrate to the graft in a process mediated by enhanced cellular motility, cell adhesion molecules of the donor endothelium, and recipient lymphocyte surface and inflammatory mediators such as "chemokines."

The next step in the acute cellular rejection of an allograft is tissue injury caused by the recipient's leukocytes that have entered the graft. The pathologic picture of allograft rejection, which includes such features as interstitial edema, focal ischemia, thrombosis, and hemorrhage, suggests that endothelial cells are the major target of the immune response. Tissue injury may be mediated by products such as cytokines secreted by "helper" T lymphocytes, so called because these products contribute to the activation of B cells, other T cells, and macrophages. Helper T cells traditionally are thought to carry the CD4 antigen; however, CD8+ helper cells also may exist. The second mechanism of allograft injury may involve cell-mediated cytotoxicity, that is, killing. Cytotoxicity involves release of granules containing perforin and other cytotoxic substances and is traditionally thought to be mediated by CD8+ cells, although CD4+ cytotoxic T cells also can be found. An important aspect of cell-mediated cytotoxicity is the very high degree of specificity, which unlike delayed-type hypersensitivity, spares "innocent bystander" cells that do not have foreign antigen.

HUMORAL REJECTION

The reaction of recipient antibodies with a vascularized organ graft is associated with a spectrum of clinical and pathologic syndromes. The influence of a humoral response on the outcome of an allograft depends on such factors as (1) whether the graft is a free tissue such as the skin or whether it is a vascularized organ, (2) whether antidonor antibodies are present in the circulation prior to transplantation or are elicited in response to the graft, (3) the isotype of the responding antibodies, and perhaps (4) the target antigen recognized by the humoral response. In some cases, antidonor antibodies appear to protect vascularized grafts against cell-mediated rejection, and indeed, sometimes potential recipients are exposed to donor blood cells with the objective of generating such antibodies.

HYPERACUTE REJECTION. *Hyperacute rejection* is defined as the immediate or very early (within 24 hours) rejection of a vascularized organ graft. Characterized histologically by interstitial hemorrhage and thrombosis, it is possibly the most explosive of immunologic reactions. Hyperacute rejection is caused by the binding of antibodies in the donor to blood vessels in a newly transplanted organ, leading to activation of the complement system, which in turn mediates severe, irreversible injury to the endothelial lining of blood vessels. To avoid this problem, the serum of a potential recipient is tested for the presence of antibodies against the donor using a "crossmatch" assay.

ACUTE VASCULAR REJECTION. *Acute vascular rejection* is typically observed weeks to months after transplantation of an organ into a recipient treated with immunosuppressive therapy. It is characterized by swelling of endothelium particularly in arterial vessels, formation of fibrin thrombi, and sometimes the influx of inflammatory cells into the blood vessel walls. This type of rejection usually resists conventional types of immunosuppression; however, responses to more heroic measures have been observed.

CHRONIC REJECTION. The most common cause of allograft failure is *chronic rejection*. Chronic rejection is observed months or years after transplantation and is characterized clinically by a slow decline in graft function that is unresponsive to immunosuppressive therapy. Chronic rejection may be mediated by humoral or cellular immune responses or by other factors.

IV

Renal Transplantation

Clyde F. Barker, M.D., Ali Naji, M.D., Ph.D.,
James F. Markmann, M.D., Ph.D.,
and Kenneth L. Brayman, M.D., Ph.D.

RECIPIENT SELECTION AND MANAGEMENT

INDICATIONS. Transplantation should be considered seriously in all patients with end-stage renal disease, since both the quality of life and survival are superior to those of dialysis. The two most common indications are glomerulonephritis and diabetes mellitus. Other common indications are pyelonephritis and hypertension, which is the most common indication in blacks. Contraindications are infection or malignancy that cannot be eradicated and predictable noncompliance with immunosuppression. Advanced age or cardiovascular disease is a deterrent.

RECIPIENT EVALUATION AND PREPARATION. The evaluation of transplant candidates should include history and physical examination; complete blood count, urinalysis, urine cultures, and serum chemistries; assays for human immunodeficiency virus, cytomegalovirus, and hepatitis B and C; chest film; electrocardiogram; coagulation profile; Pap smear; and ABO typing. Regardless of the donor source, ABO compatibility and a negative complement-dependent cytotoxicity crossmatch are mandatory.

DONOR SELECTION AND MANAGEMENT

In addition to close histocompatibility, utilization of a related donor has the advantage of decreasing waiting time on dialysis and of minimizing the likelihood of acute tubular necrosis related to cadaveric organ recovery and transport. Since the advent of cyclosporine therapy in 1983, short-term survivals of cadaveric allografts now approach those of related-donor kidneys, but long-term results still favor related donors, which are used for about 25% of kidney transplants in the United States.

Long-term allograft survival of about 95% can be expected when a related donor and recipient are HLA-identical (25% of sibling pairs). There is a progressively lower graft survival associated with one-haplotype matching or mismatches for both haplotypes. The operative mortality of about 0.05% has led to a traditional policy of accepting only perfectly healthy

---

See the corresponding chapter or part in the *Textbook of Surgery,* 15th edition, pp. 408–429, for a more detailed discussion of this topic, including a comprehensive list of references.

donors between the ages of 18 and 55 years. The fear of possible long-term deleterious effects of kidney donation, such as hypertension and renal dysfunction, have not been realized. The severe shortage of cadaver donors has led to liberalization of these criteria and to the use of living-unrelated (usually spousal) donors by some centers. Interestingly, the success of living-unrelated donor transplants is considerably better than that of cadaveric donor transplants.

Cadaver donors should be previously healthy subjects between 3 and 65 years of age who have sustained fatal head injuries or cerebrovascular accidents. Factors that preclude organ donation are generalized infections (bacterial, viral, or fungal), malignancy other than nonmetastasizing brain tumors, renal disease, severe hypertension, and advanced arteriosclerosis. Reports from European centers have generally indicated that HLA matching for cadaveric grafts has a beneficial effect, although a consensus on this issue has not been reached by centers in North America. This difference may be the greater genetic homogeneity of the European population and the uniformity of tissue typing that is performed only in the experienced laboratories of Eurotransplant. The perception that cyclosporine overrides the effects of HLA mismatching has been used to support the concept that prompt local use of poorly matched kidneys is preferable to transplantation into better-matched recipients at distant centers. However, some reports indicate that kidneys shared with distant centers do as well as those transplanted locally. In the United States, the rules of UNOS mandate national sharing of kidneys totally matched for HLA antigens. The results of such transplants are clearly superior to those of unmatched transplants, but for cadaveric kidneys of less-than-perfect match, the importance of histocompatibility remains controversial.

RECOVERY AND PRESERVATION OF CADAVERIC KIDNEYS. After declaration of brain death, the donor is brought to the operating room, where optimal respiration and circulation are maintained during the procedure. Because of the donor shortage, use of non-heart-beating cadavers is also being explored at some centers. The kidneys, ureters, aorta, and vena cava are excised *en bloc* and transferred to a basin of cold solution, where careful dissection of the renal vessels is performed. Preservation can be accomplished either by simple cooling or by continuous pulsatile perfusion. Continuous perfusion allows somewhat longer preservation. In 1987, Belzer introduced a solution containing lactobionate, raffinose, and hydroxyethyl starch that extended substantially the acceptable duration of simple cooling to 24 to 36 hours. Because pulsatile perfusion requires continuous monitoring and is more expensive, few centers now utilize this method.

THE RECIPIENT OPERATION. The iliac vessels are exposed retroperitoneally, and end-to-side anastomosis of the renal artery and vein to the external iliac artery and vein, respectively, is used most often. Urinary tract continuity is usually established by ureteroneocystostomy. Ureteropyelostomy is an alternative procedure that should be used in instances of ureteral devascularization or injury.

XENOGRAFTS

Recently, severe organ shortage has led to reconsideration of using animal donors, a strategy that proved inferior when explored for kidney transplantation in the 1960s. Several human patients have received animal heart and liver grafts in the last few years. These grafts also have failed within days to several months despite the use of improved modern immunosuppression, indicating that further research is needed before xenografts can be widely employed.

POSTTRANSPLANT MANAGEMENT

Unless the transplanted kidney has suffered ischemic damage, a brisk diuresis usually begins within minutes of revascularization. Since the transplant operation is relatively nondisruptive to intestinal function, medications and fluids usually can be given by mouth within 12 to 24 hours. A well-functioning transplant can normalize renal function tests within a few days.

Immunosuppression

AZATHIOPRINE AND STEROIDS. Rejection of renal allografts was prevented in the 1950s by whole-body irradiation, a profoundly immunodepressive procedure with a prohibitive risk of lethal infection. In the 1960s, the antimetabolite drug azathioprine was found to have a reversible and safer action than irradiation. Although adrenal corticosteroids were not sufficient to prevent rejection, they were found to be synergistic with azathioprine. In addition, brief courses of high-dose steroid therapy often can reverse acute rejection episodes.

ANTILYMPHOCYTIC ANTIBODIES. In the 1960s, a new immunosuppressive agent, antilymphocyte serum (ALS, a xenoantibody raised by repeated immunization of animals with human lymphoid cells), was found to be even more potent and somewhat more specific than azathioprine. Several problems diminished its usefulness. Even the purified globulin fraction (ALG) sometimes provoked allergic reactions, leukopenia, and thrombocytopenia. Antibody production to the heterologous protein limited its effectiveness, and repeated use and large doses or prolonged therapy often led to serious infections. Today, the most frequent indication for ALG is reversal of rejection crises, which sometimes respond even though they are resistant to large-dose steroid therapy.

The effectiveness of ALS in reversing rejection led to the introduction of monoclonal anti-T-cell antibodies, which rapidly depleted T lymphocytes from peripheral blood while having little detrimental effect on red blood cells, platelets, or granulocytes.

CYCLOSPORINE. Since its release for general use in 1983, the fungal derivative cyclosporine has been adopted as the basis of most contemporary immunosuppressive protocols.

It blocks production of the lymphokine interleukin-2 (IL-2) through inhibition of T-lymphocyte messenger RNA. Like azathioprine and unlike OKT3 and ALS, cyclosporine is most useful for prophylaxis than in the reversal of rejection. Cyclosporine has the major advantage over azathioprine of lacking bone marrow toxicity. Nephrotoxicity is its major side effect. Others include hypertension, hepatotoxicity, seizures, tremor, hypertrichosis, nausea, vomiting, and diarrhea. Patient survival also has been improved by the introduction of cyclosporine, probably because of a decreased incidence and severity of infections. Disappointingly, there is little evidence that cyclosporine has the same favorable impact on long-term results as it does on early ones. A continuing attrition in late graft survival is most likely due to chronic rejection, which apparently is not overcome by cyclosporine.

TACROLIMUS (FK506). This agent has properties similar to and possibly superior to cyclosporine. It appears to be particularly valuable for "rescue" of grafts that are failing on cyclosporine or other immunosuppressive regimens. It has been used most extensively for liver transplants.

OTHER IMMUNOSUPPRESSIVE AGENTS AND STRATEGIES. A number of new immunosuppressive agents have been discovered recently and are in preliminary clinical trials, including mycophenolate mofetil, sirolimus, deoxyspergualin, and several new monoclonal antibodies.

Blood transfusion as a method of inducing unresponsiveness appeared to be a useful strategy until the mid-1980s. Its use was largely abandoned as the beneficial effect (which was never well understood) disappeared with the improvement in results that followed the introduction of cyclosporine. Currently, several groups are exploring protocols in which bone marrow from the kidney donor is administered to produce a durable chimeric state in the recipient that could induce specific tolerance.

REJECTION

Although rejection is conveniently categorized into hyperacute, acute, and chronic forms, there are overlapping features and transitions between these categories.

HYPERACUTE REJECTION. Hyperacute rejection occurs within minutes of kidney revascularization and is evidenced by bluish discoloration of the kidney, deterioration of perfusion, and irreversible sudden cessation of function. Extensive intravascular deposits of fibrin and platelets and intraglomerular accumulation of polymorphonuclear leukocytes, fibrin, platelets, and red blood cells are seen histologically, along with accumulation of polymorphonuclear leukocytes in the peritubular and glomerular capillaries. Refractory to immunosuppressive or anticoagulant therapy, hyperacute rejection is usually correlated with the presence of preformed circulating antibodies against donor antigens. Since in the modern era these antibodies can be identified by a pretransplant leukocyte crossmatch, this form of rejection is now rarely seen.

ACUTE CELLULAR REJECTION. Acute cellular rejection occurs most commonly during the early weeks following transplantation. Findings include weight gain, rising blood urea nitrogen and creatinine, and deterioration of flow and tubular function on radionuclide scans. Transcutaneous allograft biopsy may be required to confirm the diagnosis, especially if early posttransplant function has been impaired by ischemic damage.

Microscopic signs of acute rejection include the adherence of lymphocytes to the endothelium of peritubular capillaries and venules, progressing to disruption of these vessels, tubular necrosis, and interstitial infiltrates. As a result of a recent international conference at Banff, widely accepted criteria are used for semiquantitative analysis of rejection and the development of standardized nomenclature.

Prompt institution of antirejection therapy (steroids, ALS, OKT3) is necessary to prevent permanent damage to the allograft. Steroid-resistant rejection, which occurs in 30% to 50% of patients, responds to ALG or OKT3 in an additional 30% of cases. During the 1970s (prior to the introduction of cyclosporine), a progressive improvement in patient survival occurred in most centers. This was the result of the realization that overly intense immunosuppression and repeated courses of antirejection therapy were dangerous. Recognition that eventual loss of some grafts could not be avoided allowed earlier transplant nephrectomy and reinstitution of dialysis. A later successful transplant and a live patient were found preferable to serious infection and even death from immunosuppression given with little likelihood of forestalling inevitable rejection of a compromised graft.

CHRONIC REJECTION. Chronic rejection is the usual cause of late deterioration of renal allografts, although other causes such as recurrent disease (glomerulonephritis, diabetes, oxalosis) and renal artery stenosis always should be considered. The typical course is gradual, progressive loss of renal function. It may begin after years of stable function but is more often seen in patients who have had multiple early and incompletely reversed episodes of acute rejection. Glomerular changes are also seen. Clinical manifestations include proteinuria, microscopic hematuria, hypertension, and fluid retention with progressive uremia. Histologic evidence of protracted humoral injury is marked by arterial intimal fibroproliferative lesions. Also seen are increased mesangial matrix and mesangial proliferation. The glomerular basement membrane is thickened, and focal deposition of IgM, IgG, and complement may be identified.

Antirejection therapy is ineffective, and large-dose steroid, ALS, or OKT3 therapy should not be risked, since these may cause opportunistic infection or other serious sequelae. A prompt biopsy is warranted in cases of unexpected or precipitous deterioration in stable function, since episodes of late acute cellular rejection can sometimes be reversed. With judicious fluid and electrolyte control, patients with chronic rejection often can be maintained for months to years before returning to dialysis.

COMPLICATIONS OF RENAL TRANSPLANTATION

Complications occurring in the first few hours or days after transplantation are commonly related to technical mishaps.

VASCULAR COMPLICATIONS. Arterial occlusion, as a cause of early postoperative oliguria or anuria, should be considered if an established diuresis suddenly ceases. Although radioisotopic scanning and arteriography can be used to confirm the diagnosis, immediate reoperation without delay for diagnostic studies may allow the only chance for salvaging the graft. Renal transplant artery stenosis may be confused with rejection, since both may cause hypertension and diminished renal function. Although renal transplant artery stenosis is a relatively unusual cause of decreased renal function, a high index of suspicion should be maintained, since it is correctable by operation or by percutaneous transluminal angioplasty.

URINARY TRACT COMPLICATIONS. The most common cause of sudden cessation of urinary output in the immediate postoperative period is presence of a blood clot in the bladder or urethral catheter. More serious causes of urinary obstruction (2% to 5% in most series) should be investigated simultaneously with consideration of vascular occlusion, acute tubular necrosis, and rejection.

Devascularization of the ureter during donor nephrectomy is a serious problem and may cause ureteral necrosis and urinary fistula within the first few days or weeks following operation. Analysis of fluid obtained from wound drains or needle aspiration for urea, ultrasound, radioactive scans, cystograms, and antegrade pyeloureterography are other helpful studies. Treatment consists of reconstruction of the ureteroneocystostomy or ureteropyelostomy using the patient's own ureter.

ACUTE TUBULAR NECROSIS (ATN). In the absence of vascular or ureteral problems, initial nonfunction of cadaver kidneys may be attributed to ATN (incidence of 5% to 30%). Oliguria in the early transplant period should be treated with boluses of fluid for exclusion of hypovolemia. The impact of ATN is adverse, since it indicates some ischemic damage and it may interfere with the early diagnosis and treatment of rejection. The nephrotoxic potential of cyclosporine is heightened with ATN, which causes some surgeons to sharply lower the dose or avoid its use completely during ATN.

NONTECHNICAL COMPLICATIONS. *Infection,* the most common complication of immunosuppression, occurs in 30% to 60% of patients during the first posttransplant year. Despite more cautious use of immunosuppression over the last decade, it is the major cause of death in half of the 5% to 10% of patients who die during the first year.

Bacterial infections are the most common infections during the first month after transplant, and the urinary tract, respiratory system, and wound are the most prevalent sites. These infections usually respond to prompt antibiotic therapy. It is important to exclude the possibility of infection before antirejection therapy, since immunosuppression should be decreased rather than intensified in this situation.

The period between the first and sixth months after transplantation, usually the time of most intense immunosuppression, is the most common time for *opportunistic infections.* Cytomegalovirus (CMV), a member of the herpes family, is a ubiquitous agent that infects most individuals at some time in their lives. It causes clinically silent or mild infection in healthy individuals, and the latent virus and seropositivity persist for life. Seronegative recipients who receive a kidney from a seropositive donor often develop symptomatic illness, which varies in severity from mild fever and malaise to a debilitating syndrome marked by leukopenia, hepatitis, interstitial pneumonia, arthritis, central nervous system changes, gastrointestinal ulceration and bleeding, renal insufficiency, bacterial or fungal infection, and even death. Fortunately, both the incidence and severity of CMV disease appear to be diminished in cyclosporine-treated patients. Prophylactic acyclovir or ganciclovir decrease the incidence of CMV, and in established CMV disease, ganciclovir (DHPG) is quite effective. Other opportunistic infections such as *Pneumocystis carinii* pneumonia, aspergillosis, blastomycosis, nocardiosis, toxoplasmosis, cryptococcosis, and tuberculosis are more likely to occur in transplant recipients than in nonimmunosuppressed patients.

GASTROINTESTINAL COMPLICATIONS. Ulceration and perforation of the gastrointestinal tract are not uncommon following transplantation, with the colon being especially vulnerable. Pancreatitis and infectious gastrointestinal complications such as *Candida* stomatitis and esophagitis, pseudomembranous colitis, and CMV ulceration are also common.

HYPERPARATHYROIDISM. Secondary hyperparathyroidism from chronic renal failure usually subsides after a successful transplant. However, it persists *(tertiary hyperparathyroidism)* in about 5% of patients with normally functioning allografts. In cases in which significant hypercalcemia and elevated parathyroid hormone levels continue for more than 6 to 12 months despite normal renal function, the authors advocate total parathyroidectomy and autotransplantation of a portion of one gland.

TUMORS. Immune deficiency is associated with an increased risk of neoplasia. In transplant recipients, incidence of *de novo* malignancy is approximately 100 times greater than that in normal age-matched populations. Cancers common in the general population (breast, colon, prostate) are not increased. The most common neoplasms are squamous cell carcinomas of skin and lip. Transplant recipients have 350 times the normal incidence of lymphomas. Compelling evidence that *de novo* lymphomas may begin as lymphoproliferative lesions induced by viruses stems from the finding of Epstein-Barr virus in the genome resembling infectious mononucleosis. During the stage of polyclonality, cessation of immunosuppression and the use of antiviral agents may cause regression of the lesions. Tumors that are initially polyclonal may develop the monoclonality characteristic of true B-cell lymphomas, which then do not regress following cessation of immunosuppression and usually have a fatal outcome.

RESULTS OF RENAL TRANSPLANTATION AND SOCIOECONOMIC CONSIDERATIONS

Between 1951 and 1966, renal allografts had only a 63% 1-year functional survival in sibling recipients and only 35% with the use of cadaver donors. The introduction of cyclosporine is credited with a striking improvement, but other changes in practice also have contributed to the present results. The 1-year survival of cadaveric grafts is now nearly 85%. The still better results with living-related donors and their longer persistence continue to justify their use, especially in the case of HLA-identical sibling recipients (96% 1-year graft survival).

Patient survival after transplantation has improved even more dramatically than has graft survival. In 1967, the 1-year patient survival was only 36% with cadaveric grafts, and by 1981, it was 90%. Thus improvement (which actually began before the use of cyclosporine) was mainly attributable to a striking fall in the incidence of severe infections related to a general policy of decreasing the intensity of immunosuppression. The release of cyclosporine further improved graft survival while lowering susceptibility to infection. One-year patient survivals of 95% to 98% are now reported by many centers.

One disappointing aspect of the results of renal transplantation is evident from examining long-term outcome of cadaveric grafts. Despite the striking improvements in short-term survival, there is a continuing attrition of cadaveric grafts after 1 year which, despite cyclosporine, has remained almost constant at 7% per year. The importance of histocompatibility remains obvious when long-term graft survival is examined. Of kidney transplants performed now, only 40% of cadaveric donor grafts can be expected to survive 10 years, while 80% of HLA-identical sibling grafts will survive that long.

SOCIOECONOMIC CONSIDERATIONS IN TREATMENT OF END-STAGE RENAL DISEASE

Although transplantation is expensive, it is not as expensive as chronic dialysis. Transplantation costs $38,000 and, if successful, about $4000 per year thereafter. Despite the high initial cost, the lower subsequent expenses of patients with functioning grafts compare so favorably with those of patients on maintenance hemodialysis ($20,000 per year for life) that the costs of transplantation, even including failed grafts, are recouped in about 3 years. Other important advantages of transplantation are better rehabilitation and quality of life.

The evolution of renal transplantation from an experimental approach to a highly successful clinical therapy represents one of the remarkable medical achievements of this century. End-stage renal disease, an entity that 40 years ago was uniformly fatal, can now be treated with greater success than can most malignancies. Since many victims of kidney disease are relatively young, the achievement of a successful transplant in this group is one of the most satisfying in medical practice.

V

Vascular Access Procedures for Renal Dialysis (Including Peritoneal Dialysis)

Carl E. Haisch, M.D., and James Cerilli, M.D.

VASCULAR ACCESS

Without adequate hemoaccess, the development of hemodialysis would not have been possible. Hemoaccess is required when frequent access to the vascular system is required, a high-flow system is needed, the ability to withstand multiple needle punctures is required, or highly sclerotic solutions are administered. The most common use of arteriovenous fistulas, shunts, or grafts is hemodialysis.

External shunts have been used extensively in the past but now are used in selected situations, such as in trauma patients requiring dialysis for acute renal failure. For acute access in patients requiring hemodialysis, the most common catheter placement is in the subclavian, internal jugular, external jugular, or femoral vein. This is performed with a single- or double-lumen catheter that can be used for dialysis from weeks to months depending on the configuration of the catheter. A soft Silastic double-lumen catheter placed via the internal jugular vein can be used for as long as a year. Catheters that are somewhat stiff and are placed into the subclavian vein can cause subclavian vein stenosis or thrombosis in up to 50% of patients who have had the catheters in place longer than 2 weeks. Patients who do have subclavian vein stenosis can have balloon dilatation performed, with improvement in up to 50% of those patients in whom it was attempted. A tight subclavian vein stenosis produces unsuccessful placement of a long-term fistula or jump graft.

The "gold standard" for long-term access is the Brescia-Cimino radial artery to cephalic vein arteriovenous fistula. A natural fistula has the best patency and the least incidence of infection. It is placed in a number of configurations, including end artery to end vein, side artery to side vein, side artery to

See the corresponding chapter or part in the *Textbook of Surgery,* 15th edition, pp. 429–436, for a more detailed discussion of this topic, including a comprehensive list of references.

end vein, and end artery to side vein. A significant amount of the flow for a Brescia-Cimino fistula comes from the palmar arch, so one must be certain that there is adequate collateral flow from the ulnar artery. An Allen test is performed to be certain that the palmar arch is open and that the steal syndrome does not occur. Other natural fistulas can be placed, including ulnar artery to basilic vein, antecubital vein–to–brachial artery, and brachiobasilic fistula. All these should be attempted before nonautogenous material is considered.

The leading complication of these fistulas is thrombosis. The patency rate at 1 year is 65%. Most of the losses occur in the first 2 to 3 months, with few losses thereafter.

Prosthetic grafts for access are used in patients who have exhausted all superficial veins for access. The types are radial artery to cephalic vein at the elbow, forearm loop between the brachial artery and antecubital vein, upper-arm loop between the axillary artery and vein, and leg graft between the superficial femoral artery and saphenous vein. When these sites have been exhausted, grafts that use more central vessels may be used, including a loop on the chest, axillary vein to axillary artery, a necklace axillary artery to axillary vein, axillary artery in the arm to subclavian vein or internal jugular vein in the neck, or axillary artery to iliac vein. The patency rate for most of the grafts is approximately 80% at 1 year. The forearm straight graft between the radial artery and the cephalic vein has the lowest patency, with a rate of approximately 35%.

The leading complication with all these grafts is thrombosis. The venous outflow tract develops intimal hyperplasia. There has been much interest in following these grafts with color Doppler ultrasound. If a 50% stenosis occurs, half the patients with this grade stenosis clot the graft within 6 months. This sort of graft surveillance entails earlier intervention and therefore a decreased incidence of thrombosis and increased graft longevity. The treatment of this complication is bypass with a segment of graft, a patch over the stenosis, or balloon dilatation using a balloon that will tolerate approximately 17 atm. of pressure. Infection is the second most common complication and can be treated with local wound care, placement of a skin flap, or removal of the graft. These sorts of local care produce a graft salvage of approximately 25% to 50%.

PERITONEAL DIALYSIS

Chronic ambulatory peritoneal dialysis (CAPD) uses a Silastic tube placed into the peritoneal cavity. This tube places a dialysis fluid into the abdominal cavity, and the semipermeable peritoneal membrane passes solutes and fluids out of the body into the peritoneal cavity. A large amount of fluid may be extracted if a dialysate fluid high in dextrose is used (4.5%). Electrolyte disturbances can be corrected by adding or deleting the particular electrolyte from the dialysate fluid.

CAPD is indicated in patients (1) desiring home dialysis, (2) with no available sites for vascular access, (3) with repeated infections of vascular access sites, (4) with an unstable cardiovascular system, (5) with diabetes, who would benefit from a constant insulin infusion from the peritoneal cavity, (6) above 65 years of age, (7) with bleeding difficulties in which heparin is contraindicated, such as duodenal ulcer, (8) who wish to avoid blood transfusions, (9) with AIDS, and (10) who are small children. Contraindications are few. If there is an obliterated peritoneal space, lack of diaphragmatic integrity, or poor peritoneal clearance, CAPD cannot be used. The relative contraindications include respiratory insufficiency, diffuse abdominal malignancy, a large hernia, or low back pain caused by degenerative disk disease.

The catheter for peritoneal dialysis can be placed percutaneously or surgically, and there are some reports of placing the catheter using laparoscopy. The leading complication is infection, either peritonitis or Dacron cuff infection of the catheter. The source of infection can be skin, dialysis fluid, bowel flora, or ascending infection from fallopian tubes in females.

The catheter functions for 1 year in 85% of patients. The leading reason patients do not remain on CAPD is infection.

Both CAPD and hemodialysis have specific indications for individual patients. However, transplantation still is considered the therapy of choice for a large number of patients.

VI

Principles of Therapeutic Immunosuppression

Angus W. Thomson, Ph.D., D.Sc.,
Suzanne T. Ildstad, M.D.,
and Richard L. Simmons, M.D.

Transplantation of solid organs has become the treatment of choice for end-stage renal, hepatic, cardiac, and pulmonary disease. After Alexis Carrel described the technique for vascular anastomosis in 1902, technical challenges for transplanting kidneys and other solid-organ allografts were for the most part resolved. Subsequent advances that allowed solid-organ transplantation to become clinically feasible were due to the development of immunosuppressive agents that could prevent or control rejection. Management of rejection requires an understanding of the complexity of the immune system and the cells and other factors involved in the rejection response.

CONCEPTUAL APPROACHES TO IMMUNOSUPPRESSIVE THERAPY

Lymphocytes and *macrophages* constitute the heart of the immune system. The rejection reaction begins when T-lympho-

---

See the corresponding chapter or part in the *Textbook of Surgery*, 15th edition, pp. 437–455, for a more detailed discussion of this topic, including a comprehensive list of references.

cytes recognize foreign antigens present on cells of the transplanted tissue. The most potent of these antigen-presenting cells (APCs) are the dendritic leukocytes. The immunologic specificity for differentiating self from non-self resides in the lymphocytes, which are activated by the recognition of major histocompatibility complex (MHC) locus or transplantation antigen differences.

Stimulation of a resting lymphocyte by the antigen causes it to transform into a large, active cell that secretes intercellular chemical communicators called *cytokines* (many are also known as *interleukins*), effective across short distances that amplify the response and activate other cells. Manipulation of this complex of events offers many opportunities for immunosuppression in the attempt to halt or prevent the rejection response. Immunosuppression is less effective after the lymphocyte has responded to the foreign antigen, and the immune response is far more difficult to control after activation.

Current immunosuppressive agents act in a nonspecific manner to suppress the entire immune response. Because of their mechanism of action, they have associated toxic and side effects such as an increase in opportunistic infections and an increased occurrence of malignancy. Effective general immunosuppression may allow the graft to survive but also may cripple the host response to infections or prevent other proliferating cells, such as bone marrow and intestinal mucosal cells, from maintaining a safe population. Infections with cytomegalovirus and *Pneumocystis carinii*, which do not present a life-threatening problem to the normal patient, frequently become lethal to the transplant patient.

At present, clinical immunosuppression relies on three general approaches. The *first* is simply to reduce the number of circulating lymphocytes by destroying them with corticosteroids or antiserum. The *second* uses an inhibitor of antigen-induced lymphocyte activation (cyclosporine or tacrolimus [formerly FK506]) to interrupt cytokine gene expression. The *third* uses a variety of metabolic inhibitors to interfere with lymphocyte proliferation. Although the latter agents are biochemically specific, they do not distinguish between dividing lymphocytes and other proliferating cells.

THE BIOLOGY OF ANTIGRAFT IMMUNITY

The development of the lymphoid system begins with a pluripotential stem cell in the liver and bone marrow of the fetus. With maturation of the fetus toward term, the bone marrow becomes the primary site for lymphopoiesis. The marrow produces T-lymphocytes, B-lymphocytes, and macrophages, cells critical to the immune response. The thymus is the *primary lymphoid organ* in which the *T-lymphocyte* is matured, or *educated*, and released to stock the *peripheral lymphoid tissues* such as lymph nodes, the spleen, and the gut. It is in the thymus that T-lymphocytes acquire their subset differentiation markers (CD4, CD8, and so on), which influence their ultimate functional role in the immune system. Another subpopulation that descends from the stem cell is the *B-cell line.* The primary lymphoid organ that produces B cells in mammals is unknown, whereas in birds it is the bursa of Fabricius. Interleukin 4 (IL-4), IL-5, and IL-6 have been identified as lymphokines that stimulate the proliferation and maturation of activated B cells. Both T- and B-lymphocytes acquire their immune specificity during early development. Fully competent clones of small lymphocytes are waiting to respond to foreign antigens. An individual lymphocyte can recognize only one of a few closely related antigens. *Macrophages,* which also have an integral role in the immune response, are derived from the same pluripotent stem cells as the intraepithelial cells such as keratinocytes and tissue macrophages. They function to process antigen and present it to lymphocytes and to produce cytokines, soluble factors that regulate the immune response. The most potent APCs, however, are the rarer bone marrow–derived dendritic cells. These are distributed ubiquitously throughout the body and can migrate and convey antigen from nonlymphoid to lymphoid tissue, where they present antigen to T cells.

The T cells, B cells, and macrophages have unique roles in orchestrating the immune response. It is a very tightly controlled network, the majority of communication mediated by cytokines. B cells synthesize antibody, and the subpopulations of T cells have several different activities. Certain T-effector cells can lyse foreign cells directly, whereas others become killer (cytotoxic CD8+) cells. In addition, there are T-helper (Th; CD4+) and T-suppressor (CD8+) cells that function to activate or suppress, respectively, the response to a specific antigen. Because each of these T-cell subpopulations expresses both the T-cell (CD3) receptor and their own unique receptor antigen (CD4 or CD8), individual subpopulations can be depleted, enriched, or modulated by the use of antiserum or monoclonal antibody (mAb) immunosuppressive therapy. OKT3, an mAb directed against the CD3/T-cell receptor (TcR) complex, is used clinically in episodes of acute solid-organ graft rejection. An additional potential target for immunosuppressive therapy is the B7 family (B7-1, B7-2) of co-stimulatory molecules expressed on APCs. These molecules interact with CD28 on the T-cell surface and provide a crucial *second signal* for CD4+ T-cell activation.

Cell-to-Cell Interactions

Once confronted with an antigen, the response of the lymphocytes is complex. Multiple cell-to-cell interactions are required to produce the immune response. APCs, T cells, B cells, and cytokines all have a role. Critical to this response are the *professional APCs*—dendritic cells and macrophages—which act in a nonspecific manner to bind antigen and present it to T and B cells. Certain complex antigens may first need to be partially digested by phagocytic cells before the antigenic information can be presented to the lymphocyte for self and non-self recognition. In addition, activated APCs produce and secrete IL-1, IL-6, and IL-12, cytokines that function to further amplify the response and stimulate T- or B-lymphocyte activation.

The recognition of foreign cells is a complex process. One class of antigens on the surfaces of the graft cells stimulates certain T cells (Th cells, CD4+) to divide. The proliferating cells do not destroy the graft; rather, they activate another group of T cells (cytotoxic), which in turn damage the graft. Th cells are necessary for the development of the cell-mediated cytolytic activity of cytotoxic (CD8+) T cells. Th cell proliferation is an important site of amplification of the immune response, and these actively dividing cells are particularly vulnerable to antimetabolites. The activities of the Th cells are one of the major targets of clinical immunosuppression using drugs or mAbs. Studies on mouse CD4+ Th cells have defined two functional subsets on the basis of their pattern of cytokine synthesis. Th1 cells secrete IL-2 and interferon-gamma (IFN-γ); Th2 cells secrete IL-4, IL-5, and IL-10. Th1 cells induce macrophage activation, whereas Th2 cells control antibody-mediated responses. One subset of these Th cells can regulate the activities of the other.

Although the T- and B-cell systems have been presented as independent of each other, they cooperate to enhance immunity against a specific antigen. T cells develop *cellular immunity* in response to transplantation antigens, and in addition, Th cells assist clones of B cells to produce specific antibody against the graft antigens. Finally, some T cells act as suppressors for antibody formation. After immunity has been acquired, additional cellular cooperation contributes to destruction of the graft during the rejection episode.

As lymphocytes transform from resting to dividing cells, they pass through distinct phases common to all cells. Susceptibility to the commonly used immunosuppressive agents varies over the different cell phases. The small lymphocyte is in the resting or G_0 phase. Antigenic stimulation activates the cell and moves it into the first gap (or G_1) phase of the proliferative cycle. After the cell becomes committed to divide, DNA synthesis (S phase) occurs. The gap (G_2) between S phase and the final mitosis (M phase) is relatively short. After mitosis has occurred, the cells enter into the G_1 phase again, and the cell cycle is complete.

Differentiation appears to progress with cell division, and with each successive cycle, the cells become more and more capable of eliminating the activating antigen. After successive divisions, B cells become plasma cells, which are the most efficient producers of specific antibody. A similar progression occurs among T cells. T-cell activation occurs through the TcR complex (CD3), IL-2, and the IL-2 receptors (IL-2R)—also potential targets for therapeutic intervention. Activated T cells secrete IL-2, a cytokine that functions as a T-cell growth factor. The IL-2 then binds to IL-2R on resting T cells and stimulates cell mitosis and DNA synthesis via activation of the inositol phosphate pathway with protein kinase C. When the antigenic stimulus is no longer present, IL-2 is no longer produced, and T-cell activation and proliferation cease. Continued presence of antigen causes amplification of the T-cell response through IL-2. The presence of IL-2R for activation suggests a mediator-receptor system with negative feedback control. An understanding of the process of the activation of the T cell via the

IL-2–IL-2R receptor pathway allows a more focused approach for targeted immunosuppression.

Much of the susceptibility of lymphocytes to immunosuppression follows from the cellular changes produced by immune stimulation. The many biosynthetic events that occur make the lymphocytes vulnerable to errors and inhibitions caused by structural analogs, termed *antimetabolites*. *Alkylating agents* such as cyclophosphamide and *radiation* produce crosslinkages and breaks in DNA strands, which interfere with cell differentiation and division.

Graft Rejection

Graft rejection requires the participation of various combinations of immunologically specific and nonspecific cells. Three types of graft rejection are encountered. *Acute rejection* is the most common. It is mediated primarily by T-lymphocytes and first occurs between 1 and 3 weeks following solid-organ transplantation. *Hyperacute rejection* occurs during the first 1 to 2 days following transplantation and is mediated primarily by preformed cytotoxic antibody. *Chronic rejection* occurs over months and is probably caused by both T- and B-cell–mediated responses.

CLINICAL IMMUNOSUPPRESSION

Until the advent of cyclosporine, clinical immunosuppression relied primarily on agents or procedures with antiproliferative activity. These include the antimetabolites, alkylating agents, toxic antibiotics, and irradiation, all of which are used as cytoreductive agents in cancer chemotherapy. The introduction of cyclosporine and the mAb OKT3 radically changed the principles of therapeutic immunosuppression.

Adrenal Corticosteroids

Adrenal corticosteroids are the immunosuppressive agents used most commonly in clinical practice. Glucocorticoids have many diverse anti-inflammatory actions, which make them potent immunosuppressants. A profound decrease in the blood lymphocyte count occurs within the first 6 hours of steroid administration. Glucocorticoids cause emigration of recirculating T cells from the intravascular compartment to the lymphoid tissues with less effect on the distribution of B cells. Steroids also inhibit cytokine gene transcription in macrophages and the production and the effect of T-cell cytokines, which amplify the responses of the lymphocytes and macrophages. In addition, the ability of macrophages to respond to lymphocyte-derived signals such as migration inhibition factor and macrophage-activation factor is also blocked by steroids.

Toxic effects associated with the use of steroids include hypertension, weight gain, peptic ulceration, gastrointestinal bleeding, euphoric personality changes, cataract formation, hyperglycemia, pancreatitis, and osteoporosis with avascular necrosis of the femoral head and other bones.

Antiproliferative Agents

Antiproliferative agents inhibit the full expression of the immune response by preventing the differentiation and division of the immunocompetent lymphocytes after their encounter with antigen. They act in one of two ways: either they structurally resemble needed metabolites, or they combine with certain cellular components, such as DNA, and thereby interfere with molecular function. Alkylating agents (e.g., cyclophosphamide) and certain antibiotics include those compounds which combine with DNA and other cellular components. Because of their toxic effects, their use has been limited to bone marrow transplantation and as occasional substitutes for azathioprine.

Antimetabolites

The antimetabolites have a structural similarity to cell metabolites and either inhibit enzymes of that metabolic pathway or are incorporated during synthesis to produce *faulty* molecules. They include *purine, pyrimidine,* and *folic acid* analogs that are most effective against proliferating and differentiating cells. These drugs are given at the time of transplantation when the immunocompetent cells are first stimulated and are continued for the life of the graft.

Purine Analogs

Until recently, the purine analog *azathioprine* (Imuran) was the most widely used immunosuppressive drug in clinical organ transplantation. Azathioprine is 6-mercaptopurine (6-MP) plus a side chain to protect the labile sulfhydryl group. In the liver, the side chain is split off to form the active compound 6-MP. Full metabolic activity occurs in the cell with the addition of ribose-S_6-phosphate from phosphoribosyl pyrophosphate to form 6-MP ribonucleotide. The structural resemblance of this molecule to inosine monophosphate is obvious, and 6-MP ribonucleotide inhibits the enzymes that begin to convert inosine nucleotide to adenosine and guanosine monophosphate, thereby interfering with nucleic acid synthesis. The biologic activity of azathioprine and 6-MP is greatest when nucleic acid synthesis is most active (S phase). They inhibit the development of both humoral and cellular primary immunity by interfering with the differentiation and proliferation of the responding lymphocytes. The toxicity of azathioprine follows the same mechanisms and includes bone marrow suppression, causing leukopenia. Toxic effects in the liver also can result. Promising new purine biosynthesis inhibitors for therapy of organ rejection include mizoribine and mycophenolate mofetil (Cellcept).

T-Cell–Directed Immunosuppressants

CYCLOSPORINE. The discovery of the immunosuppressive properties of cyclosporine in 1972 contributed enormously to the development of the field of organ transplantation. It represented a completely new class of clinically important immunosuppressive agents. Many of its suppressive effects on T cells appear to be related to the inhibition of TcR-mediated activation events. It also inhibits cytokine production by Th cells *in vitro* and arrests development of mature CD4+ and CD8+ single-positive T cells in the thymus. Cyclosporine (Sandimmune) is a cyclic peptide produced by a fungus. It is nearly insoluble in aqueous solutions, and absorption from the gastrointestinal tract is slow and incomplete. There is a well-characterized enterohepatic cycle, and excretion of the drug is primarily through the bile. The mechanism of action of cyclosporine is relatively specific for T-lymphocytes. Other inflammatory cells are much less sensitive to its immunosuppressive effects.

Cyclosporine selectively inhibits activated T-lymphocytes and prevents these cells from manufacturing and/or releasing IL-2 and other cytokines. In addition, resting T-lymphocyte activation by IL-2 is blocked by cyclosporine. Since IL-2 is necessary for the expansion of activated clones of T cells, cyclosporine effectively inhibits the immune responses to grafted antigens without eliminating any of the clonal repertoire. Many kidney and other solid-organ transplantation trials have shown that cyclosporine induces potent immunosuppression without myelosuppression. The adverse effects of cyclosporine include hirsutism, tremor and other neurotoxic effects, hypertension, hyperkalemia, nephrotoxicity, hepatotoxicity, and diabetogenicity. The principal toxic effect is nephrotoxicity.

TACROLIMUS (FORMERLY FK 506). Tacrolimus is a potent new immunosuppressive agent that is also produced by a fungus. Its immunosuppressive effects are approximately 100 times greater than those of cyclosporine *in vitro*. Tacrolimus functions to (1) inhibit IL-2 production, (2) inhibit mixed-lymphocyte culture cellular proliferation, which is mediated by Th cells, (3) inhibit the generation of cytotoxic T cells, and (4) inhibit the appearance of IL-2R on human lymphocytes. *In vivo*, tacrolimus has been demonstrated to prolong the survival of MHC-disparate skin, cardiac, renal, hepatic, and small bowel allografts. It was approved in 1994 as an immunosuppressive agent for liver allograft recipients. Its adverse effects are similar to those of cyclosporine.

Lymphocyte Depletion Measures

A number of clinically important immunosuppressive agents are effective because they deplete the host of lymphocytes. As the mechanism of action of these agents becomes better understood, a more sophisticated classification system may evolve; for the present, however, antilymphocyte globulin (ALG), radiation, and mAb therapy appear to act by relatively nonselective lymphocyte depletion or inactivation.

ANTILYMPHOCYTE GLOBULIN (ALG). ALGs are produced when lymphocytes are injected into animals of a different species. ALG administration interferes most with the cell-mediated reactions—allograft rejection, tuberculin sensitivity, and the graft-versus-host reaction. ALG has a definite but lesser effect on T-cell–dependent antibody production. Lymphocytes coated with ALG are either lysed or cleared from the blood by reticuloendothelial cells in the liver and spleen. ALG may be administered prophylactically, during the early posttransplant period, or used effectively to reverse ongoing rejection. Allergic reactions to the antiserum itself are the most common clinical problem associated with the use of ALG. Urticaria, anaphylactoid reactions, and serum sickness, including joint pain, fever, and malaise, all follow development of immunity to the heterologous globulin. These reactions are reduced, however, in the presence of the other immunosuppressive drugs used in renal transplantation.

MONOCLONAL ANTIBODY (OKT3). In 1975 Kohler and Milstein developed the technology for somatic cell hybridization *(hybridoma formation)*, which could establish immortalized cell lines that each secrete a single, or *monoclonal, antibody* (mAb) in limitless supply. Subsequently, mAbs have been generated that react with T cells in general (OKT3, anti-CD3) and various T-cell subsets (OKT4, anti-CD4, OKT8, anti-CD8). OKT3, first used clinically in 1980, has become the most useful therapeutic mAb. It is used to treat established episodes of acute kidney, liver, heart, or heart-lung rejection. The prophylactic potency of regimens including OKT3 in renal transplantation also has been demonstrated. OKT3 binds to a site associated with the TCR (CD3) and functions to modulate the receptor and inactivate T-cell function. After prolonged use, OKT3 becomes less effective due to the production of antibody that binds to and effects the removal of circulating OKT3.

RADIATION. Radiation was probably the first agent used clinically to produce immunosuppression. Most of the immunosuppressive effects of irradiation are caused by changes produced in nucleic acids. DNA is particularly vulnerable; so, consequently, is cell replication. The effectiveness of radiation depends on the phase of the cell cycle. Cells in the M or G_2 phase are most sensitive to irradiation. The timing of radiation must be planned carefully for the desired immunosuppressive effect.

Other Immunosuppressive Approaches

BLOOD TRANSFUSION. Many studies have shown improved kidney graft survival with the use of allogeneic blood transfusions before transplantation, and some form of transfusion protocol became part of the preoperative regimen for most patients in renal failure who were awaiting a graft. For circumventing sensitization, azathioprine administered at the time of transfusion reduces the rate of sensitization to 5%. The exact mechanism by which transfusions exert a beneficial effect is unknown, but the following have been suggested: (1) clonal deletion/inactivation, (2) induction of suppressor/

regulatory cells, and (3) induction of blocking/anti-idiotypic antibodies.

CONSEQUENCES OF IMMUNOSUPPRESSION
Infection

An increased incidence of bacterial, fungal, and viral infections is observed in patients who receive nonspecific immunosuppressive agents. Because of its nonspecific method of action, immunosuppression understandably increases the risk of infection. Infection is the most common complication of immunosuppression, and overall it is the most common cause of death in transplant recipients. Most of the deaths early in the history of kidney transplantation occurred in the first few posttransplant months as a result of highly pathogenic bacterial infections. More recently, improved antibiotics and greater skill in immunosuppression therapy have shifted the spectrum of organisms. There has been a relative increase in lethal infection caused by opportunistic organisms that are normally weakly pathogenic. Antibiotics eradicate the more aggressive bacteria, but opportunistic fungal, protozoal, and viral organisms remain free to colonize the susceptible transplant patient.

FUNGAL AND PROTOZOAL. The opportunistic organisms, which are normally eliminated by cellular defense mechanisms, can now proliferate with the relative T-cell depression. Fungi are prominent opportunists. *Candida albicans* infections are probably the most common. *Aspergillus* species are probably the second most common cause of fungal infection and typically produce upper lobe pulmonary cavities. *Rhizopus oryzae, Histoplasma capsulatum,* and *Cryptococcus neoformans* also invade the lung, and *C. neoformans* occasionally causes meningitis. *Pneumocytis carinii,* more commonly seen in patients undergoing cancer chemotherapy, usually causes an alveolar infiltrate with disproportionate dyspnea and cyanosis.

VIRAL. Viral infections appear to be almost ubiquitous in kidney transplant recipients. The herpes group of DNA viruses is most commonly present. Cytomegalovirus infection also has become a serious clinical problem with potentially lethal consequences.

Malignancy

The incidence of *de novo* malignancy is increased in recipients of transplants, but the rate is not sufficiently high to contraindicate the transplant procedure. The rate of development of malignancy in patients surviving renal transplantation may be as high as 30 times that in a similar normal population. The most frequent cancers include lymphomas, reticulum cell sarcomas, and squamous and basal cell carcinomas.

EXPERIMENTAL IMMUNOSUPPRESSION

The currently available immunosuppressive agents have revolutionized the field of transplantation. However, because they act in a nonspecific manner to suppress all aspects of immune function, associated toxic effects result. Consequently, investigative efforts have been directed at finding an improved, more specific method of immunosuppression. The complexity of the immune response gives rise to the hope that many potential points of vulnerability in activation and deployment of the cells responsible for the rejection reaction exist. Potential approaches include (1) more specific mAbs, e.g., to activated T cells that bear the IL-2R alpha chain (anti-IL-2R mAbs), (2) anti-intercellular adhesion molecule Abs, (3) co-stimulatory molecule blockade, e.g., of B7 molecules on APCs using the CTLA4Ig fusion protein, (4) anticytokine mAbs, (5) immunosuppression by specific antigens, (6) donor-specific transplantation tolerance, and (7) generation of specific regulatory cells to halt the rejection reaction. The goal of each of these approaches is to induce donor-specific transplantation tolerance yet maintain host immunocompetence.

VII

Organ Preservation
Folkert O. Belzer, M.D., and James H. Southard, Ph.D.

The objective of organ preservation is to preserve viability for a period of time that will allow maximal use of all suitable cadaveric organs. These include liver, pancreas, kidneys, heart, lungs, and small bowel. The time of preservation currently needed for optimal use of organs on a national basis is about 24 to 36 hours. Within that time, most organs can be tissue matched with the recipient (if needed, as in the case of the kidney), the recipient prepared, and the organ shipped to the recipient's hospital. The incidence of delayed graft function or primary nonfunction with the need for retransplantation is usually not the result of poor preservation if the times are kept within these limits. This degree of preservation is available for kidney, liver, and pancreas when preserved with the University of Wisconsin solution (UW solution). However, the heart and lung are best preserved for only about 4 to 8 hours.

The method most often used to preserve organs is simple cold storage. This involves flushing out the blood from the vascular system. This is now often accomplished *in situ* because most organ donors are used for multiple organs. Once removed from the body, the organs are usually "back table flushed" with the preservative at about 4° C and stored at 4° C until transplanted. This method of preservation (cold ische-

See the corresponding chapter or part in the *Textbook of Surgery*, 15th edition, pp. 455–461, for a more detailed discussion of this topic, including a comprehensive list of references.

mia) is successful because of hypothermia, which slows down catabolic reactions that lead to functional and structural tissue degradation. In addition, during cold ischemia, ATP is catabolized and membrane ion pumps cease operation. Thus the cells of cold-stored organs gain water and volume. Tissue edema is suppressed by impermeants in the cold storage solution. The most suitable impermeant appears to be anionic, such as lactobionate, which effectively prevents cell swelling in all tissues examined to date. Lactobionate is a key component of the UW solution. In addition to suppression of cell swelling, preservatives are effective by providing the cells with cofactors or substrates that facilitate regeneration of functions upon transplantation (reperfusion). Glutathione appears important because of its antioxidant properties and suppression of oxygen free-radical injury to the reperfused organs.

Simple cold storage is successful for only a finite amount of time; probably the limits have been reached for most organs and are around 3 days. For longer-term preservation and better quality, continuous perfusion is the method of choice. This method is used clinically only for the kidney and only in about 20% of transplants. This method, however, gives better early graft function and also may improve long-term outcome in kidney transplant patients. Perfusion is done by continuously pumping a perfusate (UW gluconate) through the kidney at 4° to 8° C and at a low pressure (40 to 50 mm. Hg). This method continuously delivers oxygen and substrates to the organ, stimulates metabolism (ATP synthesis), and allows the organ to remain viable for up to 5 to 7 days.

Current methods for preserving the kidney, liver, and pancreas are sufficient, and very few organs are wasted because of lack of sufficient preservation capabilities. The heart and lung are more difficult to preserve, although it is unclear exactly why. In the future, methods to preserve these organs need to be developed.

VIII

Liver Transplantation
Pierre A. Clavien, M.D., Ph.D.,
and Allan D. Kirk, M.D., Ph.D.

Liver transplantation has evolved in the past decade from an experimental procedure to an accepted, effective therapy for end-stage liver diseases. Continued improvements in peri-

---

See the corresponding chapter or part in the *Textbook of Surgery*, 15th edition, pp. 461–473, for a more detailed discussion of this topic, including a comprehensive list of references.

operative management and operative technique are being realized with significant improvements in outcome.

INDICATIONS FOR TRANSPLANTATION

The success of orthotopic liver transplantation (OLT) is closely tied to the rational selection of patients most likely to benefit from the procedure. The most important prognostic factor affecting survival is the medical condition of the recipient at the time of OLT. The specific indications for liver transplantation are becoming more standardized.

Several diseases are now accepted as amenable to cure by transplantation. Cholestatic diseases of the liver, including primary and secondary biliary cirrhosis and primary sclerosing cholangitis, are the most successfully treated diseases by OLT. Operative survival is greater than 90%, and 5-year survival is approximately 80%. Several metabolic diseases are treated successfully with OLT, including alpha$_1$-antitrypsin deficiency, Wilson's disease, hemochromatosis, Crigler-Najjar syndrome, tyrosinemia, primary hyperoxaluria, and familial homozygous hypercholesterolemia. OLT for alcoholic cirrhosis is becoming an increasingly accepted procedure. Survival of grafts and patients is not significantly different from that of other favorable indications, and disease recurrence (return to heavy alcohol use) is approximately 12%. Extensive preoperative evaluation is required, and patient selection is critical. Another rapidly increasing indication for OLT is hepatitis caused by the hepatitis C virus. Transplantation is pursued for symptomatic infection only. Reinfection at almost 90% with active recurrent hepatitis occurring in approximately 50% may temper current enthusiasm for this indication. Fulminant hepatic failure clearly is an appropriate setting for OLT if cerebral edema and other end-organ dysfunctions are reversible. Despite the dramatic disease progression, these patients have very acceptable results from OLT (5-year survival of 60%).

Transplantation for chronic hepatitis B virus (HBV) cirrhosis remains a controversial topic primarily due to the discouraging reinfection rate of over 80%, a high rate of clinical hepatitis recurrence (60% at 1 year), and high related mortality (30% at 1 year and 52% at 5 years). Although generally contraindicated, transplantation may be appropriate in the setting of a specific clinical trial involving antiviral prophylaxis for viral DNA–negative patients. Transplantation for primary and metastatic cancer has been associated with high recurrence of tumor. Only selective, localized, and asymptomatic primary liver tumor may represent a reasonable indication.

The most common indication for OLT in children is biliary atresia. The general course of action is early (neonatal) Kasai portoenterostomy, with transplantation reserved for those children developing hepatic insufficiency despite a Kasai. The remaining standard indications for pediatric transplantation also occur in the adult population.

DONOR SELECTION

Immediate function of a transplanted liver is imperative. Failure of a graft to function at all after a technically successful transplantation is known as *primary nonfunction* (PNF). The only treatment for this condition is retransplantation within 24 to 72 hours. Factors contributing to the development of PNF include parenchymal insufficiency unrecognized at the time of harvest, graft injury during the harvest or cadaver resuscitation, preservation injury, or prolonged cold ischemia (>24 hours with UW solution), prolonged rewarming time (>90 minutes), and reperfusion injury after implantation. Several factors aid in the prediction of PNF. The most widely noted is the estimated parenchymal fat content. Expert retrieval of a donor liver is critical for a successful OLT, with particular care taken to optimize the preharvest resuscitation of the heart-beating cadaver. Procurement of the organ involves complete mobilization of the liver, with great attention paid to the vascular supply and preservation of aberrant hepatic arteries. Once mobilization is completed, perfusion with cold UW solution is initiated.

THE OPERATION

Few surgical procedures require the fastidious attention to technical detail required in liver transplantation. Technical errors are translated directly into infectious complications or marginal biliary function. Thus transplantation should be performed only by surgeons proficient in the procedure. Implantation begins with the suprahepatic caval anastomosis, followed by the infrahepatic caval anastomosis. The operation then proceeds to the portal anastomosis. Following all venous connections, the liver is reperfused. Anastomosis of the hepatic artery is the final vascular step in the procedure. The biliary reconstruction remains an area of debate. Options include Roux-en-Y choledochojejunostomy, or choledochocholedochostomy with or without externalized T-tube stents. Postoperative management in the ICU is similar to that following any major procedure. Liberal use of the Doppler ultrasound to evaluate the hepatic artery is mandatory with early graft dysfunction.

IMMUNOLOGIC MANAGEMENT

Many concepts of immunologic management following OLT must be considered separately because established concepts of donor-host interaction following kidney or heart transplantation do not apply to OLT. HLA matching is currently not temporally feasible before liver transplantation. Although HLA matching decreases the cellular rejection rate, it increases the disease recurrence rate for viral and autoimmune diseases. Similarly, the lymphocytotoxic crossmatch is not used prospectively before liver transplantation. Hyperacute rejection is rarely seen even in the face of ABO incompatibility.

As with other allografts, T-cell-mediated destruction of the liver is inevitable without immunosuppressive therapy. The primary targets for T-cell recognition are HLA antigens on the biliary epithelium and vascular endothelium. This rejection, termed *acute cellular rejection,* develops in most cases within the first 6 weeks. More than half of patients develop at least one episode of acute rejection. Symptoms are nonspecific and often include mild intermittent fever and general malaise with alteration in liver tests. The diagnosis should be confirmed by liver biopsy. Most episodes (90%) are readily reversible given prompt recognition and initiation of antirejection therapy.

Chronic rejection, in contrast, occurs over a period of months to years and often is refractory to treatment. Histologically, it appears as a paucity of bile duct epithelium without a significant lymphocytic infiltrate. An obliterative vasculopathy also can occur with parenchymal fibrosis. The time course, histology, and refractory nature of chronic rejection suggest that the mechanisms of graft destruction involve several limbs of the immune system, and the resulting exposure to soluble factors, including fibrogenic cytokines, eventually takes its toll on the fragile epithelium. Chronic rejection often requires retransplantation.

Manipulation of the immune system is required to avoid graft loss from rejection, although maintenance immunosuppression after liver transplantation can be comparatively low, with many patients weaned to little or no immunosuppression over a period of years. Generally, immunosuppression includes cyclosporine and prednisone with or without azathioprine. A recent addition to liver transplant pharmacology has been the drug tacrolimus (FK506). This agent has a similar mechanism of action as cyclosporine and has thus been used as a replacement for this drug.

The importance of viral infection, particularly CMV, in liver transplant patients cannot be overstated. *De novo* infection or latent viral reactivation of pathogens is directly related to the intensity of the immunosuppressive regimen employed. Most transplant centers have incorporated antiviral prophylaxis with ganciclovir, acyclovir, and antiviral immune globulin into their protocols.

OUTCOMES

Diseases treated by OLT are by definition terminal with few exceptions and, as such, are lethal without hepatic replacement. Operative survival now exceeds 90% for first grafts. Retransplant-free survival has steadily improved in the past 10 years and is now 73% at 1 year for all transplants. The 5-year survival reflecting transplantation before ganciclovir is approximately 60%, and improvements of 2% to 3% per year have been made each year since 1987. Predicted actuarial 5-year survival for transplants performed in 1994 is over 70%. The likelihood of cure is associated with the primary liver disease. Metabolic and cholestatic diseases are generally resolved, as are the physiologic disorders of alcoholic cirrhosis. Unfortunately, viral infections remain generally uncured by liver replacement. Obviously, no extrahepatic malignancy can be cured by OLT, and the potential for cure in patients with intrahepatic malignancy is solely related to the presence or absence of metastatic disease at the time of recipient hepatectomy.

The quality of a patient's life following OLT is the most important issue in judging the validity of the procedure. Successful transplantation allows a return to a normal active lifestyle free from the metabolic and hematologic complications of hepatic failure or portal hypertension. Currently, 60% of patients undergoing OLT return to work within the first year.

Despite these good results, the procedure involves considerable morbidity. Most patients have some complication that deviates from an ideal recovery. All patients also accept the trade of their liver disease for the "disease" of immunosuppression. This factor, however, is less intrusive for liver transplant patients than for other solid organ recipients, given their reduced need for immunosuppression. Negative outcomes are generally remedied by prompt recognition of problems and aggressive correction.

Several complications deserve particular attention. Primary nonfunction presents as a complete lack of liver function from the time of reperfusion. The patient develops encephalopathy, increased intracranial pressure, coagulopathy, hyperbilirubinemia, and hypertransaminasemia. Aggressive supportive therapy and retransplantation are required within 72 hours. Hepatic artery thrombosis remains a complication, especially in children. This presents as a rapid rise in serum transaminase levels. Failure to restore flow causes graft loss. Stricture or stenosis of the hepatic artery generally presents with a lesser degree of metabolic change later in the postoperative course. Another cause of dearterialization is bile leak resulting from necrosis of the hepatic duct. An additional vascular complication that is less frequent but equally devastating is early thrombosis of the portal vein. Any suspected change in hepatic function requires immediate evaluation of the hepatic vasculature by Doppler ultrasound followed by either re-exploration or a confirmatory arteriogram. Biliary complications suggest vascular compromise. Both leaks and strictures can occur regardless of the method of reconstruction. Percutaneous or endoscopic management is generally considered an acceptable first alternative, but reoperation should not be avoided for appropriate lesions at the expense of hepatic function or cholangitis.

IX

Pancreas Transplantation
Hans W. Sollinger, M.D., Ph.D., and Stuart J. Knechtle, M.D.

HISTORICAL ASPECTS

1959	Brooks and Gifford: Pancreas transplantation in a large animal model.
1960–1970	Dejode, Howard, Reemtsma, Merkel, Lillehei, Largiader, Bergan: Technical development of pancreas transplantation in animals.
1966	Kelly, Lillehei: First pancreas transplant in man.
1973	Gliedman: Exocrine drainage to ureter.
1974	Groth: Exocrine drainage to small bowel.
1977	Dubernard: Duct injection with polymers.
1982	Sollinger: Bladder drainage.

INDICATIONS FOR PANCREAS TRANSPLANTATION

Pancreas transplantation is performed in three groups of patients with insulin-dependent diabetes mellitus.

Pancreas Transplantation Alone

The procedure is performed in patients who do not have renal failure.

ADVANTAGES. (1) None or few secondary diabetic complications; (2) good surgical risk; (3) early diabetic complications potentially reversible.

DISADVANTAGES. (1) Major surgical procedure; (2) side effects of immunosuppressive therapy; (3) difficulty diagnosing rejection due to poor monitoring tests.

Pancreas Transplantation After a Successful Kidney Transplant

ADVANTAGES. Same immunosuppression as kidney transplant.

DISADVANTAGES. (1) Major surgical procedure; (2) dia-

See the corresponding chapter or part in the *Textbook of Surgery,* 15th edition, pp. 473–477, for a more detailed discussion of this topic, including a comprehensive list of references.

betic complications already advanced; (3) difficulty diagnosing rejection due to poor monitoring tests.

Simultaneous Pancreas-Kidney Transplantation

ADVANTAGES. (1) One surgical procedure; (2) same immunosuppression; (3) good results.

DISADVANTAGES. Already advanced diabetic complications.

ORGAN PROCUREMENT AND PRESERVATION

The pancreas can be procured alone or in combination with the liver. In the United States, combined pancreas-liver procurement has become increasingly frequent for meeting the demand for both liver and pancreas grafts. After *in situ* flushing with Belzer-UW (University of Wisconsin) solution, both organs are removed *en bloc* and divided *ex vivo*. The portal vein is divided midway between the pancreas and the liver, and the arterial blood supply of the pancreas is reconstructed with an iliac artery Y-graft. Belzer-UW solution is the best preservation solution, as demonstrated by a low rate of vascular thrombosis and graft pancreatitis. Three-year graft survival is 10% to 20% better in grafts preserved with UW solution compared with other solutions. The maximal preservation time with the use of UW solution is approximately 30 hours.

SURGICAL TECHNIQUE

The pancreas may be transplanted as a whole organ (currently preferred technique) or as a segment (body and tail). Three surgical techniques are most commonly used. They differ in the way exocrine pancreas secretions are managed.

Enteric Drainage: Anastomosis of Pancreatic Duct to Bowel

ADVANTAGES. (1) No metabolic problems; (2) no urinary problems.

DISADVANTAGES. (1) High rate of septic intra-abdominal complications; (2) difficult to make diagnosis of rejection.

Duct Occlusion: The Pancreatic Duct is Injected with Polymers

ADVANTAGES. (1) Surgically simple; (2) low infection rate.

DISADVANTAGES. (1) High thrombosis rate; (2) high fistula rate; (3) difficult to make diagnosis of rejection.

Bladder Drainage and Anastomosis of Pancreatic Duct to Bladder

ADVANTAGES. (1) Safe, low infection rate; (2) urinary amylase used to make diagnosis of rejection; (3) best results.

DISADVANTAGES. (1) Metabolic acidosis; (2) urinary problems: hematuria, urinary tract infection, urethritis.

Currently, bladder drainage is the most popular technique. Worldwide more than 85% of all pancreas transplants are performed with bladder drainage.

DIAGNOSIS OF REJECTION

The early diagnosis of pancreas allograft rejection is difficult. Methods and laboratory tests for the diagnosis of rejection are as follows:

Methods	Comments
Serum glucose	Specific but late marker
Urinary amylase	Early marker; specific; large fluctuations difficult to interpret
	Only possible with bladder drainage
Serum anodal trypsinogen	Specific early marker; not widely available; difficult test
Pancreas biopsy (percutaneous)	Technically difficult; yield is only 50%; possible complications
Pancreas biopsy (transcystoscopic)	Requires general anesthesia; special expertise necessary; 85% specificity
Nuclear perfusion scan	Useful confirmatory test when used in conjunction with other tests
Ultrasonography, computed tomography, magnetic resonance imaging	Not proven to be useful in diagnosis of rejection

INFLUENCE ON METABOLIC AND SECONDARY DIABETIC COMPLICATIONS

Benefits that may be provided by a well-functioning pancreas transplant are (1) insulin independence, (2) nearly normal blood glucose tolerance test result, (3) normalization of HgA$_1$ C, (4) prevention of progression of diabetic nephropathy, (5) improvement of peripheral and autonomic neuropathy, and (6) improvement in microcirculation.

Not all these beneficial effects of pancreas transplantation on secondary diabetic complications have been proved. No study has conclusively demonstrated a beneficial effect of pancreas transplantation on diabetic retinopathy.

X

Cardiac and Cardiopulmonary Homotransplants
R. Morton Bolman III, M.D.

CLINICAL CARDIAC TRANSPLANTATION

Originally introduced in 1967 by Barnard, clinical cardiac transplantation has recently enjoyed a great increase in popularity owing to the availability of the immunosuppressive agent cyclosporine. Approximately 1500 procedures have been performed each year from 1986 through 1989 as a result of this growth.

Recipient Selection

Individuals from newborn age up to the age of 60 years can be considered candidates for cardiac transplantation. They experience symptoms of Class IV congestive heart failure (NYHA) and must have exhausted all conventional medical and surgical options. Fixed, irreversible deficits in extracardiac organ function contraindicate transplantation, since they would not be expected to be corrected by improved cardiac function. Psychosocial screening is important for ensuring proper compliance with prescribed medical regimens after transplantation. From a hemodynamic standpoint, the most critical determinant of operative risk is the pulmonary vascular resistance. If the pulmonary vascular resistance is greater than 5 to 6 Wood units and cannot be pharmacologically reversed with manipulations in the catheterization laboratory that could be duplicated at the time of transplantation, orthotopic transplantation would have a substantial operative risk. Patients must harbor no active malignancy or infection, and active peptic ulceration is a contraindication as well (Table 1).

Donor Selection

The criteria for cardiac donor selection are outlined in Table 2. Individuals up to the age of 55 and occasionally 60 years with demonstrable normal function of the heart and absence of severe coronary artery disease can be suitable donors. Useful on-site screening tests include electrocardiography and echocardiography. Donor and recipient must be ABO-compatible, and a prospective crossmatch is not necessary provided

---

See the corresponding chapter or part in the *Textbook of Surgery*, 15th edition, pp. 478–487, for a more detailed discussion of this topic, including a comprehensive list of references.

TABLE 1. Recipient Selection Criteria for Heart Transplantation

Age newborn to 60 years
Irremediable cardiac disease—Class IV NYHA
Normal function or reversible dysfunction of kidneys, liver,
    lungs, central nervous system
Pulmonary vascular resistance less than 6–8 Wood units or
    pharmacologically reversible
Absence of:
    Active malignancy or infection
    Recent pulmonary infarction
    Severe peripheral or cerebrovascular disease

the recipient is reactive to 10% or less of a panel of randomly
selected HLA types (panel-reactive antibodies less than 10%).
Donor and recipient weight should be matched to within 20%
to 50%. Cardiac allografts can be procured at a distance,
provided the period of graft ischemia is 4 hours or less between cross-clamping the aorta in the donor and restoring
perfusion in the recipient. Donor hearts are preserved with 1
liter of crystalloid cardioplegia coupled with copious topical
cooling.

The Operation

The recipient operation is not initiated until the donor heart
has been visualized by the procurement team and found to
be suitable for transplantation. At that point, the recipient is
placed under anesthesia and made ready for transplantation.
The recipient heart is removed as the donor heart arrives, and
implantation ensues with left and right atrium, pulmonary
artery, and aorta being anastomosed between donor and recipient. Careful hemostasis is mandatory because the complications attending excessive bleeding are potentially severe in
the immunosuppressed host.

Immunosuppression

Prophylaxis against allograft rejection in most centers consists of "triple therapy," the combination of cyclosporine, aza-

TABLE 2. Donor Selection Criteria for Heart Transplantation

Age less than 60 years
Minimal pressor support
Negative cardiac history
Normal electrocardiogram
Normal echocardiogram
ABO compatibility
Size within 20%–50% of recipient
Negative T-cell crossmatch if panel-reactive antibodies 10% or
    greater
Negative serologic tests for hepatitis, HIV infection

thioprine, and prednisone. This regimen has been associated with the lowest reported incidence of cardiac rejection and has yielded excellent rates of survival and a low incidence of infection.

Another approach being employed at some centers is that of "induction therapy" utilizing the murine monoclonal antibody OKT3, followed by administration of cyclosporine, azathioprine, and prednisone. Prednisone can then be discontinued in some of these individuals.

Complications

ACUTE ALLOGRAFT REJECTION. Diagnosis of cardiac rejection rests on the judicious application of the endomyocardial biopsy guided by clinical indicators such as cardiac arrhythmia, hypotension, and fever. The endomyocardial biopsy remains the standard despite the proposal of numerous noninvasive methods. Rejection is treated with 3 days of pulse methylprednisolone followed by rebiopsy.

INFECTION. All patients who are cytomegalovirus seronegative before transplantation receive exclusively cytomegalovirus-negative blood and blood products. All patients receive nystatin (Mycostatin) and high-dose acyclovir for 3 months and trimethoprim-sulfamethoxazole indefinitely following the transplant procedure. Perioperative wound prophylaxis consists of a second-generation cephalosporin and vancomycin coupled with copious intraoperative vancomycin irrigation. This regimen, coupled with a low incidence of rejection experienced as the result of triple therapy has yielded a very low incidence of serious infection. For example, none of the author's patients has had mediastinitis or a sternal wound infection.

TRANSPLANT CORONARY DISEASE. A dreaded sequela of cardiac transplantation is that of transplant coronary artery disease. This entity continues to plague cardiac transplant recipients and will become an increasing problem with the passage of time. Olivari has reported the University of Minnesota's experience in this regard. Defined as any decrease in luminal coronary artery diameter, transplant coronary artery disease findings were demonstrated in 8% of patients at 1 year, 24% at 2 years, and 29% at 3 years. This phenomenon is thought to represent a manifestation of chronic rejection, and close surveillance is required in the form of yearly coronary angiography. Treatment consists of percutaneous transluminal coronary angioplasty or, if severe, retransplantation.

Clinical Outcomes

In 163 patients transplanted at the University of Minnesota since the introduction of triple therapy in 1983, actuarial patient survival of 78% at 5 years has been observed. Eighty-six per cent of patients are free of rejection at 1 year after transplantation, by far the lowest reported incidence in the literature.

Cardiac Transplantation Summary

Since its inception in 1967, cardiac transplantation has progressed steadily, and today this procedure has earned its rightful place in the treatment of end-stage heart disease. Improved patient selection, coupled with effective and safe immunosuppressive strategies, has restored health to patients formerly doomed to a premature death. Serious problems remain, which include a shortage of donor organs and the problem of transplant coronary artery disease, currently the number one factor limiting long-term survival.

CARDIOPULMONARY TRANSPLANTATION

Recipient Selection

Certain patients have diseases of the heart and lungs that require replacement of these organs. Recipient selection criteria are outlined in Table 3. The most common indications for this procedure are primary pulmonary hypertension and Eisenmenger's syndrome. Patients should be severely limited by their disease and unable to work or attend school, and most are on supplemental oxygen therapy. These individuals must fulfill all the other criteria for transplantation as outlined in the section on heart transplantation.

Donor Selection

A small percentage of donors suitable for transplantation (10% to 20%) also have lungs that can be transplanted. Criteria for suitable cardiopulmonary donors are listed in Table 4. In addition to normal cardiac function, the heart-lung donor must have normal gas exchange with low airway pressures. The chest radiograph should be normal and pulmonary secretions minimal. Donor and recipient are matched according to ABO type as well as on the basis of results of an HLA antibody screen. Size matching is also important. Current techniques of preservation allow successful transplantation following up to 4 hours of *ex vivo* preservation. Most programs employ the technique of cardioplegic arrest of the heart coupled with pulmonary artery flushing with a modified Euro-Collins' solution, supplemented by copious topical cooling.

TABLE 3. Recipient Selection Criteria for Cardiopulmonary Transplantation

Age less than 50 years
End-stage pulmonary vascular or parenchymal disease
   associated with severe right ventricular compromise and/or
   severe tricuspid regurgitation
Absence of:
   Other nonreversible organ dysfunction or disease
   Major prior thoracotomy or sternotomy
   High-dose steroid therapy

TABLE 4. Donor Selection Criteria for Cardiopulmonary Transplantation

Close size match—donor smaller than or same size as recipient

Satisfactory gas exchange—arterial $Po_2 > 400$ mm. Hg on Fio_2 of 1.0

Normal lung compliance—peak airway pressure of 30 mm. Hg with normal tidal volume

Clear chest radiograph

Absence of purulent pulmonary secretions

The Operation

The recipient is placed on cardiopulmonary bypass when word is received that the donor is stable and the organs are satisfactory. Cardiopulmonary bypass is then begun and the heart removed. Pedicles of pericardium containing the phrenic nerves are isolated, and windows are created bilaterally through the posterior pericardium to allow passage of the donor lungs to their respective pleural cavities. The diseased lungs are then removed, and hemostasis is secured in the posterior mediastinum. The trachea is isolated and transected just above the carina. The donor heart-lung block is then passed into the chest, and implantation proceeds with anastomoses of trachea, right atrium, and aorta.

Immunosuppression

Recipients of cardiopulmonary allografts receive triple therapy similar to that of heart transplant recipients with a few modifications. Corticosteroid therapy is administered perioperatively for 24 hours and then withheld for the ensuing 14 days for optimization of airway healing. Antilymphocyte globulin is administered for 3 to 5 days, during which cyclosporine levels are maintained deliberately at subtherapeutic levels for maintenance of normal renal function. After 14 days, prednisone is begun at a low dose, and maintenance therapy consists of triple-drug immunosuppression as outlined previously.

Complications

REJECTION. Most recipients experience an episode of rejection within the first 2 weeks. Heart and lungs do not necessarily reject synchronously; therefore, the heart biopsy is not a reliable means of monitoring lung rejection. Diagnosis of lung rejection rests on clinical grounds supplemented by transbronchial biopsy. Symptoms may include fever, breathlessness, malaise, and signs of decreased oxygenation and radiographic infiltrates. Treatment is with pulse corticosteroid therapy for a period of 3 days followed by reassessment.

INFECTION. Prophylaxis of infection in heart-lung recipients is identical to that described for the heart transplant recipient. Most infections following cardiopulmonary transplantation are pulmonary, and any evidence of infection warrants urgent evaluation and treatment.

BRONCHIOLITIS OBLITERANS. The most serious complication that occurs in recipients of cardiopulmonary transplantation is bronchiolitis obliterans. Thought to represent a form of chronic rejection analogous to transplant coronary artery disease, this entity can occur a few months following transplant. It occurs in 30% to 50% of cardiopulmonary recipients, and attempts to reverse its course in most cases have proved futile.

Clinical Outcomes

Since the pioneering work of Reitz, investigators have continued to develop the techniques of cardiopulmonary transplantation, including refined patient selection and improved postoperative management. Comparing patients transplanted between March 1981 and February 1986 with patients transplanted subsequent to that period, one notes that improvements have been demonstrated in short-term and long-term survival, with decreased incidence of bronchiolitis obliterans in the later group as well. Improved results are attributed to the routine employment of triple-drug immunosuppression and more aggressive surveillance for rejection and infection, including routine application of bronchoscopy with bronchoalveolar lavage and transbronchial biopsy.

Cardiopulmonary Transplantation Summary

Owing to severe restrictions in donor availability, relatively small numbers of these procedures have been performed in the United States each year. Despite this, gratifying results in those who do well have inspired further efforts in the field. Cardiopulmonary transplantation remains a therapeutic option for selected individuals for whom no other conventional or transplant alternative is available. Intensive research continues in the area of chronic rejection of the heart-lung allograft. This remains the single greatest impediment to long-term survival in these patients.

XI

Lung Transplantation

R. Sudhir Sundaresan, M.D.,
and Joel D. Cooper, M.D.

Lung transplantation has undergone dramatic growth recently as a treatment for end-stage lung disease. It was employed initially as a "rescue" maneuver in debilitated patients after they developed ventilator dependency and almost uniformly met with failure. However, with improvements in recipient and donor selection criteria, lung preservation techniques, operative techniques, and immunosuppression, lung transplantation currently enjoys considerably better success.

INDICATIONS FOR LUNG TRANSPLANTATION

1. Obstructive lung disease [chronic obstructive pulmonary disease (COPD) and alpha₁-antitrypsin deficiency emphysema]
2. Cystic fibrosis (CF)
3. Restrictive lung disease [idiopathic pulmonary fibrosis (IPF)]
4. Pulmonary vascular disease [primary pulmonary hypertension (PPH) and Eisenmenger's syndrome]

PREOPERATIVE CONSIDERATIONS IN LUNG TRANSPLANTATION. Lung transplantation is offered to certain patients with clinically and physiologically severe lung disease, where other medical or surgical therapy is ineffective or unavailable, and where life expectancy is estimated at less than 24 months. The patient must be ambulatory with the potential to participate in a cardiopulmonary rehabilitation program and demonstrate compliance for future follow-up and therapy. Contraindications to lung transplantation include the acutely unstable patient, significant disease of other organ systems, uncontrolled sepsis or neoplasm, current smoking status, significant psychological or social problems, and demonstrated noncompliance with treatment.

CHOICE OF TRANSPLANT PROCEDURE. Both single and bilateral lung transplantation can be applied to obstructive lung disease, restrictive lung disease, and pulmonary vascular disease. However, in cystic fibrosis patients (and any patients with diffuse bilateral pulmonary sepsis), bilateral lung replacement must be performed to obviate the septic complications that would ensue from retention of one septic native lung in an immunosuppressed patient.

THE LUNG TRANSPLANTATION PROCEDURE. Single lung transplantation is accomplished through a posterolateral thoracotomy, while bilateral lung replacement is achieved using a bilateral sequential single lung technique through a

---

See the corresponding chapter or part in the *Textbook of Surgery*, 15th edition, pp. 487–497, for a more detailed discussion of this topic, including a comprehensive list of references.

transverse thoracosternotomy incision ("clam shell") approach. Cardiopulmonary bypass is necessary in all lung transplants for pulmonary vascular disease. Otherwise, bypass is used on a selective basis when insufficient ventilation, oxygenation, or perfusion is encountered intraoperatively. The technique of lung implantation has become standardized, with the order of anastomoses being bronchus, artery, and then vein.

POSTOPERATIVE MANAGEMENT. Lung transplant recipients are monitored postoperatively in the intensive care unit. Pain control is achieved initially using an epidural catheter and later by patient-controlled analgesia and oral agents. Mechanical ventilation with positive end-expiratory pressure (PEEP) is used except in single lung transplants for emphysema. Oxygenation is optimized by minimizing fluid administration, aggressive use of diuretics, PEEP, chest physical therapy and posturing, and frequent bronchoscopies. Weaning from mechanical ventilation is usually accomplished within 2 to 3 days of transplantation. Infection control must include the following:

1. In CF patients, antibiotics are directed at the recipient's organisms based on preoperative culture and sensitivity data.

2. Otherwise, antibiotic prophylaxis consists of cefazolin 1 gm. IV every 8 hours and is modified based on donor bronchial washings.

3. Prophylaxis for opportunistic pathogens including herpes, *Pneumocystis,* and *Candida.*

4. CMV prophylaxis when CMV-negative recipients receive CMV-positive grafts.

IMMUNOSUPPRESSION. Most use a triple-drug protocol combining cyclosporine, azathioprine, and steroids.

SURVEILLANCE OF THE LUNG TRANSPLANT RECIPIENT. Surveillance is necessary because these immunosuppressed patients are at ongoing risk of rejection and septic complications despite their appearing clinically well and physiologically stable. Surveillance includes clinical follow-up, regular pulmonary function testing (focusing on FEV_1), regular chest radiographs, and fiberoptic bronchoscopy with bronchoalveolar lavage (BAL) and transbronchial lung biopsy (TBLB). BAL is useful in identifying graft infection, while TBLB is necessary to document acute rejection and to differentiate rejection from CMV infection. Open-lung biopsy is necessary occasionally when these studies are inconclusive.

LUNG ALLOGRAFT REJECTION. Acute lung allograft rejection is characterized by nonspecific symptoms (malaise, low-grade fever), a slight decline in oxygenation and spirometry, and a hilar or basal infiltrate on chest radiograph. Its presence is confirmed by TBLB, and the usual treatment is short-term high-dose corticosteroids (methylprednisolone 500 to 1000 mg. daily for 3 days, sometimes along with an increase in the oral prednisone dose). Monoclonal antibodies (OKT3) or antithymocyte globulin is used in severe or refractory cases.

Chronic lung allograft rejection manifests as a clinical syndrome of chronic graft dysfunction now referred to as *bronchiolitis obliterans syndrome* (BOS). The typical histologic finding is obliterative bronchiolitis (dense fibrosis that obliterates the bronchioles). The predominant functional abnormality is airflow obstruction, as evidenced by serial decline in the FEV_1. The resulting fibrosis is irreversible, so there is no satisfactory treatment for established BOS. Since BOS is presumed to arise from chronic rejection, the treatment in most centers is empirical and consists of augmented immunosuppression. A few patients stabilize, but most afflicted recipients progress steadily with this disease and succumb to it or to opportunistic infections induced by the augmented immunosuppression.

BRONCHIAL ANASTOMOTIC COMPLICATIONS. These were formerly very frequent and a serious impediment to progress in lung transplantation. Their incidence is now dramatically decreased. Failure of bronchial anastomotic healing usually represents an ischemic complication. Reoperation is rarely necessary, and the majority of these are managed conservatively with a combination of early drainage followed later by bronchoscopic débridment and dilatation and/or stent placement.

SURVIVAL FOLLOWING LUNG TRANSPLANTATION. Actuarial survival data for the reported international experience shows a 1-year survival of 70% and a 5-year survival of 43%. The 3-year actuarial survival by type of transplant shows a slight (but not significant) survival advantage for patients undergoing bilateral compared with single lung replacement. Survival does not differ significantly among the various diagnostic groups.

FUNCTIONAL RESULTS. In general, the functional outcome of lung transplantation has been excellent and sustained in all the diagnostic groups for those recipients who do not develop BOS.

XII

Autotransplantation
R. Randal Bollinger, M.D., Ph.D.

Autotransplantation is the transfer of an organ, a part of an organ, a tissue, or cells from one site to another in the same individual. Autotransplantation has several practical advantages over *allotransplantation* (transfer between individuals of the same species) or *xenotransplantation* (transfer between individuals of different species). Immunologic rejection does not occur, the donor is at all times readily available, and prolonged preservation is usually unnecessary in the case of auto-

---

See the corresponding chapter or part in the *Textbook of Surgery*, 15th edition, pp. 497–506, for a more detailed discussion of this topic, including a comprehensive list of references.

transplants. Because of these advantages, autotransplantation was used earlier, more successfully, and more widely by all surgical specialties than were other forms of transplantation.

SKIN GRAFTS

Skin grafts are used to cover wounds where insufficient skin is available to permit immediate (primary) or delayed (secondary) suture closure. A *pedicle graft* is never separated from its blood supply, since revascularization at the recipient site is allowed to develop before the original blood supply is finally severed. A *free graft* is completely separated from its vascular, nervous, and lymphatic connections during the transplantation procedure. A *full-thickness* skin graft is a free graft including the entire epidermis and dermis, whereas a *partial* or *split-thickness* graft from 0.30 to 0.45 mm. in thickness includes all the epidermis and a variable part of the dermis. *Anastomosed free grafts,* in which the small arteries and veins supplying a graft are reanastomosed to small vessels at the recipient site, have gained popularity as microsurgical techniques have improved. Full-thickness skin grafts are used when pigment matching, resistance to contraction, or growth of a child are important considerations in wound healing. Split-thickness skin grafts survive better than do full-thickness grafts on compromised surfaces, such as granulating wounds contaminated with bacteria, because split-thickness skin is more richly supplied with open blood vessels on its underside. Since only a part of the dermis is taken, the donor site heals spontaneously by epithelial outgrowth from the remaining epithelial islands, sweat glands, and hair follicles. The wound to be skin grafted must be clean and well vascularized but free from bleeding. Meshing or perforation of the graft prevents serum accumulation beneath it. If the recipient site is free of debris, if bleeding is controlled, and if motion between the graft and its bed is prevented by a pressure dressing or plaster splint, the approximation necessary for fibrin adhesion and subsequent capillary invasion will be achieved.

NERVE AUTOGRAFTS

Nerve autografts are used to repair unsuturable defects in major peripheral nerves. Wallerian degeneration occurs in the distal damaged nerve and the donor graft before reinnervation can occur. The Schwann cells, endoneural tubes, and connective tissue survive in the form of conduits through which the axons may regenerate to reach viable end organs at a rate of 1 mm. per day in free grafts and 1.5 mm. per day in revascularized nerve grafts. Thick nerves undergo central ischemic necrosis, so thin nerves are used, either alone or in groups known as *cable grafts.*

MUSCULOSKELETAL AUTOGRAFTS

MUSCLE. Nonvascularized muscle transplants rapidly undergo ischemic necrosis, resorption, and replacement by fibrous tissue. Transfer of an entire muscle group without division of its neurovascular supply has been used to restore function in the distribution of an adjacent damaged nerve, for example, radial nerve and muscle transfer for ulnar palsy. Transplanted whole muscle can survive and be reinnervated 5 months after microneurovascular anastomosis.

BONE. The bulk of the bone implanted as a conventional free autograft does not survive transplantation. All but the most superficial cells of cortical grafts die of ischemia, leading to bone resorption and replacement in a process termed *creeping substitution.* More cells survive in the case of cancellous bone, which has an open structure that facilitates diffusion of nutrients and ingrowth of osteoclasts and osteoblasts. Excellent local blood supply, broad contact with recipient bone, and complete immobilization contribute to success. Infection, scarring, and irradiation of the tissues are responsible for failure. Cancellous bone for the reconstruction of major skeletal defects is obtained from the iliac crest or the metaphyseal ends of long bones. Cortical grafts are derived from the ribs, the central and proximal portions of the fibula, and the diaphysis of long bones.

CARTILAGE. Autotransplantation of cartilage from the costochondral junctions is used primarily in facial reconstruction. Cartilage heals to adjacent tissue by formation of a fibrous or fibrocartilaginous scar. Grafts from adults do not grow, and portions frequently undergo slow resorption.

TENDON. Autografts of tendon are used to replace damaged or destroyed tendons in the hands and feet in order to restore motion and strength. Free tendon grafts are taken from the palmaris longus, the flexor digitorum superficialis of the ring finger, the triceps, the plantaris, or the extensor digitorum communis tendons of the toes.

COMPOSITE-TISSUE AUTOGRAFTS. Transfers of entire functional units rather than individual components of the musculoskeletal system include toe-digital transfers and the iliac, rib, or fibular osteocutaneous neurosensory flaps. Osteocutaneous transplantation allows simultaneous reconstruction of both bone and skin defects with provision of sensation in the transplanted skin. Doppler flowmetry is used to monitor blood flow to the composite graft in the perioperative period.

VASCULAR AUTOGRAFTS

Both autogenous arteries and veins are used to replace destroyed or obstructed sections of major arteries. Although femoral, popliteal, upper extremity, and neck veins have been used, the greater saphenous vein has proved to be the most satisfactory arterial replacement. The wall is strong yet is flexible and easily sutured. The diameter is sufficiently great (minimum of 4 mm.) for avoidance of thrombosis, and nourishment is provided by the intraluminal blood flow. The smooth, natural endothelial lining is less thrombogenic than is any known synthetic surface, particularly when placed across joints. Moreover, the lining surface heals itself and may sequester white cells to fight infection. Autografts heal even when placed into the infected bed of a previous synthetic graft. Saphenous vein is ordinarily harvested from the same leg for femoropopliteal bypass and from the opposite leg for repair of vascular trauma to the lower extremity. The vein is reversed to prevent obstruction by the valves. In cases of *in situ* saphenous vein bypass, the vein may be left in its bed, all branches ligated, all valves internally disrupted, and flow reversed by suturing the vein proximally to the femoral artery and distally to a tibial or peroneal artery.

The internal mammary artery is a preferred source of blood for partially occluded coronary arteries, and the splenic artery may be rotated down to the left renal artery to bypass proximal renal stenosis. Infected prostheses, mycotic aneurysms, and infected arterial repairs can be managed successfully by excision and replacement with autografts from the iliac arteries. Autografting for repair of diseased or damaged veins has been much less successful than is arterial replacement, primarily because of early graft thrombosis in low-pressure, low-flow venous systems.

ENDOCRINE AUTOGRAFTS

Every endocrine gland has been autotransplanted experimentally, providing identification of several technical requirements for success: delicate handling of the tissues, prevention of ischemia by cooling or placement in an appropriate medium, and implantation of small fragments. The oxygen and nutrients in interstitial fluid around a subcutaneous, intramuscular, or renal capsular implant will maintain an endocrine graft until revascularization occurs if the fragments are no more than 1 mm. thick. Although thyroid, pituitary, ovary, adrenal, testis, pancreas, and parathyroid have all been autografted in humans, only the last four are often transplanted therapeutically today.

Autotransplantation in the form of orchidopexy is the treatment of choice for an undescended testis. Autotransplantation of segmental pancreas grafts or of isolated islet cells may prevent diabetes after pancreatectomy in more than half of cases. Since parathyroid hormone replacement is not available and medical therapy for hypoparathyroidism is complicated, preservation and autografting of excised parathyroid tissue are essential for preventing the deficiency symptoms of tetany, psychological disturbances, convulsions, coma, and death. Parathyroid glands are cut into 1-mm. pieces and reimplanted into pockets in the sternocleidomastoid muscle. When all glands are removed for diffuse parathyroid hyperplasia, implantation of fragments into the forearm muscles facilitates subsequent removal of more tissue under local anesthesia if hyperparathyroidism persists. Cryopreserved parathyroid tissue functions normally when autografted for treatment of hypoparathyroidism. Hyperplastic adrenal tissue may be autotransplanted for treatment of Cushing's disease, but autotransplantation of adrenal medulla for treatment of intractable Parkinson's disease has been abandoned because of postoperative morbidity.

URINARY AUTOGRAFTS

KIDNEY. Renal autotransplantation and extracorporeal reconstruction permit salvage of some kidneys that cannot be repaired *in situ*. Hypothermic pulsatile perfusion improves preservation and permits *ex vivo* microvascular surgery on the kidney before reimplantation. The kidney may be returned to its original site or grafted to the iliac vessels with use of allotransplantation techniques. The ureter may be reimplanted into the bladder or preserved intact during the autografting. Renal autografting has been employed for extensive renovascular disease from fibrous dysplasia, atherosclerosis, or abdominal aortic aneurysms; for repair of traumatic arterial injuries; for excision of renal cell carcinoma involving both kidneys or a solitary kidney; and for kidneys with diseased or damaged ureters too short for reimplantation.

URETER AND BLADDER. Autotransplantation of the bladder in the form of a vesicopsoas hitch or a bladder flap is the treatment of choice for injury or disease in the distal third of the ureter. Up to 18 cm. of distal ureter can be replaced with bladder by combining a tubular pedicle graft of bladder and the superior suturing of posterior bladder to psoas tendon. Autotransplantation of a segment of ileum currently provides the most successful replacement conduit for proximal ureter or excised bladder. Alternative reconstructions include suturing one ureter to the other ureter (transureteroureterostomy), the skin (cutaneous ureterostomy), or the sigmoid colon (ureterosigmoidostomy). A contracted bladder can be enlarged successfully by autotransplantation of a segment of ileum and cecum, an augmentation ileocecocystoplasty.

GASTROINTESTINAL AUTOGRAFTS

The gastrointestinal tract is ideally suited for autotransplantation. The mesentery provides a long, natural vascular pedicle for attached grafts, and the vascular arcades provide easily anastomosed arteries and veins for free grafts. Small intestinal autografts are used widely to replace the colon after proctocolectomy for inflammatory bowel disease. Stomach, jejunum, colon, or free intestinal segments are used to replace the hypopharynx and esophagus following extirpation of carcinomas of the larynx, pharynx, or esophagus; ingestion of caustic substances; or severe head and neck trauma. Stomach remains the most frequently used autograft for esophageal reconstruction and may be transposed into the neck and sutured to the base of the tongue after pharyngolaryngectomy.

Many other tissues have found limited but effective use as autotransplants, including the greater omentum, hair, tongue, teeth, fasciae latae, whole joints, and even the entire heart. Experimental autotransplantation studies have preceded and supported the ultimate feasibility of many allotransplantation procedures currently in clinical use.

21

IMMUNOBIOLOGY AND IMMUNOTHERAPY OF NEOPLASTIC DISEASE; MELANOMA; SOFT TISSUE SARCOMAS; TUMOR MARKERS

I

Immunobiology and Immunotherapy of Neoplastic Disease

H. Kim Lyerly, M.D., and Cohava Gelber, Ph.D.

THE IMMUNOLOGIC BASIS FOR CELLULAR IMMUNOTHERAPY

Tumor cells encode distinct antigens (tumor associated antigens, or TAAs, and tumor specific antigens, or TSAs) that are recognized by components of the immune response that can eradicate the growing tumor. Recent knowledge acquired from animal experiments shed light on how cytotoxic T-lymphocytes (CTLs) recognize an antigen on a cell. Investigation on the molecular level of antigen processing and presentation revealed that CTLs can detect antigens derived from cell surface–associated proteins, as well as proteins that localize to the cytoplasm, the nucleus, or anywhere within the cell.

Endogenously synthesized proteins were shown to be degraded within the cytoplasm into 9- to 10-amino-acid-long peptides. These peptides were then transported to the endocytoplasmic reticulum and associated with newly synthesized MHC Class I molecules. Certain peptides could fit within the MHC Class I molecule and were then transported to the cell surface as a complex. It was this complex, consisting of a 9- to 10-amino-acid peptide within an MHC Class I molecule that was presented to, and recognized by CD8 + CTLs. Alterations of normal genes leading to their overexpression, to the production of novel fusion proteins, or to simple amino acid substitutions in these peptides were sufficient to be recognized by CTLs as foreign and thus facilitate their elimination. Methods to identify and isolate genes encoding for TAAs or TSAs recognized by CD8 + CTLs have been developed, proving that tumor cells do express genetically defined TAAs or TSAs.

See the corresponding chapter or part in the *Textbook of Surgery*, 15th edition, pp. 507–515, for a more detailed discussion of this topic, including a comprehensive list of references.

Tumor antigens expressed on spontaneous malignancies may be auto or self antigens. For example, several of the identified melanoma-specific antigens such as MAGE and MART are also expressed in normal melanocytes and in other tissues. It is not altogether clear why, but the fact is that while tolerance is maintained to self antigens expressed on normal tissue, when such antigens are expressed on tumor cells, they induce an immune response. The immune response induced against the self antigen expressed on the tumor cells could very well crossreact with normal tissue expressing the same antigen and lead to autoimmunity. While clear manifestations of autoimmunity in animals treated with active or adoptive immunotherapy have not yet been observed or reported, it is suspected that development of increasingly potent immune therapy protocols may lead to autoimmune manifestations, and as in other instances in clinical medicine, a risk/benefit assessment will have to be made in each case.

In summary, the biological basis of immune-based therapy against cancer has become strongly supported by basic research in defining how the cellular immune response identifies cells as foreign and the identification of TAAs or TSAs as discussed above. It appears that the lack of demonstrable immunity of most human forms of cancer may not reflect lack of TAAs or TSAs but rather that tumors have elaborated mechanisms to prevent the induction of effective antitumor immune responses. The purpose of tumor immunotherapy is to direct the immune system to the TAA capable of mediating tumor rejection. Two approaches that have received increasing consideration and are discussed in this chapter are adoptive and active immunotherapy.

ADOPTIVE IMMUNOTHERAPY

Adoptive immunotherapy refers to the adoptive transfer of specific immunologic components, usually cellular components, for the treatment of cancer. It is most readily recognized in the form of non-antigen-specific effectors, which include lymphokine-activated killer (LAK) cells or tumor-infiltrating lymphocytes (TILs), as established by Rosenberg and colleagues. LAK cells, generated by short-term culture of peripheral blood lymphocytes in the presence of high concentrations of interleukin 2 (IL-2), lyse transformed target cells and have minimal lytic activity for most normal tissues. Up to 10^{11} *in vitro*–generated LAK cells have been administered in a single intravenous infusion to cancer patients. Treated patients experienced only minor constitutional symptoms and no pulmonary compromise, demonstrating the safety of systemically administering large numbers of *in vitro* activated lymphocytes. Therapeutic trials also have combined short courses of high-dose systemic IL-2 administration with LAK cell transfer to promote LAK function and viability with apparent enhanced efficacy. The shortcomings of LAK and IL-2 therapy included a larger degree of toxicity, including pulmonary, renal, and hepatobiliary, with a significant proportion of patients requiring intensive care unit admissions and a 2% to 5% treatment-related mortality. Despite this, response rate remained relatively low.

In an effort to increase the efficacy of the cellular component of the therapy, more effective effector cells were sought. One such therapy using *in vitro* expanded lymphocytes derived from a tumor infiltrate (TIL) has been evaluated in clinical trials. In humans, TIL cell lines have been generated by mincing tumor specimens and culturing eluted lymphocytes with high concentrations of IL-2. TIL lines can be expanded to 10^8 to 10^{11} cells over 3 to 8 weeks in culture, and some lines appear to function as T cells with lytic specificity for autologous but not allogeneic tumor targets, whereas others function as LAK cells and lyse both autologous and allogeneic tumor targets. Adoptive transfer of 5×10^{10} TIL cells alone has not been associated with significant toxicity, and administration of 5×10^{10} TIL cells with concurrent systemic IL-2 has caused toxicities that are attributable to the IL-2.

These clinical studies of adoptive immunotherapy relied on non-antigen-specific LAK and TIL cells, because specific TAAs recognized by the cytotoxic effector cells had not yet been identified. Nonetheless, they have established the feasibility and safety of this approach and demonstrated *in vivo* biological effects of transferred effector cells. Other types of effector cells, including cells from draining lymph nodes, and *in vivo* primed cells also have been evaluated in the era prior to the clear elucidation of defined TAAs.

ACTIVE IMMUNOTHERAPY

In addition to adoptive immunotherapy, active immunotherapy has emerged as another modality of immunotherapy and has received increasing attention. Specific active immunotherapy (SAI) differs dramatically from the nonspecific immune-based trials that have been utilized previously, in that the objective is not to generally stimulate the immune system or nonspecifically stimulate one component of the immune system. Rather, SAI refers to the specific induction of a component of the immune system that affects the rejection of a particular tumor type. Several different approaches in experimental animal studies in the 1970s formed the basis for human clinical trials of SAI against human cancers. Although several thousand patients have been injected with a variety of tumor cell preparations in this country and elsewhere during the past 25 years, the complexity of the studies has made it difficult to definitively assess the value of this approach to cancer therapy. Nonetheless, a number of clinical trials have suggested a therapeutic benefit of SAI. Most of these trials have two features in common: (1) a therapeutic effect was not seen or, if seen, has not been confirmed independently, and (2) no acceptable information was provided regarding the presence of tumor antigens in the vaccines and the immune response of patients to these antigens. Skin tests for delayed-type hypersensitivity (DTH) to whole tumor cells, cell extracts, or cell-mediated cytotoxicity assays were performed in a number of trials, but the difficulty of defining specificity limits the usefulness of these assays. Therefore, a solid foundation for future progress has not been provided by most of these clinical studies. These studies suggest that a review of traditional response criteria is needed and perhaps focus not on response rates but on disease stabilization, time to relapse, survival, and quality of life.

Because of the lack of clinical success in these trials, active immunotherapy remained confined to clinical trials, usually in melanoma and renal cell carcinoma. However, recent advances in gene transfer have steered to a new direction of active immunotherapy, based on gene modification of the tumor cells in an effort to enhance their ability to elicit a tumor-specific immune response. Furthermore, advances in the understanding of the role of dendritic cells in the initiation of T-cell responses and practical methods to isolate dendritic cells will likely lead to their use in active immunotherapy for cancer in the future.

II

Melanoma
Craig L. Slingluff, Jr., M.D., and H. F. Seigler, M.D.

Melanoma is a neoplastic disorder arising on the skin, mucous membranes, meninges, and ciliary body of the eye. This malignancy is increasing in incidence more rapidly than any other malignant disorder.

PRECURSOR FACTORS

The one environmental factor that is associated with the development of this disease is ultraviolet irradiation. A genetic predisposition appears to be an important component of this disease. Individuals with fair skin, red or blonde hair, and blue or green eyes are at greater risk for the development of melanoma than are individuals with dark skin, brown eyes, and brown or black hair.

CLINICOPATHOLOGIC FEATURES

The four histopathologic types of mucocutaneous melanoma include lentigo maligna melanoma, superficial spreading melanoma, acral lentiginous melanoma, and nodular melanoma. Lentigo maligna melanoma occurs most commonly

---

See the corresponding chapter or part in the *Textbook of Surgery*, 15th edition, pp. 515–528, for a more detailed discussion of this topic, including a comprehensive list of references.

in older individuals and on sun-exposed areas of the body. Superficial spreading melanoma usually grows for a period of time in a horizontal direction and does not have a metastatic potential. Once vertical growth has been realized, a systemic potential exists. Acral lentiginous melanoma presents on the glabrous skin, subungual areas, and mucous membranes. Nodular melanoma demonstrates vertical growth from its inception and is associated with a less favorable prognosis.

PROGNOSTIC FACTORS

The three most predictive prognostic indicators for mucocutaneous melanoma include the level of invasion, tumor thickness, and ulceration. Patients with tumor thickness of less than 1.0 mm. have a less than 10% metastatic potential and usually can be cured by simple excision alone. Patients with intermediate-thickness melanoma ranging from 1.0 to 4.0 mm. have approximately a 30% to 45% risk of spread and are best managed by excision of the primary tumor with adequate tissue borders and, in selected cases, elective lymph node dissection. Patients with tumor thickness exceeding 4.0 mm. have a high risk of systemic element to their disease and are best managed by excision and careful follow-up. The likelihood that these patients will develop metastatic disease is approximately 70%.

CHOICE OF BIOPSY

If the lesion is small and in a nonstrategic area, the preferred biopsy is excision of the pigmented area with subcutaneous fat submitted with the cutaneous elements. This permits the pathologist to assess accurately ulceration, tumor thickness, and level of invasion. If the primary lesion is large and in a strategic area, incisional biopsy including the area of greatest vertical growth should be selected. Shave biopsies, curettage, and electrocoagulation should not be performed.

SURGICAL MANAGEMENT OF THE PRIMARY LESION

Once the histopathology has been confirmed by adequate biopsy, surgical management of the primary lesion can be planned accurately. For those lesions with Level I and Level II invasion and tumor thickness less than 1.0 mm., excision with 1.0- to 2.0-cm. margins is adequate. In most areas, this permits primary wound closure. Patients with invasive melanoma with intermediate or thick tumor measurements can be managed adequately by excision with 2.0 cm. of normal tissue around the primary site and primary closure when possible. The ultimate disease-free interval and patient survival are not predicted by the surgical margins. Clinical outcome is predicted by the prognostic variables rather than by the margin of excision.

SURGICAL MANAGEMENT OF REGIONAL DISEASE

A substantial number of patients can survive long term after therapeutic resection of regional lymph nodes. On the other hand, the therapeutic role of resecting clinically negative nodes remains unclear. Elective lymph node dissection (ELND) has long been in the armamentarium of surgeons managing melanoma. Since regional lymph nodes are the first sites of metastases from melanoma in over 60% of cases, it is rational to suspect that resection of regional nodes early might have therapeutic value. However, the operation can be associated with significant morbidity. While some surgeons do not consider ELND to have a role in melanoma, others believe that it has a limited role, primarily in patients who have an intermediate-thickness melanoma (1.5 to 4.0 mm.) without evidence of metastatic disease, have a single nodal basin draining the site of the primary lesion, and have no other contraindications to the procedure.

SURGICAL CONSIDERATIONS FOR DISTANT DISEASE

For the most part, only those patients with documented solitary metastases to distant sites benefit from surgical removal of the metastatic deposit. The common areas of distant metastatic disease include the lung, brain, adrenal gland, and small intestine. Surgical removal of the solitary metastasis coupled with systemic therapy is associated with increased disease-free interval as well as improved quality of life. Patients with multiple metastatic lesions are best managed by systemic therapy, with little benefit gained from surgical intervention.

HORMONAL ASPECTS OF MELANOMA

The presence of estrogen receptors on malignant melanocytes has been evaluated extensively. At the present time, it appears that pigmented lesions have a false-positive estrogen receptor, as determined by biochemical analysis. The estradiol-binding component in melanoma most probably represents an artifact, and true estrogen receptors are probably absent with this tumor. If the patient is diagnosed with melanoma during pregnancy, there is a greater likelihood that first-order lymph nodes will be involved than if she is not pregnant at the time of initial diagnosis. Additionally, the disease-free interval is shorter for patients with pregnancy and melanoma occurring simultaneously. Ultimate patient survival is essentially the same between the pregnant and nonpregnant patient populations. Patients with a past history of melanoma do not appear to have increased risk if they become pregnant at a later date.

COMBINED-MODALITY TREATMENT FOR MELANOMA

Conventional systemic chemotherapy for melanoma is associated with approximately a 40% response rate. Only 10% of patients will experience complete resolution of their disease. More recently, high-dose chemotherapy with autologous bone marrow reconstitution has increased the drug response rate, although defined disease-free interval and ultimate patient survival are yet to be determined. Both prophylactic and therapeutic isolated limb perfusions are associated with a prolonged disease-free interval and increased patient survival. The addition of hyperthermia also seems to improve the effectiveness of this therapeutic modality. Interferon, tumor necrosis factor, and monoclonal antibodies have yet to show clear therapeutic potential. Recombinant interleukin-2 administered in association with either lymphokine-activated lymphocytes or expanded tumor-infiltrating lymphocytes has been associated with a 25% to 40% response rate. This new therapeutic modality must be considered experimental, and ultimate disease-free interval and improved patient survival are not yet defined. Specific active immunotherapy using melanoma vaccines has its greatest effect in patients with either small tumor burdens or in the adjuvant mode.

Soft Tissue Sarcomas
Jonathan J. Lewis, M.D., Ph.D., and Murray F. Brennan, M.D.

Soft tissue sarcomas are rare and unusual neoplasms. The annual incidence in the United States is approximately 5000 to 6000, and they account for 1% of adult malignancies and 15% of pediatric malignancies.

PREDISPOSING FACTORS. These include the genetic syndromes of neurofibromatosis, familial adenomatous polyposis, and the Li-Fraumeni syndrome. Ionizing radiation and lymphedema are established, uncommon antecedents to the development of soft tissue sarcoma. Chemical carcinogens have been implicated widely, but the data to support their association are less well founded. The tumor suppressor genes best studied in sarcomas are *p53* and *RB1*, and inactivation of both genes is involved in the tumorigenesis of several sarcomas.

HISTOPATHOLOGY AND PROGNOSTIC FACTORS. The

See the corresponding chapter or part in the *Textbook of Surgery,* 15th edition, pp. 528–534, for a more detailed discussion of this topic, including a comprehensive list of references.

histologic subtypes most commonly found are liposarcoma, malignant fibrous histiocytoma (MFH), and leiomyosarcoma. In general, a specific histologic diagnosis appears to be of secondary importance because biologic behavior is currently best predicted based on histologic grade. Current staging systems focus on histologic grade, the size of the primary tumor, and the presence or absence of metastasis. For therapeutic planning, the broad categories of low (Grades I or II) or high (Grades III or IV) grade suffice. Low-grade lesions are assumed to have a low (<15%) risk of subsequent metastasis and the high-grade lesions a high (>50%) risk of subsequent metastasis.

DIAGNOSIS AND MANAGEMENT. Generally, in an adult any soft tissue mass that is symptomatic or enlarging, any mass that is larger than 5 cm., or any new mass that persists beyond 4 weeks should be biopsied. An incisional biopsy is usually preferred with a longitudinal incision (extremity lesions) to facilitate subsequent wide local excision. At the time of definitive resection, the previous scar should be excised *en bloc* together with the tumor. Patients with intra-abdominal or retroperitoneal sarcomas often experience nonspecific abdominal discomfort and gastrointestinal symptoms before diagnosis. The diagnosis is usually suspected on finding a soft tissue mass on abdominal CT or MRI scan. Fine-needle aspiration biopsy has no role in the routine diagnostic evaluation of these patients, and in most patients exploratory laparotomy should be performed and the diagnosis made at operation.

Surgery remains the dominant modality of curative therapy for all soft tissue sarcomas. Wherever practical, function- and limb-sparing procedures should be performed. The surgical objective should be complete removal of the tumor with negative margins and maximal preservation of function. Where possible, tumors should be excised with 2 to 3 cm. of normal tissue because of the propensity for local, unappreciated spread. Adjuvant radiation has been demonstrated to improve local control. Adjuvant chemotherapy has not been proven to be efficacious. In retroperitoneal and visceral lesions, surgery remains the dominant modality of therapy because of the current inability to deliver adequate doses of radiation without serious damage to normal tissue.

Despite optimal multimodality therapy, at least one third of patients develop recurrent disease. Patients with isolated local recurrence should undergo re-resection. The results of re-resection are good, and two thirds of these patients experience long-term survival. Adjuvant radiation therapy should be administered after surgery. For extremity lesions, the most common site of metastasis is the lung. Patients whose primary tumors are controlled or controllable, who have no extrathoracic disease, who are medically fit for thoracotomy, and in whom complete resection of all lung disease appears possible should undergo thoracotomy with the intent of resecting all disease. Patients with unresectable pulmonary metastases or extrapulmonary metastatic sarcoma have a uniformly poor prognosis and are best treated with systemic chemotherapy.

IV

Tumor Markers
Jeffrey A. Norton, M.D., and Douglas L. Fraker, M.D.

IDEAL TUMOR MARKER

The potential utility of tumor markers includes screening, diagnosis, prognosis, assessment of therapeutic efficacy, and detection of residual or recurrent disease. A successful screening test to detect cancer in the general population or at-risk individuals must possess a high sensitivity for early lesions for the detection of disease in asymptomatic patients with small, curable tumor burdens. The best example of a marker for screening is the use of plasma levels of calcitonin following provocative testing with calcium and/or pentagastrin for detecting surgically curable C-cell carcinoma or medullary thyroid carcinoma *in situ* in patients from kindreds with familial multiple endocrine neoplasia Type 2A. Interestingly, this test very recently has been further improved by the measurement of the *ret* oncogene in these individuals.

A second application for tumor markers is as an unequivocal diagnostic modality. Again, the best examples of this application are the hormone markers of endocrine tumors, in which the diagnosis depends on measurement of the marker in serum or staining of the tumor for the marker by immunohistochemistry. A third application for measurement of tumor markers at the time of diagnosis is the yield of prognostic information by some markers. For example, in patients with colorectal cancer, the prognosis worsens with greater serum levels of carcinoembryonic antigen (CEA) at the time of initial diagnosis. Finally, circulating tumor markers reflect treatment efficacy and follow-up for recurrent disease. In these settings, measurement of marker levels may influence such management decisions as continuing or discontinuing therapy or performing imaging studies or surgical therapy to detect recurrent disease.

Unfortunately, at present, no ideal tumor markers exist. The characteristics of individual tumor markers such as specificity, sensitivity, and correlation of marker level with tumor burden and type of disease define the actual clinical utility for each marker in individual patients with specific tumors.

TYPES OF TUMOR MARKERS

Circulating tumor markers can be categorized by functional and biochemical characteristics into tumor antigens, enzymes, hormones, and other markers of tumor or host origin. Tumor

---

See the corresponding chapter or part in the *Textbook of Surgery*, 15th edition, pp. 534–553, for a more detailed discussion of this topic, including a comprehensive list of references.

antigens are defined by immunogenic structural characteristics and can be subcategorized by historical, biochemical, and distributional features as oncofetal antigens and polyclonal- or monoclonal-defined antigens. Oncofetal antigens are compounds produced during normal development by the placental-fetal complex and are also produced by neoplastic tissue. This group contains the original and most prevalent tumor markers, including carcinoembryonic antigen, alpha-fetoprotein (AFP), and beta-human chorionic gonadotropin (β-HCG). A second and rapidly enlarging group of tumor markers consists of tumor-associated antigens that are detected by polyclonal or monoclonal antibodies directed against tumor extracts or cell lines. Tumor-associated antigens include carcinoma antigen (CA) CA 125, CA 19-9, CA 50, CA 242, and CA 15-3.

Enzymes and hormones initially were identified by bioactivity as catalysts of specific chemical reactions or biological effects from binding specific receptors, respectively. Although they were measured formerly by cumbersome biological assay techniques, immunoassay techniques now exist to quantitate minute amounts of essentially all enzymes and hormones used as tumor markers. Enzymes produced in excess amount by the tumor or the tumor-bearing host can be used as circulating markers and include neuron-specific enolase (NSE) and acid phosphatase. Hormones and hormone degradation products are specific and sensitive serum markers for a wide number of endocrine tumors. Chromogranin A is a secretory granule protein that may be shed into the circulation in patients with neuroendocrine tumors. Prostate-specific antigen is a marker specific for prostatic tissue that increases in patients with prostatic cancer.

Carcinoembryonic Antigen and Colorectal Cancer

Carcinoembryonic antigen (CEA) is a glycoprotein (molecular weight 180 kd) consisting of a single polypeptide chain with a variable carbohydrate content. In general, serum levels lower than 2.5 ng. per ml. are normal and concentrations greater than 5 ng. per ml. are elevated. CEA is a classic example of a tumor marker that, although widely used, is not an ideal marker because of low specificity and sensitivity. Both malignant and nonmalignant diseases may elevate serum levels of CEA. Although CEA is associated primarily with colorectal cancer, serum levels also may be elevated in patients with cancer of the pancreas, stomach, lung, breast, thyroid, and ovary. The lack of specificity is further proven by nonmalignant conditions that also may elevate serum CEA levels: gastrointestinal disorders (including peptic ulcer disease, gastritis, pancreatitis, and inflammatory bowel disease), hepatobiliary diseases (including cirrhosis, hepatitis, and obstructive jaundice), and nonmalignant pulmonary disease (bronchitis and emphysema), as well as benign prostatic hypertrophy and renal failure.

Carcinoembryonic antigen has been studied as a marker of colorectal tumors since the 1960s. Although CEA is not colorectal tumor–specific, the highest concentrations in tissue and serum are found in patients with colorectal carcinoma. Serum CEA determinations are not useful in screening normal populations of adults for colorectal cancer. Elevated CEA levels occur in only 5% of patients with localized, surgically curable colon cancer and in 65% to 90% of patients with either distant or locally advanced disease. Screening of patients with conditions such as ulcerative colitis or polyposis coli that predispose them to colorectal cancer also has been unsuccessful because these diseases may produce elevated serum levels of CEA.

Several reports have indicated that the preoperative serum CEA concentration before definitive resection of primary colorectal cancer is an independent prognostic parameter of subsequent survival; that is, the higher the serum CEA level, the poorer the prognosis of an individual with colorectal cancer.

Elevated serum levels of CEA indicate recurrent colorectal cancer usually 4 to 6 months before it is clinically evident. In general, serum CEA levels are elevated in approximately two of three patients before any other evidence of recurrent colon or rectal cancer. Serum CEA levels need not have been raised preoperatively to be elevated postoperatively as a marker of tumor recurrence. Because there is no effective nonsurgical therapy for nonimagable colorectal carcinoma, a second-look exploratory procedure with resection of recurrent disease has been used by many groups. Results of CEA-initiated second-look procedures vary among different groups, with one group reporting being able to remove all tumor in 70% of patients and others finding no benefit. This strategy of reoperation can provide cure for a small percentage of patients (10% to 30%) and can document recurrent colorectal carcinoma in most patients (80%), who can then graduate to other therapies.

Potential improvement in selection of patients and results for CEA-initiated second-look operative procedures may be achieved through better preoperative demonstration of the location and extent of disease. A new method is the use of radiolabeled antibody to CEA and external scintigraphy for detecting the exact location and extent of recurrent tumor. Patients with localized, resectable, locally recurrent disease or liver disease can then be selected for a second-look operation.

Serum levels of CEA correlate fairly well with disease extent in patients with colorectal cancer. Serum levels usually rise with progression and fall with disease regression, but once markedly elevated, they do not always correlate directly with tumor burden. Serum CEA levels have been used to follow the response to chemotherapy in patients with metastatic colorectal cancer. In patients with metastatic colorectal carcinoma who had elevated serum CEA levels and responded to chemotherapy, 89% showed a decrease in serum CEA level. In patients who had progressive disease despite chemotherapy, 90% had an increase in serum CEA level compared with pretreatment level.

Alpha-Fetoprotein and Hepatocellular Carcinoma

Alpha-fetoprotein (AFP), the first oncofetal antigen discovered, is a useful tumor marker for primary hepatocellular carcinoma (HCC) and nonseminomatous germ cell tumors of the testis. Abnormal serum levels of AFP usually occur in malignant neoplasms but may occur in benign diseases of endodermally derived organs, including hepatitis, inflammatory bowel disease, ataxia telangiectasia, and hereditary tyrosinemia. However, highly elevated serum levels of AFP (greater than 500 ng. per ml.) are present almost exclusively in primary HCC and nonseminomatous testicular tumors. Eighty per cent of patients with HCC have elevated serum levels of AFP. Patients with other malignant tumors also may have elevated serum levels of AFP. Twenty per cent of patients with gastric or pancreatic cancer and 5% of patients with colorectal or lung cancer also have significant elevations (greater than 5 ng. per ml.).

In 1983, a case report published in *Lancet* demonstrated the feasibility of screening a population at high risk for development of HCC with serial serum levels of AFP. Other investigators have tried to use serum AFP levels to detect HCC in at-risk populations, with disappointing results. Serum AFP levels may be normal in 35% to 50% of patients with biopsy-proven HCC. In a minority of patients with HCC, serum levels of AFP fall despite continued tumor growth, and other patients have elevated levels of AFP and nonmalignant diseases of the liver. However, in the presence of cirrhosis, a serum AFP level greater than 500 ng. per ml. is diagnostic of HCC.

Serum levels of AFP in patients with HCC may be of prognostic value. The subgroup of patients who have HCC and normal serum levels of AFP have a relatively good prognosis. In these patients, the primary factor predicting better prognosis may be the absence of cirrhosis. Normal serum AFP levels are more common in patients without underlying cirrhosis. A rapid AFP doubling time is also associated with a poorer prognosis.

Serial measurement of serum AFP level can be helpful before and after presumably curative surgical therapy in patients with HCC. However, the serum levels of this tumor marker do not always show the presence of recurrent HCC. HCC may be recurrent despite normal serum AFP levels. There is variation in AFP synthesis in different parts of the same tumor. The tumor's ability to secrete AFP may change with growth. It may be that "recurrences" of the tumor within the liver are really new primary tumors with different characteristics.

If specific chemotherapy is effective, serum AFP levels fall continuously, indicating tumor regression and effective treatment. If serum AFP levels demonstrate a continued rise despite antitumor treatment, the tumor is resistant to the treatment, and an alternative regimen should be used. Monitoring of serum AFP levels in patients with HCC can avoid prolonged ineffective use of potentially toxic chemotherapy.

Alpha-Fetoprotein and Human Chorionic Gonadotropin in Testicular and Gynecologic Cancer

The characteristics of AFP were described in the preceding section. Human chorionic gonadotropin (HCG) is a placental

hormone that is also a tumor marker for gestational trophoblastic neoplasms and nonseminomatous testicular cancer. It is
a glycoprotein consisting of two distinct noncovalently bound
subunits. Many immunoassay kits for the measurement of
HCG are commercially available. The sensitivity of these
assays is in the range of 1 unit per ml. or 0.2 ng. per ml. The
upper limit of normal for circulating HCG is less than 5 to 8
units per ml. for women and less than 3 units per ml. for men.

The application of HCG as a circulating tumor marker
ranges from the prototype of an ideal tumor marker for gestational trophoblastic neoplasia and a valuable tool in testicular
cancer to a less well-defined role in other gynecologic malignancies, uroepithelial tumors, and a spectrum of other solid
tumors. HCG is highly sensitive for the diagnosis of choriocarcinoma and a trophoblastic neoplasm following evacuation
of a molar pregnancy. In testicular cancer, 70% to 75% of
nonseminomatous tumors and 10% of pure seminomas are
associated with elevated serum HCG levels. If both serum
HCG and AFP levels are measured, 89% of patients with
nonseminomatous testicular cancer have an elevation of one
or both markers. Serum HCG and AFP levels are very useful
as markers for detecting the response to therapy and for
detecting persistent or recurrent testicular cancer. In addition,
the serum levels of both AFP and HCG are inversely proportional to outcome in patients with testicular cancer.

Serum HCG elevations have been detected in a small proportion of patients with nontrophoblastic, nontesticular neoplasms (60 of 828, 7.2%). Specifically, 20% of patients with
bladder cancer and between 13% and 36% of patients with
gynecologic cancers, including cervical, endometrial, and vulvar cancer, and 5% of patients with ovarian cancer have elevated serum HCG levels. In addition, with newer techniques
used to detect the free beta subunit of HCG and the beta core
fragment of HCG, 77% of patients with ovarian and other
gynecologic neoplasms have elevated serum HCG levels.

CA 125 and Ovarian Cancer

CA 125 is a carbohydrate epitope on a glycoprotein carcinoma antigen that is useful as a serum marker for ovarian
cancer. A murine monoclonal antibody was raised against a
cultured cell line established from a patient with a serous
papillary adenocarcinoma of the ovary. Immunoassay kits are
available for measurement of CA 125; normal serum levels
are less than 35 units per ml., since only 1% of normal subjects
have a value greater than 35 units per ml.

CA 125 antigen is abnormally elevated in the serum of 80%
of patients with nonmucinous epithelial ovarian carcinoma.
Serum levels of CA 125 correlate directly with tumor bulk.
Elevated levels of CA 125 in the sera of patients with occult
recurrent disease precede other clinical signs of recurrent
ovarian carcinoma. Serum levels of CA 125 are also elevated
in a high percentage of patients with fallopian, endometrial,
and endocervical carcinoma.

CA 19-9 and CA 50 in
Gastrointestinal Cancer

CA 19-9 is a carbohydrate antigen that is identified by a monoclonal antibody raised versus a colorectal cancer cell line. Sera from patients with colorectal, pancreas, and gastric cancer can neutralize binding of this monoclonal antibody to its specific cell extracts, suggesting that CA 19-9 is present in the sera of these patients with cancer. The antigen is present in normal fetal tissues, including salivary and lacrimal glands, conjunctivae, bronchi, pancreas, esophagus, stomach, small intestine, and gallbladder, but is absent in the fetal colon. The carbohydrate epitope may be present in the pancreas, salivary gland, endocervix, and gallbladder of normal adults.

Sensitive immunoassay kits are currently available for measurement of CA 19-9. A study of healthy subjects indicated that normal serum levels of CA 19-9 were less than 35 units per ml. CA 19-9 is a serum marker for the management of patients with gastric, pancreatic, and colorectal cancer. Patients with pancreatitis also may have an elevation of serum CA 19-9 levels. However, in patients with pancreatitis, the serum levels of CA 19-9 seldom exceed 100 units per ml., and patients with pancreatic cancer have higher levels of this marker (73% greater than 100 units per ml.). In the management of patients with gastric and colorectal cancer, serum CA 19-9 levels appear to offer no advantage over serum CEA levels.

CA 50 is a carbohydrate antigen closely related to CA 19-9 defined by monoclonal antibodies to a colorectal cancer cell line. CA 50 has the same determinants as does CA 19-9, but it also has a unique carbohydrate moiety that lacks a fucose residue and is not associated with CA 19-9 activity. Serum levels of CA 50 can be detected in approximately 5% of the population who are Lewis antigen–negative. Serum levels of CA 50 less than 17 units per ml. are normal.

The utility of CA 50 parallels that of CA 19-9. CA 50 antigen is not detectable in normal tissue except the pancreas. CA 50 levels are not elevated in normal serum, but levels are increased in a few patients (less than 12%) with benign liver disease and inflammatory bowel disease and in patients with sclerosing cholangitis. Circulating CA 50 is elevated in a significant proportion of patients with colorectal, gastric, liver, biliary, pancreatic, prostatic, lung, and breast cancer. The clinical utility of CA 50 and its comparison with other markers such as AFP, CEA, and CA 19-9 need further study.

CA 15-3 and Breast Cancer

CA 15-3 is a glycoprotein antigen that serves as a marker for breast cancer. It is identified by two specific monoclonal antibodies that recognize different epitopes on an identical antigen. CA 15-3 is both a differentiation antigen and a milk-related antigen because its production is increased during cell differentiation and it is present in breast milk. The mean value of CA 15-3 in the sera of normal subjects is 13.3 ± 6 units per ml., and over 90% of normal individuals have levels less than 22 units per ml.

Initial clinical studies suggest that CA 15-3 serum levels may help in the management of patients with breast cancer. The percentage of patients who have elevated serum levels of CA 15-3 increases with more advanced stage breast cancer. In addition, 66% of patients with breast cancer who have normal serum levels of CEA have elevated serum levels of CA 15-3. CA 15-3 may be elevated in some patients with cancer besides breast cancer.

Prostate-Specific Antigen, Prostatic Acid Phosphatase, and Prostate Cancer

Prostate-specific antigen (PSA) is a glycoprotein specific for prostatic tissue with utility as a tumor marker for prostatic cancer. More than 90% of normal men have detectable serum levels of PSA (1.1 ± 0.7 ng. per ml.), and the normal range for men is less than 2.5 ng. per ml.

PSA is a very sensitive marker for prostatic cancer; 96% of patients with very early stage lesions (Stage A) and 100% of patients with more advanced disease have elevated serum levels of PSA. However, 86% of patients with benign prostatic hypertrophy have moderate elevations of serum PSA levels, limiting its ability as a screening test for prostate cancer. The level of the serum marker also may increase following prostatic massage, prostatic biopsy, and transurethral resection. Several recent studies of the biology and biochemistry of PSA, as well as extensive screening studies, have further delineated the utility of PSA.

Prostatic acid phosphatase is not a useful circulating tumor marker in patients with prostatic cancer. Specifically, serum prostatic acid phosphatase level is not useful as a screening test because elevations frequently occur in patients with benign prostatic hypertrophy, and serum levels are not usually elevated in patients with early prostatic cancer or small amounts of residual disease.

Neuron-Specific Enolase and Chromogranin A in APUDomas

Neuron-specific enolase (NSE) is an acidic isoenzyme of enolase. NSE was isolated initially from bovine brain and reported to be found exclusively in neural tissue. Subsequent studies indicated a high level of NSE in neuroendocrine tissues, the amine precursor uptake and decarboxylation (APUD) cells.

The development of a specific radioimmunoassay enabled measurement of NSE in the sera of normal subjects and patients with malignant disease originating from neuroendocrine tissue. Normal individuals have serum levels between 5 and 10 ng. per ml. Study of patients with different neuroendocrine tumors demonstrated elevated serum levels of NSE in patients with pancreatic islet cell tumors, gut carcinoids, adrenal tumors, neuroblastomas, medullary cancer of the thyroid, and small cell lung cancer. Because additional, more specific and sensitive tumor markers exist for most patients with endocrine tumors, serum NSE levels do not help in the management of these patients. However, recent studies suggest that circulating NSE levels may be a valuable marker for patients with small cell lung cancer because other good alternative markers are not available. Another potential application of serum NSE levels is for management of patients with seminomas, because 73% of patients have elevated levels.

Chromogranin A is a 49-kd protein that occurs in the secretory granules of most neuroendocrine cells. This protein is shed into the serum by these tumors that secrete other peptides. Measurement of serum levels of chromogranin A may be a useful tool in the management of patients with APUDomas.

22

THE BREAST
J. Dirk Iglehart, M.D.

Diseases of the breast may be disorders of function and of normal physiology or they may be due to neoplastic proliferations, either benign or malignant. Benign tumors are common and cause concern because they mimic more serious malignancies. Fibroadenomas and gross breast cysts are the most common benign tumors within the breast. Malignant tumors are neoplasms of the breast ductal and lobular epithelium and are further divided into invasive (infiltrating) and noninvasive *(in situ)* proliferations. The treatment of breast cancer has changed dramatically and continues to change today. This evolution is driven by clinical research, new drug discovery, and advances in cellular and molecular biology. It is important for surgeons to remain current in many disciplines in order to provide the best care and contribute to this advancing knowledge.

GROSS AND MICROSCOPIC ANATOMY

The mature breast rests on the pectoralis major muscle and is attached to the *superficial pectoral fascia* by *Cooper's ligaments*, suspensory ligaments that run from the overlying skin of the breast to the pectoral fascia. The axilla is invested by the *clavipectoral fascia*, which is a continuation of the fascial investments of the pectoralis minor muscle. The *lateral pectoral nerve* (also named the *medial pectoral nerve*) swings around or through the lateral margin of the pectoralis minor muscle to innervate the pectoralis major muscle. During axillary dissection, this nerve is identified and can be preserved; just anterior and deep to the lateral pectoral nerve is the *axillary vein*. The Level I lymph nodes are those lateral to the lateral margin of the pectoralis minor; the Level II nodes are under the pectoralis minor muscle, and the Level III nodes (rarely dissected) are medial to the medial margin of the pectoralis minor muscle. Division of the *intercostal brachial nerves* during axillary dissection produces anesthesia down the back of the arm and along the posterior axillary line of the chest wall. The *long thoracic nerve* runs along the medial side of the posterior axilla below the intercostal brachial nerves and enters the serratus anterior musculature of the chest wall. The *thoracodorsal nerve* innervates the latissimus dorsi muscle on the lateral side of the axilla. These two motor nerves are routinely preserved during axillary dissection.

The breast is composed of an array of successively branching ducts connecting the milk-producing lobules to the

---

See the corresponding chapter or part in the *Textbook of Surgery,* 15th edition, pp. 555–593, for a more detailed discussion of this topic, including a comprehensive list of references.

nipple and areola. The breast *lobule*, or *acinus*, is formed by multiple branchings of terminal ducts, similar in concept to alveoli in the lung. The lobule is invested in a loose connective tissue that contains migratory lymphocytes and macrophages. Surrounding the lobules and their specialized connective tissue investment are dense connective tissue and fat. Under the nipple, large subareolar ducts, or *lactiferous sinuses,* open onto the surface of the nipple through 10 to 15 separate orifices.

ABNORMAL PHYSIOLOGY AND DEVELOPMENT

GYNECOMASTIA. Hypertrophy of the male breast is a common condition that tends to occur in young males (*pubertal hypertrophy*) and in older men (*senescent hypertrophy*). Hypertrophy in older men is common and associated with both systemic illness, such as hepatic or renal disease, and with the use of certain medications, particularly cardiovascular agents. The hypertrophy is frequently unilateral and tender. In both ages, gynecomastia tends to produce a symmetrical increase in breast tissue around the areola and is rubbery and smooth. Cancer in the male breast is not tender, is asymmetrically placed in relation to the areola, and may display fixation to the chest wall or skin. Mammography of the male breast is done exactly as in females. Gynecomastia in older men is rarely treated surgically unless there is confusion about the diagnosis. In younger boys, subcutaneous mastectomy may be required for cosmetic reasons.

NIPPLE DISCHARGE. Nipple discharge is usually functional and is rarely caused by malignancy. Surgically significant discharge that needs biopsy is unilateral, comes from a single duct orifice on one nipple, and may be bloody. Discharge from multiple duct orifices or from both nipples is always benign. Cytologies of the discharge are rarely helpful. Radiographic imaging of the duct has some proponents but is not necessary. Single-duct discharge that is spontaneous and blood-tinged should be biopsied under local anesthesia with sedation after cannulization of the involved duct with a lacrimal duct probe. The vast majority of these biopsies will uncover a benign intraductal papilloma.

MASTODYNIA (PAINFUL BREASTS). Breast pain is exceedingly common, particularly in women who are in their 30s or 40s, prior to menopause. A variety of treatments can be tried, such as vitamin E, caffeine restriction, and nicotine withdrawal. However, there is no documented efficacy for these measures. The pain is frequently unilateral and involving the upper outer quadrant of the affected breast. It is usually tender to palpation. A complete examination may be combined with a mammogram. If these examinations are normal, the patient should be counseled that breast pain is common, functional, and not a sign of breast cancer. It is usually self-limited, although it commonly relapses.

FIBROCYSTIC DISEASE, CYSTIC MASTITIS. The term *fibrocystic disease* should be reserved for the women whose breasts are fibrous, nodular, and painful. Frequently, these patients will form gross breast cysts that require aspiration. Dense tissue, benign microcalcifications, and architectural distortions make mammography difficult in these women. Many physicians feel that the term *fibrocystic disease* should be abandoned because there is no increased risk of cancer in these patients. However, for the patient with painful and cystic breasts, it is helpful to recognize the disability that this disease does produce.

DIAGNOSIS OF BREAST DISEASE

RISK FACTORS FOR BREAST CANCER. Risk assessment is an important part of an active practice in breast diseases. The most important risk factor used every day in clinical practice is age. Breast cancer is very uncommon in women under the age of 30 but is probably the most common diagnosis of a new breast mass in a woman over the age of 60. The age-adjusted incidence of breast cancer continues to rise throughout life. Family history is most important when primary relatives (mothers, sisters, and daughters) have breast cancer, particularly if these primary relatives had cancer when they were young or if it was bilateral. A history of breast cancer, either invasive or noninvasive, greatly increases the subsequent risk of breast cancer. This is particularly true for the ipsilateral breast that has been preserved during primary therapy and for the contralateral breast in women treated by mastectomy for their first cancers. Recently, two genes that cause cancer in families have been identified. These genes, *BRCA1* and *BRCA2*, together cause fewer than 5% of all breast cancers. However, it is possible to test for predisposing mutations in these genes and provide very accurate predictions for a small number of women.

Physical Examination

Visual inspection of the breast may disclose edema and erythema, termed *peau d'orange*, which is the hallmark of inflammatory carcinoma. Visible skin changes involving the nipple and areola may be a sign of Paget's disease. In this condition, intraductal carcinoma within subareolar ducts invades across the epidermal-epithelial junction and enters the epidermal layer of the skin on the nipple, producing a dermatitis that originates on the nipple and secondarily encompasses the areola. Masses are characterized by their size, shape, consistency, location, and fixation to the surrounding breast tissue, skin, or chest wall. Fine-needle aspiration can be performed to determine whether it is solid or cystic (fluid-containing). Cyst fluid is commonly turbid and dark green or amber in color. If the mass disappears after withdrawal and the fluid is not bloody, the diagnosis of a functional cyst is made. If the mass is solid, breast biopsy must be performed to exclude a carcinoma.

Breast Imaging (Mammography and Ultrasonography)

The mammogram is the most sensitive and specific test that can be used in addition to physical examination. Mammographic features of malignancy are density abnormalities (including masses, asymmetries, and architectural distortions) and microcalcifications. Densities with indistinct margins, stellate borders, or significant architectural distortion of the surrounding parenchyma are most likely to be malignant. Microcalcifications are very small and never palpable unless associated with a density abnormality that is palpable on physical examination.

Screening mammography is probably beneficial if the studies are obtained annually after the age of 50 years. Benefit may extend to those between the ages of 40 and 50 years, but increased survival has been difficult to demonstrate for women in this group. In women with a personal or family history of breast cancer, the benefits of early and continued screening are likely to be greater.

Ultrasonography is indicated as a complement to mammography or physical examination but has no proven benefit in screening. The principal utility of ultrasonography is to distinguish solid from cystic masses.

BENIGN BREAST MASSES

Breast Cysts

Cysts are fluid-filled epithelial cavities that vary in size from microscopic to large and palpable masses. Formation, enlargement, and regression of cysts are influenced by ovarian hormones. The incidence of large cysts peaks after the age of 35 years, is rare in women before the age of 25 years, and sharply declines after menopause. The diagnosis of a cyst is made by needle aspiration or by ultrasonography. The relationship of cysts to carcinoma is not great, and the finding of a gross cyst should not be the subject of great concern to the patient or physician. Biopsy is reserved for those lesions which do not disappear completely after aspiration, for those which recur multiple times after aspiration, or when the fluid withdrawn is clearly bloody.

Fibroadenoma and Related Tumors

Fibroadenoma is the most common benign solid tumor in the female breast and the most common breast tumor in young women. It is a solid tumor containing a proliferation of fibrous stroma and a variable proliferation of epithelium-lined ducts or spaces. In young women (under the age of 30 years), the differential diagnosis of a breast mass is usually between cyst and fibroadenoma. The two entities are distinguished by needle aspiration, which yields no fluid in the case of fibroadenoma. In older women, cancer must be added to the list of possibilities if aspiration reveals a solid mass.

Fibroadenomas have no malignant potential, although they may be related to a group of tumors of stromal elements termed *cystosarcoma phyllodes* or *phyllodes tumors*. Phyllodes tumors are commonly benign but may be malignant, behaving much like soft tissue sarcomas elsewhere in the body. The treatment for fibroadenoma is excision of the tumor without the necessity for much margin of normal breast tissue.

Breast Abscesses and Infections

Infections and abscesses usually occur around the nipple and areola, presumably originating in large subareolar lactiferous sinuses. The treatment is usually conservation and consists of administration of antibiotics. Incision and drainage are reserved for the unusual case that cannot be controlled with antibiotics. Chronic, recurrent subareolar mastitis may respond to excision of the subareolar ductal tissue when the process is quiescent.

Papilloma

Solitary intraductal papillomas are true benign polyps of the breast ducts. They are usually located in the large ductal spaces underneath the nipple and are the most common cause of a bloody nipple discharge. *Papillomatosis* is a term in common usage but refers to epithelial hyperplasia and not to true polyp formation as in solitary or multiple papilloma.

MALIGNANT TUMORS OF THE BREAST

Pathology of Breast Cancer

Malignancies of the breast are broadly divided into epithelial tumors of cells lining breast ducts and lobules and nonepithelial malignancies of the supporting breast stroma. A second important division of epithelial malignancies is between noninvasive and invasive cancer. The noninvasive malignancies are of ductal origin *(intraductal carcinoma)* or arise in lobules *(lobular carcinoma in situ)*. These are true carcinomas *in situ* and are distinguished by the fact that they do not invade the basement membrane of the ductal or lobular structures. As with carcinoma *in situ* elsewhere in the body, these lesions may coexist with invasive disease in the same malignant tumor. Most pathologists utilize the classification proposed by the World Health Organization and outlined in the fascicles of the Armed Forces Institute of Pathology.

Ductal Carcinoma *In Situ*, Intraductal Carcinoma

In health, the breast ducts are lined by two or three cell layers of epithelium. In ductal carcinoma *in situ*, the ducts become swollen with malignant cells, which may grow in solid sheets or in a cribriform or papillary manner. Because they are confined to the basement membrane, angiogenesis is retarded, and the center may undergo necrosis with production of the "comedo" appearance. This necrotic debris may calcify, which produces the fine stippled or branching calcifications seen on high-quality mammography.

Lobular Carcinoma *In Situ*, Lobular Neoplasia

This *in situ* proliferation is confined to the breast lobules and causes their expansion. Central necrosis is not a feature of this malignancy, and calcifications do not occur. Because of this, lobular carcinoma *in situ* does not form a recognizable abnormality on mammography. Lobular carcinoma *in situ* is found incidentally during evaluation of biopsy material performed for unrelated masses or mammographic findings. This disease may not invariably progress to invasive cancer and is frequently multicentric and bilateral. Because of its low malignant potential, some refer to lobular carcinoma *in situ* as *lobular neoplasia* in order to distinguish it from more malignant proliferations.

Infiltrating Ductal Carcinoma

This is the most common malignant tumor in the breast recognized after biopsy. The term *ductal* refers to its origin from ductal epithelium, and it is commonly found coexisting with intraductal carcinoma. The term *infiltrating* refers to the fact that it has invaded beyond the basement membrane of the breast duct and is found in the surrounding stroma. This tumor accounts for at least 70% of the invasive carcinomas of the breast.

Invasive Lobular Carcinoma

As the name implies, the origin of the infiltrating cell is probably from the epithelium lining of the breast lobules. Invasive lobular carcinoma constitutes between 3% and 15% of all invasive breast cancers. Clinically, lobular carcinoma behaves very similarly to its ductal counterpart.

Less Common Forms of Ductal Carcinoma

These tumors are a heterogeneous group and display different morphologic patterns. In general, these variants appear more differentiated and have an improved prognosis. An exception is medullary carcinoma of the breast, which is probably a ductal carcinoma characterized by bizarre and anaplastic tumor cells surrounded by an intense infiltrate of lymphocytes. Tubular carcinoma, characterized by small, well-formed ductal structures, and colloid or mucinous carcinoma, which produces lakes of mucin surrounding islands of tumor cells, both impart a better prognosis to their host than does the average ductal carcinoma.

Staging Breast Cancer

The most widely used method for staging breast carcinoma in the TNM (tumor, nodes, metastasis) system proposed by the American Joint Committee on Cancer and the International Union Against Cancer. Clinicopathologic staging is done after completion of surgery and pathologic examination of the primary site and regional lymph nodes. Table 1 displays estimates of the survival rates for various categories of breast cancer after modern therapy.

Current Surgical Therapy for Invasive Breast Cancer

Primary surgical therapy of breast cancer has undergone remarkable evolution during the past 25 years. In 1970, radical mastectomy was the standard procedure for both invasive and noninvasive breast cancers. By 1980, the modified radical mastectomy (MRM) had replaced radical operations, and reconstructive surgery was commonplace. During the 1980s, the results of several randomized trials that compared mastectomy to wide excision of the primary cancer and radiation (*breast conservation, breast preservation, lumpectomy*) were published. By 1990, breast-conserving surgery was firmly established as an alternative to mastectomy for operable breast cancers. During the 1990s, surgeons have questioned the role of axillary dissection and have proposed strategies to limit the extent of the axillary operation. Investigators have pushed the indications for lumpectomy by giving preoperative chemotherapy to shrink large primary cancers, thus allowing local excision to clear operative margins. During the later half of this decade, investigators will no doubt capitalize on the discovery of *BRCA1* and *BRCA2* and experiment with preventive mastectomies in patients who carry mutations in these genes. In each of these cases, the evolution of prospective clinical trials and clinical research methodology will provide a measure of quality control and credibility that has not been possible in previous decades. The surgical treatment of breast cancer is a paradigm for clinical research and for translational research that converts biological principles into clinical practice.

CONSERVATIVE SURGERY FOR OPERABLE BREAST CANCER. Seven prospective clinical trials have randomized more than 4500 patients to various surgical strategies, all of which include a mastectomy arm and a breast-preserving arm consisting of lumpectomy and breast radiotherapy (RT). Endpoints of these studies are local failure, distant failure, and survival. All studies except the NCI (USA) randomized trial required histologically negative margins for the lumpectomy specimen. Whole-breast radiation after surgical removal of the primary tumor was designed to deliver between 45 and 50 Gy. (4500 and 5000 rads) in all these trials. All the studies required axillary dissection, and adjuvant chemotherapy was prescribed for most node-positive patients. Follow-up times from 8 to more than 10 years have elapsed in all these studies,

TABLE 1. Breast Cancer Survival Estimates, 1996

Staging Category	Disease-Free Survival at 5 Years	Overall Survival at 5 Years
Stage 1: $T < 1$ cm	>90%	>95%
Stage 1: 1 cm $< T <$ 2 cm	>80%	>80%
Stage 2: $N = 0$	~80%	>80%
Stage 2: $N = 1-3$	~50%	~60%
Stage 2: $N \geq 4$	~30%	~40%
Stage 3a	~30%	~40%
Stage 3b	~30%	~40%
Stage 4	~10%	~20%

allowing firm conclusions to be drawn. In 1990, an NIH consensus conference was held and reviewed all the available data regarding breast conservation. Based on the results of randomized clinical trials, the conference concluded that MRM, MRM with delayed or immediate reconstruction, and wide excision to negative margins and postoperative RT are equivalent treatments in terms of overall breast cancer survival.

The following guidelines are a reasonable reflection of treatment practice in 1996. It is probably accurate to quote a 1% ipsilateral breast recurrence rate to candidates who are considering breast conservation. The chance of surviving breast cancer is not affected by choosing either mastectomy or lumpectomy and RT. Complication rates from breast radiation are low (between 2% and 5%) and consist of spontaneous rib fracture, transient pericarditis for left-sided cancers, some distortion of the breast and tissues around the wide excision, and a higher incidence of seroma formation and difficulty with wound healing. If an axillary dissection is performed, axillary radiation should not be routine unless there are many positive nodes or gross disease remains. Radiopaque clips should be placed within the lumpectomy defect to assist planning therapeutic radiation. No attempt should be made to approximate the deep tissues within the lumpectomy defect. If meticulous hemostasis is obtained, the wound will fill with serous fluid and slowly contract over a period of several weeks. The specimen that is removed should be oriented and ink applied before it is bisected. If a histologically positive margin is found, a reoperation to remove more tissue frequently will achieve a clear margin and allow conservation of the breast. Waiting for 2 or 3 weeks for healing and wound contracture makes the second operation technically easier and can be combined with the axillary dissection if indicated and not performed at the first operation. A gross or histologically positive margin is the only unerring contraindication to recommending breast conservation. Extensive intraductal carcinoma may be associated with a higher recurrence rate but does not negate lumpectomy and RT as long as a negative margin can be obtained.

THE MANAGEMENT OF NONINVASIVE (IN SITU) CARCINOMA

Special attention to the subject of noninvasive carcinoma is necessary because of its increasing recognition and the controversy surrounding the proper treatment of ductal and lobular carcinoma *in situ*. With the current emphasis on screening mammography, the incidence of these malignancies is increasing; their treatment should be curative.

DUCTAL CARCINOMA IN SITU (DCIS, INTRADUCTAL CARCINOMA). Treatment recommendations for patients with intraductal carcinoma are based on consideration of several issues, including (1) occult invasive cancer coexisting with the *in situ* lesion, (2) multicentricity of intraductal carcinoma, (3) the occurrence of disease in the contralateral breast, and (4) the natural history following diagnosis by biopsy. If the intraductal tumor is small and totally removed with clear surgical margins, the patient may be a candidate for wide excision without additional treatment. This is particularly true for papillary or cribriform lesions that do not display marked comedo necrosis, back-to-back ductal proliferations, and high-grade cytology. For larger lesions and for those with higher-grade histology, postoperative RT to the breast is the standard treatment recommendation. For patients with more extensive lesions that are multifocal and involving surgical margins, total mastectomy may be required. For high-grade malignancies with extensive comedo necrosis, a modified central axillary node dissection seems reasonable; in these cases, the chance of unrecognized invasive disease may be as high as 25%, and the incidence of axillary metastases approaches 10%.

The rate of ipsilateral recurrent breast cancer after treatment of a localized intraductal malignancy by excision only is probably twice the rate if the tumor was treated by excision plus radiation to the breast. However, for very small lesions of low histologic grade, the risk is sufficiently small to make excision alone reasonable. The National Surgical Adjuvant Breast and Bowel Project has concluded a trial that compared excision alone to excision plus postoperative radiation for localized intraductal carcinomas excised to clear margins. Axillary node dissection was not required in the amended protocol. After a short follow-up, 16.4% of patients treated by excision only recurred in the ipsilateral breast compared with 7.0% of the patients receiving postoperative radiation. Of greater significance, distant disease and mortality were no different and very small in this study.

In contrast to lobular carcinoma *in situ*, discussed below, DCIS does not convey increased risk to the contralateral breast over and above the risk inherent for any woman who has had one breast cancer. An average risk of contralateral cancer in the range of 0.5% to 1% per year is a reasonable figure to quote in counseling patients with either invasive cancer or DCIS, even when the noninvasive cancer is diffuse and multicentric.

LOBULAR CARCINOMA *IN SITU* (LCIS). LCIS is a relatively rare lesion that is more common in younger, premenopausal women. This lesion predisposes to eventual breast cancer, either noninvasive or invasive and both ductal and lobular in type. Haagensen reported a 21% actuarial probability of developing carcinoma at the end of 35 years of follow-up for patients treated by observation only. This risk of cancer is shared equally by both ipsilateral and contralateral breasts. A conservative approach to LCIS is probably most commonly practiced among surgical oncologists in North America and around the world. There is no reason to recommend mirror-image biopsy, an older strategy that has little to offer. The only reasonable alternative to observation is bilateral mastectomy, which seems extreme for most patients.

ADJUVANT THERAPY FOR OPERABLE BREAST CANCER

Adjuvant systemic therapy refers to the use of cytotoxic chemotherapy, hormonal therapy, or immunotherapy given after surgery that has been done with a curative intent for apparently localized breast cancer. After two decades of intense investigation involving thousands of women who participated in clinical trials, summary conclusions are now possible. Individual studies began by randomizing patients with positive lymph nodes (Stage II patients) to receive chemotherapy or observation only after definitive surgery (usually modified radical mastectomy in the earlier studies). In the 1980s, randomized studies were begun that included or concentrated on node-negative patients (generally Stage I patients). In parallel to these chemotherapy trials, older hormone treatment trials used oophorectomy as the hormonal manipulation in the treatment arm of randomized, prospective trials. Newer hormone adjuvant trials have used tamoxifen (an estrogen agonist/antagonist agent) in comparison with a control arm. Overview analysis of all published randomized trials has been done and allows conclusions to be drawn.

Most modern adjuvant regimens use drugs in combination. One common combination is cytoxan, methotrexate, and 5-fluorouracil (CMF). A more intense combination substitutes doxorubicin (Adriamycin) for methotrexate (CAF). Less intense combinations drop the cyclophosphamide (MF). In the overview analyses, these combinations were responsible for a reduction in the annual odds of recurrence of about 25% and a reduction in the annual odds of dying of about 18%. These benefits extended to both node-positive and node-negative patients and to patients older than age 50 as well as those less than age 50. In other words, the magnitude of benefit is constant across all patient and stage categories. In those patients with a higher intrinsic chance of treatment failure, a constant reduction in odds of recurrence or death leads to a larger absolute benefit.

Similar effects were found when oophorectomy or tamoxifen was compared with no-treatment control groups. Tamoxifen therapy was more effective for hormone-receptor-positive cancers and in women who were older than age 50. In contrast, oophorectomy was done in the past for premenopausal women. For tamoxifen, the proportional reduction in the odds of recurrence or death was almost identical for node-positive (28% reduction in recurrence, 18% reduction in odds of death) and node-negative women (26% for recurrence, 17% for survival). However, there was a steady trend toward improved benefits with longer durations of treatment (<1 year versus 2 years versus >2 years). For node-positive, hormone-receptor-positive patients, tamoxifen is an ideal adjuvant treatment that can be used sequentially with adjuvant chemotherapy. Generally, tamoxifen is given after chemotherapy is completed. For node-negative women with receptor-positive cancers, tamoxifen is an ideal treatment with or without chemotherapy. Oophorectomy is rarely used as an adjuvant treatment; tamoxifen is at least as effective as any other hormone stratagem to which it has been compared.

The current approach to the treatment of patients with operable breast cancer is summarized in Table 2. The recommendations are not a consensus statement but are a series of reasonable options for guiding physicians who are counseling

TABLE 2. Recommendations for Adjuvant Treatment Outside Clinical Trials

Menopausal Status	Axillary Nodes	Tumor Characteristics*	Recommended Treatment
Premenopausal	Positive	Favorable or unfavorable	Combination chemotherapy ± tamoxifen
Premenopausal	Negative	Favorable	No data to support adjuvant chemotherapy
Premenopausal	Negative	Unfavorable	Combination chemotherapy ± tamoxifen
Postmenopausal	Positive	ER/PR +	Tamoxifen ± chemotherapy
Postmenopausal	Positive	ER/PR –	Chemotherapy may be offered
Postmenopausal	Negative	Favorable	Tamoxifen may be offered for ER/PR + cancers
Postmenopausal	Negative	Unfavorable	Chemotherapy ± tamoxifen may be offered

*Favorable tumor characteristics include size ≤1 cm, ER or PR positive, good nuclear and histologic grade (1 or 2). Unfavorable tumor characteristics include size ≥2 cm, ER or PR negative, and poor nuclear and histologic grade (3). Combination chemotherapy is usually CMF or CAF for patients at high risk or recurrence and CMF or MF for patients at lower risk.

patients. The recommendations also provide a framework for understanding current practice. These recommendations are always changing, and clinicians who care for breast cancer must continue to seek new information.

I

Reconstructive and Aesthetic Breast Surgery
Gregory S. Georgiade, M.D.

Reconstructive and aesthetic breast surgery has an increasingly important role for the female patient. Aesthetic surgery of the breast consists of a number of procedures.

Augmentation mammaplasty is the most common aesthetic breast operation. This procedure for enlarging the volume of the breast mound can be accomplished by insertion of a saline-filled prosthesis in the submammary or subpectoral area with use of an inframammary, circumareolar, transareolar, periumbilical, or axillary surgical approach. The outer surface of the Silastic prostheses can be smooth-walled or microtextured to produce a roughened exterior wall. The microtextured types have become quite popular because there are indications that there is a considerable decrease in scar contracture around prostheses with these irregular configurations of the outer shell, which disrupt the linear contractures that occur with smooth-walled prostheses.

Reduction mammaplasty is the second most common procedure. Breast hypertrophy with associated ptosis creates a severe functional deformity with associated mastodynia, shoulder and back pain, and skin excoriations. Reduction mammaplasty can be performed by use of a number of techniques. A vertical, superior, or inferior-based dermal pedicle can be used to move the nipple-areola complex and reduce the amount of breast tissue from the base of the breast. The contour of the basic breast mound that contains the nipple-areola complex can be maintained, and reduction of the breast volume can be achieved by excision of measured quantities of breast tissue in a semicircular manner around the central core of breast tissue. This procedure can be performed with or without the use of an inferior dermal pedicle.

Ptosis of the breast is recognizable as an aesthetic problem with varying degrees of deformity depending on the position of the nipple on the breast mound. Mild ptosis can be im-

---

See the corresponding chapter or part in the *Textbook of Surgery*, 15th edition, pp. 594–598, for a more detailed discussion of this topic, including a comprehensive list of references.

proved many times by an augmentation mammaplasty. In the more severe cases, if there is sufficient volume of breast tissue, the nipple-areola complex can be elevated on a dermal pedicle, and the excess tissues are then excised in the infra-areola area.

Reconstruction of the breast following ablative surgery can be accomplished at the time of the initial modified radical mastectomy or simple mastectomy, or reconstruction can be performed at a later date. Patients undergoing radiation therapy or chemotherapy should not undergo reconstruction until therapy has been completed.

A common procedure, whether immediate or delayed, involves the creation of a pocket beneath the pectoralis major and serratus anterior muscles with extension of the undermining beneath the rectus fascia. A standard saline-filled Silastic implant or a tissue expander with a reservoir is inserted at the initial stage. When an acceptable breast mound has been attained, the final prosthesis is inserted, and the nipple-areola complex is reconstructed by use of a full-thickness skin graft from the groin for the areola and nipple sharing or a local chest flap for the nipple reconstruction with subsequent tattooing as needed on the nipple. Extensive loss of breast skin or underlying pectoralis musculature necessitates use of a latissimus dorsi musculocutaneous flap based on the thoracodorsal artery. The other alternative for larger defects is a rectus abdominis musculocutaneous flap based on the superior epigastric artery. A free microvascular rectus abdominis musculocutaneous flap also should be considered when simpler types of reconstructions are not available and in situations in which a large amount of breast coverage is needed and can be supplied only with large abdominal flaps.

In summary, during the last decade, a number of highly reliable techniques have been developed that allow correction of many different types of breast abnormalities. This allows improvement in many aesthetic abnormalities of the breast and reconstruction of extensive breast deformities after ablative surgery for breast malignancies. As these techniques have improved, the satisfaction of the patient and the aesthetic results also have improved.

23

THE THYROID GLAND

I

Physiology
H. Kim Lyerly, M.D.

The thyroid gland functions primarily to produce thyroid hormone for development and regulation of metabolism. Thyroid hormone production is under the regulation of the anterior pituitary hormone thyrotropin, or thyroid-stimulating hormone (TSH), and by a system of autoregulation within the thyroid gland. The thyroid hormones are the iodinated amino acids thyroxine (T_4) and 3,5,3'-triiodothyronine (T_3). In the thyroid, they are an integral part of thyroglobulin (Tg), in which they are synthesized and stored. In the plasma, they circulate as free amino acids in reversible equilibrium with the thyroid hormone–binding proteins; however, they have an effect on metabolism only when they are in the free form. Free thyroid hormones are able to penetrate cells to induce and stimulate oxygen consumption; increase body heat and the rates of metabolism of carbohydrates, fats, and proteins; and stimulate the feedback mechanism with the pituitary gland. Iodine is necessary for the synthesis of thyroid hormones. The inorganic iodine is reduced to iodide ion in the gut, where most is absorbed from the small intestine and is cleared from plasma by the thyroid. The thyroid actively transports and concentrates iodide in the thyroid follicular cell and the colloid at a rate of about 2 μg. per hour.

Iodide remains free only briefly before being oxidized to a highly reactive form that binds to tyrosine residues in thyroglobulin (Tg). After its synthesis and intracellular transport, exophytic vesicles discharge their content into the follicle, and Tg accumulates in the lumen. The iodination reaction of Tg is catalyzed by thyroid peroxidase (TPO), which is interrupted by the thiocarbamide group of drugs (such as propylthiouracil). After being bound to tyrosine residues in the thyroglobulin, iodide proceeds to be part of T_4 and T_3 via monoiodotyrosine (MIT) and diiodotyrosine (DIT).

The normal thyroid contains approximately 8000 μg. of iodine, only about 1% being inorganic iodide. T_4 constitutes approximately 35% of the total amount of thyroid hormone; T_3, 5%; DIT, 25%; and MIT, 25%. Approximately 1% of the hormone in the thyroid store is released to the circulation each day after being separated in the cell by acid proteases and peptide enzymes. The thyroid gland has a storage reserve of approximately 3 weeks.

See the corresponding chapter or part in the *Textbook of Surgery,* 15th edition, pp. 599–611, for a more detailed discussion of this topic, including a comprehensive list of references.

The concentration of total thyroxine is 30 to 50 times the concentration of T_3. However, only 0.03% of the total serum T_4 and 0.3% of the total serum T_3 is present in the unbound or biologically active form. The major serum thyroid hormone–binding proteins are thyronine-binding globulin (TBG), thyroxine-binding prealbumin (TBPA), and albumin (ALB). Hormone-binding proteins are the principal intravascular factors influencing total hormone concentration, which is normally maintained at a level appropriate for the concentration of carrier proteins to maintain a constant free hormone level. Various factors may cause changes in the concentration of TBG. Because alterations in TBG may alter the total hormone concentration independent of the metabolic status of the body, free hormone, rather than the total hormone, is a more accurate indicator of the thyroid hormone–dependent metabolic state.

Although T_4 is the principal secretory product of the thyroid gland, the principal active hormone in metabolic regulation is triiodothyronine (T_3). Thyroid hormones have numerous metabolic effects. Enhancement of the basal metabolic rate (BMR) as reflected by increased oxygen consumption is one of the classic actions of thyroid hormone. An optimal amount is necessary for balanced growth and maturation, and many of the effects of thyroid hormones on carbohydrate metabolism appear permissive with respect to the effects of other hormones. Thyroid hormone stimulates both lipogenesis and lipolysis. Thyroid hormone characteristically lowers the level of serum cholesterol by enhanced excretion in the feces and conversion of cholesterol to bile acids. Hypothyroidism is associated with altered lipoprotein metabolism, including an increase in serum concentrations of intermediate-density lipoprotein and low-density lipoprotein (LDL) cholesterol. The generalized metabolic response increases the demand for vitamins and cofactors, and there is a magnified catecholamine effect produced by excess thyroid hormone.

MECHANISMS OF THYROID REGULATION

The principal regulatory mechanisms of the thyroid gland are the hypothalamic-pituitary-thyroid control system and the intrathyroidal autoregulatory system. The former is represented by the pituitary thyrotropin TSH, which stimulates many aspects of thyroid activity, particularly thyroid hormone synthesis and secretion, and thyroid hormones inhibit the secretion of TSH by the pituitary.

Thyroid-Stimulating Hormone (TSH)

TSH is a glycoprotein hormone that has a major role in thyroid growth. Iodide deficiency and excessive treatment of hyperthyroidism with blockers of iodide binding to thyroglobulin lead to increased TSH secretion and thyroid enlargement.

Thyrotropin-Releasing Hormone (TRH)

TRH is a tripeptide (pyroglutamyl-histidylproline amide) produced by the supraoptic and paraventricular nuclei of the hypothalamus that provides tonic stimulation of TSH-producing cells within the pituitary.

Autoregulation of Thyroid Function

Although TSH is the primary regulator of the activity of the thyroid gland, it is most prominent in adaptation to conditions of iodine deficiency or excess. In humans, the Wolff-Chaikoff block (acute block of iodide binding) is induced by an elevation of the plasma iodide concentration followed by a progressive inhibition of iodide binding to tyrosyl residues in thyroglobulin. In addition, administration of potassium iodide to a patient with Graves' disease or a normal subject causes a prompt reduction in the release of iodine-containing compounds from the gland and a prompt decrease in serum thyroid hormone levels and a reduction of the hypervascularity.

II

Hyperthyroidism
H. Kim Lyerly, M.D.

Hyperthyroidism is caused by increased levels of thyroid hormone with a loss of the normal feedback mechanism controlling the secretion of thyroid hormone. Common types of hyperthyroidism include diffuse toxic goiter (Graves' disease) and toxic adenoma or toxic multinodular goiter (Plummer's disease). One must distinguish between hyperthyroidism due to Graves' disease or due to single or multiple adenomas of the thyroid. Graves' disease is a systemic autoimmune syndrome with variable expression that includes goiter with hyperthyroidism, exophthalmos, pretibial myxedema, and acropachy. Any or all of these features may be present, since Graves' disease reflects disturbances of immunity not yet clearly defined. In contrast, an adenoma may be viewed as benign neoplasia associated with excess secretion of thyroid hormone and is thus a localized disease.

See the corresponding chapter or part in the *Textbook of Surgery*, 15th edition, pp. 611–623, for a more detailed discussion of this topic, including a comprehensive list of references.

GRAVES' DISEASE

Approximately 36 females and 8 males per 100,000 of female and male populations develop Graves' disease. A hereditary component of Graves' disease has been recognized. Graves' disease may be found with other autoimmune conditions in the same individual and within families. Although the origin of Graves' disease remains obscure, current evidence suggests that it is an autoimmune disorder caused by thyroid-stimulating immunoglobulins (TSIs) that have been produced against an antigen in the thyroid. These polyclonal immunoglobulins appear to be directed to thyroid-stimulating hormone (TSH) receptors and can be detected by sensitive and specific radioreceptor assays.

The symptoms and signs of hyperthyroidism are a history of irritability, weight loss, heat intolerance, and emotional instability and the physical findings of goiter, exophthalmos, and other eye signs. These features may be more subtle in the elderly or chronically ill. The eye features of Graves' disease include a continuum from mere stare and lid lag to complete visual loss from corneal or optic nerve involvement.

Laboratory examinations are now available to confirm the diagnosis; hyperthyroidism is usually confirmed by measuring circulating thyroid hormone concentrations of total thyroxine (TT_4). Hyperthyroidism in Graves' disease is managed with a number of strategies. The thyroid hypersecretion can be controlled by reducing the functional mass of thyroid tissue by surgical removal of a large part of the gland or by destruction of most of the gland with radioiodine. Thyrotoxicosis also can be controlled with antithyroid drugs to reduce the secretion of thyroid hormone and by drugs that block beta-adrenergic receptors. Most methods cause a reduction of the net secretion of thyroid hormone to euthyroid levels.

Thyrotoxicosis is effectively controlled by antithyroid drugs, and trials with antithyroid drugs are used in most patients to control signs and symptoms. They have relatively mild and infrequent side effects, are easy to use, have predictable therapeutic actions, and are inexpensive. In most patients, thyroid function returns to normal within several weeks to several months. Unfortunately, these agents may succeed in inducing a permanent remission in only a small minority of adults and in approximately 20% of children. In addition, prolonged use of these agents is limited due to toxic side effects such as rash, liver dysfunction, neuritis, arthralgia, myalgia, lymphadenopathy, psychosis, and the occasional development of irreversible agranulocytosis (<1 in 200). Beta-receptor blockade, while effectively controlling some of the major effects of thyrotoxicosis, has not been effective as a sole means of therapy.

Radioiodine (^{131}I) therapy may be considered for nearly all patients with thyrotoxicosis except newborns, pregnant females, or when it is precluded by a low iodine uptake. Treatment is highly effective, although hypothyroidism requiring thyroid replacement is common. Potential complications of radiotherapy including thyroid carcinoma and congenital abnormalities in future offspring have not been demonstrated; however, there is still reluctance to treat children and women of childbearing age with radioiodine. Symptoms improve in most patients in 6 to 8 weeks, and most parameters of hyperthyroidism return to normal by 10 to 12 weeks. Because of the inherent delay in achieving a therapeutic response with ^{131}I, ancillary treatment with a beta-adrenergic–blocking drug is often desirable. The primary drawback of radioiodine treatment is the high incidence of subsequent hypothyroidism. Depending on the therapeutic strategy, permanent hypothyroidism occurs in as many as 50% to 80% of patients.

Although most patients with Graves' disease are treated with radioiodine or antithyroid drug therapy, a significant percentage of patients require surgical therapy. Indications for subtotal thyroidectomy for Graves' disease include (1) intolerance or noncompliance with antithyroid drug therapy and (2) contraindications to radioiodine therapy. Conditions in patients who undergo subtotal thyroidectomy include Graves' disease occurring in children and adolescents, in women who are potential mothers, in patients under the age of 20 unlikely to undergo remission because of a large goiter, and in those who do not experience a remission, as indicated by persistent thyromegaly or the need for continued antithyroid medication beyond 1 or 2 years.

Surgical management of hyperthyroidism is directed toward removal of sufficient thyroid tissue to render the patient euthyroid and is accomplished in 95% to 97% of patients. Control of hyperthyroidism is immediate, and the need for drug therapy and the genetic hazards associated with radioiodine therapy are avoided. Surgical risks are minimal but include recurrent laryngeal nerve injury, hypoparathyroidism, and permanent hypothyroidism.

Subtotal thyroidectomy should be performed after thyrotoxicosis is controlled medically. Propylthiouracil is used to inhibit thyroid hormone synthesis and limit peripheral conversion of T_4 to T_3. Thyroidectomy performed immediately after control of thyrotoxicosis is associated with a risk of thyroid crisis, and it is preferable to wait approximately 2 months after a patient is euthyroid.

Thyrotoxic patients are usually treated with iodide and iodine (Lugol's solution, which is a combination of potassium iodide, 10 gm. per 100 ml., and iodine, 5 gm. per 100 ml.) for 10 days before operation to decrease the vascularity of the gland. Preoperative preparation with Lugol's solution without propylthiouracil to control the thyrotoxicosis is now uncommon, and operation must be scheduled before thyroid escape from iodine control occurs after 10 days of treatment. Thyroid hormone, rather than iodine, also can be used to reduce the vascularity of the gland treated with propylthiouracil, because adequate doses of thyroid hormone suppress the TSH increase associated with propylthiouracil and decrease the thyroid vascularity stimulated by that mechanism. Beta-adrenergic blockade alone has been prescribed for preoperative preparation but is used more commonly as an adjunct to thioamides, particularly if the patient at the time of operation is not euthyroid.

Subtotal thyroidectomy effectively and immediately controls thyrotoxicosis. The incidence of recurrent disease is inversely related to the incidence of hypothyroidism and is 1% to 5%. Within 1 to 2 years, hypothyroidism may develop in 5% to 50% of patients, with a slight additional increase in subsequent years. The incidence of hypothyroidism can be related to the estimated weight of the thyroid remnant. The incidence is 45% or higher with a remnant weight of 2 to 4 gm., compared with an incidence of less than 20% when a remnant of 8 to 10 gm. is left. The autoimmune nature of the disease also influences the overall rate of hypothyroidism. Patients with high titers of antibodies and lymphocytic infiltration of the thyroid tissue are more likely to develop postoperative hypothyroidism. Postoperative hypothyroidism is effectively treated with thyroid replacement.

Hyperfunctioning adenomas are often first recognized on a thyroid scan, where they appear as "hot" nodules. Often the patient is still euthyroid, because even though the adenoma is hypersecreting independently of the pituitary feedback system, suppression of thyroid secretion from the normal gland maintains a physiologic net secretion rate of thyroid hormone. Only when the normal gland can no longer be suppressed and the adenoma continues to increase its secretion rate of thyroid hormone does laboratory or clinical evidence of hyperthyroidism appear.

There is no evidence that drugs such as propylthiouracil exert a direct, permanent effect on thyroid function, so cessation of therapy inevitably is followed by relapse. Ablation of the neoplasm or neoplasms by surgery or radioiodine is the only course to be offered these patients.

III

Thyroiditis
H. Kim Lyerly, M.D.

The term *thyroiditis* refers to infiltration of the thyroid gland by inflammatory cells, caused by a diverse group of infectious and inflammatory disorders. Inflammation of the thyroid may be organ-specific or part of a multisystem process and may be acute and self-limiting or chronic and progressive. The term *autoimmune thyroid disease* defines a group of conditions characterized by the presence of circulating thyroid antibodies and immunologically competent cells capable of reacting with certain thyroid constituents. However, it does not imply that these antibodies or cells necessarily have any causal relationship to the thyroid disease. These autoimmune thyroid dis-

---

See the corresponding chapter or part in the *Textbook of Surgery*, 15th edition, pp. 623–626, for a more detailed discussion of this topic, including a comprehensive list of references.

eases are Hashimoto's disease (lymphocytic thyroiditis), primary myxedema, and juvenile, fibrous, focal, and painless varieties of thyroiditis.

Hashimoto's disease is the most common cause of goitrous hypothyroidism in adults and sporadic goiter in children. In Hashimoto's disease, thyroid tissue damaged by immunologic factors is replaced by lymphocytes, plasma cells, and fibrosis. Antithyroid antibodies are present in the serum of patients with Hashimoto's disease, directed against elements in the thyroid cell or colloid such as thyroglobulin, a second colloid antigen (other than thyroglobulin), microsomes, and perhaps to a cell surface antigen. No antibodies to the TSH receptor of the cell surface (as seen in Graves' disease) have been associated with Hashimoto's disease.

Symptoms of hypothyroidism in association with a painless, firm goiter are frequent presenting complaints; however, patients may be euthyroid. The diagnosis of Hashimoto's disease begins by documenting hypothyroidism with thyroid function tests. Routine tests for thyroglobulin and microsomal antibodies should be performed to confirm the diagnosis of Hashimoto's disease, since the presence and the titer of these antibodies correlate with the severity and extent of the autoimmune process.

There is no specific treatment for Hashimoto's disease. Patients are usually followed medically, and replacement therapy with T_4 is begun in patients with hypothyroidism that is symptomatic or associated with a goiter that is causing pressure symptoms. Early initiation of thyroid hormone therapy has been recommended by many to prevent further thyroid enlargement and reduce the risk of myxedma, especially in postpartum patients.

PAINLESS THYROIDITIS

This syndrome, increasingly described over the past decade and referred to as *silent* or *painless thyroiditis* but most accurately as *lymphocytic thyroiditis with spontaneous resolving hyperthyroidism*, is now recognized as a distinct entity. It presents either sporadically or in the postpartum period. Clinical features mimic those of subacute thyroiditis (SAT) but without the neck pain. Hyperthyroidism, which is usually self-limiting, develops abruptly in a patient in whom the thyroid is painless and only slightly enlarged, has low radioactive iodine uptake, and histologically demonstrates lymphocytic infiltration without the characteristic giant cell and granulomatous changes seen in SAT. Differentiation from SAT appears worthwhile, because with long-term follow-up it is clear that whereas few patients with SAT have a recurrence or progress to permanent thyroid disease, this is not the situation with the painless thyroiditis syndrome.

DE QUERVAIN'S (SUBACUTE OR GIANT CELL) THYROIDITIS

Subacute thyroiditis (SAT) represents approximately 1% of all cases of thyroid disease and is the most common cause of an anterior neck mass and pain in the thyroid gland. Although a causative agent is rarely demonstrated, it often follows upper respiratory tract infections, suggesting that it is due to a viral infection.

The course of SAT consists of several clinical stages, the first of which begins with acute pain in the thyroid gland. Compression of the esophagus may occur, and the patient has dysphagia or odynophagia. Hyperthyroidism is observed in this first stage of the disease, and the syndrome lasts for several weeks to several months. Graves' disease and the thyrotoxic phase of SAT are differentiated by thyroid scan; patients with Graves' disease have diffuse increased uptake, whereas patients in the thyrotoxic phase of SAT demonstrate diffuse decreased uptake. SAT differs from Hashimoto's disease in that SAT is not consistently associated with antithyroid antibodies. This condition remits spontaneously after a variable period from a few days to a few months and relapses occasionally before the disease remits permanently. The treatment consists of analgesics such as aspirin or ibuprofen in mild cases. Steroids are effective in controlling symptoms in the more severe cases. Spontaneous recovery is observed in over 90% of patients after 3 to 6 weeks; however, up to 30% of patients go on to a hypothyroid phase caused by extensive destruction of follicular cells. Most of these patients regain normal thyroid function in 4 to 6 weeks, but in up to 10% of patients, hypothyroidism is permanent.

ACUTE SUPPURATIVE THYROIDITIS

This is a rare condition of the thyroid gland that is usually due to bacterial infections such as *Streptococcus*, *Staphylococcus*, and *Pneumococcus* and, rarely, *Salmonella* or *Bacteroides*. Symptoms occur with an acute onset and characteristically include tenderness, enlargement, warmth, erythema, and neck pain exacerbated by neck extension and swallowing. Thyroid function is usually normal, as is the RAIU, although should an abscess develop, it will be observed as an area of decreased uptake on the thyroid scan. Although the clinical characteristics of acute suppurative thyroiditis are usually straightforward, differentiation from de Quervain's thyroiditis is important. Primary treatment of suppurative thyroiditis consists of appropriate antibiotics against the causative organism.

IV

Nodular Goiter and Benign and Malignant Neoplasms of the Thyroid
George S. Leight, Jr., M.D.

Nodular goiter refers to a thyroid gland at least twice the normal 20-gm. weight that has enlarged due to one or more nodules. The incidence of clinically detectable nodular thyroid disease is approximately 4.2% in the U.S. population, although it approaches 50% in autopsy surveys. Nodular enlargement of the thyroid results from excessive replication of thyroid epithelial cells that form new follicles with variable morphology and function. This may result from a deficiency of iodine in the diet causing decreased thyroid hormone production and increased TSH secretion, which accelerates the process. Other goitrogenic agents, including dietary goitrogens, medications, malnutrition, inherited defects in thyroid hormone synthesis, and growth-stimulating antibodies, also may play a role.

Although frequently asymptomatic, an enlarging goiter can cause tracheal or esophageal compression, resulting in dysphagia, cough, respiratory compromise, or a feeling of fullness in the neck. These symptoms may be more common with substernal goiters because of the limited space for expansion. CT scan is useful to document the degree of compression of neck structures. Although the risk of malignancy is low, surgical treatment becomes necessary when compressive symptoms develop. The goal of surgical therapy is to remove all abnormal nodular thyroid tissue, since all nodules potentially contain autonomously growing cells with the potential to cause recurrent goiter. Nodules that grow despite thyroid hormone therapy are autonomous and are associated with a higher risk of malignancy. Needle biopsy should be performed, with surgical resection of those lesions which are suspicious or definitely malignant. The vast majority of substernal goiters can be removed through a cervical approach.

BENIGN NEOPLASMS

Thyroid adenomas are benign neoplasms arising from follicular tissue and are considered distinct etiologically from the multiple adenomas that occur in multinodular goiter. True adenomas may be the product of clones of follicular cells with very high individual growth rates. The most common lesion

See the corresponding chapter or part in the *Textbook of Surgery*, 15th edition, pp. 626–637, for a more detailed discussion of this topic, including a comprehensive list of references.

is a follicular adenoma, which is usually surrounded by a well-defined capsule. Most papillary lesions are considered to be malignant. Adenomas usually grow slowly and are typically asymptomatic. The most important factor in the management of thyroid adenomas is their differentiation from malignant thyroid lesions. Once it can be established by needle biopsy that a nodule is a benign adenoma, the patient is usually followed closely. Adenomas that continue to enlarge progressively cause compressive symptoms or cause thyrotoxicosis and should be considered for surgical resection.

MANAGEMENT OF THYROID NODULES

A solitary thyroid nodule is a clinically discrete nodule in a normal-sized or diffusely enlarged gland. A solitary nodule (4.7%) or a dominant nodule in a multinodular gland (4.1%) has a higher risk of being malignant than the multiple palpable nodules of a multinodular gland (1%). The challenge to the clinician is to select from the large group of patients with thyroid nodules the 5% of patients whose nodules harbor thyroid cancer. Evaluation begins with a careful history and physical examination. Characteristics of a nodule suggestive for malignancy include firm texture, irregularity, fixation to surrounding structures, and enlarged ipsilateral cervical lymph nodes. Fine-needle aspiration biopsy (FNAB) is accepted as the most precise diagnostic screening procedure for differentiating benign from malignant thyroid nodules. The important factors for a satisfactory test include a representative specimen from the nodule and an experienced cytologist to interpret the findings. Sensitivity of FNAB in a large series was 92% with a specificity of 74%; patients selected for operation based on suspicious or malignant cytology demonstrated a yield of cancer of 45%, with only 2.5% missed carcinomas. Although FNAB is the best current method for diagnosing thyroid carcinoma, false-negative diagnoses do occur, and it is mandatory that patients with persistent thyroid nodularity have repeat periodic aspirations.

THYROID CARCINOMA

Thyroid carcinomas are a heterogeneous group of tumors that show considerable variability in biologic behavior, histologic appearance, and response to therapy. Clinically detectable thyroid carcinoma is rare, representing 1% of all malignancies; approximately 11,000 patients per year are treated in the United States for thyroid carcinoma. The annual mortality is only 6 per million population, or 1050 patients, reflecting the favorable prognosis for most thyroid carcinomas. The cause of thyroid carcinoma remains to be established, although irradiation is an established etiologic factor and several oncogenes have been identified that seem to play a role in pathogenesis. The prognosis in most patients with well-differentiated thyroid carcinoma is quite favorable, although several factors that influence recurrence and survival have been identified. Some of these factors are related to the host (age and sex), some are intrinsic to the tumor (histologic type and grade), and others reflect the relationship between the host and the tumor (size, extent of invasion, local or distant metastases). To quantify the importance of these factors, several prognostic index systems (AGES, AMES, MACIS) have been devised to assess overall risk. The significance of these systems is to help determine the extent of operative and postoperative therapy required to achieve an optimal result.

PAPILLARY CARCINOMA

Although the primary management of papillary carcinoma is surgical excision, the extent of resection and indications for regional lymph node dissection remain controversial. There is consensus that the minimum operation for documented or suspected papillary carcinoma is total lobectomy and isthmectomy. In patients with a history of cervical irradiation, total thyroidectomy should be performed because of the higher incidence of multifocal neoplasms. Some surgeons prefer to treat low-risk patients with lobectomy and isthmectomy, while others recommend total thyroidectomy for all patients with papillary carcinomas larger than 1.5 cm. when the operation can be performed safely. As the extent of thyroidectomy increases, the risk of complications (recurrent nerve injury, hypoparathyroidism) also increases. Following total thyroidectomy, radioactive iodine can be used to identify and treat local or distant metastases, and the overall recurrence rate is lower in these patients. Cervical lymph node metastases do increase the risk of recurrence in the neck but have a minor detrimental effect on survival. When total thyroidectomy is performed, the central neck nodes are removed with the operative specimen. In patients with palpably enlarged lateral cervical nodes, removal by modified radical neck dissection is indicated.

FOLLICULAR CARCINOMA

Pathologically, the two types of follicular carcinoma are the low-grade encapsulated (microinvasive) type and the high-grade angioinvasive (macroinvasive) type. The vast majority of patients with follicular carcinoma have this microinvasive type, which rarely metastasizes and has an excellent prognosis. The macroinvasive tumor frequently disseminates hematogenously, with bone, lung, liver, and CNS as the most frequent sites. If an unequivocal diagnosis of follicular carcinoma can be made on frozen section, total thyroidectomy should be performed for lesions larger than 1 cm. It remains controversial whether complete thyroidectomy should be done for microinvasive follicular carcinomas diagnosed only by permanent section, although some experienced surgeons elect to follow these patients. Macroinvasive tumors are usually large with extension into surrounding structures. These patients are best treated with total thyroidectomy. Numerous studies have demonstrated that the lowest recurrence and death rates in patients with well-differentiated thyroid carcinoma occur in those treated with both ^{131}I and thyroid hormone suppression.

V

Multiple Endocrine Neoplasia Syndromes

Terry C. Lairmore, M.D., and Samuel A. Wells, Jr., M.D.

Tumors of the endocrine system most often develop within a single gland. There are inherited disorders, however, which are characterized by the development of neoplasms in multiple endocrine glands. Multiple endocrine neoplasia Type 1 (MEN 1) consists of parathyroid hyperplasia, pancreatic islet cell neoplasms, and adenomas of the anterior pituitary. Multiple endocrine neoplasia Type 2A (MEN 2A) consists of medullary thyroid carcinoma (MTC), pheochromocytomas, and parathyroid hyperplasia, while MEN 2B consists of MTC, pheochromocytomas, mucosal neuromas, and a distinctive marfanoid habitus.

MULTIPLE ENDOCRINE NEOPLASIA TYPE 1

Genetic Studies

Genetic linkage studies and studies using deletion mapping in tumor DNA have localized the MEN 1 locus to the long arm of chromosome 11. The pattern of allelic deletions in MEN 1 is consistent with a two-mutational model of oncogenesis in which "two hits" are required to inactivate both copies of a tumor suppressor gene, as demonstrated for other inherited neoplasms (notably retinoblastoma). At the time of this writing, the specific MEN 1 mutation(s) has not been identified.

Clinical and Pathologic Features

The gene for MEN 1 is transmitted with near 100% penetrance, but with variable expressivity, such that each affected individual exhibits some but not necessarily all of the components of the syndrome. The most common abnormality in MEN 1 is parathyroid hyperplasia, which occurs in approximately 90% to 97% of patients, followed by pancreatic islet cell neoplasms (30% to 80%) and pituitary adenomas (15% to 50%).

See the corresponding chapter or part in the *Textbook of Surgery*, 15th edition, pp. 638–646, for a more detailed discussion of this topic, including a comprehensive list of references.

PARATHYROIDS. The characteristic parathyroid lesion is chief cell hyperplasia of all four glands. The diagnosis is made by measurement of serum calcium and parathyroid hormone levels. In patients with MEN 1, biochemical evidence of hyperparathyroidism usually precedes the clinical onset of an islet cell or pituitary neoplasm by several years. Symptomatic patients develop renal stones or nephrocalcinosis. Skeletal complications of hyperparathyroidism occur but are uncommon.

Patients with MEN 1 and parathyroid hyperplasia have been managed by subtotal ($3\frac{1}{2}$ gland) parathyroidectomy in an attempt to render them normocalcemic. However, persistent or recurrent hypercalcemia in MEN 1 patients treated in this manner has been as high as 30% to 40%. Alternatively, patients with multiglandular hyperplasia can be treated by total parathyroidectomy with autotransplantation of parathyroid tissue into the forearm. Advantages of this procedure include a lower incidence of recurrent hypercalcemia and management of recurrent disease by excision of grafted tissue under local anesthesia.

PANCREAS. The most common clinical pancreatic islet cell lesion in patients with MEN 1 is gastrinoma. Clinically, patients present with a severe peptic ulcer diathesis following autonomous gastrin hypersecretion. Gastrinomas associated with MEN 1 account for 20% of all cases of the Zollinger-Ellison syndrome (ZES). The diagnosis of gastrinoma is made by documentation of gastric acid hypersecretion (greater than 15 mEq. per liter) and elevated fasting levels of serum gastrin (greater than 100 pg. per ml.). Gastrinomas that develop in patients with MEN 1 are usually malignant. Because of the multicentricity and small size of these neoplasms, the true gastrinoma may not be localized preoperatively by computed tomographic (CT) scanning, angiography, or portal venous sampling.

In patients with unresectable or metastatic gastrinoma, H_2-receptor antagonists and proton pump inhibitors such as omeprazole effectively control acid hypersecretion and its attendant complications. Resection of gastrinomas larger than 2 to 3 cm. that are identified on radiographic studies is indicated to control the tumoral process, but operation is rarely curative in patients with MEN 1. Gastrinomas have an indolent course in many patients, and with aggressive medical therapy and surgery to limit tumor progression, affected individuals may enjoy long survival.

The second most common pancreatic islet cell neoplasm in patients with MEN 1 is insulinoma. The insulinomas are usually smaller than 2 cm. and multiple in contrast to those which occur sporadically, where approximately 80% are solitary. Patients commonly present with recurrent symptoms of neuroglycopenia: sweating, dizziness, confusion, or syncope. The diagnosis of insulinoma is made by documenting symptomatic hypoglycemia concomitant with inappropriately elevated plasma levels of insulin and C-peptide during a supervised 72-hour fast. There is no ideal medical therapy for insulinoma; therefore, these lesions are most often treated by surgical resection (subtotal pancreatectomy). Often, surgically treated patients become asymptomatic with normoglycemia. Approximately 10% of insulinomas occurring in patients with MEN 1 are malignant.

Other pancreatic islet cell neoplasms, such as glucagonoma, somatostatinoma, and tumors secreting vasoactive intestinal peptide or pancreatic polypeptide, occur rarely in association with MEN 1.

PITUITARY. Pituitary neoplasms occur in 15% to 50% of patients. Most of these tumors are prolactin-secreting adenomas. Pituitary tumors cause symptoms either by hypersecretion of hormones or compression of adjacent structures. Pituitary tumors, either functioning or nonfunctioning, may require ablation by surgery or irradiation. Bromocriptine, a dopamine agonist and an inhibitor of prolactin secretion, has been used to treat prolactinomas medically.

MULTIPLE ENDOCRINE NEOPLASIA TYPES 2A AND 2B

Genetic Studies

The MEN 2A and MEN 2B syndromes are inherited in an autosomal dominant pattern; however, MEN 2B in particular may occur sporadically or arise as a new mutation with autosomal dominant transmission in subsequent generations. The identification of germline mutations in the *ret* protooncogene (which encodes a receptor tyrosine kinase signal transduction molecule) in patients with the MEN 2A and MEN 2B has led to the use of DNA-based predictive testing to identify patients who have inherited the mutation before they manifest clinical or biochemical evidence of MTC.

Clinical and Pathologic Features

MEDULLARY THYROID CARCINOMA. In patients with MEN 2A or MEN 2B, MTC virtually always occurs as bilateral, multicentric foci of tumor in the middle and upper portions of each thyroid lobe. A diffuse premalignant proliferation of C cells in the thyroid glands of patients with familial MTC has been described and termed *C-cell hyperplasia* (CCH). The presence of bilateral MTC or microscopic evidence of CCH in areas of the thyroid adjacent to macroscopic foci of MTC strongly suggests the presence of familial disease.

Calcitonin (CT) is a sensitive plasma tumor marker for the presence of MTC in preoperative screening or postoperative evaluation. Provocative testing with calcium gluconate and pentagastrin and measurement of plasma CT by radioimmunoassay is an extremely sensitive way to detect MTC when it is clinically occult and is the method of choice for screening kindred members at risk for MEN 2A before the mutations at the DNA level are identified. Measurement of CT after calcium/pentagastrin stimulation remains the most important method for detecting persistent or recurrent MTC postoperatively.

The surgical treatment of MTC is total thyroidectomy, with removal of the nodes in the central compartment of the neck.

Patients with macroscopic lymph node metastases should undergo ipsilateral modified neck dissection in addition to total thyroidectomy. Medullary thyroid carcinoma often has an indolent biologic course, and although early metastases to cervical lymph nodes may occur, it may remain confined to the neck for many months or years. In patients with persistently elevated CT levels postoperatively and disease apparently confined to the neck, reoperation and meticulous superior mediastinal and bilateral lymph node dissection under magnification to remove all tumor in the neck may achieve normalization of plasma CT levels in 28% to 36% of patients.

PHEOCHROMOCYTOMA. The pheochromocytomas in patients with MEN 2A and MEN 2B usually appear in the second or third decade of life. Approximately 60% to 80% are bilateral, and they are nearly always benign. Patients with MEN 2A or MEN 2B develop adrenal medullary hyperplasia before the development of pheochromocytomas. When symptomatic, the adrenal lesions produce severe pounding frontal headaches, episodic diaphoresis, palpitations, vague feelings of anxiety, and paroxysmal hypertension.

The diagnosis of pheochromocytoma in patients with MEN 2A and MEN 2B is made biochemically by measurement of the urinary excretion of catecholamines and catecholamine metabolites (epinephrine, norepinephrine, metanephrines, and vanillylmandelic acid). Patients with elevated levels of one or more components of the 24-hour urine catecholamine determinations should be evaluated further by computed tomography of the adrenal glands. If pheochromocytoma is detected, a bilateral subcostal or midline incision should be performed with exploration of both adrenal glands, the sympathetic chain, and the organ of Zückerkandl. Patients with bilateral pheochromocytomas should have both adrenal glands removed. Although a matter of some controversy, in patients with unilateral pheochromocytoma and a palpably normal contralateral gland at operation, it is acceptable policy to perform a unilateral adrenalectomy.

PARATHYROIDS. Hyperfunction of the parathyroid glands in patients with MEN 2A is the most variable component of the syndrome. The parathyroid lesions in patients with MEN 2A consist primarily of generalized chief cell hyperplasia, and typically there is multiple gland enlargement. The diagnosis of hyperparathyroidism rests on the finding of hypercalcemia (serum calcium greater than 10.5 mg. per 100 ml.) and an inappropriately elevated parathyroid hormone (PTH) level. Although some surgeons perform a subtotal (3½ gland) parathyroidectomy in patients with parathyroid hyperplasia and MEN 2A, the authors perform total parathyroidectomy with autograft of parathyroid tissue into the forearm musculature. In patients without hypercalcemia undergoing thyroidectomy for MTC, grossly normal parathyroid glands should be left in place.

DNA TESTING AND PROPHYLACTIC THYROIDECTOMY IN PATIENTS WITH MEN 2A. Although very sensitive and specific, provocative testing with calcium and pentagastrin is associated with bothersome side effects that have caused some kindred members to refuse repetitive testing.

Predictive DNA testing based on linked genetic markers is highly accurate, but the analysis is labor-intensive and requires a suitable pedigree structure and collection of DNA from affected and unaffected kindred members for genotyping.

The recent identification of germline mutations in the *RET* proto-oncogene in patients with MEN 2A, MEN 2B, and familial MTC has made direct DNA testing the preferred method of screening kindred members at risk. Direct genetic testing may be performed at any age and requires collection of a single peripheral blood sample for rapid preparation of a small amount of genomic DNA. The ability to detect mutations at the base-pair level has simplified the management of these patients by allowing the performance of prophylactic thyroidectomy in patients who have inherited a disease-specific mutation and by identifying those individuals who do not require further testing.

24

THE PARATHYROID GLANDS

Gerard M. Doherty, M.D., and Samuel A. Wells, Jr., M.D.

The physiologic role of the parathyroid glands is the endocrine control of calcium homeostasis. This function is mediated through the production of parathyroid hormone (PTH). The major clinical disorders affecting the parathyroids involve either over- or undersecretion of PTH—hyper- or hypoparathyroidism. *Primary hyperparathyroidism* occurs when the normal feedback control of serum calcium is disturbed and there is overproduction of PTH. *Secondary hyperparathyroidism* develops most commonly in patients with renal disease; there is a defect in mineral homeostasis causing a compensatory increase in gland function. Occasionally, a hyperplastic compensatory gland develops autonomous function, a condition referred to as *tertiary hyperparathyroidism.* Hypoparathyroidism is seen most frequently as a surgical complication of either the thyroid or parathyroid glands.

EMBRYOLOGY AND ANATOMY

The superior parathyroids arise from the fourth branchial pouch along with the lateral thyroid. The inferior parathyroids develop from the third branchial pouch in conjunction with the thymus. Although the four glands are identified most commonly on the posterior aspect of the upper and lower lateral thyroid lobes, they may be found anywhere from the musculature of the pharynx to the deep mediastinum, spanning the origin and the end of migration of their respective *branchial pouch* structures. Ectopic superior glands tend to migrate posteriorly along the esophagus and into the mediastinum. Inferior glands are found most commonly in association with the thymus. There are nearly always at least four parathyroids. Five glands are found approximately 4% of the time.

The parathyroid glands tend to be flat and ovoid in shape and are yellow-brown in color. Normally they measure 2 x 3 x 7 mm. with a combined weight of 90 to 200 mg. The arterial supply is most commonly from a branch of the inferior thyroid artery; the venous drainage is highly variable. On histologic examination, they are composed of a parenchyma of hormonally active cells and a stroma composed primarily of adipocytes. The functional significance of the various cell types remains unclear, although the chief cell appears to be the predominant type.

See the corresponding chapter or part in the *Textbook of Surgery,* 15th edition, pp. 647–664, for a more detailed discussion of this topic, including a comprehensive list of references.

PHYSIOLOGY

The parathyroid glands are critical in the normal control of calcium homeostasis. PTH and vitamin D are the major regulators of calcium and phosphate metabolism. *Calcium* is a critical constituent of all body fluids and is intimately involved in a number of physiologic processes ranging from blood coagulation to bone formation. It represents a major cellular messenger and is critical in muscle contraction and membrane repolarization. Calcium in the inorganic form is absorbed from the upper small intestine. On a regular diet, approximately 1 gm. is ingested daily. The calcium in the extracellular fluid is constantly being exchanged with that in the exchangeable bone pool, the intracellular fluid, and the glomerular filtrate. Normal plasma calcium measures about 9 to 10.5 mg. per 100 ml. (4.5 to 5.2 mEq. per liter) and is about equally divided between an ionized, or metabolically active, and a protein-bound phase. Total serum calcium is affected by the concentration both of albumin, the major calcium-binding protein, and of hydrogen ion, which displaces calcium from albumin.

Plasma phosphate measures 2.6 to 4.3 mg. per 100 ml. and varies inversely with the calcium such that the product of their concentrations is constant and measures between 30 and 40.

The primary agents responsible for *regulation of calcium metabolism* are PTH, vitamin D, and calcitonin. Their major actions are summarized in Table 1. Briefly, a reduction in serum ionized calcium increases secretion of PTH, which secondarily stimulates hydroxylation of 25(OH)-vitamin D to metabolically active 1,25(OH)$_2$-vitamin D$_3$ in the kidney. Through their actions on bone, renal reabsorption, and intestinal absorption,

TABLE 1. Actions of Major Calcium-Regulating Hormones

	Bone	Kidney	Intestine
Parathyroid hormone	Stimulates resorption of calcium and phosphate	Stimulates reabsorption of calcium and conversion of 25(OH)D$_3$ to 1,25(OH)$_2$D$_3$; inhibits reabsorption of phosphate and bicarbonate	No direct effects
Vitamin D	Stimulates transport of calcium	Inhibits reabsorption of calcium	Stimulates absorption of calcium and phosphate
Calcitonin	Inhibits resorption of calcium and phosphate	Inhibits reabsorption of calcium and phosphate	No direct effects

these hormones act to increase serum calcium. Calcitonin's action actually tends to reduce serum calcium, although it has never been demonstrated to be important in the control of serum calcium in man.

PARATHYROID DISORDERS

Primary Hyperparathyroidism

The *incidence* of hyperparathyroidism is approximately 25 per 100,000, and 50,000 new cases occur annually. The incidence increases markedly with age, and it is especially common in postmenopausal women.

ETIOLOGY. The etiology of hyperparathyroidism is unknown. A sustained stimulus to PTH production, such as the renal calcium leak that occurs with age, has been postulated but never proved. There appears to be an association with low-dose ionizing radiation to the neck, usually in childhood. Recent studies have suggested the presence of chromosomal deletions in some parathyroid adenomas, although the implications of this finding remain to be determined.

PRESENTATION. Whereas in the past most patients presented with severe bone or renal disease, as a result of increased routine screening for calcium and phosphate, approximately half of patients today are *asymptomatic*. When carefully questioned, however, many of these patients describe symptoms or associated conditions that can be related to hyperparathyroidism. The most frequent symptoms in 100 sequential patients evaluated in the authors' clinic are shown in Table 2. The earliest complaints are nonspecific and include muscle weakness, anorexia, nausea, constipation, and polyuria. *Renal complications* are generally the most serious. Of patients presenting with nephrolithiasis, approximately 5% to 10% have hyperparathyroidism. Although renal stones may be removed, calcification of the renal parenchyma (nephrocalcinosis) seldom improves even after parathyroidectomy. Some abnormality in renal function is detectable in 80% to 90% of patients with hyperparathyroidism. *Hypertension* with its complications (heart failure, arterial hemorrhage, and renal insuffi-

TABLE 2. Presenting Symptoms in 100 Patients with Primary Hyperparathyroidism

Symptoms	Percentage of Population
Nephrolithiasis	30
Bone disease	2
Peptic ulcer disease	12
Psychiatric disorders	15
Muscle weakness	70
Constipation	32
Polyuria	28
Pancreatitis	1
Myalgia	54
Arthralgia	54

ciency) has been associated with hyperparathyroidism. The relationship is unknown, although it appears related to the degree of renal impairment. The hypertension may or may not improve in patients after parathyroidectomy.

Symptomatic *bone disease* develops in 5% to 15% of patients. In its most severe form, it is referred to as *osteitis fibrosa cystica,* a disease entity that is characterized by bone pain and secondary fractures. Radiologic findings include subperiosteal resorption most evident on the radial aspect of the middle phalanx of the second and third fingers and a mottled cystic appearance to the skull. Osteoclastomas or "brown tumors" may be present. In general, bone and renal diseases tend not to occur in the same patients, and patients with bone disease often have a higher serum calcium and larger, more rapidly growing tumors.

Gastrointestinal manifestations including associations with peptic ulcer, pancreatitis, and cholelithiasis have been reported but not confirmed by all investigators. Their relationship with hyperparathyroidism remains controversial. The hypercalcemia is also associated with neurologic and psychiatric disturbances ranging from depression and anxiety to psychosis and coma. These abnormalities may resolve following parathyroidectomy.

Abnormal calcium deposition in hyperparathyroidism is associated with the development of chondrocalcinosis and pseudogout. Vascular calcification, skin necrosis, and band keratopathy of the cornea all occur. Muscle weakness and fatigue also may develop.

Diagnosis

The laboratory diagnosis of hyperparathyroidism depends on the documentation of an elevated *serum calcium* in conjunction with an elevated PTH. Normal values for calcium range from about 9.0 to 10.5 mg. per 100 ml. Because of variations in serum protein and pH, the measurement of ionized calcium is the more accurate determination. This technique is still somewhat cumbersome but is becoming more readily available clinically.

On release from the parathyroid, *PTH* is cleaved into a biologically active amino-terminal fragment and an inactive carboxy-terminal fragment. The carboxy-terminal fragment has a longer half-life and has been more useful for radioimmunoassay determinations. An elevated PTH is diagnostic of hyperparathyroidism only in the presence of an elevated serum calcium.

Half of patients with hyperparathyroidism have hypophosphatemia, the normal range being about 2.5 to 4.5 mg. per ml. They also often have a *hyperchloremic metabolic acidosis* as a result of increased bicarbonate excretion. The chloride:phosphate ratio, when elevated (greater than 33), is highly suggestive of hyperparathyroidism. In patients with bone disease, the *alkaline phosphatase* is frequently elevated.

Less Common Manifestations

Hyperparathyroidism can occur in a familial form both as an isolated disease and in association with multiple endocrine neoplasia (MEN) Types 1 and 2. MEN 1 is characterized by parathyroid hyperplasia, pituitary adenomas, and pancreatic islet cell neoplasms. Type 2 consists of medullary thyroid carcinoma, pheochromocytoma, and parathyroid hyperplasia. Familial hypocalciuric hypercalcemia and severe neonatal hyperparathyroidism are related disorders caused by mutations in the calcium-sensing receptor gene. People heterozygotic for the abnormality have an elevated calcium set point with high serum calcium, normal urine calcium, and slightly elevated serum PTH (familial hypocalciuric hypercalcemia). No treatment is necessary. Infants with two abnormal gene copies have severe neonatal hyperparathyroidism and require parathyroidectomy.

Parathyroid Carcinoma

Parathyroid carcinoma is rare, representing less than 1% of patients with hyperparathyroidism. The diagnosis is made on the basis of histologic evidence of local invasion or metastases. Characteristically, the serum concentrations of calcium, PTH, and alkaline phosphatase are markedly elevated when compared with levels in patients with benign parathyroid tumors. In half of patients, the parathyroid carcinoma is palpable. The majority of patients are symptomatic, and both the kidneys and the skeleton are commonly affected. Treatment involves radical resection of the involved gland, the ipsilateral thyroid, and the adjacent soft tissues and regional lymph nodes. Neither chemotherapy nor radiotherapy offers any benefit, and the 10-year survival is less than 20%.

Hyperparathyroid Crisis

Occasionally, hyperparathyroid patients may become acutely ill with urgent symptoms that can prove fatal. Serum calcium is almost always markedly elevated in the range of 16 to 20 mg. per 100 ml., and the symptoms are similar to those seen in *severe hypercalcemia* accompanying other diseases. They include rapidly developing muscle weakness, nausea, and vomiting, weight loss, fatigue, and confusion. The evolution of this syndrome appears to involve uncontrolled PTH secretion followed by hypercalciuria, polyuria, dehydration, and subsequent worsening hypercalcemia. Initial management is similar to that for other causes of acute hypercalcemia. Diuresis is initiated, first with normal saline infusion and then, when adequate hydration is ensured, by the addition of furosemide. A number of other agents are available if the free calcium in the serum remains elevated (Table 3). Definitive therapy in the case of hyperparathyroidism involves neck exploration and resection of the hyperfunctioning tissue.

TABLE 3. Agents Used in the Treatment of Hypercalcemia

Agent	Dosage	Administration	Comment
Calcitonin	2–6 MRC units/kg. 10–20 MRC units	Subcutaneous, every 6–8 hr. Intravenous, hourly	Nausea and vomiting are side effects. Allergy is the only contraindication. Onset of calcium-lowering effect is rapid.
Mithramycin	25 μg./kg.	Intravenously over 1 hr. in 100 ml. 0.9% saline or 5% dextrose	Contraindications are renal or hepatic dysfunction. Calcium-lowering effect occurs within 24 hr. Drug is useful when diuretic and intravenous saline are contraindicated. Nausea and vomiting are side effects.
Glucocorticoids	Prednisone 40–50 mg./day Prednisolone phosphate 40 mg.	Oral Intramuscularly or intravenously every 8 hr.	Lag period may be 7–10 days. Glucocorticoids are safe for short-term use. Alternate-day oral program may be used for long-term use.
Orthophosphate	1–2 gm./24 hr.	Oral	Dose adjustment for renal impairment. Soft tissue calcification may occur. Intravenous phosphate is not recommended.
Gallium nitrate	200 mg./sq.m./day × 5 days	Intravenous	Inhibits bone resorption. Can have nephrotoxicity.

Modified from Purnell D. C., and van Heerden J. A.: Management of symptomatic hypercalcemia and hypocalcemia. World J. Surg., 6:702, 1982.

Secondary Hyperparathyroidism (Renal Osteodystrophy)

Secondary hyperparathyroidism develops as a result of the metabolic alterations in chronic renal failure patients on dialysis. Phosphate retention and hyperphosphatemia in conjunction with a decrease in the renal production of $1,25(OH)_2$-vitamin D_3 reduce serum calcium and cause secondary hyperparathyroidism. In addition, aluminum from the dialysate and phosphate binder medications accumulates in the bone and contributes to the osteomalacia. Conservative therapy involves dietary calcium and vitamin D supplementations and phosphate restriction.

Differential Diagnosis

The *differential diagnosis* of hypercalcemia is listed in Table 4. No single test, short of neck exploration, establishes the diagnosis of hyperparathyroidism. In hospitalized patients, malignancy is the most common cause. Generally, these patients can be divided into two groups: (1) those with hematologic malignancy (25%) who appear to have hypercalcemia caused by cytokine release in lytic bone metastases stimulating osteoclasts and (2) those with solid tumors that produce parathyroid hormone–related protein (PTHrP) causing similar calcium homeostasis changes as in hyperparathyroidism.

Of the other more common causes, *artifactual elevations* due to laboratory error occur and usually can be eliminated by repeating the test. Hyperthyroidism, the milk-alkali syndrome, hypervitaminosis D and A, and immobilization can be excluded by a careful history and physical examination. In patients with sarcoidosis or multiple myeloma, immunoglobulin levels are usually elevated, and there are characteristic radiologic findings.

TABLE 4. Diseases Causing Hypercalcemia

Hyperparathyroidism
Malignancy
  Hematologic
  Solid (PTHrP producer)
Hyperthyroidism
Multiple myeloma
Sarcoidosis and other granulomatous diseases
Milk-alkali syndrome
Vitamin D intoxication
Vitamin A intoxication
Paget's disease
Immobilization
Thiazide diuretics
Addisonian crisis
Familial hypocalciuric hypercalcemia
Neonatal severe hyperparathyroidism

Localization

Approximately 95% of patients with primary hyperparathyroidism are cured at the initial neck exploration by an experienced surgeon. No study has yet demonstrated that preoperative *localization* reduces either the length of operation or the incidence of complications. Many surgeons believe that these techniques should be reserved for patients undergoing re-exploration after a failed initial procedure, and they will be discussed in that context.

Treatment

The increasing percentage of patients with primary hyperparathyroidism who present with asymptomatic disease has raised the question of conservative, nonoperative management. A National Institutes of Health Consensus Development Conference reviewed the data on this subject in 1990. The panel agreed that operation is indicated for all patients with symptoms. The indications for operation in asymptomatic patients were outlined (Table 5), and the panel mandated semiannual follow-up for patients not operated on. In addition, operation was recommended for patients in whom medical surveillance was neither desirable nor suitable, as when the patient requests surgery, consistent follow-up is unlikely, coexistent illness complicates management, or if the patient is less than 50 years of age. More complete resolution of this question requires a randomized, controlled trial, and until that time, the only curative treatment is surgical therapy. The complication rate is less than 3% and includes injury to the superior and recurrent laryngeal nerves and the development of hypocalcemia.

TABLE 5. Indications for Operative Treatment of Asymptomatic Patients with Primary Hyperparathyroidism

On initial evaluation:
- Markedly elevated serum calcium
- History of an episode of life-threatening hypercalcemia
- Reduced creatinine clearance
- Presence of kidney stone(s) detected by abdominal radiograph
- Markedly elevated 24-hr. urinary calcium excretion
- Substantially reduced bone mass as determined by direct measurement

During monitoring of an asymptomatic patient, these developments:
- Typical symptoms of the skeletal, renal or GI systems
- Sustained serum calcium > 1.0–1.6 mg./100 ml. above normal
- Significant decline in renal function (> 30% decline in creatinine clearance)
- Nephrolithiasis or worsening calciuria
- Significant decline in bone mass (to less than 2 SD below age/gender/racial matched mean)
- Significant neuromuscular or psychologic symptoms
- Inability or unwillingness of patient to continue medical surveillance

Parathyroid exploration is performed under general anesthesia through a transverse cervical incision. The thyroid lobes are elevated, the recurrent laryngeal nerve and inferior thyroid artery are visualized, and all four (or more) parathyroids are identified. The upper glands are usually located dorsally on the upper surface of the thyroid lobe. The inferior glands are usually more anterior and may be found anywhere from the neck to the mediastinum along the course of migration of the thymus.

An assiduous primary operation is essential. A second exploration because of failure to find the gland initially is more difficult, and damage to the recurrent nerve is more likely. If no parathyroid is found after meticulous exploration of the neck and removal of the thymic pedicle, which usually can be done through the cervical incision, the thyroid lobe on that side should be palpated carefully and even removed as a last resort. To ensure that the parathyroids have been identified, small biopsies should be taken of each gland. If, after diligent exploration of the neck, no abnormal parathyroid can be found, a decision must be made regarding *mediastinotomy*. This is required in only 1% to 2% of patients. Most surgeons would delay at least 2 to 4 weeks after the initial procedure if the serum calcium remains elevated. The mediastinum is usually explored through a median sternotomy. Glands most often are located in association with the thymic remnant, but they may even be found in the posterior mediastinum.

Operative management depends on the number of enlarged glands. The most reliable index of abnormality is determination of gland size. If only one gland is enlarged, its resection is curative in nearly all patients. If two or three glands are enlarged, they are resected, although this is associated with recurrent hypercalcemia in approximately 10% of patients over a prolonged period of follow-up. The management of patients with *parathyroid hyperplasia* or generalized enlargement of four glands is more difficult. Standard therapy of subtotal (3½ gland) parathyroidectomy has been associated with recurrent hyperparathyroidism in 0% to 16% and permanent hypoparathyroidism in 45%. Because of these less than satisfactory results, the authors have elected to manage these patients by total parathyroidectomy and heterotopic autotransplantation, particularly those patients with familial parathyroid hyperplasia (MEN 1).

TABLE 6. Gland Enlargement in 100 Patients with Primary Hyperparathyroidism

Number of Glands Enlarged	Number of Patients
1	65
2	15
3	10
4	10

From Wells, S. A., Leight, G. S., and Ross, A. J.: Primary hyperparathyroidism. *In* Ravitch, M. M., et al. (Eds.): Current Problems in Surgery. Chicago, Year Book Medical Publishers, 1980.

RECURRENT HYPERPARATHYROIDISM. If *recurrent hypercalcemia* develops after neck exploration and the initial diagnosis was correct, most patients have a missed adenoma, although inadequately excised hyperplastic tissue also can occur. It is in this setting that *localization procedures* are indicated. High-resolution, real-time ultrasonography, computed tomography, magnetic resonance imaging, and technetium sestamibi subtraction scanning may all prove useful. If one or more of these studies proves negative, selective angiography and venous sampling for PTH also may help to localize the lesion. Arteriography has been associated with serious neurologic complications, and both invasive techniques require special expertise.

Reoperation by an experienced surgeon is associated with resolution of the hypercalcemia in approximately 90% of patients, although 10% to 15% become permanently hypocalcemic. Resected parathyroid tissue should be viably cryopreserved at all reoperations for delayed autotransplantation if necessary.

MANAGEMENT OF SECONDARY HYPERPARATHYROIDISM. Although medical management of *secondary hyperparathyroidism* is generally effective, occasionally patients develop refractory hypercalcemia or bone pain and fractures. Patients can be managed by subtotal parathyroidectomy or total parathyroidectomy with autotransplantation.

PARATHYROID TRANSPLANTATION. Reoperation for recurrent hyperparathyroidism is accompanied by a significant increase in the risks of both recurrent laryngeal nerve injury and permanent hypoparathyroidism. This situation most frequently arises after subtotal parathyroidectomy for parathyroid hyperplasia, either primary or secondary. The technique of *total parathyroidectomy with heterotopic autotransplantation* was developed to circumvent this dilemma. Approximately 20 to 25 pieces of finely sliced parathyroid are autografted into the forearm musculature or viably frozen in cases in which there is uncertainty about the amount of remaining parathyroid. If the patient becomes hypercalcemic after the transplant, a few pieces can be removed from the arm under local anesthesia. If the patient becomes hypocalcemic, pieces of frozen tissue similarly may be reimplanted.

Hypoparathyroidism

The most common cause of *hypoparathyroidism* is injury to the glands during thyroid surgery, but it also occurs as a complication of neck exploration for hyperparathyroidism. Idiopathic lack of function has been reported, primarily in children, but it is extremely rare. In newborns it may be due to prenatal suppression as a consequence of maternal hyperparathyroidism. The major signs and symptoms are a direct consequence of the hypocalcemia that causes neuromuscular excitability. Patients first develop numbness and paresthesias followed by anxiety, depression, and confusion. This may progress to frank tetany with carpopedal spasm, tonic-clonic convulsions, and laryngeal stridor, which may prove fatal. Physical examination reveals contraction of the facial muscles on tapping the facial nerve anterior to the ear (Chvostek's sign). Trousseau's sign is carpal spasm produced by occluding blood flow to the forearm for 3 minutes. The treatment of acute hypocalcemia is intravenous administration of calcium gluconate or calcium chloride. Vitamin D and oral calcium are used for long-term management.

25

THE PITUITARY AND ADRENAL GLANDS

John A. Olson, Jr., M.D., Ph.D.,
and Samuel A. Wells, Jr., M.D.

PITUITARY

Anatomy

The anterior pituitary comprises 80% of the pituitary, and together with the posterior lobe, it fills approximately three-fourths of the sella turcica ("turkish saddle"). This fossa is bordered anteriorly, posteriorly, and inferiorly by the sphenoid bone and laterally by the cavernous sinus through which travel the carotid arteries and cranial nerves III, IV, and VI. The arterial supply to the hypothalamic-pituitary region is complex and arises from three sources: the inferior hypophyseal artery, the superior hypophyseal artery, and the middle hypophyseal artery. Capillary portions of the superior hypophyseal arteries drain from the hypothalamus into the hypophyseal portal system, which constitutes the principal blood supply to the anterior pituitary and serves as the medium through which releasing hormones from the hypothalamus reach the pituitary.

Cell types of the anterior pituitary are now classified by their secretory products: lactotropes produce prolactin (PRL), somatotropes produce growth hormone (GH), adrenocorticotropes produce adrenocorticotropic hormone (ACTH), thyrotropes produce thyroid-stimulating hormone (TSH), and gonadotropes produce follicle-stimulating hormone (FSH) and luteinizing hormone (LH).

The posterior pituitary includes the posterior lobe, the pituitary stalk, and the median eminence. Antidiuretic hormone (ADH) and oxytocin are synthesized in supraoptic and paraventricular nuclei of the hypothalamus and are released from the posterior pituitary into the capillary circulation.

Physiology

The anterior pituitary secretes ACTH, PRL, GH, TSH, LH, and FSH. ACTH controls cortisol production by the adrenal cortex. GH indirectly regulates growth of muscle and longitudinal growth of bones and also directly regulates intermediary metabolism to raise blood glucose during stress. PRL promotes lactation in women and also regulates progesterone synthesis in the ovary and testosterone synthesis in the testis. TSH stimulates synthesis and release of thyroxine by the

---

See the corresponding chapter or part in the *Textbook of Surgery,* 15th edition, pp. 665–701, for a more detailed discussion of this topic, including a comprehensive list of references.

thyroid. LH and FSH control the sex steroid production and gametogenesis by the gonads. Stimuli that promote release of ACTH, GH, TSH, LH, and FSH are synthesized in the hypothalamus and are known as *releasing hormones*. PRL is under tonic inhibition by hypothalamic dopamine. Target gland hormones, in turn, participate in feedback control of the anterior pituitary and hypothalamus.

Antidiuretic hormone (ADH) and oxytocin are the two principal hormones secreted by the posterior pituitary. Antidiuretic hormone stimulates Na^+, Cl^-, and water reabsorption by the kidney. Stimuli for ADH release include a rise in plasma osmolality above 285 mOsm. or a decrease in circulating blood volume by 5% or more. Oxytocin stimulates uterine contraction during labor and elicits milk ejection during lactation.

EVALUATION AND DIAGNOSIS OF PITUITARY DISEASE

Diagnosis of Suspected Pituitary Disease

CLINICAL AND LABORATORY ASSESSMENT. Pituitary tumors account for 10% to 15% of intracranial neoplasms and are classified as microadenomas (diameter < 10 mm.) or macroadenomas (diameter > 10 mm.). Prolactinomas, nonsecreting adenomas, and GH-producing adenomas are the most frequent pituitary tumor types, while ACTH-producing adenomas, gonadotrope adenomas, and TSH-producing adenomas are uncommon. Other sellar or parasellar tumors include craniopharyngiomas, germ cell tumors, and metastatic lesions.

Sellar masses may produce headache as well as signs and symptoms related to compression of nearby cranial nerves. ACTH-producing tumors produce signs and symptoms of hypercortisolism (Cushing's syndrome). Prolactinomas cause galactorrhea and hypogonadism. GH-secreting tumors cause gigantism in children and acromegaly in adults. LH- or FSH-producing adenomas cause infertility and sexual dysfunction. Conversely, patients may develop total or selective hypopituitarism from untreated pituitary adenomas, from pituitary radiation or surgery, or from head injury.

Direct ACTH measurement with two-site IRMA is now the preferred test to identify ACTH-dependent causes of Cushing's syndrome. Normal levels are above 5 pg. per ml., while lower levels suggest ACTH-independent hypercortisolism. A random serum PRL level is sufficient to accurately diagnose prolactinoma in the majority of cases. A level above 300 μg. per liter is virtually always associated with a prolactinoma, and a level of 150 μg. per liter in a nonpregnant patient is usually caused by a prolactinoma. Random serum GH levels are not helpful in the diagnosis of GH excess, although serum IGF-1 is a useful screening test for this disorder. Sensitive TSH IRMA is used in conjunction with serum T_4 or free T_4 index to evaluate central (pituitary) hypothyroidism.

Biochemical assessment of posterior pituitary function is indirect. The syndrome of inappropriate antidiuretic hormone secretion (SIADH) is characterized by euvolemic hyponatremia with an inappropriately concentrated urine. SIADH is generally a diagnosis of exclusion after other causes of euvolemic hyponatremia, including hypothyroidism and adrenal insufficiency, have been excluded. Deficiency of antidiuretic hormone (diabetes insipidus) is suggested by prolonged polyuria and polydipsia, and it is confirmed by a combination of high plasma osmolality (>285 mOsm.) and low urine osmolality (<200 mOsm.) following water deprivation. Correction of diabetes insipidus following exogenously administered ADH differentiates central versus nephrogenic diabetes insipidus.

NEURO-OPHTHALMOLOGIC EVALUATION. All patients with visual complaints and suspected pituitary lesions should have neuro-ophthalmologic evaluation. Bedside testing with confrontation may detect gross field cuts only.

DIAGNOSTIC IMAGING AND LOCALIZATION. High-resolution MRI with intravenous gadolinium contrast is the diagnostic modality of choice for radiologic localization of pituitary disease. When MRI is not available or is contraindicated (i.e., metal in the body, pacemakers), fine-section (1.5 mm.) coronal CT with intravenous contrast is an acceptable alternative.

Inferior petrosal sinus sampling (IPS) assists in the evaluation of patients with acromegaly or Cushing's syndrome by localizing ACTH-secreting pituitary tumors that are undetectable by MRI or CT.

Diagnosis and Management of Specific Pituitary Disorders

PROLACTINOMA. Prolactinomas are the most common functioning pituitary tumors, representing 30% to 60% of all pituitary neoplasms. Most are diagnosed in women. Microadenomas are diagnosed in 10% to 40% of women with amenorrhea alone and are found in 30% of women with amenorrhea and galactorrhea. Several medical conditions and medications also may cause hyperprolactinemia, and most are discernible by history, physical examination, and routine laboratory tests. A pregnancy test is mandatory in all female patients with hyperprolactinemia. Measurement of plasma PRL levels is central to the diagnosis of a PRL-secreting tumor, and the degree of hyperprolactinemia correlates with tumor size. Most asymptomatic microprolactinomas remain stable over time and require only observation. Symptomatic microprolactinomas and macroprolactinomas require treatment with bromocriptine. Surgical therapy also should be considered when medical therapy is ineffective.

NONFUNCTIONING ADENOMA. Clinically nonfunctioning adenomas are the second most common pituitary tumor, representing 30% to 40% of surgically removed lesions. These tumors are diagnosed when they cause symptoms from encroachment on adjacent structures, including loss of vision, headache, hydrocephalus, and fifth or sixth nerve palsies. Many so-called nonfunctioning adenomas in fact secrete very low levels of LH, FSH, and glycoprotein hormone alpha subunit. Evaluation of these patients includes measurement of basal prolactin, IGF-1, LH, FSH, TSH, and alpha subunit levels. Transsphenoidal resection is the primary treatment of nonfunctioning adenomas.

GH-PRODUCING ADENOMA. GH-secreting adenomas are the third most common pituitary adenoma and cause acromegaly. Gigantism results when GH excess occurs prior to epiphyseal plate closure in children and is much less common than acromegaly. Over 99% of cases of acromegaly are due to a primary pituitary adenoma. Currently, measurement of serum IGF-1 concentration is the best screening test for acromegaly. Definitive testing with glucose suppression of GH release should follow. Tumors are localized with MRI, CT, or IPS. Treatment for acromegaly is achieved most rapidly by transsphenoidal excision of the adenoma.

ACTH-PRODUCING ADENOMA. Hypercortisolism, or Cushing's syndrome, is characterized by central obesity, moon facies, purple striae, proximal myopathy, amenorrhea, fatigue, and psychiatric abnormalities. ACTH-producing pituitary adenomas (Cushing's disease) cause up to 75% of cases of Cushing's syndrome. Laboratory evaluation of hypercortisolism is described subsequently in the adrenal section. Tumors are localized with MRI, CT, or IPS. Transsphenoidal resection of corticotrope microadenomas is the preferred management for Cushing's disease. All patients undergoing pituitary resection for Cushing's disease require administration of stress-dose steroids.

GONADOTROPIN-PRODUCING ADENOMA. Gonadotrope adenomas usually produce headaches or visual abnormalities. Diagnosis of these tumors requires biochemical measurement of FSH, LH, alpha and beta subunits, as well as testosterone. Anatomic localization is performed with MRI or CT. Treatment is transsphenoidal resection.

TSH-PRODUCING ADENOMA. These tumors are the rarest pituitary adenomas (<1%) and produce symptoms of a enlarging sellar mass as well as hyperthyroidism. Treatment is transsphenoidal resection.

Other Tumors and Conditions

CRANIOPHARYNGIOMA. Craniopharyngiomas represent 3% to 5% of intracranial neoplasms. These tumors usually affect children and produce symptoms of increased intracranial pressure. Evaluation includes pituitary function tests, visual field testing, and imaging with CT. Transfrontal resection is the treatment of choice for craniopharyngioma. Morbidity and mortality is high, and tumors recur frequently.

PITUITARY APOPLEXY. Pituitary apoplexy follows sudden hemorrhage into or infarction of a pituitary tumor. Symptoms include sudden severe headache, meningismus, loss of vision, and extraocular nerve palsies. Acute pituitary apoplexy is a neurosurgical emergency.

SHEEHAN'S SYNDROME. Pituitary necrosis and subsequent hypopituitarism may occur rarely following postpartum hemorrhage and hypovolemia. Treatment is appropriate pituitary hormone replacement.

EMPTY SELLA SYNDROME. An empty sella turcica results from arachnoid herniation through an incomplete diaphragm sellae. Primary empty sella syndrome occurs in obese, multiparous, hypertensive women who experience headaches but have no underlying neurologic disorders. Secondary empty sella syndrome is observed in patients with otherwise benign CSF hypertension and in patients with a loss of pituitary function due to apoplexy or surgical therapy. No treatment is necessary for the primary condition, while correction of the underlying cause is necessary for the secondary form.

ADRENAL

Anatomy

The adrenal glands are bilateral retroperitoneal organs located on the superomedial aspect of the upper pole of each kidney. Each adrenal is composed of a cortex and medulla. The adrenal glands are highly vascular and derive their blood supply from branches of the inferior phrenic artery, the aorta, and the renal artery. Right adrenal gland venous effluent drains to the inferior vena cava through a wide but short central vein. The left adrenal vein usually empties primarily into the left renal vein. The adult adrenal cortex is composed of an outer zona glomerulosa, a middle zona fasciculata, and an inner zona reticularis. The adrenal medulla is smaller than the cortex and contributes approximately 10% of the total gland weight.

Physiology

Three major biosynthetic pathways lead to the production of glucocorticoids, mineralocorticoids, and adrenal androgens. Mineralocorticoids are synthesized in the outer zona glomerulosa, while glucocorticoids are synthesized in the inner zonae fasciculata and reticularis. Cortisol is the principal glucocorticoid in man and is regulated by pituitary-derived ACTH under most conditions. Cortisol regulates the intermediary metabolism of carbohydrates, proteins, and lipids and possesses profound anti-inflammatory and immunosuppressive properties. Cortisol also retards wound healing and produces osteopenia. Aldosterone is the major mineralocorticoid in man. Aldosterone stimulates sodium retention and potassium and hydrogen ion secretion by the distal convoluted tubule of the kidney to expand intravascular volume. The renin-angiotensin system and plasma potassium are the principal regulators of aldosterone. Adrenal androgens are normally produced in small amounts and have little overall effect on development of fetal tissues or the later development of the gonads and secondary sexual characteristics.

Diseases of the Adrenal Cortex

CUSHING'S SYNDROME. In 1932, Harvey Cushing described eight patients with central obesity, glucose intolerance, hypertension, plethora, hirsutism, osteoporosis, nephrolithiasis, menstrual irregularity, muscle weakness, and emotional lability. Today, the most common cause of this syndrome is iatrogenic due to chronic administration of synthetic corticosteroids for other disorders. Endogenous hypercortisolism in all cases is due to increased adrenal production of cortisol, which may be ACTH dependent (80% to 90%) or independent (10% to 20%).

ACTH-dependent Cushing's syndrome is most often due to an ACTH-secreting pituitary adenoma (Cushing's disease). Ectopic ACTH-producing nonendocrine tumors constitute the remaining 10% to 20% of cases of ACTH-dependent Cushing's syndrome. Small cell carcinoma of the lung is the most common cause of the ectopic ACTH syndrome.

ACTH-independent Cushing's syndrome is due to an autonomously hypersecreting adenoma, an adrenal carcinoma, or bilateral adrenal cortical hyperplasia. Most patients with ACTH-dependent Cushing's syndrome have adrenal adenomas. Adrenocortical carcinoma may present with rapidly progressive Cushing's syndrome, often accompanied by virilizing features. Pituitary-independent adrenal hyperplasia is rare.

Measurement of cortisol in a two to three consecutive 24-hour collections of urine is the best screening test for Cushing's syndrome. A single random plasma cortisol level is not helpful in establishing a diagnosis of Cushing's syndrome. The low-dose dexamethasone suppression test is confirmative: 1 mg. of dexamethasone is administered orally at 11:00 P.M. and plasma cortisol is obtained at 8:00 A.M. the following day. In normal individuals, the plasma cortisol level is suppressed to less than 3 to 5 μg. per 100 ml., while very few individuals with Cushing's syndrome demonstrate suppression of plasma cortisol to below 3 μg. per 100 ml. Determination of basal ACTH by immunoradiometric assay (IRMA) is the next test. Suppression of the absolute level of ACTH below 5 pg. per ml. is nearly diagnostic of adrenocortical neoplasms. ACTH levels in Cushing's disease may range from the upper limits of normal (15 pg. per ml.) to 500 pg. per ml. Highest plasma levels of ACTH (more than 1000 pg. per ml.) have been observed in patients with ectopic ACTH syndrome. Standard high-dose dexamethasone suppression testing and the metyrapone test subsequently identify pituitary from ectopic ACTH syndrome.

Pituitary adenomas are best visualized with gadolinium-enhanced MRI of the sella turcica. Patients with ACTH-independent Cushing's syndrome require thin-section CT or MRI of the adrenal, both of which identify adrenal abnormalities with over 95% sensitivity.

Bilateral inferior petrosal sinus sampling can delineate unclear cases of Cushing's disease from other causes of hypercortisolism. Simultaneous bilateral petrosal sinus and peripheral blood samples are obtained before and after peripheral intravenous injection of 1 μg. per kg. CRH. A ratio of inferior petrosal sinus to peripheral plasma ACTH of 2.0 at basal or of 3.0 following CRH administration is 100% sensitive and specific for pituitary adenoma.

Treatment of Cushing's syndrome involves removing the

cause of cortisol excess, either a primary adrenal lesion or ectopic and pituitary lesions secreting excessive ACTH. The treatment of choice for Cushing's disease is transsphenoidal resection of the pituitary tumor, which is successful in 80% or more of cases. Treatment of ectopic ACTH syndrome involves removal of the primary lesion. Removal of the adrenal tumor and affected gland is the primary approach to primary causes of Cushing's syndrome. All patients who undergo adrenalectomy for primary adrenal causes of Cushing's syndrome require perioperative and postoperative glucocorticoid replacement, since the contralateral gland is suppressed.

ALDOSTERONISM. In 1955, Jerome Conn described a 34-year-old woman with hypertension, generalized weakness, and polyuria who was cured by resection of a right adrenal cortical adenoma. Aldosteronism is a syndrome of hypertension and hypokalemia caused by hypersecretion of the mineralocorticoid aldosterone. An aldosterone-producing adrenal adenoma (Conn's syndrome) is the cause of primary aldosteronism in two-thirds of cases and is one of the few surgically correctable causes of hypertension. Idiopathic bilateral adrenal hyperplasia (IHA) causes 30% to 40% of cases of primary aldosteronism. Adrenocortical carcinoma and autosomal dominant glucocorticoid-suppressible aldosteronism (GSA) are rare causes of primary aldosteronism. Secondary aldosteronism is a physiologic response of the renin-angiotensin system to renal artery stenosis, cirrhosis, congestive heart failure, and normal pregnancy. The adrenal functions normally.

Aldosterone-mediated retention of sodium and excretion of potassium and hydrogen ion by the kidney causes hypokalemia and moderate diastolic hypertension. Edema is characteristically absent. The laboratory diagnosis of primary aldosteronism requires demonstration of hypokalemia, inappropriate kaliuresis, and elevated aldosterone with normal cortisol. Upright plasma renin activity of less than 3 ng. per ml. corroborates the diagnosis. Confirmation of primary aldosteronism involves determination of serum potassium, plasma renin activity, and a 24-hour urine collection for sodium, cortisol, and aldosterone following 5 days of a high-sodium diet. Patients with primary hyperaldosteronism do not demonstrate aldosterone suppressibility following salt loading. The captopril test and the plasma aldosterone-to-renin ratio test are other useful tests to define the appropriateness of the plasma renin activity for a given level of aldosterone. After the diagnosis of primary aldosteronism is made, distinction must be made between an aldosteronoma and IHA. Patients with an aldosteronoma show diurnal variation in plasma aldosterone that parallels cortisol and is unaffected by postural changes. Conversely, in patients with IHA, plasma aldosterone levels do not exhibit diurnal variation and are elevated 33% or more by postural changes.

High-resolution adrenal CT should be the initial step in localization of an adrenal tumor. CT localizes APA in 90% of cases overall, and the presence of a unilateral adenoma >1 cm. on CT and supportive biochemical evidence of an aldosteronoma are generally all that are needed to make the diagnosis of Conn's syndrome. Uncertainty regarding aldosteronoma versus IAH following biochemical testing and noninvasive localization may be settled definitively by bilateral adrenal venous sampling for aldosterone and cortisol. Simultaneous adrenal vein blood samples for aldosterone and cortisol are taken; a ratio of aldosterone to cortisol is greater than 4:1 for a diagnosis of aldosteronoma or less than 4:1 for IHA.

Surgical removal of an aldosterone-secreting adenoma through a posterior approach or the newer laparoscopic approach results in immediate cure or substantial improvement of hypertension and hyperkalemia in over 90% of patients with Conn's syndrome. IHA is treated with spironolactone, triamterene, amiloride, or nifedipine, and adrenalectomy is indicated only when symptomatic hypokalemia is refractory to medical therapy.

CONGENITAL ADRENAL HYPERPLASIA. The congenital adrenal hyperplasias (CAH) result from inherited defects of one or several of the enzymes necessary for cortisol biosynthesis that lead to ACTH overproduction, secondary hyperplasia of the adrenal cortex, and shunting of cortisol precursors into adrenal androgen pathways. Prenatal CAH in females produces pseudohermaphrodism, while variable degrees of salt wasting occur in both sexes. Postnatal CAH causes virilization of females and isosexual precocity of males. Both sexes experience rapid somatic growth, an advanced bone age, early closure of epiphyses, and short stature. These syndromes are caused by deficiencies in 21-hydroxylase, 11-beta-hydroxylase, 3-beta-hydroxydehydrogenase, or side-chain-cleaving enzyme. Treatment involves recognition and appropriate glucocorticoid and mineralocorticoid replacement as well as timely surgical correction of genital malformations.

ADRENOCORTICAL CARCINOMA. Adrenocortical carcinoma is a rare but aggressive malignancy, and most patients with this cancer present with locally advanced disease. Syndromes of adrenal hormone overproduction may include rapidly progressive hypercortisolism, hyperaldosteronism, or virilization. Large (>6 cm.) adrenal masses that extend to nearby structures on CT scanning likely represent carcinoma. Complete surgical resection of locally confined tumor is the only chance for cure of adrenocortical carcinoma. Definitive diagnosis of adrenocortical carcinoma requires operative and pathologic demonstration of nodal or distant metastases. Any adrenal neoplasm weighing more than 50 gm. should be considered malignant. Often, patients with adrenocortical carcinoma present with metastatic disease, most often involving the lung, lymph nodes, liver, or bone. Palliative surgical debulking of locally advanced or metastatic adrenocortical carcinoma may provide these patients with symptomatic relief from some slow-growing, hormonally productive cancers. The prognosis for patients with adrenocortical carcinoma is poor.

ADRENAL INSUFFICIENCY. In 1855, Thomas Addison described 11 patients with primary adrenal insufficiency, including 5 patients with tuberculous destruction of the adrenal glands. Acute adrenal insufficiency is an emergency and should be suspected in stressed patients with a history of either adrenal insufficiency or exogenous steroid use. Signs and symptoms include fever, nausea, vomiting, severe hypotension, and lethargy. Characteristic laboratory findings of adrenal insufficiency include hyponatremia, hyperkalemia, azotemia, and fasting or reactive hypoglycemia. The rapid ACTH stimulation test is the best test of adrenal insufficiency. Synthetic ACTH (250 µg.) is administered intravenously, and plasma cortisol levels are measured at 0, 30, and 60 minutes later. Normal peak cortisol response should exceed 20 µg. per 100 ml.

Treatment of adrenal crisis must be based on clinical suspicion before laboratory confirmation is available. Intravenous volume replacement with normal or hypertonic saline and dextrose is essential, as is immediate intravenous steroid replacement therapy with 4 mg. dexamethasone. Thereafter, 100 mg. hydrocortisone is administered intravenously every 6 to 8 hours and is tapered to standard replacement doses as the patient's condition stabilizes. Subsequent recognition and treatment of the underlying cause, particularly if it is infectious, usually resolve the crisis. Mineralocorticoid replacement is not required until intravenous fluids are discontinued and oral intake resumes.

Patients who have known adrenal insufficiency or have received supraphysiologic doses of steroid for at least 1 week in the year preceeding surgery should receive 100 mg. hydrocortisone the evening before and the morning of major surgery followed by 100 mg. hydrocortisone every 8 hours during the perioperative 24 hours.

ADRENAL MEDULLA

Physiology

Cells of the adrenal medulla secrete dopamine, norepinephrine, and epinephrine. These catecholamines profoundly alter the cardiovascular system, smooth and skeletal muscle activity, metabolism, and blood flow within the liver, spleen, lung, and brain. Catecholamines are metabolized in liver and kidney to methoxyhydroxyphenylglycol (MHPG), vanillylmandelic acid (VMA), normetanephrine, and metanephrine that are measurable in the urine.

Diseases of the Adrenal Medulla

PHEOCHROMOCYTOMA. Pheochromocytomas are functional adrenal tumors that arise from neuroectodermal cells of the adrenal medulla or in certain extra-adrenal sites. Pheochromocytomas are rare tumors but are found with increased frequency in screened hypertensive populations and in individuals with multiple endocrine neoplasia Types IIa and IIb, von Recklinghausen's neurofibromatosis, and von Hippel–Lindau disease. The "rule of tens" has been applied to pheochromocytoma: Tumors are bilateral in 10%, extradrenal in 10%, familial in 10%, multicentric in 10%, malignant in 10%, and occur in children in 10% of cases. The organ of Zuckerkandl is the most common extra-adrenal site of pheochromocytoma. All symptoms of pheochromocytoma are attributable to excessive circulating catecholamines. Elevation of the blood pressure, which may range from mild hypertension to a dramatic hypertensive crisis, is the most consistent manifestation. This hypertension is sustained in roughly half of patients, is paroxysmal in a third, and is absent in one-fifth. Other symptoms include palpitations, anxiety, and tremulousness.

Analysis of catecholamines and their metabolites in a single 24-hour urine collection is the best test to make or exclude the diagnosis of pheochromocytoma. CT and MRI are the two radiologic modalities of choice to localize pheochromocytomas. Functional nuclear imaging with ^{131}I-metaiodobenzylguanidine (^{131}I-MIBG) is another important technique used to localize pheochromocytoma and may be superior to CT and MRI in detecting small functional foci of tumor located outside the adrenal.

Preoperative preparation of the patient with pheochromocytoma centers on blood pressure control and optimization of fluid balance. Blood pressure control is obtained through alpha-adrenergic blockade with phenoxybenzamine hydrochloride for 1 to 3 weeks prior to operation. Beta-adrenergic blockade with propranolol is indicated for tachycardia greater than 140 beats per minute, arrhythmia, and primarily epinephrine-secreting tumors. Propranolol should not be given until adequate alpha blockade has been established.

Formerly, an anterior approach through either a midline incision or bilateral subcostal incisions was used exclusively to resect pheochromocytomas. Today, CT, MRI, and nuclear scans permit preoperative localization of tumor in 95% or more of cases so that the surgical approach may be more directed using either a posterior or laparoscopic approach.

THE INCIDENTAL ADRENAL MASS

The increased availability and use of abdominal CT has led to the detection of incidental adrenal masses with rising frequency. Evaluation decisions must weigh the prevalence of adrenal tumor types and the consequences of a missed diagnosis. Pheochromocytoma has a comparatively high prevalence, and the consequences of a missed diagnosis may be great; therefore, all patients with incidental adrenal masses should be screened by measurement of 24-hour urine levels of catecholamines, metanephrine, and VMA. Hypertensive patients with incidental masses should have serum potassium determination and, if low, should be tested for aldosteronism. Routine biochemical screening for hypercortisolism and hyperandrogenism in patients with incidental adrenal masses is not indicated. Masses that appear cystic may be aspirated under CT guidance. Fine-needle aspiration biopsy may be of value in patients with known extra-adrenal malignancy; however, it is not indicated in the evaluation of primary adrenal neoplasms and is contraindicated if pheochromocytoma is suspected. Adrenalectomy is recommended for lesions >6 cm. secondary to high malignant potential for lesions of this size.

ADRENALECTOMY

Surgical approaches to the adrenal glands include the anterior transabdominal approach, a combined thoracoabdominal procedure, the posterior flank approach, and laparoscopic adrenalectomy. Either adrenal may be removed using any of these approaches, and the choice of approach depends on the suspected pathology and size of the adrenal lesion. Small tumors that are localized with confidence by radiologic imaging and are likely benign may be resected using a posterior or laparoscopic approach. Large masses and those which may harbor malignancy generally should be resected using an anterior approach to adequately explore the entire abdomen and gain sufficient exposure for safe resection. Very large adrenocortical carcinomas, usually 10 to 15 cm., often require a thoracoabdominal approach for *en bloc* resection with involved adjacent structures.

26

THE ESOPHAGUS

I

Historical Aspects and Anatomy
Mark B. Orringer, M.D.

HISTORICAL ASPECTS

Modern surgical treatment of esophageal disease is the product of refinements in both anesthetic and operative techniques and methods of assessing normal and abnormal anatomy and physiology. Chevalier Jackson pioneered the use of the rigid esophagoscope in the early 1900s, and LoPresti and Hilmi (1964) developed the flexible fiberoptic esophagoscope. Before the availability of anesthetic techniques that would permit operations on the intrathoracic esophagus, resection of the cervical esophagus for carcinoma by Billroth (1871) and Czery (1877) and reconstruction of the cervical esophagus with a skin tube by Mikulicz (1886) were surgical milestones. Turner (1933) performed the first successful transmediastinal blunt esophagectomy for carcinoma and established alimentary continuity with an antethoracic skin tube. With the advent of endotracheal anesthesia, transthoracic esophagectomy and an esophagogastric anastomosis were first carried out successfully in Japan by Ohsawa (1933) and in the United States by Marshall (1937) and Adams and Phemister (1938). Ivor Lewis (1946) popularized the right-sided transthoracic esophagectomy for carcinoma. Techniques of esophageal replacement with stomach, jejunum, and colon were then refined. Orringer and Sloan (1978) repopularized the technique of transhiatal esophagectomy without thoracotomy. Surgical milestones in the treatment of benign esophageal disease include primary repair of congenital esophageal atresia (Haight, 1943); the addition of esophagomyotomy to resection of pulsion diverticula (Allen and Clagget, 1965; Belsey, 1966); cardioesophagomyotomy for achalasia (Heller, 1913; Zaaijer, 1923; Ellis, 1969); antireflux operations to create a functional distal esophageal sphincter mechanism (Nissen, 1961; Belsey, 1967; Hill, 1967); and combined esophageal-lengthening Collis gastroplasty and fundoplication procedures to better control reflux in patients with esophageal shortening (Pearson, 1971; Orringer and Sloan, 1976, 1978; Henderson, 1977). Important developments in objective diagnostic studies to assess esophageal function include esophageal manometry (Code, 1958; Vantrappen, 1958), the intraesophageal pH electrode (Tuttle and Grossman, 1958), provocative pH reflux testing (Kantrow-

---

See the corresponding chapter or part in the *Textbook of Surgery,* 15th edition, pp. 702–707, for a more detailed discussion of this topic, including a comprehensive list of references.

itz, 1969; Skinner and Booth, 1970), and 24-hour distal esophageal pH monitoring (Johnson and DeMeester, 1974).

ANATOMY

The esophagus is 25 cm. (10 in.) long. It begins at the cricopharyngeal or upper esophageal sphincter (UES), 15 cm. from the upper incisor teeth. The UES is the narrowest point of the gastrointestinal tract (14 mm.) and is a *bow* of muscle connecting the lateral borders of the cricoid cartilage. The cervical esophagus lies anterior to the prevertebral fascia, behind and more to the left of the trachea (and is therefore best approached surgically from the left side). The thoracic esophagus enters the posterior mediastinum behind the aortic arch and great vessels, curves slightly to the left of the trachea, passes behind the left mainstem bronchus and pericardium, and enters the diaphragmatic hiatus at the level of the T11. Its lateral boundaries are the thin right and left parietal pleurae. The abdominal esophagus is 1 to 2 cm. long and joins the stomach at the *cardia*, or esophagogastric (EG) junction (40 cm. from the upper incisors). The esophagus is normally lined by squamous epithelium except for the distal 1 to 2 cm., which contains columnar epithelium. The squamocolumnar epithelial junction (or Z-line) typically occurs at the EG junction.

The esophagus has no serosa and is surrounded by fibroareolar adventitia. It has outer longitudinal and inner circular muscle layers, both of which are striated in the upper third and nonstriated (smooth) in the distal two-thirds. The esophageal *arterial blood supply* is from the superior and inferior thyroid arteries, four to six aortic esophageal arteries, and intercostal, bronchial, inferior phrenic, and left gastric collateral arteries. The aortic esophageal arteries terminate in fine capillary networks before entering the muscle layer. *Sympathetic innervation* is from the cervical sympathetic ganglia, upper thoracic and splanchnic nerves, and the celiac ganglion. Intrinsic autonomic innervation is from Meissner's plexus in the submucosa and Auerbach's plexus between the circular and longitudinal muscle layers. *Parasympathetic* innervation is from the vagus nerves, which in the neck give rise to the external and internal laryngeal nerves. The external laryngeal nerve innervates the cricothyroid muscle and part of the inferior pharyngeal constrictor. The internal laryngeal nerves provide sensory innervation of the pharyngeal surface of the larynx and base of the tongue. The recurrent laryngeal nerves provide parasympathetic innervation to the cervical esophagus and UES, and their injury may therefore cause both hoarseness and UES dysfunction with secondary aspiration on swallowing. The vagus nerves send fibers to the thoracic esophagus. At the diaphragmatic hiatus, the left vagus lies anterior to the esophagus and the right posterior. Esophageal carcinomas metastasize along extensive submucosal lymphatics and to the internal jugular nodes in the neck, paratracheal nodes in the superior mediastinum, subcarinal nodes in the midchest, paraesophageal nodes in the lower mediastinum and inferior pulmonary ligament, and perigastric and left gastric artery lymph nodes.

II

Physiology
Mark B. Orringer, M.D.

The esophagus functions to transport swallowed material from the pharynx into the stomach. Secondarily, gastroesophageal reflux (GER) is prevented by the lower esophageal sphincter (LES) or distal high pressure zone (HPZ), and air entry into the esophagus with inspiration is prevented by the upper esophageal sphincter (UES). Esophageal manometry documents intraesophageal pressure phenomena: the amplitude and length of the UES and LES, the extent and duration of relaxation of the sphincters with swallowing, and the characteristics of esophageal peristaltic activity. The intraesophageal pH electrode permits objective documentation of the degree of abnormal gastroesophageal reflux present, and 24-hour distal esophageal pH monitoring has further characterized patterns of gastroesophageal reflux.

The act of *swallowing* begins with voluntary movement of the tongue, which initiates an involuntary peristaltic wave that rapidly traverses the pharynx and reaches the UES, producing relaxation that is followed by a postdeglutitive contraction. The UES is approximately 3 cm. in length and has resting pressures of 16 to 118 mm. Hg (mean approximately 40 mm. Hg). Its duration of relaxation with swallowing is 0.5 to 1.2 seconds. Contraction of the UES after the relaxation phase produces an intraluminal pressure often twice as high as resting pressures and lasts 2 to 4 seconds. As the swallowed bolus enters the esophagus, a *primary* progressive peristaltic wave is activated and propels the swallowed material from the pharynx into the stomach in 4 to 8 seconds. Normally, a progressive peristaltic contraction (primary wave) follows 97% of all wet swallows. Pressures within the esophageal body, like those in the chest, are maximally negative (-5 to -10 mm. Hg) during deep inspiration and highest (0 to 5 mm. Hg) during expiration. Esophageal peristaltic pressure ranges from 20 to 100 mm. Hg, and contractions last between 2 to 4 seconds. If the entire swallowed bolus of food does not empty from the esophagus into the stomach, *secondary* peristaltic waves are initiated by the local distension. These contractions, like the primary waves, are progressive and sequential but

See the corresponding chapter or part in the *Textbook of Surgery*, 15th edition, pp. 707–711, for a more detailed discussion of this topic, including a comprehensive list of references.

begin in the smooth muscle segment of the esophagus (near the level of the aortic arch) and continue until retained intraesophageal contents empty into the stomach. *Tertiary* contractions are simultaneous, incoordinated, nonprogressive, mono- or multiphasic waves that occur throughout the esophagus and are responsible for the "corkscrew" appearance of esophageal spasm on barium swallow examination. Increased resting pressures within the body of the esophagus and abnormal motor function are seen with conditions causing obstruction, either mechanical or functional.

Manometric studies have demonstrated a *functional* LES that is 3 to 5 cm. in length and serves as a barrier against abnormal GER. Since there is no demonstrable *anatomic* lower esophageal sphincter (LES), this valve mechanism is more accurately referred to as the LES *mechanism* or the *distal esophageal HPZ*. Normal resting pressure within the HPZ ranges from 10 to 20 mm. Hg, but *no absolute HPZ value per se indicates either competence or incompetence of the LES mechanism.* HPZ pressures of 0 to 5 mm. Hg and lengths of 2 cm. or less are more likely to be associated with incompetence of the LES and secondary GER. Within 1.5 to 2.5 seconds after a swallow is initiated, distal HPZ relaxation occurs and lasts 4 to 6 seconds. A postdeglutitive contraction then occurs, generating pressures of 25 to 35 mm. Hg for 7 to 10 seconds, after which HPZ tone returns to resting levels. Esophagoscopy, the barium swallow examination, and the acid perfusion (Bernstein) test are poor and inconsistent indicators of GER. The intraesophageal pH electrode provides the most sensitive means of demonstrating abnormal acid reflux. Of the parameters measured with 24-hour distal esophageal pH monitoring, documentation of pH <4 for >4% of the day is most indicative of abnormal GER.

III

Disorders of Esophageal Motility
Mark B. Orringer, M.D.

Functional disorders of the esophagus, which include abnormalities of motility, are conditions that interfere with the normal act of swallowing or produce dysphagia in the absence of intraluminal organic obstruction or extrinsic compression. As a general rule, a barium swallow, esophagoscopy, and esophageal function tests, including manometry and intraesophageal pH reflux testing, constitute the minimal evalua-

---

See the corresponding chapter or part in the *Textbook of Surgery*, 15th edition, pp. 712–728, for a more detailed discussion of this topic, including a comprehensive list of references.

tion of the patient with a suspected disorder of esophageal motility.

UPPER ESOPHAGEAL SPHINCTER (UES) DYSFUNCTION (OROPHARYNGEAL DYSPHAGIA OR CRICOPHARYNGEAL DYSFUNCTION)

A number of abnormalities of the central and peripheral nervous systems, metabolic and inflammatory myopathy, gastroesophageal reflux, and unknown factors result in difficulty propelling liquid or solid food from the oropharynx into the upper esophagus. Standard esophageal manometric techniques fail to characterize these abnormalities adequately due to limitations of this equipment in recording the rapid sequence of events that occurs with normal deglutition in a unique asymmetrical sphincter that changes position with laryngeal excursions during swallowing. Other nonmotor causes of upper esophageal dysphagia, such as carcinoma, caustic stricture, cervical vertebral bone spurs, and thyromegaly, must be excluded. *Globus hystericus,* indicating a purely psychological basis for a patient's complaint of cervical dysphagia, is a diagnosis of exclusion, made only after ruling out significant esophageal disease.

UES dysfunction characteristically produces cervical dysphagia, expectoration of saliva, intermittent hoarseness, and weight loss. The barium esophagogram may be normal or show UES spasm with a typical posterior cricopharyngeal *bar* at the level of C7 or T1 or a pharyngoesophageal (Zenker's) diverticulum. Esophageal manometry and acid reflux testing may demonstrate abnormalities of thoracic esophageal peristalsis or an incompetent lower esophageal sphincter. Treatment varies with the cause of UES dysfunction and may include periodic esophageal dilatations or a cervical esophagomyotomy through the abnormal UES in the patient with incapacitating cervical dysphagia and aspiration, for example, after a midbrain bulbar stroke.

DISORDERS OF THE BODY OF THE ESOPHAGUS

Achalasia

Achalasia, a Greek term, means "failure of relaxation" and refers to the failure of the LES in these patients to relax normally with swallowing. Achalasia, however, involves the entire body of the esophagus not only the LES. In South America, the etiology of achalasia is Chagas' disease, a parasitic infestation by the leishmanial forms of *Trypanosoma cruzi,* which destroys the ganglion cells of Auerbach's plexus, resulting in motor dysfunction and progressive dilatation of the esophagus, colon, ureters, and other viscera. In Europe and North America, however, the etiology is obscure, the condition frequently following a variety of physically or emotionally stressful situations. Regardless of the etiology, degeneration of the ganglion cells of Auerbach's plexus is invariably found. Patients present with a *classic triad* of dysphagia, regurgitation, and weight loss. Retrosternal pain is more characteristic of esophageal spasm, not achalasia. Achalasia is a premalignant esophageal lesion, middle third squamous cell carcinoma developing as a late complication in nearly 10% after 15 to 25 years.

The barium esophagogram shows mild esophageal dilatation early to a massively dilated sigmoid-shaped megaesophagus in advanced achalasia. The radiographic hallmark is the distal "bird beak" taper of the EG junction. The chest x-ray shows a characteristic *double mediastinal stripe* (the dilated esophagus) and a posterior mediastinal air-fluid level on a lateral view. Manometric criteria of achalasia are (1) failure of the distal esophageal HPZ to relax reflexly with swallowing and (2) lack of progressive peristalsis throughout the length of the esophagus. Esophagoscopy is indicated to assess for possible carcinoma, retention esophagitis, or a distal stricture from reflux esophagitis developing after prior forceful dilatations or esophagomyotomy. Because achalasia is incurable, its treatment is *palliative*. In the early stages of the disease, sublingual nitroglycerin before meals, long-acting nitrates, and calcium channel blockers improve swallowing. Forceful pneumatic balloon dilatation relieves dysphagia in 65% to 77% with a perforation rate of 1% to 5%. If pneumatic dilatation fails, it may be repeated a second time, but then a 7- to 10-cm. distal esophagomyotomy through the LES is recommended for recurrent symptoms. Many advocate addition of a partial, nonobstructing fundoplication (e.g., a Belsey 240-degree wrap) to prevent the subsequent development of gastroesophageal reflux. Esophagomyotomy relieves dysphagia in 85% with a perforation rate of 1%. Newer, unproven approaches include botulinum toxin injection of the LES and video-assisted thoracoscopic or laparoscopic esophagomyotomy.

Diffuse Esophageal Spasm (DES)

Patients with this hypermotility disorder complain of chest pain and/or dysphagia as a result of repetitive, simultaneous, high-amplitude esophageal contractions. Patients are characteristically anxious, and the chest pain mimics coronary artery disease. A history of irritable bowel syndrome, pylorospasm, spastic colon, or other functional gastrointestinal complaints is common, and gastroesophageal reflux, gallstones, peptic ulcer disease, and pancreatitis can all trigger DES. Underlying psychiatric disease is common. A cardiac evaluation is indicated to exclude coronary artery disease. The classic radiographic appearance of DES on barium esophagogram is a "corkscrew" esophagus caused by segmental contractions of the circular muscle and is not always seen. DES represents functional bowel disease and is best treated by avoidance of stress and *trigger* foods or drinks, psychiatric counseling, treatment of associated GER, antispasmodics, H$_2$ blockers, nitrates, calcium channel blockers, or periodic esophageal dilations with mercury-weighted tapered bougies. Surgery—a left transthoracic long esophagomyotomy from the level of the aortic arch to the LES—should be reserved only for those with incapacitating chest pain or dysphagia, but long-term relief is achieved in more than 50%.

Scleroderma (Systemic Sclerosis)

This collagen vascular disease is characterized by induration of the skin, fibrous replacement of the smooth muscle of internal organs, and progressive loss of visceral and cutaneous function. Disruption of normal esophageal peristalsis is common and is a major diagnostic sign of the disease, particularly in patients with Raynaud's phenomenon. Fibrous replacement of esophageal smooth muscle produces loss of distal HPZ tone and GER. Normal peristalsis in the distal two-thirds of the esophagus is replaced by weak, simultaneous nonpropulsive contractions. Patients must wash slow-passing food through the esophagus with water and experience severe reflux symptoms. Contact between refluxed gastric acid and the esophageal mucosa is prolonged because the atonic lower esophagus clears refluxed gastric acid poorly. Accelerated reflux esophagitis may occur. Treatment is an aggressive antireflux medical regimen and periodic esophageal dilatations as needed. Intractable esophagitis may necessitate an esophageal-lengthening Collis gastroplasty–fundoplication procedure or a transhiatal esophagectomy and cervical esophagogastric anastomosis for a severe reflux stricture.

IV

Diverticula and Miscellaneous Conditions of the Esophagus
Mark B. Orringer, M.D.

Esophageal diverticula are epithelial-lined mucosal protrusions from the esophageal lumen that are classified according to their location, the extent of the esophageal wall thickness that accompanies them, and their mechanism of formation. Most are acquired and occur in adults. A *true* diverticulum contains all layers of the normal esophageal wall (mucosa, submucosa, and muscle). A *false* diverticulum consists of mucosa and submucosa protruding through the muscle layer.

See the corresponding chapter or part in the *Textbook of Surgery,* 15th edition, pp. 729–735, for a more detailed discussion of this topic, including a comprehensive list of references.

Pharyngoesophageal (Zenker's) diverticula occur at the junction of the pharynx and esophagus; *parabronchial* (midesophageal) diverticula, near the tracheal bifurcation; and *epiphrenic* (supradiaphragmatic) diverticula, within the distal 10 cm. of the esophagus. *Pulsion* (e.g., Zenker's and epiphrenic) diverticula result from elevated intraluminal pressure forcing mucosa and submucosa to herniate through the esophageal muscle; they are false diverticula. *Traction* (e.g., parabronchial) diverticula result from external inflammation in mediastinal lymph nodes that adhere to the esophagus and pull the entire wall toward them as they heal and contract; they are true diverticula.

PHARYNGOESOPHAGEAL (ZENKER'S) DIVERTICULUM

This is the most common esophageal diverticulum. It is an acquired *pulsion* diverticulum that occurs between 30 and 50 years of age. A Zenker's diverticulum arises within the inferior pharyngeal constrictor at a point of potential weakness (Killian's triangle) between the oblique fibers of the thyropharyngeus muscle and the horizontal cricopharyngeus muscle or upper esophageal sphincter (UES). For a variety of reasons, a derangement in the complex neuromotor series of events during swallowing results in unusually elevated pharyngeal pressure, and mucosa and submucosa herniate through the anatomically weak area above the UES. Typical symptoms are cervical dysphagia, regurgitation of undigested food or pills consumed hours earlier, a cervical gurgling sensation on swallowing, choking, and recurrent aspiration. The diagnosis is established with a barium esophagogram. In most symptomatic patients, surgery is indicated to prevent malnutrition or pulmonary sepsis. The degree of UES motor dysfunction, *not the size of the pouch,* determines the severity of symptoms. Currently, the most popular operation is a *cricopharyngeal myotomy,* which divides the UES, thereby relieving the obstruction distal to the pouch. Most pouches 2.5 cm. or less in diameter require no additional treatment. Larger pouches are resected or may be suspended from the prevertebral fascia (diverticulopexy). Complications include salivary fistula from the operative site and recurrent laryngeal nerve injury, both in less than 2%. Endoscopic division of the UES (Dohlman procedure) is popular in Europe. Regardless of the approach, *so long as the obstruction distal to the pouch is relieved,* recurrence is rare and results excellent.

MIDESOPHAGEAL (TRACTION) DIVERTICULUM

These are characteristically associated with mediastinal granulomatous disease (e.g., tuberculosis, histoplasmosis), small (1 cm. or less), asymptomatic, found incidentally on a barium esophagogram, and rarely require treatment. They have a blunt, tapered tip that points upward to the adjacent lymph node to which they are adherent, in contrast with the large, round, relatively narrow-mouthed pulsion diverticula.

EPIPHRENIC DIVERTICULUM

These occur within the distal 10 cm. of the esophagus, are pulsion diverticula, and result from elevated intraluminal pressure, most often in association with either esophageal motor dysfunction (spasm) or occasionally a mechanical distal obstruction (e.g., stricture). Associated esophageal pathology—hiatal hernia with gastroesophageal reflux, diffuse esophageal spasm, achalasia, reflux esophagitis, and carcinoma—is common. Symptoms include dysphagia, regurgitation, and retrosternal pain from diffuse esophageal spasm. Mildly symptomatic patients with pouches less than 3 cm. often require no treatment. Those with progressive dysphagia and chest pain or anatomically dependent or enlarging pouches are surgical candidates. The surgical approach is a left thoracotomy, resection of the pouch, and a long extramucosal esophagomyotomy from beneath the aortic arch to the esophagogastric junction. The distal extent of the esophagomyotomy is controversial, but most favor carrying the incision through the LES and onto the stomach for 1.0 to 1.5 cm. A partial fundoplication (e.g., modified Belsey repair) is then done to prevent gastroesophageal reflux. A 360-degree fundoplication is more likely to produce functional obstruction after a long esophagomyotomy and is not advocated here.

MISCELLANEOUS CONDITIONS

Sideropenic Dysphagia (Plummer-Vinson or Paterson-Kelly Syndrome)

This syndrome is characterized by dysphagia due to a cervical esophageal web and chronic iron deficiency anemia. Patients are typically elderly, edentulous, malnourished women with glossitis and spoon-shaped fingernails (koilonychia). Treatment is esophageal dilation and correction of the nutritional deficiency. This is a premalignant lesion, 10% of patients developing squamous cell carcinoma of the hypopharynx, oral cavity, or esophagus.

Schatzki's Ring (Distal Esophageal Web)

A Schatzki's ring is a short annular constriction occurring precisely at the esophagogastric junction proximal to a sliding hiatal hernia and identified with a barium esophagogram. When the ring diameter is 13 mm. or less, dysphagia is likely. Histologically, slight submucosal fibrosis is seen beneath the squamocolumnar epithelial junction. A Schatzki's ring indicates *only* that there is a hiatal hernia but *not* that there is either gastroesophageal reflux or esophagitis. Many patients with symptomatic rings have no reflux symptoms and respond well to intermittent esophageal bougienage. Those with dysphagia as well as reflux symptoms require dilation and an antireflux medical regimen. For severe dysphagia or refractory reflux symptoms, intraoperative dilation combined with an antireflux operation is indicated. Resection of the ring alone,

without repair of the associated hiatal hernia, should not
be done.

Mallory-Weiss Syndrome (Emetogenic Mucosal Laceration)

Forceful emesis may cause a distal esophageal mucosal tear
that presents as either melena or hematemesis. This may occur
with alcoholism, pregnancy, peptic ulcer disease, bowel obstruction, drug withdrawal, food poisoning, and so on. Barium esophagogram is rarely diagnostic. Esophagoscopy often
fails to identify the tear. In more than 90%, the bleeding stops
with nasogastric decompression and iced saline gastric lavage.
Persistent hemorrhage warrants an upper abdominal approach, long proximal gastrotomy, and oversewing of the
mucosal tear at the cardia. Results are excellent and recurrent
bleeding rare.

Esophagoscopy
Mark B. Orringer, M.D.

Esophagoscopy is among the most vital diagnostic tools in
the assessment of esophageal symptoms from any cause. This
procedure, particularly in association with dilation of a stricture, is one of the most dangerous operations performed, a
perforation resulting in major morbidity and mortality.

INDICATIONS AND CONTRAINDICATIONS

Diagnostic esophagoscopy is indicated in the assessment of
dysphagia, refractory reflux symptoms, odynophagia, hematemesis, occult blood loss, atypical chest pain, and established
pathology (e.g., esophagitis, tumor, stricture); abnormalities
identified with barium esophagogram; and postoperative
problems (e.g., anastomotic stricture, tumor recurrence). Therapeutically, esophagoscopy is used for dilation and biopsy of
strictures, removal of foreign bodies, placement of endolumi-
nal prostheses, sclerotherapy and laser photocoagulation, or
tumor debulking. Safe esophagoscopy requires adequate patient sedation and anesthesia. Relative contraindications are
recent myocardial infarction, severe cervical spine deformities,
and large thoracic aortic aneurysm.

See the corresponding chapter or part in the *Textbook of Surgery*, 15th
edition, pp. 736–744, for a more detailed discussion of this topic,
including a comprehensive list of references.

GENERAL PRINCIPLES

Elective esophagoscopy should not be performed without a prior barium esophagogram visualized by the endoscopist. The esophagogram identifies the level and extent of the abnormality and unsuspected pathology, for example, a Zenker's diverticulum, which may complicate the procedure. Barium esophagogram findings are related to anatomic landmarks that are used to approximate the level at which the abnormality will be seen endoscopically:

1. The cricopharyngeus sphincter occurs at the level of the C7 or T1 vertebral bodies, approximately 15 cm. from the upper incisor teeth at esophagoscopy.
2. The angle of Louis (sternomanubrial junction) aligns with the tracheal bifurcation and the fourth thoracic vertebral body, approximately 25 cm. from the incisors at esophagoscopy.
3. The esophagogastric junction is located 40 cm. from the upper incisors endoscopically, at the level of the eleventh or twelfth thoracic vertebrae.

Most esophagoscopies can be performed with the flexible fiberoptic esophagoscope using topical anesthesia of the posterior tongue and pharynx and mild sedation. The rigid esophagoscope is best for evaluating lesions at or just below the cricopharyngeus sphincter, removal of foreign bodies, dilation of certain high-grade stenoses, and obtaining larger and more adequate biopsies.

The consistent use of a standardized grading system for endoscopic reflux esophagitis (a number have been proposed) provides a more objective description of the pathologic changes seen and more meaningful evaluation at different times and by different endoscopists. One such classification by Skinner and Belsey is Grade I, distal mucosal erythema; Grade II, mucosal erythema with superficial linear ulcerations; Grade III, mucosal erythema, ulceration, and submucosal fibrosis—a dilatable "early" stricture; Grade IV, extensive ulceration and fibrous panmural stenosis.

Two questions might be answered about every esophageal stricture: (1) Is the stricture benign or malignant, and (2) if benign, can the stricture be dilated? Both questions are answered by esophagoscopy, which is a mandatory part of the evaluation of every stricture. As a general rule, comfortable swallowing requires that esophageal dilatation be achieved to the range of a 46 French or larger bougie. Strictures should not only be biopsied but also brushed for cytologic evaluation, since this combination establishes the diagnosis of carcinoma in 95% of cases.

Perforation, the leading and most serious complication of esophagoscopy, occurs in 1% to 2%, most often just proximal to the upper esophageal sphincter in the neck, then just above the esophagogastric junction, and least often at the level of the aortic arch.

Pain or fever after esophageal instrumentation represents an esophageal perforation until proven otherwise and is an indication for an immediate esophagogram so that expeditious treatment can be instituted. If no perforation is identified with a water-soluble agent (Gastrografin), dilute barium should be used for better detail. Cervical or high thoracic esophageal perforations are drained through a cervical incision; the upper two-thirds of the thoracic esophagus are approached through a right thoracotomy; distal third perforations and those at the esophagogastric junction are approached through a left thoracotomy.

VI

Tumors of the Esophagus
Mark B. Orringer, M.D.

BENIGN ESOPHAGEAL TUMORS AND CYSTS

LEIOMYOMAS. Esophageal leiomyomas, the most common benign esophageal neoplasms, are smooth muscle tumors that occur between 20 and 50 years of age and are multiple in 3% to 10% of patients. More than 80% occur in the middle and lower thirds of the esophagus. They may present as a calcified mediastinal mass. Most are asymptomatic, but tumors larger than 5 cm. produce dysphagia, vague retrosternal pressure, or pain. Leiomyomas characteristically appear on barium esophagogram as a smooth concave defect with intact mucosa and sharp borders and abrupt sharp angles where the tumor meets the normal esophageal wall. Esophagoscopy is indicated to exclude carcinoma, but if a leiomyoma is suspected, a biopsy of the mass should *not* be performed so that subsequent extramucosal resection is not complicated by scarring at the biopsy site. Symptomatic leiomyomas or those larger than 5 cm. should be excised, and submucosal enucleation is the procedure of choice. Results of resection are excellent; recurrence is rare. Asymptomatic or small leiomyomas may be followed with periodic barium esophagograms and esophageal ultrasonography, since they grow slowly and the likelihood of malignant degeneration is low.

ESOPHAGEAL CYSTS. Esophageal cysts arise as diverticula of the embryonic foregut and contain stratified squamous and simple columnar ciliated epithelium as well as fat and smooth muscle. Esophageal duplication cysts are lined by squamous epithelium and have submucosal and muscle layers; the latter may interdigitate with the outer longitudinal muscle layer of the normal esophagus. Three-quarters of duplication cysts present in childhood, over 60% occur along the right side of the esophagus, and they are frequently associated with vertebral anomalies (e.g., Klippel-Feil deformity or spina

---

See the corresponding chapter or part in the *Textbook of Surgery*, 15th edition, pp. 744–758, for a more detailed discussion of this topic, including a comprehensive list of references.

bifida) and abnormalities of the spinal cord. More than 60% of congenital esophageal cysts present in the first year of life with either respiratory or esophageal symptoms. Adults remain asymptomatic until bleeding or infection in the cyst causes enlargement with secondary dysphagia, choking, or retrosternal pain. The barium esophagogram shows a smooth extramucosal esophageal mass that may communicate with the esophageal lumen. Because of the potential for bleeding, ulceration, perforation, or infection, excision of the cyst is recommended. Extramucosal enucleation has excellent long-term results, and there is no recurrence if the initial excision is complete.

PEDUNCULATED INTRALUMINAL POLYPS. Benign esophageal polyps are rare. They arise in the cervical esophagus, develop progressively longer pedicles, may intermittently extrude into and even out of the mouth, and may cause intermittent dysphagia asphyxiation, hematemesis, or melena. Histologically, they consist of vascular fibroblastic tissue with varying amounts of fat. Despite their size, they are easily overlooked at esophagoscopy. Resection through a lateral cervical esophagotomy is curative.

MALIGNANT TUMORS OF THE ESOPHAGUS AND CARDIA

In the United States, the incidence of esophageal carcinoma is 6 cases per 100,000 population per year. Alcohol and tobacco are strong etiologic factors, but gastroesophageal reflux causing Barrett's mucosa is responsible for adenocarcinoma now being seen in epidemic proportions. The following esophageal lesions are premalignant: achalasia, reflux esophagitis, Barrett's esophagitis, radiation esophagitis, caustic burns, Plummer-Vinson syndrome, leukoplakia, esophageal diverticula, and familial keratosis palmaris et plantaris (tylosis).

PATHOLOGY. Worldwide, approximately 95% of esophageal carcinomas are squamous cell carcinomas (SCC), the majority being advanced (Stage III or IV) and occurring in 60- to 70-year-old men. In the United States, adenocarcinoma is becoming the most frequent type of esophageal carcinoma. SCC is most common in the upper and middle thoracic segments, adenocarcinoma in the distal third. Esophageal cancer is notoriously aggressive, infiltrating locally, invading adjacent intramural lymphatics and lymph nodes, and metastasizing widely by hematogenous spread. Extraesophageal tumor extension is present in 70% of cases at the time of diagnosis. Overall 5-year survival for treated tumors is 5% to 12%, 3% with lymph node metastases and 42% without. Patients with a columnar-lined lower esophagus (Barrett's metaplasia) have been estimated to be 40 times more likely to develop adenocarcinoma that the general population. The finding of dysplasia in Barrett's mucosa is an ominous prognostic sign of impending malignant degeneration. *Severe dysplasia* is synonymous with carcinoma *in situ* and is an indication for esophagectomy. Other rare types of esophageal malignant tumors include anaplastic small cell (oat cell carcinoma), adenoid cystic carcinoma, malignant melanoma, and carcinosarcoma.

PRESENTATION AND DIAGNOSIS. Progressive dysphagia is the predominant symptom, followed by weight loss, odynophagia, chest pain, and occasionally, hematemesis. A complaint of progressive dysphagia warrants *both* a barium esophagogram and esophagoscopy to rule out carcinoma. A stricture seen on barium esophagogram should be both biopsied and brushed for cytologic assessment, since the combination of these two studies establishes the diagnosis of carcinoma in 95% of cases. The CT scan is an essential part of preoperative staging of the tumor. A standardized TNM classification is used for staging.

TREATMENT. Since in the vast majority of patients local tumor invasion or distant metastases preclude cure, treatment of esophageal carcinoma is primarily palliative, that is, restoring the ability to swallow comfortably in the most simple and expeditious manner possible. Neither chemotherapy, radiation therapy, nor surgery for esophageal carcinoma has achieved significant and consistent long-term survival. Endoscopic laser resection or transoral intubation of obstructing esophageal tumors using any of a number of available prosthetic tubes may re-establish a passage for saliva, but comfortable swallowing of food is often not achieved, and the average survival with unresected esophageal cancer is less than 6 months.

For most patients with localized esophageal carcinoma, resection provides the best palliation. *Transthoracic* esophagectomy and an intrathoracic esophagogastric anastomosis provide excellent palliation but may be associated with major morbidity, including respiratory insufficiency from combined thoracic and abdominal incisions and intrathoracic anastomotic leak, which carries a 50% mortality from the resultant mediastinitis. Worldwide operative mortality figures ranging from 15% to 40% are common. With *transhiatal* esophagectomy (THE), the thoracic esophagus is resected through upper midline abdominal and cervical incisions, the stomach is pulled into the posterior mediastinum in the original esophageal bed, and a *cervical* esophagogastric anastomosis is performed. This procedure avoids the morbidity of a thoracotomy, and a cervical anastomotic leak is relatively easily managed by opening the neck wound for drainage and packing. Operative mortality is approximately 5%. Survival is equal to that achieved with standard transthoracic esophageal resection. Advocates of "radical" esophagectomy (extensive *en bloc* resection of the esophagus and contiguous tissues and lymph nodes) have not demonstrated consistently superior survival with this approach. Recently conducted nonrandomized phase II trials of combined preoperative chemotherapy (primarily with cisplatin and 5-FU) and radiation therapy prior to esophagectomy have yielded encouraging results that have justified prospective trials that are now under way.

VII

Perforation of the Esophagus
André Duranceau, M.D.

ETIOLOGY. Esophageal perforations are caused by endoscopic manipulations in 58% of all patients. Spontaneous perforations and external traumas are, respectively, responsible for 15% to 20% of all disruptions. Pathologic conditions affecting the esophageal wall are responsible for the other ruptures.

PATHOPHYSIOLOGY. Laceration of the posterior pharyngoesophageal junction is the most frequent location of endoscopic trauma. The esophageal body is perforated by attempts at deep biopsies of the esophageal wall or by dilation. Postemetic perforation is the result of a sudden increase in intraesophageal pressures when the glottis and the upper esophageal end are closed. Direct trauma by penetrating injuries or blunt trauma to the chest or abdomen may mimic the barotrauma of postemetic rupture. Esophageal disease may result in esophageal wall destruction and disruption.

SYMPTOMS AND SIGNS. Pain is the main symptom recorded when the esophagus has been perforated; it is either an unrelenting pain that follows endoscopic manipulations or dilations or an excruciating chest pain that follows straining or vomiting efforts. Dyspnea, epigastric pain, the hypersonority and/or dullness of hydropneumothorax, hypotension, and signs of sepsis are the most frequently reported signs and symptoms. Subcutaneous emphysema is present usually if the perforation is cervical.

DIAGNOSIS. The diagnosis is based on a strong degree of suspicion in view of the clinical presentation. The plain chest film is suggestive in 90% of reported disruptions: widening of the mediastinum; air in the mediastinum with pleural effusion occurs rapidly. Over 75% of patients show a left pleural effusion. The definitive diagnosis is obtained using a hydrosoluble contrast substance. The use of CT scan is helpful mostly to define and localize complications around the esophagus and in the pleural cavity. Esophagoscopy is rarely needed to diagnose an esophageal perforation.

TREATMENT. Etiology, time delay between rupture and diagnosis, and location of the perforation affect management and results. Conservative management is rare when the leak is contained in a stable patient and without evidence of sepsis. Early operation remains the mainstay of management. Extensive débridement of all nonviable tissue in the mediastinum and the pleural cavity is followed by clear identification of the perforation. Primary repair of the laceration is usually reinforced by healthy, well-vascularized tissue (stomach, mus-

---

See the corresponding chapter or part in the *Textbook of Surgery,* 15th edition, pp. 759–767, for a more detailed discussion of this topic, including a comprehensive list of references.

cle, pleura). When there has been a long delay since the
perforation, when the degree of mediastinitis is extensive, and
when sepsis decreases the chances of survival, consideration
must be given to resection with creation of an esophagostomy,
a gastrostomy, and a jejunostomy. Further reconstruction is
planned in a stable patient. Alternative procedures that have
been proposed include exclusion of the perforated esophagus
and drainage of the contaminated space or a directed fistulization on an intraesophageal T-tube with periesophageal
drainage.

RESULTS. Survival should near 95% when primary repair
is completed within 24 hours of rupture. Morbidity and mortality increase with late repair or with failure of the initial
repair resulting in uncontrolled sepsis.

VIII

Hiatal Hernia and Gastroesophageal Reflux

André Duranceau, M.D., and Glyn G. Jamieson, M.D.

Hiatal hernia and symptomatic gastroesophageal reflux are
the most frequent clinical conditions seen in the esophageal
clinic and laboratory. While nearly 50% of the adult population is found to have a hernia, 11% to 15% of these patients
will complain of daily to monthly heartburn.

Normal anatomic and physiologic integrity of the esophagus constitutes the best protection against reflux disease. With
every swallow, a continuous peristaltic wave traverses the
esophagus to push the bolus toward the stomach. At the
gastroesophageal function, the tissue organization of the specialized smooth muscle creates an asymmetrical high-pressure
zone responsible for lower esophageal sphincter (LES) activity.
This LES relaxes with the oncoming peristaltic wave. After
meals, short, transient LES relaxations occur, unrelated to
peristalsis, and allow reflux episodes in normal individuals as
well as in pathologic reflux disease.

PATHOPHYSIOLOGY

Patients with gastroesophageal reflux disease show a low
LES tone, and the potential for reflux is linearly related to this
resting pressure. Increasing reflux damage on the esophageal
mucosa is usually accompanied by a weaker sphincter. In the

See the corresponding chapter or part in the *Textbook of Surgery*, 15th
edition, pp. 767–784, for a more detailed discussion of this topic,
including a comprehensive list of references.

esophageal body, the peristaltic wave remains normal when early reflux damage exists. With increasing damage however, loss of peristalsis, failed peristalsis, and weaker contractions increase, allowing impaired clearance and longer exposure to the refluxate. More damage occurs when the reflux liquid contains acid and alkaline secretions mixed with pancreatico-duodenal enzymes. Refluxing patients are often tense and overweight individuals. Fatty food, smoking, and drinking are major factors affecting the integrity of their esophagogastric function.

INVESTIGATION

SYMPTOMS. Heartburn and regurgitations are the typical symptoms of reflux disease. They are made worse by lying down or bending. Dysphagia and painful swallowing are usually caused by mechanical or functional obstruction from reflux damage. Abnormal contractions can easily mimic cardiac pain. Hematemesis and melena suggest severe disease. Asthma, oropharyngeal dysphagia, and recurrent atypical chest pain may be associated with reflux disease, but only if they correlate with esophageal mucosal damage.

RADIOLOGY. Seeing reflux of barium into the esophagus by itself does not mean that reflux disease is present. Radiology helps to define the anatomic abnormalities associated with reflux. Abnormalities in mucosal pattern, ulcers, and strictures are determined with a good sensitivity. Radiology defines and classifies the presence or absence of a hiatal hernia. Type I is the small sliding hernia. Type II is a paraesophageal hernia, with the gastroesophageal junction in a normal position. Type III hernia is an association of Types I and II where the gastroesophageal junction is displaced into the chest. Type IV is typically the massive Type III hernia with another abdominal organ alongside the herniated stomach.

ESOPHAGOSCOPY AND ESOPHAGEAL BIOPSIES. These constitute the best way to report visual damage to the esophageal mucosa. Linear erosions, ulcers, strictures, and metaplasia are the most objective evidence of mucosal damage. On esophageal biopsies, acute inflammation and erosions, ulcers, fibrosis, and the specialized columnar mucosa of Barrett's epithelium are unequivocal documentation of reflux damage.

MANOMETRY. The most frequent physiologic abnormality seen with reflux disease is a low LES tone. The lowest sphincter pressure or an absent tone at the gastroesophageal junction tends to be seen in patients with the worst mucosal damage. Esophageal body contractions are usually normal when minimal mucosal damage exists. Functional deterioration is observed with progressing damage to the esophageal wall.

MONITORING ACID AND BILE. Twenty-four-hour acid pH monitoring and fiberoptic quantification of bile exposure measure and correlate reflux episodes with symptoms. Increased exposure is usually correlated with greater mucosal damage.

MANAGEMENT

MEDICAL TREATMENT. The great majority of patients seen with small hiatal hernias and occasional reflux symptoms require symptomatic treatment only. More intensive therapy must always be based on accurate investigation and staging of the disease.

1. *Modification of lifestyle:* Reduce weight, decrease fat intake, avoid chocolate, mint, coffee, and LES-weakening medications. Exclude tobacco and alcohol.

2. Protect the esophageal mucosa by simple antacids, alginates, or cytoprotectors. H_2-receptor antagonists are useful for lesser degrees of reflux disease. Proton pump inhibitors are used when the esophagitis is severe and resistant to receptor antagonists.

3. Improve esophageal function by prokinetic agents (cisapride, domperidone) in an effort to recreate better LES pressures and improve esophageal emptying. A major effort at reducing weight to a normal height/weight ratio must be sought during the 6-month to 1-year treatment period.

SURGICAL TREATMENT. An operation is indicated when esophageal symptoms and damage persist following a well-supervised period of medical treatment. The massive hernias (Types II, III, and IV) must be corrected surgically. Surgical treatment aims to restore a normal anatomy with a normal tension-free intra-abdominal length of esophagus and an improved high-pressure zone at the LES level. This is usually obtained by creating a total fundoplication or a partial fundoplication around the intra-abdominal esophagus. If more esophageal damage is present, a gastroplasty to elongate the esophagus must be created prior to adding the fundoplication. Control of reflux disease and mucosal damage is obtained in over 80% of patients.

IX

Corrosive Strictures of the Esophagus
James L. Talbert, M.D.

Despite an enhanced public and legislative awareness, caustic ingestions remain a significant health problem in the United States, affecting between 5000 and 26,000 citizens annually. The incidence is bimodal in age distribution, with over

---

See the corresponding chapter or part in the *Textbook of Surgery*, 15th edition, pp. 784–789, for a more detailed discussion of this topic, including a comprehensive list of references.

75% of injuries involving children younger than 5 years and a much lower secondary peak occurring in late adolescence and early adult life. The ingestion is almost always accidental in the young child, who all too frequently has been enticed by chemical solutions that have been carelessly placed in familiar soft drink containers or by crystalline caustics that resemble sugar or candy exposed in jars or cans. In the older patient, the event is usually linked to a suicide attempt. Immediate surgical attention is essential in such cases because of the high potential for inflicting serious damage to the airway and upper gastrointestinal tract. The agents most frequently involved are alkaline caustics (lye), acid or acidlike corrosives, and household bleaches. However, severe localized esophageal burns also can result from the ingestion of Clinitest tablets, which are used for testing sugar in the urine and contain significant amounts of anhydrous sodium hydroxide, or from swallowing small, disk-shaped (button) alkaline batteries, which may become entrapped in the esophagus of a young child.

Caustic injury is manifest by oral pain, drooling, excessive salivation, and inability or refusal to swallow or drink, in association with visible erythema, blistering, or ulceration of the lips, oral mucosa, tongue, and pharynx. The presence of hoarseness, stridor, and dyspnea suggests laryngeal injury, whereas substernal, back, or abdominal pain and rigidity may signify mediastinal or peritoneal perforation. However, reported series have repeatedly emphasized that the absence of symptoms or identifiable oropharyngeal burns does not exclude the possibility of esophageal injury.

The most important element in the successful management of a corrosive burn of the esophagus is immediate verification of the etiologic agent and accurate assessment of the depth and extent of injury. Induced vomiting and gastric lavage are usually contraindicated because they may compound the original injury and potentially cause laryngeal damage. As soon as an appropriate period of time has elapsed to allow gastric emptying and stabilization of the patient, esophagoscopy should be performed expeditiously, preferably within the first 12 to 48 hours, to confirm the extent and severity of the burn. In children this procedure is best accomplished under general anesthesia. The only exceptions to this approach are those patients in whom esophageal or gastric perforation or impending airway obstruction is evident. The primary goal of the endoscopist is to confirm the presence or absence of a caustic burn. Regardless of the mode of treatment, clinical reports have increasingly emphasized that in the presence of a full-thickness esophageal injury, there is an inherent high potential for stricture formation. In those patients who sustain only superficial injuries, as manifest by erythema, edema, or blistering, the prognosis appears excellent, even without any specific treatment. However, the identification of ulcerations, especially when circumferential, warrants special concern.

The changing spectrum of ingested caustics over the past 30 years has involved a variety of substances with differing potentials for injury, and there has been no large, well-controlled reference series of patients comparable with that used nationally for randomized, coordinated trials of childhood cancer treatment. Therefore, the management of this condition has remained controversial, with advocates espousing both pharmacologic and mechanical modification of wound healing, either separately or in combination.

Pharmacologic management of esophageal burns has been predicated on the use of steroids to modify the inflammatory response to injury and antibiotics to control secondary bacterial infection. However, a recent report by Anderson and colleagues of a controlled trial involving 60 children treated over an 18-year period failed to substantiate any statistical benefit of steroid administration in preventing stricture formation. Because the reflux of acidic gastric secretions may exacerbate the injury to the esophageal mucosa and further increase the likelihood of stricture formation, the administration of H_2 blockers or therapeutic doses of antacids also has been recommended for 6 to 8 weeks.

An alternative method involves mechanical modification of wound healing through the placement of intraluminal Silastic stents, either by mouth under fluoroscopic guidance or in concert with a gastrostomy. Whether stents are employed with or without systemic antibiotics and steroids, several reports have indicated success in decreasing the incidence of residual significant scarring and stricture formation, even in the presence of severe circumferential esophageal mucosal injury. However, this treatment may not always prove feasible, because it may entail intense monitoring and require a prolonged period of hospitalization for at least 3 weeks, depending on the type and configuration of the stent.

Early complications may include perforation of the esophagus or stomach, demanding immediate celiotomy or thoracotomy; development of airway obstruction, requiring insertion of a tracheostomy; and development of a tracheoesophageal fistula, necessitating bipolar exclusion of the esophagus by proximal and distal division and closure in the neck and abdomen in conjunction with a cervical esophagostomy, gastrostomy, and tracheostomy. With identification of full-thickness necrosis of the esophagus and stomach, as may be incurred by the ingestion of concentrated solutions of alkalies or acids, emergency esophagectomy, gastrectomy, and even duodenectomy may be required to prevent lethal complications such as overwhelming sepsis and/or tracheoesophageal and aortoenteric fistulas.

Stricture formation is usually manifest within the first few months but may be delayed until considerably later. When stenosis ensues, dilation should be attempted through the passage of bougies, either antegrade by mouth or retrograde through a previously constructed gastrostomy. An alternative method of dilation that has proved especially helpful in managing complicated or persistent strictures involves the inflation of an intraluminal, Gruntzig-type balloon optimally positioned under fluoroscopic monitoring by means of an endoscopically directed guidewire. When a stricture proves refractory to all forms of dilation, esophageal reconstruction must be undertaken, most frequently interposing either a segment of colon or a reversed antiperistaltic gastric tube, based proximally on the greater curvature of the stomach and receiving its blood supply from the left gastroepiploic artery. Either of these techniques has been demonstrated in children to provide excellent long-term function and allow normal growth and development, but recently, the alternative of gastric transposition also has gained increasing favor.

Late complications of corrosive burns of the esophagus include the development of achalasia or hiatal hernia as a consequence of progressive intramural scarring and contraction, as well as a thousand-fold increase in the frequency of esophageal cancer as a consequence of malignant degeneration in the previously injured tissues.

27

LAPAROSCOPIC SURGERY

Steve Eubanks, M.D., and Philip R. Schauer, M.D.

The modern era of laparoscopic surgery has evoked remarkable changes in approaches to surgical diseases. The trend toward minimally invasive surgery has prompted general surgeons to scrutinize virtually all operations for possible conversion to laparoscopic techniques. The rate at which such drastic changes have occurred is unprecedented in surgical history.

The inauspicious origins of modern laparoscopic surgery combined with the rapid dissemination of reports in the lay media led to a problem-filled infancy for this field of surgery. *Laparoscopic cholecystectomy* had become a widely recognized term prior to its report in a peer-reviewed journal. The validity of the claims of dramatic patient benefits was verified and serves as the basis by which laparoscopy has survived and flourished despite such an unusual beginning.

The adolescence of laparoscopic surgery has included the addition of numerous respected surgical investigators who have begun to establish the basic science foundation essential for the endurance of this rapidly advancing type of surgery. The pendulum of surgical opinion continues to swing with gradually decreasing sweeps as the appropriate application of laparoscopy to specific diseases and operations is established. Laparoscopy is certain to maintain an important place in the armamentarium of the general surgeon. The integration of laparoscopic training into the conventional surgical residency has provided the foundation for the safe propagation of minimally invasive surgery.

The history of modern endoscopy spans nearly a century of development. Laparoscopy can be characterized as an area of medicine in which innovative surgeons, scientists, and engineers apply existing and emerging technologies to clinical problems. The driving force behind this "movement" has been the motivation of surgeons to avoid unnecessary injury to their patients while accomplishing diagnostic or therapeutic tasks within a body cavity. The roots of modern endoscopy are within cystoscopy, which was commonly performed in the late 1800s with a rigid scope developed by Maximillian Nitze in 1879. Most scholars credit Georg Kelling (1866–1945) of Dresden, Germany, with performing the first laparoscopy. Hans Christian Jacobaeus (1879–1937) of Stockholm, Sweden, was instrumental in establishing laparoscopy and thoracoscopy as clinically valuable. The first laparoscopic operation in the United States was performed at Johns Hopkins Hospital in 1911.

Mühe of Boblinen, Germany, performed the first totally laparoscopic cholecystectomy in 1985. Muhe presented his

---

See the corresponding chapter or part in the *Textbook of Surgery*, 15th edition, pp. 791–807, for a more detailed discussion of this topic, including a comprehensive list of references.

work for the first time at the Congress of the German Surgical Society in April of 1986. His initial report was largely ignored. However, by March of 1987, he had accumulated a personal experience of 94 cases. In 1987, Philip Mouret, in Lyon, France, performed a laparoscopic cholecystectomy and a few months later showed a videotape of his technique to Dubois in Paris. Within 1 year, leaders in Europe, including Dubois, Perissat, Cuschieri, and Nathanson, and in the United States, including McKernan, Saye, Reddick, and Olsen, perfected the technique and are responsible for the unprecedented and rapid world-wide expansion of this procedure. In the United States alone, laparoscopic cholecystectomy grew from a handful of operations in 1988 to over one-half million by 1993.

Many specialty fields, including thoracic surgery, pediatric surgery, gynecology, urology, orthopedics, plastic surgery, and otorhinolaryngology, are now applying modern endoscopic techniques to their respective fields. Current studies will help determine which laparoscopic procedures have significant benefit over conventional procedures, particularly regarding the cost/benefit ratio. Unanticipated complications, such as bile duct injuries during laparoscopic cholecystectomy and esophageal perforations during laparoscopic Nissen fundoplication, have arisen, which have provoked serious debate regarding appropriate training for this new technology.

The fundamental advantage of laparoscopic surgery over open surgery is that it reduces the postoperative morbidity and perhaps mortality that is specifically related to the adverse physiologic responses to surgery. Multiple clinical studies have compared open cholecystectomy with laparoscopic cholecystectomy and have clearly demonstrated a significant reduction in postoperative pain, hospital stay, perioperative morbidity, and convalescence. Studies of the physiologic changes of laparoscopic surgery substantiate the benefits of laparoscopic surgery and contribute to the understanding of the fundamental relationship between injury and recovery.

The major differences between open and laparoscopic surgery are the method of access, CO_2 pneumoperitoneum, and the degree of tissue injury. Two factors, reduced tissue injury and CO_2 pneumoperitoneum, most likely account for the important beneficial as well as adverse physiologic changes associated with laparoscopy. Reduced retraction and manipulation of abdominal viscera may be important secondary factors, especially with respect to postoperative gastrointestinal function. In general, the physiologic effects of CO_2 pneumoperitoneum are detrimental and occur transiently during the intraoperative period. Conversely, the beneficial response to reduced tissue injury affects the entire period from injury to complete recovery. The balance of these physiologic responses to the laparoscopic method should serve as the foundation for the overall benefit of laparoscopic surgery.

Insufflation of the abdomen with CO_2 has been the dominant method of laparoscopic access for many decades. Gas embolism is a potentially lethal complication of any gas used to produce pneumoperitoneum; a rapidly absorbed gas such as CO_2 is less likely to result in a persistent air lock obstructing right ventricular outflow. The main disadvantage of CO_2 is that it readily dissolves into solution and becomes biologically reactive, potentially producing many adverse effects.

CO_2 pneumoperitoneum may affect hemodynamics by entirely different mechanisms, primarily involving the mechanical effects of increased intra-abdominal pressure and the physiologic effects of absorbed CO_2. Increased intra-abdominal pressure may impair venous return, thus reducing preload and leading to a reduced cardiac output. The reduction in cardiac output may vary with the magnitude and duration of the operation as well as with the patient's hydration status. Distinct from pressure effects, the CO_2 gas may be absorbed systematically and lead to hemodynamic changes related to hypercarbia. CO_2 absorption/excretion may be affected by a variety of factors, including patient pulmonary function and ventilator settings. Factors other than pneumoperitoneum coexist during laparoscopic procedures that may significantly alter hemodynamic responses. These factors include placement of the patient in the Trendelenburg or reverse Trendelenburg positions, the patient's volume status, the patient's cardiac and pulmonary function, obesity, and type and dose of anesthetic agents.

Most clinical studies indicate that the hemodynamic effects of CO_2 pneumoperitoneum cause an increase in heart rate, mean arterial pressure, systemic vascular resistance, and central venous pressure and a decrease in cardiac output. Although rare, potentially lethal dysrhythmias may be caused by hypercarbia or abdominal pressure effects. Increases in cardiac workload may predispose patients with coronary disease to myocardial infarction. The effect of CO_2 insufflation on pulmonary function may produce impairments in oxygenation, ventilation, and pulmonary compliance and increased airway resistance.

The list of operations performed by laparoscopic techniques frequently undergoes expansion. Those operations which are performed routinely using laparoscopy include cholecystectomy, diagnostic laparoscopy, staging for malignancy, colon resection, appendectomy, antireflux operations, small bowel resection, adhesiolysis, hernia repair, and splenectomy. Operations that are technically feasible to perform by laparoscopic techniques but which, for various reasons, have yet to receive widespread acceptance include adrenalectomy, pancreatic resection, gastrojejunostomy, operations for ulcer disease, esophagomyotomy, gastric resection, treatment of rectal prolapse, and diagnostic laparoscopy for trauma. Procedures that are not performed routinely laparoscopically (or performed only in an experimental setting) include the Whipple procedure, major hepatic resection, and bypass of aortoiliac disease. Further revisions of the lists of those procedures which are best performed by laparoscopic techniques are certain to occur. Factors such as cost-effectiveness, outcomes, complications, and technical feasibility will guide the future direction of laparoscopic surgery.

28

ABDOMINAL WALL, UMBILICUS, PERITONEUM, MESENTERIES, OMENTUM, AND RETROPERITONEUM

Kevin M. Sittig, M.D., Michael S. Rohr, M.D., Ph.D., and John C. McDonald, M.D.

ABDOMINAL WALL

The abdominal wall is a complex musculoaponeurotic structure that is attached to the vertebral column posteriorly, the ribs superiorly, and the bones of the pelvis inferiorly. It is derived embryonically in a segmental metameric manner, and this is reflected in its blood supply and innervation. The abdominal wall protects and restrains the abdominal viscera, and its musculature acts indirectly to flex the vertebral column. The integrity of the abdominal wall is essential to the prevention of hernias, whether they are congenital, acquired, or iatrogenic.

Anatomy, Innervation, Lymphatic Drainage

The abdominal wall is composed of nine layers. From superficial to deep they are (1) skin, (2) tela subcutanea (subcutaneous tissue), (3) superficial fascia (Scarpa's fascia), (4) external abdominal oblique muscle, (5) internal abdominal oblique muscle, (6) transversus abdominis muscle, (7) endoabdominal (transversalis) fascia, (8) extraperitoneal adipose and areolar tissue, and (9) peritoneum. The plane between the internal oblique and transversus abdominis muscles can properly be considered a neurovascular plane because it contains the segmental arteries, veins, and nerves that supply the abdominal wall. The anterior primary rami of thoracic spinal nerves T7 to T12 and lumbar nerve L1 supply the abdominal wall in a segmental, sequential manner from superiorly to inferiorly. The main trunks of the nerves are found in the neurovascular plane. The anterior cutaneous rami pierce the rectus sheath anteriorly to supply the anterior skin.

The transversalis fascia is poorly named and often misunderstood. It more properly should be called the *endoabdominal fascia,* for it is a continuous lining of the abdominal cavity. Where this fascia lies in direct relation to certain muscles, it is given a special name. Over the psoas muscle, it is called the *psoas fascia.* Where it lies deep to the transversus abdominis muscle, it is properly called the *transversalis fascia.* The

---

See the corresponding chapter or part in the *Textbook of Surgery,* 15th edition, pp. 809–823, for a more detailed discussion of this topic, including a comprehensive list of references.

integrity of the endoabdominal fascia is absolutely essential for the integrity of the abdominal wall. If this layer is intact, no hernia exists.

The lymphatic supply of the abdominal wall allows a simple pattern. Above the umbilicus, the lymphatic pathways drain into the ipsilateral axillary lymph nodes. Below the umbilicus, they drain into the ipsilateral superficial inguinal lymph nodes. Omphalocele may be seen in the newborn and represents a defect in closure of the umbilical ring. The herniated viscera are usually covered with a sac composed of amnion. Gastroschisis is a defect of the abdominal wall that is located lateral to the umbilicus. It is due to failure of closure of the body wall in which abdominal viscera protrude through the defect. No sac is present to cover the herniated intestine.

Omphalomesenteric Duct Remnants

Remnants of the omphalomesenteric (vitelline) duct may present as abnormalities related to the abdominal wall. An umbilical polyp is a small excrescence of omphalomesenteric duct mucosa that is retained in the umbilicus. Such polyps resemble umbilical granulomas except that they do not disappear after silver nitrate cauterization. Appropriate treatment is excision of the mucosal remnant. Umbilical sinuses are due to the continued presence of the umbilical end of the omphalomesenteric duct. The morphologic features of the sinus tract can be delineated readily with a sinogram. Treatment is excision of the sinus. Persistence of the entire omphalomesenteric duct is heralded by the passage of enteric contents from the umbilicus. This is seen in the early neonatal period and should be treated promptly with laparotomy and excision of the duct to avoid intussusception or volvulus.

Urachal Anomalies

The urachus is a fetal structure that connects the developing bladder to the umbilicus. The urachus normally is obliterated by the time of birth. It may persist, causing a vesicoumbilical fistula manifested by the drainage of urine from the umbilicus. Proper treatment is excision of the fistula after distal urinary obstruction has been excluded. A persistent urachal sinus results when the umbilical end of the urachus does not obliterate normally. It may become infected and should be excised totally. Cystic remnants of the urachus may persist between the bladder and umbilicus when urachal obliteration is incomplete. These cysts may become symptomatic at any time and present as lower abdominal masses or, occasionally, abscesses. They should be excised completely.

Omphalitis

Infection of the umbilicus may occur in infants and adults. It is generally an innocuous disease due to poor hygiene and is treated with appropriate cleansing and local care to the umbilicus. However, in the neonatal period, omphalitis may be the result of bacterial infection and potentially may be associated with serious sequelae such as portal vein thrombosis. In neonates, treatment should include systemic antibiotics.

Rectus Sheath Hematoma

Extravasation of blood into the rectus sheath that causes a hematoma is rarely a life-threatening illness. However, it may mimic other abdominal diseases and must be considered in the differential diagnosis to avoid unnecessary laparotomy. Patients with rectus sheath hematomas most often give a history of receiving anticoagulant drugs for various conditions. When the hematoma develops, it ordinarily occurs at the level of the semicircular line of Douglas, where the inferior epigastric artery enters the rectus sheath.

Abdominal Wall Tumors

Benign tumors of the abdominal wall may arise from any of the elements contained within the abdominal wall. Desmoid tumors of the abdominal wall are benign fibrous tumors arising from the musculoaponeurotic abdominal wall. They should be excised widely to prevent local recurrence.

Primary malignancies of the abdominal wall are uncommon. Any of the cutaneous neoplasms may affect the abdominal wall and are treated in the same manner as skin cancers elsewhere. The abdominal wall is occasionally the site of metastasis from primary malignancies located elsewhere.

PERITONEUM

The peritoneal cavity is a potential space containing the abdominal viscera. The peritoneum provides a frictionless surface over which the abdominal viscera can move freely, and the mesothelial lining secretes fluid that serves to lubricate the peritoneal surfaces. Normally, there is about 100 ml. of clear, straw-colored fluid present in the peritoneal cavity of the adult. The quality and quantity of this fluid may change with various pathologic conditions. Peritoneal dialysis is possible because of bidirectional transport across the peritoneal membrane. By adjusting the composition of the dialysate, excess water, sodium, potassium, and products of metabolism can be removed from the bloodstream. In addition, a variety of drugs can be removed with peritoneal dialysis. Normally, there is a balance between fluid secretion and absorption in the peritoneal cavity. Ascites occurs when either the secretion rate increases or the absorption rate decreases disproportionate to the other. This fluid may be a transudate or exudate, and its composition is determined by the etiology of the ascites.

Accumulation of lymph within the peritoneal cavity is usually the result of trauma or tumor involving lymphatic structures. It differs from other fluid accumulations in the peritoneal cavity in that it has bacteriostatic properties, making infection less likely. Uninfected bile is a mild irritant to the peritoneal cavity. It causes an increased production of peritoneal fluid, resulting in bile ascites or choleperitoneum. Patients with this condition may be relatively well as long as the fluid remains sterile, exhibiting only a mild jaundice from absorption of bile pigments. Infected bile, however, causes a severe peritonitis and necessitates urgent surgical therapy. Blood is not an irritating substance in the peritoneal cavity. The most common cause of hemoperitoneum is trauma to the liver or spleen. Urine collections within the peritoneal cavity are generally due to trauma to the urinary tract. Pneumoperitoneum is usually secondary to perforation of the gastrointestinal tract or to recent operation. It may follow alveolar rupture in patients on mechanical ventilators. Treatment is directed to the underlying cause of the pneumoperitoneum.

Peritonitis

Peritonitis is inflammation of the peritoneum. *Primary peritonitis* refers to inflammation of the peritoneal cavity without a documented source of contamination. It occurs more commonly in children than in adults and in females more than in males. Children with nephrotic syndrome and, less commonly, systemic lupus erythematosus are particularly susceptible to primary peritonitis. In recent years, the bacterial flora has changed from gram-positive to gram-negative organisms. Thus the distinction between primary and secondary peritonitis is more difficult to make by peritoneal aspirate alone.

MESENTERY AND OMENTUM

The greater and lesser omenta and the intestinal mesentery are rich in lymphatics and blood vessels. In response to intraperitoneal inflammation, the omentum provides the major source of peritoneal macrophages and aids in removal of foreign material and bacteria. Torsion or infarction of the omentum, like mesenteric cysts or omental cysts, is best treated by excision.

RETROPERITONEUM

The retroperitoneum is an actual space located between the peritoneal cavity and the posterior body wall. Anteriorly, this space is bounded by the posterior parietal peritoneum and the spaces between the leaves of the small and large bowel mesenteries. Posteriorly, it is bounded by the vertebral column and the psoas and quadratus lumborum and tendinous portions of the transversus abdominis muscles. Several disorders that lend themselves to surgical treatment can be approached by an extraperitoneal or retroperitoneal exposure. This approach has many advantages over the more commonly used transabdominal approach. It is sound judgment to choose retroperitoneal or extraperitoneal exposure over transabdominal exposure when technically feasible. Many intra-abdominal abscesses are localized in such a way that a part of the limiting wall is the parietal peritoneum. Such abscesses, when recognized, are best evacuated through the retroperitoneal portion of the abscess, thereby avoiding contamination of the general peritoneal cavity.

Retroperitoneal Fibrosis

This unusual disease, which has some similarities to hypersensitivity or autoimmune disease, is relatively rare. The etiology is unknown. The important clinical aspect of retroperitoneal fibrosis is that the fibrotic process frequently entraps and constricts the ureters, thereby causing obstructive uropathy. Surgical treatment of retroperitoneal fibrosis consists of freeing the encased ureters from their fibrous encapsulation. When freed, the ureters must be protected from recurrent fibrotic encasement. This has been prevented successfully by converting the ureters into intra-abdominal organs or wrapping them with omentum. Renal autotransplantation also has been used as a means to surgically treat retroperitoneal fibrosis.

Retroperitoneal Tumors

At the time of presentation, the majority of retroperitoneal tumors have invaded adjacent organs and have reached considerable size. The majority of these tumors (60% to 85%) are malignant and are of mesodermal origin (75%) and of nervous origin (24%). Successful treatment of these tumors remains primarily surgical. An *en bloc* resection of these malignancies provides the most favorable 5-year survival of 67%.

Retroperitoneal Vascular Procedures

Elective surgical procedures on the aorta and its branches are being approached more commonly from an extraperitoneal route today. The extraperitoneally exposed visceral aorta and its branches can be controlled easily for bypass, endarterectomy, splenorenal shunting, renal autotransplantation, and correction of aneurysmal disease.

29

THE ACUTE ABDOMEN

Arnold G. Diethelm, M.D., Robert J. Stanley, M.D.,
and Michelle L. Robbin, M.D.

The clinical entity known as the *acute abdomen* represents a complex arrangement of pathologic disease which, if left undiagnosed, may cause the patient's death. Because of the acuity of the illness, a careful, methodical diagnostic approach is necessary to arrive at a correct diagnosis. Rapid or quick decisions are usually not required and often are incorrect or misleading.

HISTORY

PRESENT ILLNESS. The onset of the pain is important to elucidate, as well as its location and change in character and position. Pain that is sharp, severe, and sudden in onset—waking the patient from sleep or incapacitating the patient at work—suggests a perforated viscus. The type of pain at onset and its progression later are important in the differentiation of small bowel obstruction from intestinal infarction. The former begins as a cramping intermittent type of pain, whereas the latter causes a dull constant pain. Radiation of the pain also may be helpful in the diagnosis. Pain of acute cholecystitis frequently radiates around the right costal margin to the right scapula and to the shoulder. Pain in acute pancreatitis is usually epigastric in origin with subsequent radiation along both costal margins to the back. Ureteral calculi produce pain radiating to the groin when the stone is in the cephalad portion of the ureter and perineal pain when the stone approaches the ureterovesical junction. The temporal relationship of abdominal pain to vomiting is important and may provide valuable diagnostic clues to the underlying etiologic factor. The character of the emesis, including the color and content, may be helpful in determining the location of the obstruction. Clear vomitus suggests an obstructed pylorus, whereas bile-stained emesis indicates that the obstruction is distal to the entrance of the common bile duct into the duodenum. Anorexia is usually associated with acute abdominal pain, and in patients with acute appendicitis, it may precede the onset of pain. Constipation, diarrhea, and a recent change in bowel habits are important factors in the diagnosis of patients with abdominal pain. An accurate menstrual history is especially valuable in the assessment of abdominal pain in the female, including the frequency of the cycle and the duration of the menstrual period. The type of contraception and

See the corresponding chapter or part in the *Textbook of Surgery*, 15th edition, pp. 825–846, for a more detailed discussion of this topic, including a comprehensive list of references.

its duration of use must be considered because there are specific complications for each method.

PAST ILLNESSES. The patient's medical history prior to the present illness is of special value, particularly in regard to previous surgery (e.g., appendectomy, cholecystectomy, gastric or intestinal surgery) or the previous diagnosis of an abdominal or inguinal hernia.

FAMILY HISTORY. The probability of acute abdominal pain relating to a familial disease is unlikely but may occur in some circumstances. Familial Mediterranean fever (familial recurring polyserositis) occurs in persons of Armenian or Sephardic Jewish background as an inherited autosomal recessive trait and is characterized by spontaneous attacks of abdominal pain. Sickle cell anemia in black patients is another example of a hereditary influence on the cause of abdominal pain.

PHYSICAL EXAMINATION

The important aspect of the physical examination begins with the patient's appearance, ability to answer questions, position in bed, and degree of obvious pain or discomfort. The position in bed is important regarding whether the patient lies in a supine position or on the side with the knees and hips flexed.

The abdominal examination always begins with a visual inspection of the abdomen for previous scars, hernia, obvious masses, or abdominal wall defects. The inspection should focus on the size, shape, and contour of the abdomen. Auscultation of the abdomen should include all four quadrants, with special attention given to the frequency and pitch of bowel sounds and rushes of gas audible to the examiner that correlate with the facial expression of pain by the patient. Percussion of the abdomen should begin in the quadrant free of pain and should be performed lightly so that elicitation of pain is avoided at the onset of the examination.

The presence of peritoneal irritation can be assessed either by abdominal palpation with a quick release of the examining hand (rebound tenderness) or by gently rolling the patient from side to side with the examiner's hands placed on the patient's pelvis. The pelvic examination notes the presence of cervical discharge or vaginal bleeding, and bimanual examination either confirms or excludes tenderness on uterine or adnexal palpation. A rectal examination should note the existence of pelvic tenderness or a mass and the presence of a perirectal abscess.

RADIOGRAPHIC STUDIES

The plain supine and erect radiographs of the abdomen remain the first step in the diagnostic imaging evaluation of patients with abdominal pain, although more sensitive and specific imaging methods, such as computed tomography (CT) and ultrasonography, play an increasing role in the evaluation of this complex, emergent clinical problem. Plain radiographs of the abdomen are most valuable in the evaluation of mechanical obstruction of the gastrointestinal tract. Supine and erect radiographs of the abdomen should allow the distinction between obstruction of the gastric outlet and small and large bowel obstruction.

The indications for the use of CT and ultrasonography in the evaluation of the acute abdomen have increased greatly in the past 5 years. Ultrasonography can provide rapid evaluation of liver, spleen, pancreas, and renal morphologic features. Aortic and visceral artery aneurysms, thrombi within veins, arteriovenous fistulas, and vascular anomalies all are amenable to evaluation with modern ultrasound equipment.

CLINICAL PATHOLOGIC DIAGNOSTIC STUDIES

A complete blood count and urinalysis are essential in all patients evaluated for acute abdominal pain. Additional laboratory tests that are especially helpful include a serum amylase for patients with acute pancreatitis, liver function studies for confirming the presence of acute hepatitis, and the human chorionic gonadotropin for excluding an ectopic pregnancy.

ORGAN SUBSYSTEM ANALYSIS

The etiology of acute abdominal pain can be separated according to the organ subsystem involved. The most common cause of acute abdominal pain in the gastrointestinal subsystem relates to an inflammatory or mechanical process of the stomach, small and large intestine, gallbladder, common bile duct, liver, or pancreas.

PERFORATED PEPTIC ULCER. Free perforation of peptic ulcer disease, more often resulting from duodenal ulcer than from gastric ulcer, is more common in male patients between the third and fourth decades. The pain is sudden in onset, severe, and located first in the epigastrium, later spreading over the entire abdomen. Shoulder pain is common and reflects referred pain from diaphragmatic irritation. In the presence of generalized peritonitis from a perforated ulcer, the patient usually lies in the supine position, avoiding any undue motion that might increase the abdominal pain. The patient appears acutely ill with tachypnea and tachycardia. Percussion reveals generalized abdominal tenderness, especially in the epigastric region. Palpation suggests a firm, "boardlike" abdomen with rigidity of the rectus muscles. Rebound tenderness that is present in all four quadrants and worse in the epigastric region is an important diagnostic finding. Auscultation of the abdomen soon after perforation reveals hypoactive bowel sounds that progress over time to absent bowel sounds. Important laboratory data include an elevated white blood cell count between 12,000 and 20,000 per cu. mm. with immature forms. The hematocrit is elevated, and the serum amylases may be slightly elevated but less than occurs in acute pancreatitis. Free air underneath the diaphragm in erect films is present in about 75% of patients.

ACUTE CHOLECYSTITIS. This disease occurs most commonly in women between the ages of 30 and 60 years who have had a previous history of pregnancy. The younger patients often have a family history of biliary tract disease. The illness begins with the onset of a constant dull pain in the right upper quadrant, usually several hours after a large meal. Some patients move about, attempting to relieve the pain, whereas others lie restlessly in bed. Nausea and vomiting are common, with temporary improvement in the severity of pain after an episode of emesis. The pain may subside after several hours; if so, the episode is considered to be biliary colic. If the disease process progresses to acute cholecystitis, the pain is constant and gradually worsens with chills and fever. Examination of the abdomen reveals mild to moderate distention. Bowel sounds are hypoactive to auscultation. Tenderness to palpation is maximal in the right upper quadrant. In the absence of perforation of the gallbladder with generalized peritonitis, palpation confirms the right upper quadrant tenderness to be worse with deep inspiration. Frequently a mass can be palpated along the right costal margin, which represents a distended tense gallbladder that descends with deep inspiration. Laboratory data often reveal the white blood cell count to be elevated (10,000 to 13,000 per cu. mm.); however, a normal white blood cell count may occur in the presence of severe acute cholecystitis. An elevated serum bilirubin to 2.0 or 2.5 mg. per 100 ml. may exist with uncomplicated acute cholecystitis. If, however, the bilirubin exceeds 3.0 mg. per 100 ml., common duct calculi should be considered. Ultrasonography, currently the most common imaging method used, can rapidly assess the diameter of the biliary tree, the presence or absence of biliary calculi, and the appearance of the gallbladder wall and contents as well as the surrounding structures.

ACUTE PANCREATITIS. Pancreatitis may present with sudden onset of severe epigastric pain radiating directly through to the back and around both costal margins with or without shoulder pain. Acute pancreatitis usually occurs in patients between the ages of 25 and 50 years and frequently has been preceded by a similar episode with a previous diagnosis. The onset may be rapid, with the pain becoming intolerable in 3 to 4 hours. Anorexia, nausea, and vomiting are common, and emesis rarely provides relief. Abdominal tenderness, most evident in the epigastric region, is present with both percussion and palpation. Routine laboratory tests show a leukocytosis ranging from 12,000 to 22,000 per cu. mm. The key diagnostic test is the serum amylase, which is elevated within a few hours in most patients who have the acute form of the disease. Plain radiographs of the abdomen often are nondiagnostic in patients with acute pancreatitis. CT scan and ultrasonography may confirm the clinical diagnosis or assessment of suspected complications.

ACUTE RELAPSING PANCREATITIS. Acute relapsing pancreatitis differs from acute pancreatitis in that the pain is recurrent with each exacerbation of pancreatitis and is associated with an increase in serum amylase. The patient's previous history of pancreatitis usually will confirm the diagnosis. The diagnosis can best be established by ultrasonography or a CT scan of the pancreas.

CHRONIC PANCREATITIS. Patients with chronic pancreatitis differ from those with recurrent episodes of acute pancreatitis (acute relapsing pancreatitis) in that the pain becomes constant. The history usually suggests the diagnosis from the patient's previous attacks, and radiographs of the abdomen often reveal pancreatic calcification.

ACUTE APPENDICITIS. Acute appendicitis, a common cause of abdominal pain, is especially difficult to diagnose in patients younger than age 3 and older than age 70 years. A careful history is essential in making an accurate early diagnosis. Abdominal pain first begins in the epigastrium, then gradually migrates to the periumbilical region, and finally to the right lower quadrant. Anorexia, nausea, and vomiting are common. There is localization of the pain to the right lower quadrant after 6 to 8 hours of onset with tenderness to palpation and rebound tenderness. Guarding on palpation occurs when the process has progressed to localized peritonitis. Regardless of all the presenting illnesses, the most common complaint is right lower quadrant pain, and the most frequent physical finding is right lower quadrant tenderness to palpation. Laboratory data are nondiagnostic and may be normal. The plain abdominal film findings are usually not helpful, although a visible fecalith may be diagnostic. Recent experience with ultrasonography and CT scans has shown both imaging methods to be helpful in defining the pathologic changes characteristic of appendicitis as well as its associated complications.

RENAL CALCULI. Renal or ureteral calculi may cause severe abdominal pain; however, once the calculus begins to descend in the ureter, the pain pattern varies with radiation to the groin and perineum. The pain is sudden, excruciating in severity, and may subside in a few minutes only to recur when the calculus descends in the ureter. Radiographs of the abdomen should be performed in patients in a supine position to search for a calculus. An intravenous pyelogram and urinalysis can be helpful in differentiating renal pain from that of nonrenal origin.

MECKEL'S DIVERTICULITIS. This condition involves the persistence of a portion of the vitelline duct on the antimesenteric border of the distal ileum and may cause bleeding, intestinal obstruction, and less often, acute abdominal pain from diverticulitis. An accurate diagnosis is rarely established before operation.

ACUTE DIVERTICULITIS. Acute diverticulitis of the colon may result from congenital or acquired diverticula. In most instances, the disease is a result of the acquired form of diverticula. The incidence increases with age, and the process may involve the entire colon but more commonly involves the left colon, particularly in the sigmoid. The disease presents with dull left lower quadrant pain, chills, and fever. Vomiting and anorexia are uncommon in the early phase of the illness. Examination reveals the abdomen to be slightly distended with tenderness in the left lower quadrant. A mass, often palpable just medial to the anterosuperior iliac spine, represents an inflamed, edematous, and tender sigmoid colon.

ACUTE OBSTRUCTION OF THE SMALL INTESTINE.
The first symptom of acute obstruction of the small intestine is sudden, sharp, cramping abdominal pain, usually periumbilical in location. Between episodes of colic, the patient is free of pain and may feel quite well. Nausea and vomiting occur soon after the onset of symptoms, and emesis may temporarily relieve the pain. Auscultation of the abdomen reveals hyperactive bowel sounds of increased pitch and intensity with audible rushes as peristalsis increases in frequency. Laboratory data reveal an increase in hematocrit resulting from dehydration, with the white blood cell count increased from 12,000 to 20,000 per cu. mm. Supine and erect radiographs of the abdomen are almost always diagnostic in the evaluation of patients with acute small bowel obstruction. If the level of obstruction is in the middle or distal small bowel, dilated loops of fluid- and gas-filled small bowel will be apparent, whereas the nonobstructed colon appears devoid of gas or feces.

ACUTE OBSTRUCTION OF THE LARGE INTESTINE.
Obstruction of the large intestine occurs more often in patients over the age of 40 years, is gradual in onset, and presents with constipation and abdominal distention. The most common causes of large bowel obstruction include carcinoma of the colon, acute diverticulitis, and volvulus. The abdomen appears distended and tympanitic to percussion. The diagnosis can be suggested in most instances by a supine and an upright radiograph of the abdomen. The descending and sigmoid colons are dilated to the point of obstruction, and the small intestine may be dilated if the ileocecal valve is competent.

Volvulus of the large intestine causing acute intestinal obstruction can occur in the cecum or sigmoid portion of the colon. Sigmoid volvulus is more common than is cecal volvulus and occurs more frequently in patients over the age of 65 years. The diagnosis is established by the supine and upright radiographs of the abdomen; a water-soluble contrast enema reveals the characteristic point of torsion and nonfilling of the obstructed loop of sigmoid colon. Cecal volvulus usually occurs in patients of the middle and older age groups with sudden onset of cramping right lower quadrant and epigastric pain associated with nausea and vomiting. The diagnosis is best established by supine and upright radiographs of the abdomen demonstrating a dilated cecum and ascending colon, often with the gas-distended cecum in the left upper quadrant.

ACUTE GYNECOLOGIC DISEASE

ACUTE SALPINGITIS. This disease, most commonly due to gonococcal infection, has an index of highest frequency in sexually active patients between the ages of 15 and 35 years and is rarely seen after menopause. The pain begins caudal to the umbilicus in the midline and radiates to the right and left lower quadrants. Examination of the abdomen reveals right and left lower quadrant tenderness to percussion and palpation. Bowel sounds are hypoactive. Cervical tenderness is marked to palpation on pelvic examination. A vaginal discharge is frequent, and a positive diagnosis can be established with a cervical smear and culture.

OVARIAN CYSTS. Ovarian cysts are often asymptomatic but may present with sudden pain located in the lower abdomen and in either the right or left lower quadrant, depending on the ovary involved. Pelvic examination is the key diagnostic maneuver, and a palpable mass may confirm the suspicion.

ECTOPIC PREGNANCY. Tubal pregnancy may present as an acute intra-abdominal condition with sudden lower abdominal pain that is sharp in character and persistent with or without nausea and vomiting. A missed menstrual period or an abnormally short, scanty period will have preceded the abdominal pain. The preoperative diagnosis may be established by a positive human chorionic gonadotropin test.

SUMMARY

Acute abdominal pain is a serious surgical emergency requiring the surgeon to combine the information from the history and physical examination with properly selected laboratory and radiographic studies. The indications for surgical therapy can be established in most situations, and a correct preoperative diagnosis usually will lead to a successful operation.

30

THE STOMACH AND DUODENUM

I

Historical Aspects, Anatomy, Pathology, Physiology (Including Gastrointestinal Hormones), and Peptic Ulcer Disease

Theodore N. Pappas, M.D.

GASTRIC ANATOMY AND PHYSIOLOGY

The stomach is anatomically defined at its superior margin by the gastroesophageal junction and at its inferior border by the pylorus. It lies in the upper abdomen, bounded by the spleen to the left and the liver to the right. The blood supply to the stomach is extensive, with branches coming off both the celiac and the superior mesenteric arteries. Four major arteries to the stomach include the right gastric, the left gastric, and the right and left gastroepiploic. Neural input to the stomach includes the vagus nerve, which sends the anterior (left) and posterior (right) vagus nerves for both motor and secretory function.

Histologically, the cardia, fundus, and the antrum are distinct areas, with five major cell types. These cell types are found in the gastric glands and include parietal cells, mucus-secreting cells, zymogen or chief cells, endocrine cells, and argentaffin and undifferentiated cells.

GASTRIC PHYSIOLOGY AND ACID SECRETION

Vagal stimulation occurs during cephalic-phase secretion and is responsible for direct cholinergic stimulation of the parietal cell and indirect stimulation of parietal cell via gastrin release. Gastrin-releasing peptide (GRP) is the neurotransmitter that causes the release of gastrin for vagally mediated stimulation of this hormone. Acetylcholine is the neurotransmitter that acts at the parietal cell during vagal stimulation. Gastrin and cholinergic receptors on the parietal cell are two of the three receptors that regulate gastric acid stimulation. The third is the histamine receptor, which is stimulated by locally released histamine, predominantly from mast cells. The gastrin and cholinergic receptors act through intracellular

---

See the corresponding chapter or part in the *Textbook of Surgery,* 15th edition, pp. 847–868, for a more detailed discussion of this topic, including a comprehensive list of references.

calcium to activate phosphorylase kinase, which leads to protein phosphorylation and eventual production of acid via hydrogen/potassium ATPase. In contrast, histamine receptor stimulation activates adenylate cyclase, which produces cyclic AMP, which acts through protein kinase to phosphorylate ADP, eventually driving hydrogen/potassium ATPase.

Downregulation of acid is controlled by a variety of factors, including somatostatin. Somatostatin is released locally by the D cell in the stomach to downregulate the parietal cell. In addition, somatostatin acts as a paracrine in the antrum to downregulate the release of gastrin. This regulation of gastrin release is largely a feedback mechanism that is pH-dependent, in that a pH greater than 3 causes release of gastrin, whereas a pH less than 3 causes an inhibition of gastrin.

PHYSIOLOGY OF GASTRIC EMPTYING

Gastric emptying is controlled by the anteropyloroduodenal complex. The antrum is responsible for grinding particles into very small sizes that are passed eventually through the pylorus into the duodenum. Vagal stimulation of the antrum is largely responsible for the active emptying of gastric particles smaller than 0.5 mm. The fundus acts as a storage area that accommodates for meals via a vagal mechanism. The loss of accommodation leads to the dumping syndrome when the gastric outlet has been altered by pyloroplasty or gastrojejunostomy. The control of gastric emptying is multifactorial and includes cholecystokinin, which is a physiologic inhibitor of gastric emptying. Duodenal acidification and distal gut peptides such as peptide YY are also responsible for causing a delay in gastric emptying. The migrating motor complex (MMC) is a fasting contractile pattern in the upper gut that sweeps the upper gut of residual particles that are not passed by normal motility.

THE DUODENUM

The duodenum extends from the pylorus about 20 to 30 cm. and ends at the ligament of Treitz. There are four portions of the duodenum that are supplied by blood vessels originating from the celiac and superior mesenteric artery. Histologically, the duodenum is made up of mucosa and muscle. There are many microvilli that can be seen microscopically and increase the absorptive area of the duodenum. Cells lining these villi include goblet cells that secrete mucus, Paneth cells, endocrine cells, and undifferentiated cells. The endocrine cells belong to the APUD (amine precursor uptake and decarboxylation) system, which in the duodenum includes cholecystokinin, secretin, somatostatin, gastric inhibitory polypeptide (GIP), and neurotensin. These peptides have a variety of physiologic roles in the upper gut.

PEPTIC ULCER DISEASE

The incidence of peptic ulcer disease has been decreasing over the past 40 years. Although the introduction of histamine-2 antagonists such as cimetidine in 1977 has had a dramatic effect in the treatment of peptic ulcer disease, the falling incidence for this disease occurred at a much earlier time. The cause of this decrease in the disease is uncertain. The etiology of peptic ulcer disease is largely related to acid. The acidity in peptic ulceration varies from extreme hyperacidity as in Zollinger-Ellison syndrome to hypoacidity, which is present with Type 1 and Type 4 gastric ulcers. Since acid must be present for ulceration, antacid therapy remains the cornerstone of ulcer treatment.

A number of factors have been implicated in peptic ulceration, including nonsteroidal anti-inflammatory drugs (NSAIDs), cigarette smoking, and *Helicobacter pylori*. *H. pylori* is found in almost all patients with peptic ulceration in the upper gut. Eradication of the bacterium can decrease the recurrence rate of peptic ulcer disease.

The medical management of peptic ulcer disease includes an H_2 antagonist for 6 to 8 weeks and investigation to document the presence of *H. pylori*. Patients with *H. pylori* should receive concomitant therapy for this bacterium. Care should be taken to stop all ulcerogenic drugs that contribute to the exacerbation of this disease. Operative management of peptic ulcer disease is usually considered for four indications: intractability, perforation, obstruction, and bleeding.

Intractability

Intractable peptic ulcer disease is that which does not respond to medical therapy. These patients present electively and often are best suited for a highly selective vagotomy. This offers the advantage of relatively low ulcer recurrence rate with minimal side effects of surgery. Patients with obstruction, partial obstruction, or prepyloric ulcers associated with intractability probably should be treated with an alternative form of surgical therapy.

Obstruction

Patients who present with obstruction and peptic ulcer disease routinely require operative intervention. Semielective medical management often will treat the immediate symptoms effectively, but obstruction usually recurs. This is due to chronic scarring in the area of the outlet leading to delayed gastric emptying, stasis, and recurrent ulceration. Operative intervention usually includes vagotomy, antrectomy, and Billroth I or II reconstruction.

Bleeding

Bleeding peptic ulcer disease usually is treated endoscopically prior to consideration of surgical intervention. If endoscopic intervention fails and the patient has been transfused with more than 6 units of blood, then operative intervention is considered. The purpose of operative intervention is to control the hemorrhage and perform an ulcer operation, as necessary. Bleeding duodenal ulcers usually are treated by duodenotomy or pyloroplasty and plication of the ulcer bed with the addition of a vagotomy. This can be done as vagotomy and pyloroplasty or duodenotomy plus highly selective vagotomy. Occasionally, resectional therapy is necessary for prepyloric ulcers, although nonresectional therapy should be the procedure of choice for emergent surgery.

Perforation

Perforated peptic ulcer disease requires operative intervention for two purposes. Initially, irrigation and closure of the perforation are necessary, with the addition of an ulcer operation for those patients who have an antecedent history of peptic ulcer disease. Vagotomy, pyloroplasty, and oversew of the ulcer again are probably the procedures of choice. Patching the ulcer plus highly selective vagotomy is also a reasonable alternative. Again, resectional therapy for perforated duodenal disease is not considered first-line therapy. Complications of gastric ulcer disease require slightly different operative management. Because of the possibility of gastric cancer, operative intervention should include excisional biopsy. Therefore, resectional therapy, including antrectomy, is occasionally necessary and should be incorporated in the operative management. Gastric ulcers associated with hypersecretion, such as Type 2 and Type 3 gastric ulcers, often require an ulcer operation in addition to treating the bleeding or perforation associated with gastric ulcer. Type 1 and Type 4 ulcers tend not to be hypersecretory and therefore do not always require an ulcer operation at the time that their complication is treated.

ULCER OPERATIONS AND THEIR COMPLICATIONS

Surgical treatment for peptic ulcer disease has a very long history, but recent knowledge concerning the physiology of upper gut secretion and the pathogenesis of peptic ulcer disease has changed the surgical approach, particularly in elective operations. Elective peptic ulcer surgery for intractability usually involves highly selective vagotomy. This operation involves dividing the innervation of the parietal cell mass with little impact on the active component of antral-mediated gastric emptying. This operation minimizes side effects of dumping and postvagotomy diarrhea that can occur frequently after other peptic ulcer operations. Its efficacy is limited by surgeon experience and relative contraindications, which include prepyloric ulcers and patients with high recurrence rates such as cigarette smokers. Vagotomy with antrectomy is the operation with the lowest recurrence rate (less than 2%) but the highest complication rate. Mortality is generally quoted in the 1% to 2% range, with morbidity predominantly including dumping and diarrhea. Postvagotomy dumping after vagotomy with antrectomy is common and occurs in approximately 25% of patients. Most of this dumping resolves with time, and it is unusual for patients to have protracted dumping that requires medical intervention (1% to 2% of patients after vagotomy with antrectomy). Vagotomy with antrectomy is ideally suited for patients who have risk factors for recurrence after ulcer operation.

Vagotomy with pyloroplasty is perhaps the simplest of the vagotomy operations in that it has very low morbidity and mortality with a reasonably low (10%) ulcer recurrence rate. It is used commonly in emergent situations and occasionally for elective ulcer surgery where co-morbidities prohibit a large operation such as vagotomy with antrectomy and where post-ulceration duodenal scarring makes highly selective vagotomy a poor option.

Zollinger-Ellison syndrome was defined in 1955 by investigators from Ohio State University, who noted the presence of non-beta islet cell tumors in the setting of bleeding diathesis from upper gut ulceration. It is now known that gastrinoma is the tumor that creates the Zollinger-Ellison syndrome and occurs in two settings. The sporadic tumors occur in patients who have solitary tumors, and such patients may undergo surgical resection for cure if they have localized, nonmetastatic disease. The second group consists of patients who have gastrinoma associated with multiple endocrine neoplasia (MEN 1) syndrome. These patients have multicentric disease and are very difficult to cure surgically. Patients with gastrinoma from MEN 1 syndrome and those with sporadic gastrinoma who present with metastatic disease are best palliated with Omeprazole to avoid the complications of peptic ulceration.

II

Benign Tumors of the Stomach
Mark W. Sebastian, M.D.

INCIDENCE. Benign tumors comprise 7% of premortem gastric tumors but less than 2% of true gastric neoplasms. Approximately 40% of the tumors are mucosal epithelial polyps, and another 40% are leiomyomas. All other tumors are rare.

CLINICAL PRESENTATIONS. Benign gastric tumors occur predominantly in the middle decades of life and most commonly are located in the gastric antrum or corpus. Occult loss of blood causing iron deficiency anemia is common because these tumors ulcerate their overlying mucosal epithe-

---

See the corresponding chapter or part in the *Textbook of Surgery,* 15th edition, pp. 868–875, for a more detailed discussion of this topic, including a comprehensive list of references.

lium. Deep ulcerations overlying intramural tumors are notorious for their association with overt hemorrhage. Tumors of the cardia and pylorus may cause obstruction; if pedunculated, the tumor, usually pyloric, may create intermittent obstruction due to a ball-valve effect. Frank gastroduodenal intussusception secondary to a prolapsing gastric tumor may occur.

DIAGNOSIS. Barium studies (with or without air contrast) and gastroscopy with biopsy through the fiberoptic gastroscope are the mainstay for diagnosis. However, even with biopsy, diagnosis of a specific type of polyp or hyperplastic mural tumor is an especially vexing problem, since the biopsy forceps is unable to penetrate deeply enough for an adequate sampling of the tumor for histologic examination. This is especially true with leiomyomas and other firm, rubbery mesenchymal tumors.

The indications for extirpation of the tumor are elimination of any significant clinical effects and the need to exclude a diagnosis of malignancy. Ultimately, the tumor must be excised *completely* either by endoscopic techniques or surgical excision before a final disposition can be made.

POLYPS

Almost all polyps (Greek *polypus*, "many footed") arise from the mucosal epithelium. That the nomenclature of gastric polyps is confusing is in large measure due to early attempts at presenting them as being analogous to colorectal polyps in microscopic appearance and natural history. In fact, most gastric polyps have no exact counterparts in the large bowel. Unlike colonic polyps, gastric epithelial polyps are very uncommon tumors with an incidence of 0.4% to 0.8%. The body of endoscopic literature is beginning to define distinction between the types of epithelial polyps (hyperplastic, neoplastic or adenomatous, inflammatory, fundic gland polyp) by sex, location, and endoscopic appearance. Classically, this had not been true, since distinctions of any kind by epidemiologic or endoscopic means were not possible. The median age for gastric polyps is about 65 years, with an equal gender distribution or at most a slight female predilection. The histologic appearance of a polyp cannot be predicted on the basis of location within the stomach. However, in the same patient, polyps are almost always of the same histologic type, should they be multiple.

TREATMENT. Polyps causing pain, bleeding, or gastric outlet obstruction should be removed. Total endoscopic excision is advocated so that the nature of the polyp can be firmly established. Open surgical excision is indicated when excision by endoscopic snare and cautery is judged not to be feasible, when examination of the tissue removed endoscopically is consistent with invasive malignancy, and when a sessile polyp is present that exceeds 2 cm. in diameter. Multiple polyps involving the distal stomach or a group of closely aligned polyps in the gastric corpus can be removed by resection of the segment or by wide local excision. In diffuse polyposis, a large portion of the gastric mucosal surface is involved with innumerable tumors. The decision must take into account the fact that although these polyps are benign, they may be associated with coexisting adenocarcinoma elsewhere in the stomach. A total gastrectomy may be indicated in these cases, especially when the fundus is involved, since a coexisting fundal adenocarcinoma may be masked and difficult to identify. Local wedge excision is adequate treatment for polyps that appear with focal atypia or carcinoma *in situ*. Asymptomatic polyps should be biopsied by endoscopic snare-cautery excision. Hyperplastic polyps may be observed safely and repeat endoscopy advised on an annual basis for examination not only of the polyps but also of the entire intervening gastric mucosa.

Gastric Polyps in Polyposis Syndromes

Gastric involvement occurs in 50% of patients with familial polyposis coli and the related Gardner's syndrome, in which patients also may harbor polyps in the duodenum. The gastric polyps can be adenomatous, hyperplastic, or the fundic gland hyperplasia type.

All patients confirmed as having familial polyposis coli should have gastroduodenoscopy. Any adenomas found should be eradicated by endoscopic destruction. Repeat examination should then be undertaken at 6- to 12-week intervals until no polyps remain. Thereafter, examinations every 6 months should be made.

In *Peutz-Jeghers syndrome,* hamartomatous gastric polyps occur in about 20% of the patients, with an occasional coexisting adenocarcinoma. These patients require regular endoscopic surveillance.

Generalized juvenile polyposis and the related *Cronkhite-Canada syndrome* are associated with a high incidence of gastric retention (juvenile) polyps.

Cowden's syndrome (family name of index patient) may be associated with small sessile gastric polyps, most of which are of the hyperplastic type. The feature of disseminated polyposis (oral mucosa to anus) has been emphasized recently in this autosomal dominant disease. An increased, evidently genetically determined prevalence of malignant tumors of various organs (e.g., thyroid, breast) in patients with Cowden's disease and their family members mandates careful follow-up not exclusively focused on the stomach.

HYPERPLASTIC GASTROPATHY

The general term *hyperplastic gastropathy* refers to a rare condition in which there is enlargement of the rugal folds in the stomach. The etiology of the hyperplastic process varies.

Ménétrier's disease (polyadenomes en nappe) is a process in which gastric mucosal hypertrophy may be so great that the rugae assume the appearance of convolutions of the brain. Although this gross appearance is common to all cases of Ménétrier's disease, in an individual case, either the gastric glandular elements or the superficial epithelial elements of the gastric mucosa may predominate. Thus acid secretion may be high, normal, or low; hypoproteinemia, formerly considered an essential component of the disease, may not be present.

On microscopic examination, there is a striking *foveolar hyperplasia*, accompanied by tortuosity and some degree of cystic dilatation with extension into the base of the gastric glands. The stomach is edematous and inflamed. Hyperrugosity may regress, atrophic gastritis may develop, and carcinoma of the stomach may ensue.

Ménétrier's disease may be diagnosed at any age. The etiology is unknown. Since spontaneous resolution of the acute signs and symptoms (abdominal pain, 80%; blood loss, 34%; hypoproteinemia, 40%; weight loss; edema; malnutrition) may occur, nutritional support and a period of observation are justified when the precise diagnosis has been established. Anticholinergics and also H_2 blockers may be attempted for diminishing acid secretion and tightening gastric cell junctions, but a combination of these approaches is the norm. If pharmacologic therapy fails, *total* gastrectomy and reconstruction with a long Roux-en-Y jejunal limb is the best therapy. Any remaining gastric mucosa is the focus of a significant incidence of subsequent development of adenocarcinoma. An interesting aspect of the management of patients with Ménétrier's disease is their propensity to have a hypercoagulable state, sometimes associated with gastric carcinoma, which occurs in 1% to 15% of all cases of Ménétrier's disease.

OTHER HYPERTROPHIC CONDITIONS

Other conditions associated with hyperrugosity are gastric cancer and malignant lymphoma. In *chronic hypertrophic gastritis*, there is non-neoplastic proliferation of all epithelial elements—mucus-secreting cells as well as parietal cells and chief cells. The lesion is noninflammatory, and thus the term *gastropathy* is preferred to *gastritis*. *Zollinger-Ellison syndrome* may be associated with gastric changes, showing glandular (rather than foveolar) hyperplasia of the fundic gland, grossly similar to those of Ménétrier's disease.

CYSTIC LESIONS

The most important cystic lesion is a reduplication cyst. Usually encountered in the distal stomach, it may, but does not usually, communicate with the gastric lumen. When distention of the cyst with fluid causes obstruction and/or a palpable mass, surgical removal is indicated.

PSEUDOLYMPHOMA

Extensive lymphocytic infiltration of a portion of the stomach may be associated with benign gastric ulcer. Submucosal nodules, diffuse thickening, or enlarged rugal folds should be biopsied. The infiltrate often has a follicular pattern that may be confused with *follicular lymphoma*. However, the presence of clearly reactive germinal centers throughout the lesion, including a mixed population of inflammatory cells, establishes the diagnosis of pseudolymphoma. Immunohistochemical stains for immunoglobulins show a polyclonal pattern, but the distinction from lymphoma can be extraordinarily difficult. Much of the current literature excludes the MALT lymphomas from gastric polyp classifications.

HETEROTOPIC PANCREAS

An aberrant nest of pancreatic tissue may project into the gastric lumen and occasionally cause pain from becoming inflamed or cause pyloric obstruction or hemorrhage. Usually it is found incidentally at autopsy or laparotomy. The most characteristic gross feature is a central ductal orifice that tends to umbilicate the tumor, which is submucosal in 85% of cases. Technically a hamartoma, the antral (61%) or prepyloric (24%) mass is composed of glands and intervening connective tissue. Islets of Langerhans are seen in only 30% of cases; if present, their number is generally less than in normal pancreas. From a practical point of view, most of these lesions are excised surgically because patients and physicians alike prefer surgical excision to the diagnostic uncertainty they create.

III

Lymphoma of the Stomach
Theodore N. Pappas, M.D.

Primary intra-abdominal lymphomas represent 10% to 20% of all lymphocytic lymphomas, and gastric lymphomas compose most of the primary gastrointestinal lymphomas. In contrast, primary gastric lymphomas compose less than 5% of all primary gastric tumors. Because of their common clinical presentation, gastric lymphoma and adenocarcinoma of the stomach exist in the same differential diagnosis and must be distinguished by preoperative and intraoperative evaluation.

CLINICAL PRESENTATION AND DIAGNOSTIC TESTS. Clinical presentation of gastric lymphoma is similar to the presentation of adenocarcinoma of the stomach. Patients with primary gastric lymphoma present in their midfifties, with a male-to-female ratio of 1.7:1. Around 80% of patients present with abdominal pain, which can be associated with anorexia, early satiety, weight loss, nausea, and vomiting. Less than 10% present asymptomatically. Over 40% may present with an emergent complication of their gastrointestinal lymphoma, including bleeding, perforation, and obstruction.

See the corresponding chapter or part in the *Textbook of Surgery*, 15th edition, pp. 875–878, for a more detailed discussion of this topic, including a comprehensive list of references.

On physical examination, an abdominal mass may be present. Splenomegaly occurs because of direct extension of the tumor, but massive splenomegaly and diffuse adenopathy are more consistent with diffuse lymphoma. Barium studies have been used for diagnosis of gastric masses but usually do not distinguish between adenocarcinoma and lymphoma. Whereas lesions as small as 3 to 4 cm. in the stomach can be detected by upper gastrointestinal series, 10% to 20% of patients have a completely normal upper gastrointestinal series when a primary gastric lymphoma is present. Abdominal ultrasound and endoscopic ultrasound have a relatively limited utility in the evaluation of gastric masses. Endoscopic ultrasound has been used in staging these tumors and defining wall penetration. Computed tomography (CT) characterizes gastric masses but does not distinguish between lymphoma and adenocarcinoma of the stomach.

Gastrointestinal endoscopy is essential in the diagnosis of gastric lymphoma. Visual diagnosis is correct in only half the cases appearing as superficial stellate ulcers involving large areas of the stomach where the margin between normal mucosa and the lesion is quite precise. Biopsies and cytologic examination in patients with lymphoma accurately make the diagnosis in 30% to 90% of patients. Owing to insufficient tissue, many patients require exploratory laparotomy for definitive pathologic diagnosis.

PATHOLOGY. There are five major classifications of the gross morphologic features of primary gastric lymphoma: infiltrative, ulcerative, nodular, polypoid, and combined morphology (any combination of the other four). The histologic type of primary gastric lymphoma is characterized by mucosal or submucosal lymphoid tissue with infiltration of the gastric glands by follicular cells forming characteristic lymphoid epithelial lesions. Mucosa-associated lymphatic tumors (MALT) are low-grade lesions that are associated with *Helicobacter pylori,* and eradication of *H. pylori* causes regression of the tumor.

Pseudolymphoma represents 10% of all gastric lymphomas diagnosed with ulceration and extensive fibrosis, commonly in the presence of chronic peptic ulcer disease. This benign gastric lymphomatosis is characterized by lymphoid infiltration of the gastric wall predominantly in the mucosa without evidence of nodal disease. The *sine qua non* for the histologic diagnosis is the finding of germinal centers within the gastric lesions. Pseudolymphoma may represent a premalignant lesion that can convert to malignant lymphoma; therefore, current recommended management is conservative surgical resection, and nonoperative observation is reserved for patients at high risk for surgical therapy.

TREATMENT. The current recommended treatment of primary gastric lymphoma is attempted cure with surgical resection, including total gastrectomy in the appropriate patient. Approximately 75% are able to have resection on exploration; curative resection should yield a 5-year survival of 35% to 50% for all stages. The stage of the tumor correlates well with 5-year survival (90% to 95% for Stage I; 20% to 25% for Stage IV). Surgical resection is also recommended for decreasing the complications of bleeding and perforation during adjuvant therapy.

Adjuvant therapy is recommended for all stages of primary gastric lymphoma and may include whole abdominal radiation with an increase to the stomach bed or combination chemotherapy, such as CMOPP or CHOP. Adjuvant therapy clearly improves survival, particularly in patients with nodal disease. Primary treatment with chemotherapy or radiation for varying stages of gastric lymphoma is being evaluated for efficacy compared with primary surgical therapy.

In summary, all Stage I and Stage II patients (disease confined to stomach and regional nodes) should undergo attempted curative resection followed by adjuvant chemotherapy and/or radiation therapy. Stage III and Stage IV patients with complications of bleeding, obstruction, and perforation also should undergo attempted primary resection followed by adjuvant therapy. Patients without complications with preoperative documentation of Stage III or Stage IV disease should be treated with radiation therapy and chemotherapy initially, with surgical resection reserved for persistent local disease in the stomach or for complications.

IV

The Pathogenesis, Prophylaxis, and Treatment of Stress Gastritis

Laurence Y. Cheung, M.D.

Stress gastritis occurs primarily in patients following severe burn, trauma, hemorrhagic shock, respiratory failure, or sepsis. Multiple, superficial erosions occur primarily in the fundus of the stomach. Recent endoscopic studies reported a high incidence of these gastric erosions in patients following severe trauma, major burns, and cardiac surgery. Fortunately, only a small number of these patients (2% to 5%) had significant overt bleeding.

PATHOGENESIS. Although the precise mechanisms involved in the development of stress gastritis are still unknown, current evidence supports a multifactorial etiology. Most of the factors contribute to the development of stress gastritis by reducing the stomach's ability to protect itself against acid injury rather than by increasing the amount of acid secretion.

The Presence of Luminal Acid. Although hypersecretion is

See the corresponding chapter or part in the *Textbook of Surgery*, 15th edition, pp. 878–882, for a more detailed discussion of this topic, including a comprehensive list of references.

an unlikely cause, most experimental studies have shown that some hydrogen ions are necessary for the development of stress gastritis. Almost all experimentally induced stress gastritis, under conditions resembling the clinical situations, requires low gastric luminal pH.

Ischemia. Virtually all investigators agree that one basic pathogenetic feature of stress gastritis is mucosal ischemia. Mucosal ischemia not only is caused by reduction in blood flow secondary to episodes of shock from hemorrhage or sepsis but more importantly is the result of gastric microcirculatory changes. Recent studies have shown that microcirculatory dysfunction is a significant contributing factor to prolonged mucosal ischemia following systemic insults such as hemorrhagic shock or sepsis.

PREVENTION. Since mucosal ischemia may alter a number of mechanisms by which the stomach normally protects itself against injury, vigorous efforts should be made to correct any shocklike state resulting from blood loss and/or sepsis. In addition, efforts should be made to improve ventilatory support, to correct any systemic acid-base abnormality, and to maintain adequate nutrition in these critically ill patients.

The dictum of "no acid, no ulcer" has led to the concept that maintaining neutral pH of the gastric contents may prevent development of stress gastritis in critically ill patients. In fact, titration of gastric pH with antacid has effectively prevented gastrointestinal bleeding in intensive care patients in several controlled, prospective trials. Several studies have reported that H_2-receptor antagonists and sucralfate are also useful in the prophylaxis of stress ulceration.

A recent study has shown that the enteral form of ranitidine given every 12 hours effectively provides moderate to high serum ranitidine concentration. The study also demonstrated a significant reduction (75%) in stimulated gastric acid secretion. Cost comparisons showed a significant reduction when using the enteral compound versus the parenteral route. Therefore, oral administration of ranitidine may be recommended to prevent stress gastritis in ICU patients who may tolerate oral intake of medications.

TREATMENT. The initial management in controlling gastrointestinal hemorrhage should consist of gastric lavage with chilled solutions through a large-bore nasogastric tube. Lavage of the stomach helps fragment clots and prevents gastric distention. Fortunately, most patients appear to stop bleeding following gastric lavage. In occasional patients, specific nonoperative treatment, such as endoscopic therapy or angiographic pharmacotherapy, is required.

Surgical Therapy. Persistent or recurring bleeding not responding to all nonsurgical measures is an indication for operative intervention. The operative procedures used for the control of bleeding stress ulcers have ranged from total gastrectomy to procedures of much lesser magnitude, such as pyloroplasty and vagotomy. It can be said generally that lesser procedures are associated with lower mortality rates but with a higher incidence of rebleeding. There are no prospective clinical trials to substantiate the superiority of one form of therapy over another.

V

Tumors of the Duodenum and Small Intestine

G. Robert Mason, M.D.

Approximately half the tumors of the small bowel are benign, and half are malignant. The benign tumors are relatively evenly distributed through the length of the small bowel, whereas the malignant tumors are much more common in the duodenum. The influence of carcinogenic constituents of the bile versus the immunologic defenses of the intestine deserves further investigation. Of the benign tumors, leiomyomas and adenomas are the most common, whereas among the malignancies, adenocarcinomas and lymphomas are found most frequently.

INCIDENCE. Tumors of the small bowel are estimated to comprise approximately 1% to 6% of gastrointestinal tract tumors. An incidence of 1 in 10,000 hospital admissions and 1 in 2000 general surgical procedures has been estimated. This indicates that a typical practicing general surgeon would see one such patient every decade.

SYMPTOMS. Because the numbers of small bowel tumors found at postmortem examination greatly exceed those coming to medical attention during life, the assumption is that many such tumors are asymptomatic. As tumors enlarge to compromise the passage of intestinal contents, the patient may notice postprandial cramping and epigastric and periumbilical pain. Nausea and vomiting are indications of near or total obstruction of the lumen because the content of the small bowel is generally liquid. Benign tumors present most commonly with obstruction, usually as an intussusception, except for leiomyomas, which not only are the most common small bowel tumors but most frequently present with often vigorous bleeding.

Malignant tumors may be associated with anorexia and weight loss or produce more persistent pain. Bleeding, when present, is more likely to be occult, presenting as an anemia. Periampullary tumors may interfere with normal drainage of bile or pancreatic juice, and the patient may present with painless jaundice. When a palpable gallbladder is also present, suspicion may be higher that a neoplasm is the cause (Courvoisier).

DIAGNOSIS. The presence of obviously hereditary genetic defects such as are observed in Gardner's syndrome and the Peutz-Jeghers syndrome should alert the surgeon to underlying intestinal anomalies. Duodenal lesions are visualized and

---

See the corresponding chapter or part in the *Textbook of Surgery*, 15th edition, pp. 882–887, for a more detailed discussion of this topic, including a comprehensive list of references.

biopsied most easily by fiberoptic endoscopy. Approximately half the currently reported villous adenomas of the duodenum are malignant regardless of size, so the diagnosis of benign tumor on endoscopic biopsy must be considered carefully. Radiologic studies using barium are the standard diagnostic methods for tumors of the mesenteric small intestine. The technique of passing a nasointestinal tube to a point just above a suspected lesion and instilling contrast material at that point (enteroclysis) may add further information beyond the standard small bowel series. Lesions bleeding at a rate of 1 to 2 ml. per minute may be identified more readily by angiography. Nuclear scanning with labeled red blood cells may be useful for slower rates of bleeding. A long mercury-weighted polyethylene tube also may be useful in the preoperative localization; use of rigid or fiberoptic endoscopes through the opened intestine may be diagnostic. The advantages of computed tomography, magnetic resonance imaging, and sonography are probably less than the techniques listed above.

MANAGEMENT. Surgical excision of the tumor mass and its draining lymph nodes in the mesentery is the preferred treatment of lesions of the mesenteric small bowel. The techniques of resection and anastomosis are those introduced some decades ago and are not different in these circumstances. Malignancies of the duodenum are treated in the same way as cancers of the pancreas and distal bile ducts with pancreatoduodenectomy (see Chap. 35). Resection of benign tumors of the duodenum may require some ingenuity on the part of the surgeon to avoid constriction of the pancreatic or bile ducts or duodenum or devascularization of the duodenum. The use of onlay serosal patches, Roux-en-Y loops, and ductal reimplantation is covered elsewhere. Villous adenomas of the duodenum have been managed successfully by local resection in some patients, and the surgeon may choose this alternative in selected patients, bearing in mind the incidence of malignancy in these lesions. Management of symptoms of APUD tumors such as carcinoids, gastrinomas, glucagonomas, and others may relate specifically to the end organ affected, such as the use of H_2 blockers for the Zollinger-Ellison syndrome or methysergide and antihistamines for carcinoid tumors. The use of somatostatin may supplant these agents. Lymphomas that are resectable are best treated in this manner; however, the addition of radiation therapy appears to augment the 5-year survival of these patients. Chemotherapy for advanced metastatic cancers of the gastrointestinal tract is an evolving field that indicates the benefits of multiple-drug therapy.

OUTCOME. Patients with carcinomas of the duodenum, when treated by pancreatoduodenectomy, are reported to have 5-year survival rates in the range of 25%. Patients with adenocarcinoma of the mesenteric small intestine are reported to have 5-year survival rates of 14% to 37%. Patients with lymphomas treated by excision and adjunctive radiotherapy have 5-year survivals as high as 85%, and those with carcinoid tumors without apparent metastases at the time of resection may have 5-year survivals of greater than 70%; those with metastases may expect rates of 35%. Because the growth of the tumor is very slow, it may be more appropriate to view the 10-year survival rates, which are reported as 60% and 15%, without and with known metastases at the time of original resections.

VI

Vascular Compression of the Duodenum

Bruce D. Schirmer, M.D.

The syndrome of vascular compression of the duodenum is also known as *superior mesenteric artery syndrome, cast syndrome,* and *arteriomesenteric occlusion of the duodenum.* It was first described by Rokitansky in 1842 and first treated successfully with duodenojejunostomy by Stavely in 1908.

The anatomic basis of the syndrome is obstruction of the duodenum at the point where the distal third portion of the duodenum crosses from right to left and also superior and anterior to the lumbar spine. At this site, a narrow angle of the take-off of the superior mesenteric artery and a shorter distance between the artery and the duodenum predispose patients to duodenal compression by the superior mesenteric artery. Conditions that make this angle narrower, such as weight loss, excessive lumbar lordosis, the supine position, and high fixation of the duodenum to the ligament of Treitz, each predispose to the syndrome. The condition is uncommon, occurring in less than 0.1% of patients in the hospital.

The syndrome is characterized clinically by nausea and vomiting, abdominal distention, postprandial epigastric pain, and weight loss. Symptoms may be acute or chronic and are classically relieved when patients assume the knee-chest, left lateral, or occasionally the prone position, all of which allow gravitational decompression of the duodenum. Clinical conditions associated with the acute syndrome include thin body habitus with weight loss, body casts, severe burns, bedridden victims of trauma, and anorexia nervosa. Peptic ulcer disease is prevalent in patients with more chronic symptoms. The syndrome is described in pediatric as well as adult populations.

Conditions included in the differential diagnosis are peptic ulcer, pancreatitis, biliary disease, tumors obstructing the duodenum, surgical adhesions, collagen vascular diseases, and pseudo-obstruction syndromes.

The diagnosis is usually confirmed by radiographic studies.

See the corresponding chapter or part in the *Textbook of Surgery,* 15th edition, pp. 887–892, for a more detailed discussion of this topic, including a comprehensive list of references.

An abrupt termination of barium or contrast material is seen at the third portion of the duodenum, usually associated with a "to and fro" motion of obstructed peristalsis. Angiographic studies show compression of the duodenum by the superior mesenteric artery. Relief of the obstruction with the knee-chest position further confirms the diagnosis.

Treatment of vascular compression of the duodenum should be conservative initially, to relieve the obstruction using appropriate body positioning and nasogastric suctioning to prevent aspiration. Simultaneous attention to nutritional needs should include attempts to pass a nasojejunal feeding tube as the preferred route of nutritional support, with the use of parenteral hyperalimentation if this fails. Operative treatment has been very successful when needed in the past. Two basic strategies have been employed, both successfully. In children, the most commonly performed procedure involves division of the ligament of Treitz and mobilization of the duodenum. In adults, the most commonly performed and successful (94%) procedure has been duodenojejunostomy to bypass the obstruction.

VII

Adenocarcinoma of the Stomach
Gene D. Branum, M.D. and Aaron S. Fink, M.D.

Gastric cancer has received intense scrutiny by surgeons, pathologists, radiologists, and oncologists over the past 100 years. Despite diagnostic advances and their broad application, gastric cancer in the West continues to be a disease that presents late in its course.

EPIDEMIOLOGY. The percentage of cancer deaths from gastric cancer has declined dramatically for unclear reasons. In 1994, 24,000 new cases of gastric cancer were diagnosed, with an estimated 14,000 deaths. The death rate in the United States is approximately 7.5 per 100,000, while Costa Rica had an incidence of 77.5 cases per 100,000; Russia, Japan, and Chile all had rates near 50 per 100,000.

ENVIRONMENTAL FACTORS. In the United States, the incidence of gastric cancer is highest in lower socioeconomic groups. Migrants from Japan to the United States maintain a moderate disease risk, while second-generation Japanese in the United States have a much lower risk. The decline in gastric cancer has paralleled significant improvements in food, hygiene, and santitaion, as well as general dietary improve-

See the corresponding chapter or part in the *Textbook of Surgery*, 15th edition, pp. 893–907, for a more detailed discussion of this topic, including a comprehensive list of references.

ments, including year-round availability of fresh fruits and vegetables. Gastric cancer appears to be correlated with a high intake of preserved food (i.e., foods containing high levels of salt, nitrates, and nitrites), pickled vegetables, and salt—all of which can act as gastric irritants. Nitrates and nitrites clearly can be converted to active carcinogens, the N-nitrosamines.

Striking parallels exist between regional rates of gastric cancer and *Helicobacter pylori* infection. In Central American regions, where virtually all adults are infected, gastric cancer rates are among the highest in the world. *H. pylori* infection rates based on examination of banked sera indicate that the infection rate is decreasing over time in the United States in parallel with the decrease in gastric cancer. Three important case-control studies in Great Britain, California, and Hawaii indicate increased risk of gastric cancer in individuals with positive *H. pylori* antibody titers of from 2.9- to 6-fold. *H. pylori* produces several toxins, such as ammonia and acetaldehyde, that could lead to chronic inflammation and epithelial damage. The link between *H. pylori* and gastric cancer is strengthened by the fact that *H. pylori* infection causes more than 80% of cases of chronic gastritis.

Adenomatous gastric polyps are rare but carry a distinct potential for the development of malignancy. The risk of developing cancer in adenomatous polyps is thought to be between 10% and 20% and is greatest for polyps 2 cm. or greater in diameter. The presence of an adenomatous polyp is a marker for increased risk of carcinogenesis in the remaining gastric mucosa.

Gastric surgery for benign conditions increases the risk of gastric cancer by 2- to 6-fold after 15 to 20 years. Since the increased incidence of malignancy occurs even though the most common site of gastric cancer (antrum) has been resected, the risk may actually be greater. The lesions tend to present at a more advanced stage and in older patients; routine radiologic or endoscopic examinations begun after 10 years may improve detection.

Pernicious anemia and Ménétrier's disease may lead to gastric cancer in up to 10% of affected patients.

PATHOLOGY

Gastric cancer arises most commonly on the lesser curve in the antral and pyloric regions, although the incidence of proximal cancer is increasing. Approximately 10% to 15% of tumors are diffuse in character (linitis plastica).

Lauren divided gastric cancers into intestinal and diffuse subtypes. The *intestinal-type* tumors have a glandular structure resembling colonic carcinoma, with diffuse inflammatory cell infiltration and frequent intestinal metaplasia. *Diffuse-type* tumors are composed of tiny clusters of small uniform cells. In contrast to intestinal-type neoplasms, diffuse carcinomas are more widespread through the mucosa, have less inflammatory infiltration, and have a poorer prognosis.

Broeder's histologic grading system correlates well with survival in gastric cancer. The system classifies tumors as

Grade I to IV, with Grade IV tumors representing the most anaplastic. Grade I patients have a 66% 5-year survival rate, while Grade IV patients have 11% 5-year survival rates.

Borrman's gross classification describes four types with varying degrees of malignancy. Listed in ascending order of degree of malignancy, these are Group I, circumscribed, solitary, polypoid carcinomas without ulceration; Group II, ulcerated carcinomas with wall-like marginal elevation and sharply defined borders; Group III, partially ulcerated carcinomas with marginal elevation and partial diffuse spread; and Group IV, diffuse carcinomas.

Gastric cancers spread within the gastric wall and into the regional lymphatics, as well as by direct invasion of adjacent organs such as liver, pancreas, transverse colon, or mesocolon. Hematogenous spread via the portal vein to the liver or via the systemic circulation to the lungs, bones, and elsewhere produces distant metastases. Finally, involved gastric serosa commonly sheds metastases throughout the peritoneum. The parietal peritoneum, ovary (Krukenberg's tumor), the pelvic cul-de-sac (Bloomer's shelf), and umbilical lymph node (Sister Mary Joseph's node) or supraclavicular lymph node (Virchow's node) may be involved.

The molecular and chromosomal alterations leading to the development of gastric adenocarcinoma of the stomach are under intense study. Alterations in *p53* heterozygosity have been noted in up to two thirds of gastric tumors. Changes may be linked to the *MCC* (mutated in colon cancer) and *APC* (adenomatous polyposis coli) genes. Transforming growth factor alpha and the receptor of epidermal growth factor are overexpressed in both esophageal and gastric cancer. The *C-erbB-2* oncogene also has been demonstrated in gastric adenocarcinoma; malignant transformation may involve the loss of negative feedback control of the oncogene. *K-sam* oncogene amplification has been seen in higher percentages of undifferentiated than well-differentiated carcinomas. The complexities of the interaction between fibroblast growth factor and epidermal growth factor and their interactions with environmental or inflammatory (*H. pylori*) factors remain to be elucidated.

STAGING. The current basis for gastric cancer staging in the United States is the American Joint Committee on Cancer staging classification, as published in the manual for staging of cancer.

TNM CLASSIFICATION. Gastric cancer is staged according to the characteristics of the primary tumor (T), nodal metastases (N), and presence of metastatic disease (M). The most important prognostic indicators remain the depth of penetration by the primary tumor, the presence of cancer in local regional lymph nodes, or involvement of adjacent organs. Clinical classification (cTNM) of gastric cancers is based on diagnostic and pathologic data obtained prior to any surgical resection.

Tumors are also grouped according to histopathologic type. Adenocarcinoma is the most common histopathologic type of gastric carcinoma. It may be further subdivided into intestinal, diffuse, and mixed histology based on the Lauren classification. Other histopathologic types include papillary, tubular or mucinous adenocarcinoma, signet ring cell carcinoma, squamous cell carcinoma, small cell carcinoma, and undifferentiated carcinoma (World Health Organization).

Early gastric cancer is defined as disease involving the mucosa or submucosa and, as such, may be fairly large and associated with vague abdominal symptoms and positive lymph nodes at the time of resection. Early gastric cancer represents only 10% to 15% of diagnosed cases in Europe and North America. Five-year survival after resection of early gastric cancer is quite frequent, ranging from 70% to 95% depending on the presence of nodal involvement. *Advanced* gastric cancer suggests invasion of the muscularis or beyond. These lesions are frequently associated with distant or contiguous spread, have a higher stage, and are less often cured. Advanced gastric cancer represents less than 50% of cases in Japan today, while over 80% of U.S. cases were advanced gastric carcinomas at the time of diagnosis.

SYMPTOMS/DIAGNOSIS

Symptoms of early gastric cancer are vague and unspecific. They may mimic symptoms of benign gastric ulcer disease and may either be ignored by the patient or treated medically without further evaluation. Symptoms may not be evident until a tumor is of sufficient size to interfere significantly with gastric motor activity, decrease the size of the intraluminal passageway, or cause gross or occult bleeding from an ulcerated tumor mass. Weight loss is clearly a common symptom ranging from 20% to 60%. Abdominal pain is even more variable, ranging from 20% to 95%. Nausea and anorexia were present in approximately 30%, dysphasia in 25%, and early satiety and ulcer-type pain in approximately 20%. Continuous abdominal pain generally suggests tumor extension beyond the stomach wall. Substernal or precordial pain may be associated with tumors of the cardia or gastroesophageal (GE) junction. Approximately 10% of patients will present with signs or symptoms of disseminated disease, including supraclavicular or pelvic adenopathy, ascites, jaundice, or hepatomegaly. Routine laboratory tests should include hematocrit, erythrocyte evaluation, liver function tests, and stool guaiac. In most cases of advanced disease, laboratory evidence of anemia develops; liver function tests are usually abnormal with hepatic metastasis.

The double-contrast barium meal is a sensitive and cost-effective test for the detection of even small gastric cancers. Advanced gastric cancer usually presents as a polypoid mass protruding into the gastric lumen, an ulcer crater, or a nondistensible stomach due to diffusely infiltrating carcinoma. A polypoid mass leaves little doubt as to the presence of carcinoma. Demonstration of an ulcer crater, however, may present a difficult diagnostic problem. As seen radiographically, the crater of a malignant ulcer crater lies in a mass and does not extend outside the boundary of the gastric wall. The mucosal folds do not radiate toward the center of the crater, maintaining their contour to and beyond the ulcer. Malignant ulcers are usually larger than 1 cm. and are surrounded by rigid gastric wall on fluoroscopy.

On computed tomographic (CT) scan, gastric cancer appears most often as gastric wall thickening. The CT appearance correlates with the histopathologic findings, with the tumor appearing localized, circumferential, or diffuse. When wall thickness is 2 cm. or greater, transmural extension is assured. Scans also may suggest gastric ulceration, and the lesions may be characterized as polypoid or sessile.

Staging by CT is clearly less accurate than exploration and may overstage (15% to 20%) or understage (25% to 30%) patients. Patients with CT findings of obvious metastatic disease, including liver and widespread intraperitoneal metastases, can be spared exploratory surgery, except for palliation. Patients with limited or questionable CT findings, however, should undergo exploration for accurate staging and resection.

Flexible fiberoptic endoscopy is the most accurate method of diagnosing gastric cancer presently available. Endoscopy is used in over 90% of cases with a diagnostic accuracy of around 90%. If biopsies were obtained, accuracy increased to 94%, while cytologic accuracy was 75%. Ulcerated lesions should be biopsied at least twice in each quarter at the leading or rolled edge of the ulcer and not the base, where necrotic tissue is common.

Endoscopic ultrasonography (EUS) has proven to be very accurate in the evaluation of primary lesions, although it is not as sensitive in the detection of lymph node involvement.

TREATMENT

Surgical resection remains the only potentially curative therapy in gastric cancer. Patients must be evaluated for co-morbid conditions such as cardiovascular, pulmonary, or renal disorders. Patients with profound weight loss and metabolic complications of their cancer may be at high surgical risk. Patients without obstruction or bleeding but demonstrated preoperatively to have Virchow's node, inguinal lymph nodes, obvious liver metastases, Sister Mary Joseph's node, or Bloomer's shelf should not be explored. Patients who are obstructed or bleeding should still be considered for exploration, since palliative resection may significantly improve the quality of life remaining for such patients. In patients with metastatic obstructing proximal gastric tumors, satisfactory palliation is achieved less frequently.

The location of primary tumors may be defined as the distal, middle, or proximal one third. Surgical resection of the stomach and accompanying lymph nodes may be described using the terms R0 through R4. R0 resection must be defined as palliative and implies incomplete removal of perigastric lymph nodes. R1 resection includes complete removal of perigastric nodes. R2 resection includes resection of the stomach, perigastric nodes, and lymph nodes along the named arteries of the stomach. R3 resection is R2 plus removal of the nodes of the celiac axis, while R4 resection includes R3 plus para-aortic nodes.

An adequate proximal and distal surgical margin should be 4 to 6 cm. from the edge of the primary tumor. This should be confirmed with frozen-section analysis at the time of surgery. This necessitates different resections in distal, middle, and proximal lesions. Moreover, in diffuse tumors with extensive submucosal involvement, total gastrectomy may be the only option available to achieve adequate margins and even then may be inadequate.

R1 resection of early gastric carcinoma is usually curative, and a resection of the lesion with an adequate margin as described earlier as well as perigastric lymph nodes within 3 cm. of the lesion is sufficient. Provocative reports have described endoscopic treatment of early gastric cancer using cauterization, local injection of drugs, and laser therapy. Currently, these techniques should be reserved for patients at high risk for conventional surgery due to age or concomitant medical problems.

A typical gastric resection for cancer in the United States includes subtotal gastrectomy for antral or pyloric lesions, subtotal or total gastrectomy for middle-third lesions (depending on the size and proximal extent of the tumor), and total gastrectomy with esophagojejunostomy for proximal-third, GE junction lesions. In addition, the perigastric lymph nodes along lesser and greater curvatures and the lymph nodes along the left gastric artery are typically removed. The lesser and greater omenta are resected. Only 5% of patients having gastrectomy with clear margins had an R2 dissection as previously defined.

The standard surgical operation in Japan for advanced gastric cancer is the R2 resection with removal of N1 and N2 lymph node groups. The survival rates over the past 30 years have risen from 71% to 76% in Stage II, 39% to 63% in Stage IIIA, 28% to 39% in Stage IIIB, and 2% to 10% in Stage IV disease. Analyses of survival in the Japanese literature are largely retrospective.

The surgical treatment for gastric cancer is still controversial. For the purposes of staging and for the best chance at cure, extended resection (R2) should be performed when there is gastric serosal involvement or when locoregional lymph nodes are involved. Total gastrectomy should be performed only for diffuse tumors or large tumors of the middle or proximal thirds.

A meta-analysis of prospective, randomized trials in Europe and North America failed to show that the use of adjuvant chemotherapy in advanced gastric cancer is beneficial. However, the use of mitomycin C and 5-FU or its derivative, futrafur, in Japanese trials is supported by several nonrandomized and two randomized trials.

The optimal postoperative adjuvant therapy for gastric cancer has not been developed. Needed are less toxic chemotherapeutic regimens, further evaluation of preoperative radiation and chemotherapy, and development of regimens effective against peritoneal as well as visceral metastases. The use of intraoperative radiation is undergoing evaluation, and its place in therapy has yet to be defined.

SUMMARY

Gastric cancer remains a devastating disease. With the exception of early gastric cancer, which is usually (>90%) cured with surgery alone, survival at 5 years remains 20% to 30% *at best*, especially in Western series, where early lesions make up only 8% to 10% of the total. Recent data from the United States indicate that less than 80% of patients are explored and less than 80% of those have a resection performed. The 5-year survival in patients with resection of all gross disease and clear margins ranged from 20% to 38%, indicating microscopic spread in a majority of apparently good candidates.

While a preponderance of data indicate that extended resection (R2) can be performed safely, is useful in certain stages, and is the procedure of choice for a curative procedure when there is serosal or locoregional lymph node involvement, it is doubtful that more radical operations (R3, combined resection) add any survival benefit. Current radiochemotherapy regimens are of marginal benefit, and more effective agents or combinations are needed.

The effectiveness of mass screening in high-risk populations has been demonstrated by the impressive Japanese results. Clearly, if an impact is to be made in the treatment of gastric cancer in the West, early detection and prevention are areas in which advances are needed. Investigations into the pathogenesis and molecular genetics of the disease are ongoing and will hopefully yield clinically applicable strategies in the near future.

31

THE SMALL INTESTINE

I

Anatomy
R. Scott Jones, M.D.

The small intestine extends from the pylorus to the cecum and provides the environment for digestion and absorption. The essential anatomic characteristic of the small intestine remains its large surface area produced by intestinal length, mucosal folds, villi, and microvilli.

GROSS ANATOMY

The 21-cm. duodenum combined with the jejunum measures 261 cm. and constitutes about three fifths of the entire alimentary canal. The proximal two fifths of small intestine are arbitrarily called the *jejunum*, and the distal three fifths are arbitrarily called the *ileum*.

The mesentery suspends the small intestine from the posterior abdominal wall and contains blood vessels, nerves, lymphatics, and lymph nodes as well as stored fat. The broad-based attachment of the mesenteric root stabilizes the small bowel to prevent it from twisting on its blood supply.

The superior mesenteric artery supplies blood to the small intestine. This artery arises from the abdominal aorta and courses dorsal to the neck of the pancreas and anterior to the uncinate process to enter the small bowel mesentery. The intestinal arteries branch within the mesentery and unite with adjacent arteries to form a series of arterial arcades before sending small straight arteries to the small intestine. The veins of the small intestine drain into the superior mesenteric vein, a major tributary to the portal vein.

The submucosa of the small intestine, especially in the ileum, contains aggregated lymphatic nodules called *Peyer's patches*. The lymphatic drainage from the small intestine passes first into lymph nodes close to the wall of the small intestine, then into a second set of nodes adjacent to the mesenteric arcades, and then into a third set of nodes along the superior mesenteric artery. Lymph drains into the intestinal trunk and then into the cisterna chyli.

The mucosal surface of the small intestine contains numerous circular folds called the *plicae circulares* (*valvulae conniventes* or *valves of Kerckring*). The intestinal villi, barely visible to the naked eye, are tiny, fingerlike processes projecting into the intestinal lumen.

See the corresponding chapter or part in the *Textbook of Surgery,* 15th edition, pp. 909–911, for a more detailed discussion of this topic, including a comprehensive list of references.

The small intestine receives its parasympathetic innervation from preganglionic fibers passing through the vagus nerves to synapse with neurons of the intrinsic plexuses of the intestine. Its sympathetic innervation comes from preganglionic fibers arising from the ninth and tenth thoracic segments of the spinal cord, passing to synapse in the superior mesenteric ganglion. Postganglionic fibers then pass along branches of the superior mesenteric artery. Thoracic visceral efferents mediate pain from the intestine.

MICROSCOPIC ANATOMY

The epithelium, the lamina propria, and the muscularis mucosa make up the mucosae of the small intestine. Two important structural features characterize the mucosal surface: the villi and the crypts of Lieberkühn. The villi of the jejunum, ½ to 1 mm. in length, occur in a density of 10 to 40 per sq. mm. of mucosa. Each villus contains a central lymphatic vessel called a *lacteal*, a small artery, a vein, and a capillary network. The crypts of Lieberkühn are adjacent to the bases of the villi and extend down to but not through the muscularis mucosa.

The cells responsible for absorption, the columnar epithelial cells, are characterized by a luminal brush border and a basal nucleus. The microvilli give the appearance to the brush border and are 1 μm. tall and 0.1 μm. wide. Each microvillus contains a glycocalix containing high concentrations of digestive enzymes, particularly disaccharidases. The lateral plasma membrane contains tight junctions, intermediate junctions, and desmosomes. Goblet cells are present in both the villi and the crypts, and they contain a cytoplasm filled with mucous granules.

Enterochromaffin cells reside in the crypts of the small intestine but also occur in other parts of the gastrointestinal system. These cells usually do not contact the intestinal lumen, and their secretory granules reside below the nuclei away from the lumen. This structure suggests an endocrine function. Paneth cells occur in the base of the crypts, and their function is unknown. Undifferentiated cells occur only in the crypts, particularly at their bases. These cells exhibit mitosis, multiply, and differentiate to replace lost absorptive cells. Undifferentiated cells may differentiate into an absorptive cell and migrate to the villus, remain in the crypt and continue mitotic activity, or remain in the crypt in a resting stage. The cells entering the villi migrate to the villus tips, which shed them into the lumen. This replaces the population of the intestinal epithelial cells every 3 to 7 days.

MUSCULAR LAYER AND INTRAMURAL NEURAL STRUCTURES

Two distinct layers of smooth muscle, the outer longitudinal coat and an inner circular coat, form the muscular portion of the small intestine. Intestinal smooth muscle fibers are discrete spindle-shaped structures about 250 μm. long. Nexuses approximate the plasma membranes of adjacent muscle cells to allow electrical continuity between smooth muscle cells and permit conduction through the muscle layer. There are four identifiable neural plexuses in the small intestine: the subserous plexus, the myenteric plexus between the longitudinal and circular muscle layers, the submucosal plexus, and the mucous plexus.

II

Physiology
R. Scott Jones, M.D.

DIGESTION AND ABSORPTION

CARBOHYDRATE. Dietary starch contains two glucose polymers, amylopectin and amylose. Amylase hydrolyzes amylose to maltose and maltotriose. Amylase splits amylopectin to maltose, maltotriose, and the residual branched saccharides, the dextrins. Brush border enzymes break down maltose, maltotriose, dextrins, and dietary disaccharides lactose and sucrose to constituent monosaccharides. Glucose and galactose then are actively transported into the intestinal cells against a concentration gradient. This active transport of sugars requires metabolic energy, oxygen, and small concentrations of sodium ion. Fructose enters the intestinal cell by facilitated diffusion.

PROTEIN. The stomach initiates digestion of protein by acidic environment, which denatures protein, and the presence of pepsin, which hydrolyzes protein to polypeptides. Digestion of protein is incomplete when gastric chyme enters the duodenum, where the higher pH inactivates pepsin. The pancreas secretes proteolytic enzyme precursors into the duodenum, where the intestinal enzyme enterokinase converts trypsinogen to trypsin. Trypsin also activates trypsinogen and other pancreatic proteolytic enzyme precursors. The pancreatic endopeptidases trypsin, chymotrypsin, and elastase split peptide bonds in the central portion of protein molecules, whereas exopeptidases such as carboxypeptidase remove amino acids from the C-terminal position of protein molecules. Amino peptidases split amino acids from the end-terminal position of protein molecules. Amino acids, the final product of protein digestion, then undergo absorption. Some dipeptides are absorbed. Absorptive cell carrier-mediated active transport requiring oxygen and sodium removes luminal amino acids against a concentration gradient.

See the corresponding chapter or part in the *Textbook of Surgery*, 15th edition, pp. 912–915, for a more detailed discussion of this topic, including a comprehensive list of references.

FAT. In the duodenum, the dietary triglycerides mix with biliary and pancreatic secretions that contain bile salts, pancreatic lipase, and bicarbonate ion. Bile salts produce polymolecular aggregates called *micelles*. Micelles permit solubilization of lipid in an aqueous environment to produce micellar solutions. Pancreatic lipase aided by colipase catalyzes the hydrolysis of dietary triglyceride into 2-monoglyceride and fatty acids. The bile salt, monoglyceride, and fatty acid micelles also solubilize other lipids such as cholesterol, phospholipid, and fat-soluble vitamins. An alkaline pH favors ionization of fatty acids and bile salts, which increases their solubility in micelles. When the micelles encounter the microvilli of the intestinal epithelial cells, the fatty acids and 2-monoglycerides pass into the epithelial cells by a process not requiring energy, probably diffusion. In the epithelial cells, the endoplasmic reticulum synthesizes 2-monoglycerides and fatty acids into triglyceride. Synthesized triglyceride, phospholipid, cholesterol, cholesterol esters, and lipoprotein then form chylomicrons. Chylomicrons pass from the epithelial cells into the lacteals, into the lymphatics, and then into the venous system. Medium-chain triglycerides can be absorbed without hydrolysis and pass into the portal blood rather than into the lymph. Most bile acids that form micelles are absorbed in the ileum by an active transport process.

WATER AND ELECTROLYTES. Approximately 5 to 10 liters of water enter the small bowel daily, whereas only about 500 ml. or less leave the ileum and enter the colon. Simultaneously, large quantities of water move from intestinal lumen to blood as well as from blood to intestinal lumen. Absorption of water results from osmotic gradients established by the active transport of solutes such as sodium ion, glucose, and amino acids to the cells. In the jejunum, active transport accounts for a portion of sodium absorption, whereas most jejunal sodium absorption occurs along osmotic gradients. The human ileum absorbs sodium against steep electrochemical gradients. This observation suggests a very efficient sodium transport in the ileum. The ileum also absorbs chloride against steep electrochemical gradients. Potassium is passively absorbed in the intestine according to its electrochemical gradient. The proximal small intestine absorbs calcium by active transport. Vitamin D and parathyroid hormone enhance absorption of calcium. The small intestine regulates the body pool of iron. Normal iron stores permit only a slight transfer of iron from intestinal absorptive cells to plasma. In iron deficiency, the absorptive cells effectively transfer iron into the plasma.

MOTILITY

There are several types of visible small intestine muscular activity. *Segmenting contractions* occurring regularly and rhythmically in adjacent portions of the small intestine divide and subdivide the intestinal content, mixing it and exposing it to larger areas of mucosa, which facilitates digestion and absorption. *Pendular movements* are probably the same as or a minor modification of rhythmic segmentation. *Peristalsis* consists of intestinal contraction passing aborally at a rate of 1 to 2 cm. per second throughout several centimeters of intestine. The major function of peristalsis is distal movement of intestinal chyme. During the interdigestive period, cyclically occurring contractions called the *migrating myoelectrical complex* (MMC) move aborally along the intestine to sweep or cleanse the intestine during the interdigestive period.

Two types of electrical activity occur in the small intestine. Slow-wave electrical activity called the *basal electrical rhythm* (BER) begins in the longitudinal muscle layer of the duodenum and propagates distally. The BER can occur unrelated to motor activity. Intestinal spike potentials produce motor activity. The BER coordinates spike potentials.

The intrinsic nerve supply regulates rather than initiates motor action. Sympathetic activity inhibits motor function, whereas parasympathetic activity stimulates it.

Gastrin stimulates gastric and intestinal motility and relaxes the ileocecal sphincter. Cholecystokinin stimulates intestinal motility and decreases intestinal transit time. Secretin and glucagon inhibit intestinal motility.

ENDROCRINE FUNCTION OF THE SMALL INTESTINE

The duodenum and jejunum secrete secretin, cholecystokinin, vasoactive intestinal peptide (VIP), gastric inhibitory polypeptide, motilin, and somatostatin.

IMMUNOLOGIC FUNCTION OF THE INTESTINE

The intestine produces immunoglobulin A (IgA). This immunoglobulin arises from plasma cells and, after linkage with a protein synthesized by epithelial cells, is secreted in the lumen.

III

Intestinal Obstruction
R. Scott Jones, M.D.

ETIOLOGY

Any impediment to the aboral progression of gastrointestinal luminal contents defines intestinal obstruction. Mechanical

---

See the corresponding chapter or part in the *Textbook of Surgery*, 15th edition, pp. 915–923, for a more detailed discussion of this topic, including a comprehensive list of references.

occlusion of the bowel lumen or paralysis of the intestinal muscle can produce intestinal obstruction.

MECHANICAL OBSTRUCTION

Three types of abnormalities produce mechanical obstruction: obturation of the intestinal lumen; intrinsic bowel lesions such as atresia, stenosis, or stricture; and lesions extrinsic to the bowel such as hernia or volvulus.

PARALYTIC ILEUS

Paralytic ileus, a common disorder, occurs to some extent in most patients undergoing abdominal surgery. Neural reflexes, peritonitis, and electrolyte imbalance, particularly hypokalemia, produce ileus. Ischemia of the intestine rapidly inhibits motility.

IDIOPATHIC INTESTINAL PSEUDO-OBSTRUCTION

Idiopathic intestinal pseudo-obstruction is a chronic illness characterized by symptoms of recurrent intestinal obstruction without demonstrable mechanical occlusion of the bowel. Patients with this disease have impaired motor responses to intestinal distention. Some patients have peristalsis of the esophagus with failure of the lower esophageal sphincter to relax. Heredity may influence a patient's susceptibility. Controversy exists as to whether neural abnormalities, muscle abnormalities, or both produce the disease. The symptoms include cramping abdominal pain, vomiting, distention, diarrhea, and sometimes steatorrhea. Physical examination reveals abdominal distention. Intestinal pseudo-obstruction is difficult to distinguish from mechanical intestinal obstruction.

PATHOGENESIS OF INTESTINAL OBSTRUCTION

Simple mechanical obstruction of the small intestine causes accumulation of fluid and gas proximal to the obstruction, producing distention of the intestine. One of the most important events during simple mechanical small bowel obstruction is the loss of water and electrolytes from the body. Vomiting and accumulation of water in the intestine contribute to water loss. Progressive dehydration may produce oliguria, azotemia, and hemoconcentration. If dehydration persists, circulatory changes such as tachycardia, low central venous pressure, and reduced cardiac output may cause hypotension and hypovolemic shock. Also, during intestinal obstruction, bacteria proliferate rapidly in the intestinal lumen. Small intestinal contents thus become feculent during long-standing obstruction because of the large quantities of bacteria.

STRANGULATION OBSTRUCTION

Impaired circulation of the obstructed intestine causes strangulation obstruction. Occlusion at two points along its length produces closed-loop obstruction. This type of obstruction may proceed more rapidly to strangulation than simple obstruction. Strangulation can cause loss of blood and plasma from the strangulated segment, which may be particularly severe if venous occlusion predominates. If the strangulation produces gangrene, peritonitis with its sequelae occurs. Also important in strangulation obstruction is the toxic material from the strangulated loop. Luminal fluid from a strangulated intestinal loop and the bloody, malodorous peritoneal fluid are lethal when administered to normal animals.

COLON OBSTRUCTION

Generally, obstruction of the colon produces less fluid and electrolyte disturbance than mechanical small bowel obstruction. If the patient has a competent ileocecal valve, there may be little or no small bowel distention, and the colon behaves as a closed loop. In patients with an incompetent ileocecal bowel, the signs of small bowel distention may accompany obstruction of the colon.

DIAGNOSIS OF INTESTINAL OBSTRUCTION

Abdominal pain, vomiting, obstipation, abdominal distention, and failure to pass flatus characterize intestinal obstruction. Intestinal obstruction typically produces crampy abdominal pain. After a longer period of mechanical obstruction, the crampy pain may subside because motility may be inhibited by bowel distention. Proximal intestinal obstruction may cause profuse vomiting and no abdominal distention.

PHYSICAL EXAMINATION. Tachycardia and hypotension may indicate severe dehydration or peritonitis. The abdomen is usually distended. Surgical scars should be noted because of the etiologic implication of previous surgery. Incarcerated hernias may be obscure, particularly in the obese patient. Abdominal masses should be sought. Abdominal tenderness is a characteristic finding in patients with intestinal obstruction, although localized tenderness, rebound tenderness, and guarding suggest peritonitis and the likelihood of strangulation. The bowel sounds in intestinal obstruction are usually high-pitched. Rectal examination should be done.

RADIOLOGIC EXAMINATION. Films in patients with mechanical obstruction of the small bowel usually show multiple gas-fluid levels with distended bowel. Occasionally, ordinary x-ray films fail to distinguish a colonic from a small intestinal obstruction. A barium enema identifies an obstructed colon.

LABORATORY TESTS. Any patient suspected of having intestinal obstruction should have laboratory measurements of serum sodium, chloride, potassium, bicarbonate, and creatinine. The hematocrit, white blood cell count, and serum electrolytes also should be measured.

TREATMENT OF INTESTINAL OBSTRUCTION

In many cases, the appropriate treatment for intestinal obstruction includes surgical relief of the obstruction. The mortality from intestinal obstruction with intestinal gangrene exceeds the mortality in simple mechanical obstruction. Patients with severe fluid and electrolyte imbalance and concomitant illnesses profit from supportive treatment. Intravenous therapy should begin with an infusion of isotonic sodium chloride solution. Potassium chloride infusion should begin after adequate urine is formed. After pulse, blood pressure, central venous pressure, and urinary output are normal, surgery may be considered. Antibiotics should be given during resuscitation, particularly if strangulation is suspected. Nasogastric suction empties the stomach, reducing the hazard of pulmonary aspiration of vomitus and minimizing further intestinal distention from swallowed air preoperatively. In some cases, a long intestinal tube can be passed into the intestine to deflate the bowel. There is controversy concerning the urgency for early operation on patients thought to have partial obstruction of the small bowel due to adhesions. Most patients with partial adhesive obstruction of the small bowel resolve with nasogastric suction, usually within 24 hours. Operations may be delayed under the following circumstances: (1) in patients with pyloric obstruction; (2) in patients with postoperative intestinal obstruction; (3) in infants with ileocecal intussusception (adults with intussusception should undergo operation because of the high frequency of underlying causes for the intussusception); (4) in patients with sigmoid volvulus decompressed with a sigmoidoscope or a colonoscope; (5) in patients with intestinal obstruction due to an exacerbation of Crohn's disease; and (6) in patients with chronic partial obstruction.

OPERATIVE TREATMENT FOR INTESTINAL OBSTRUCTION

Four approaches are available to provide operative relief for intestinal obstruction: (1) In simple obstruction, the obstructed segment of bowel can be freed surgically. (2) A second approach to obstructing lesions is an intestinal bypass. (3) The placement of a cutaneous fistula such as a colostomy proximal to the obstruction is a standard form of therapy. (4) Excision of a lesion with restoration of intestinal continuity by anastomosis also may be used frequently. With few exceptions, operations for intestinal obstruction should be performed under general anesthesia administered through an endotracheal tube to minimize the risk of vomiting and tracheal-bronchial aspiration of the vomitus. The criteria generally used to assess viability of the obstructed bowel are color, motility, and arterial pulsation. The approach to obstruction of the colon differs from that to obstruction of the small bowel. The method of treating obstruction of the left colon entails two or three separate operative steps, including relief of gaseous distention by colostomy proximal to the obstruction; removal of the diseased segment of colon and anastomosis, leaving the colostomy intact; and closure of the colostomy when the anastomosis is completely healed. In many cases, for example, in obstructing left colon cancer, it may be possible to resect the cancer, perform a colostomy, and then reunite the ends of the colon later, after the patient has recovered from the ill effects of intestinal obstruction. Recent reports describe treating left colon obstruction by resection and primary anastomosis with good outcome. In treating cecal or right colon obstruction due to cancer, a right colectomy and ileotransverse colostomy usually should be performed.

TREATMENT OF PARALYTIC ILEUS

Paralytic ileus is treated by nasogastric suction and intravenous fluid administration. Correction of electrolyte imbalance, particularly hypokalemia, is especially important in managing this disorder.

IV

Crohn's Disease (Regional Enteritis)
Keith A. Kelly, M.D., and Bruce G. Wolff, M.D.

Crohn's disease is a chronic, nonspecific inflammatory disease of the gastrointestinal tract of unknown etiology. It involves mainly the ileum and large intestine, most often producing symptoms of obstruction or localized perforation with fistula. Both medical and surgical treatments are palliative. Nonetheless, operative excision gives effective symptomatic relief and results in reasonable long-term benefit.

INCIDENCE AND ETIOLOGY

The incidence of Crohn's disease in the general population is about 6 to 7 per 100,000 subjects at risk. The disease is as common in men as in women and can strike persons of any age, although the peak age of onset is between the second

See the corresponding chapter or part in the *Textbook of Surgery,* 15th edition, pp. 923–933, for a more detailed discussion of this topic, including a comprehensive list of references.

and fourth decades of life. The disease is more common among persons living in temperate climates than among those living in tropical climates. Also, spouses of persons with Crohn's disease have a higher incidence of the disease than persons in the general population.

PATHOLOGY

Crohn's disease is a generalized inflammatory disorder of the gastrointestinal tract, but it is discontinuous and segmental. One of the earliest macroscopic signs of Crohn's disease is the appearance of aphthous ulcers in the mucosa of the gastrointestinal tract. As the disease progresses, the aphthous ulcers deepen and coalesce, penetrating through the entire mucosa and forming longer ulcers that may reach 1 cm. in size or larger. Islands of normal mucosa can remain in between the ulcers to give the surface of the bowel a cobblestone appearance. As the ulcers grow and the inflammation spreads, the lesions extend transmurally deep into the wall of the bowel to involve the serosa and adjacent mesentery and mesenteric lymph nodes. Noncaseating granulomas are associated with the inflammation in about 50% of patients and are a hallmark of the disease.

Two main intestinal complications develop from these lesions: obstruction and perforation with abscess or fistula to other organs. Bleeding and toxic megacolon also can develop. Long-standing lesions of the small and large intestine are premalignant. Extraintestinal manifestations of the disease are also common and include erythema nodosum and pyoderma gangrenosum, iritis, uveitis, arthritis, and pericholangitis/hepatitis.

SYMPTOMS

The most common symptoms of Crohn's disease are those from the intestinal lesions, with abdominal pain, especially of a cramping nature, topping the list. Diarrhea is frequent. The stools may contain blood, although they often do not. The patients experience abdominal distention, flatulence, nausea, vomiting, and weight loss.

The course of the disease is one of exacerbations and remission, but as the lesions mature and complications develop, the symptoms continue unabated, and the disease becomes relentlessly progressive. About 70% of patients eventually come to operation, despite medical or dietary therapy.

DIAGNOSIS

Diagnosis is based on the history, physical findings, and appropriate laboratory tests, including endoscopy and radiography. On physical examination, thickened bowel wall or an adjacent inflammatory response or abscess may be palpable in the abdomen. Proctoscopy often reveals the characteristic rectal aphthous ulcer with surrounding normal-appearing mucosa, while anoscopy can show perianal abscesses, perianal fistulas, and even rectal-vaginal fistulas. Colonoscopy will delineate the extent of the ulcerating lesions in the large intestine. Sometimes the colonoscope can be passed through the colon and into the ileum to identify the ileal lesions of the disease. Roentgenographic examination of the gastrointestinal tract using $BaSO_4$ reveals the ulcerating lesions scattered in a segmental, irregular pattern along the wall of the involved intestine.

SURGICAL THERAPY

INDICATIONS FOR OPERATION. Patients with small intestinal Crohn's disease are usually operated on because an intestinal complication of the disease, such as obstruction, perforation, or bleeding, mandates the operation. In contrast, patients with large intestinal Crohn's most often undergo operation because of intractability to medical therapy and chronic debility.

GENERAL PRINCIPLES OF OPERATION. Because Crohn's disease involves nearly the entire gastrointestinal tract in most patients, the possibility of totally excising the disease is not reasonable. Thus surgical treatment is directed at the most severe areas of involvement, including those which account for the complications of obstruction, bleeding, or perforation. The two main operative approaches are to excise the lesions or to bypass them. Currently, most surgeons advise excision rather than bypass. Bypass allows the diseased intestine to remain in place, where it can cause continuing symptoms, require treatment, and perhaps even develop malignancy. Excision is done with 3-cm. "disease-free" margins on both sides of the area of involvement. The disease-free margins are established by gross inspection. Most surgeons do not use microscopic confirmation of healthy borders. After excision, bowel continuity is restored by an enteroenterostomy.

After resection of the index segment (or segments) of intestine that has led to the operation, fistulas from the index segment to adjacent organs usually can be closed by suture of the entrance of the fistula into the adjacent segment. Resection of the adjacent segment is seldom required.

SURGICAL TREATMENT AT SPECIFIC SITES. The three most common sites requiring operation for Crohn's disease are the ileum, the colorectum, and the anorectum, with other sites needing surgical treatment less often. With ileal involvement, obtaining a 3-cm. grossly disease-free margin on the proximal and distal ends usually means resecting the adjacent ileocolic valve, the cecum, and a small portion of the ascending colon. No attempt should be made to resect the entire thickened adjacent mesentery. Intestinal continuity is then restored with an end-to-end ileal-ascending colostomy. For extensive Crohn's disease of the jejunoileum, excision or bypass of the involved segments with an anastomosis between the uninvolved proximal small intestine and the adjacent large intestine was done in the past. Today, the performance of

multiple "stricturoplasties" on the narrowed, diseased segments of bowel is usually done. The stricturoplasties are performed by making a longitudinal incision through the narrowed areas and closing these incisions in a transverse
direction. This relieves obstruction but avoids excision.

Crohn's disease involving the ileum, cecum, and ascending
colon should be removed again with 3-cm. gross disease-free
margins. An anastomosis is made between the ileum and the
transverse colon in end-to-end fashion.

The operative approach to Crohn's disease of the colorectum varies depending on the exact sites of colorectal
involvement and their severity and can include colectomy
with ileorectostomy, colectomy with ileostomy and closure of
the rectal stump, or proctocolectomy with permanent ileostomy. Sphincter-saving operations such as the continent ileostomy (Kock pouch) or the ileal pouch–anal canal anastomosis
are not often used because of the likely recurrence of Crohn's
in the ileal pouch.

Conservative operations directed at relieving symptoms
from anorectal Crohn's disease have been done with increasing frequency in recent years. Abscesses have been drained,
fissures excised, and anal fistulas opened and debrided, sometimes aided by use of a "seton" when the fistula goes through
the anal sphincter. Rectal-vaginal fistulas have been closed by
débridement and direct suture of the opening of the fistula,
followed by advancement of a rectal mucosal flap from more
orad rectum over the opening of the fistula and down to the
dentate line.

COMPLICATIONS OF OPERATION

The main early complications of operation are intestinal
obstruction from adhesions, intra-abdominal abscess, wound
infection, anastomotic leaks, bleeding from areas of operation,
phlebothrombosis and pulmonary embolism, atelectasis and
pulmonary infections, urinary retention, and enterocutaneous
fistulas. Most of these complications can be managed nonoperatively; reoperation should be required in less than 10% of
patients. Operative mortality is unusual and should be less
than 2% of patients at risk. Late complications include steatorrhea, diarrhea, gallstones, urinary stones, and the short bowel
syndrome.

OUTCOME

Operations directed at Crohn's disease are palliative. They
provide the patients with symptomatic relief but not cure.
Overall, rates of symptomatic recurrence are about 6% of
patients at risk per year or 30% at 5 years and 60% at 10
years. Recurrences usually occur at or just proximal to an
anastomosis or stoma. Mortalities from Crohn's disease cumu-
late slowly with time. The mortality rate is about twice that
of a matched control group of healthy subjects.

V

The Surgical Approach to Morbid Obesity

Walter J. Pories, M.D.

Obesity is an increasingly serious health problem in the United States. There is a direct relationship between the amount of excess weight and the incidence of morbidity and mortality from cardiovascular disease, diabetes, stroke, certain types of cancer, osteoarthritis, sleep apnea, and biliary disease. Mortality accelerates rapidly when an individual becomes 50% overweight; morbidly obese young males have a 12-fold increase in mortality. Sudden, unexplained deaths are common. Of greater immediate concern to the patients, however, and the major reason for seeking surgery are the *psychological and socioeconomic consequences* of morbid obesity. Fat people are frequently objects of public scorn and malicious ridicule. They are unable to obtain jobs and maintain satisfactory family relationships and have sharp limitations in meeting the demands of daily living due to their bulk. The morbidly obese are severely handicapped by every measure: physically, emotionally, economically, and socially.

DEFINITIONS AND DIAGNOSIS

A number of indices have been developed for the quantification of obesity. *Height and weight standards* have the virtue of clinical simplicity and continue to be widely used. The *body mass index* (BMI), defined as the weight in kilograms/(height in meters)^2 (kg/m^2), has proven to be a reliable indicator of obesity and correlates remarkably well with mortality, even though it may be misleading in muscular individuals who demonstrate a high BMI despite minimal fat. The optimal level for the BMI lies between 20 and 27. Obesity is considered *morbid obesity* when the BMI exceeds 35, a value usually equivalent to the individual's exceeding the ideal body weight (IBW) by 100 lb. or more. Some use the term *superobese* to refer to the morbidly obese who exceed their IBW by more than 200 lb. A surgical procedure is the choice of therapy for patients with a BMI > 40 if they have no co-morbidities and with a BMI > 35 if they have such concurrent diseases as diabetes and hypertension.

Obesity is a complex and still poorly understood syndrome. Morbid obesity, especially, is not simply a matter of excessive food intake compared with "normal" food requirements; it also may be caused (1) by unusually inefficient utilization of

See the corresponding chapter or part in the *Textbook of Surgery*, 15th edition, pp. 933–946, for a more detailed discussion of this topic, including a comprehensive list of references.

food, (2) by decreased energy expenditure from lessened activity, and/or (3) by altered metabolism such as a reduced thermogenic response to food or attenuated loss of heat through the thickened subcutaneous fat. Currently, most authorities concur that both genetic and environmental factors play a role and that the genetic influences appear to be stronger.

Fat is not symmetrically distributed throughout the body but is more likely to be concentrated in the abdomen in the male and on the hips in the female. Individuals with a more android distribution ("apples") are significantly more likely to have complications of their obesity than those with a gynecoid appearance ("pears").

The arguments about the control of obesity are not merely academic. Obesity is the most common form of malnutrition in the United States today. In 1993, nearly $33 billion were spent in the United States in the pursuit of diets and slimming programs, the search for new pharmaceuticals for weight control, and the management of obesity. Control of obesity, if achieved, would probably have an effect at least equal to that of controlling smoking in terms of the nation's health.

The largest price is paid by the morbidly obese; not only do they have high health care costs, but they also cannot meet their costs of daily living because they are often unemployed and indigent. It is time to recognize, as the NIH Consensus Conference on Obesity concluded, that morbid obesity is a serious, disabling, and common disease and that morbid obesity, like other diseases, deserves treatment and insurance coverage for that therapy.

THE NONOPERATIVE TREATMENT OF MORBID OBESITY

THE FAILURE OF DIETING. Although *dieting* remains the most useful method of weight control for individuals who are mildly or moderately overweight, it is almost always ineffective for the morbidly obese. In most cases, even when massively obese patients are aided by groups such as Weight Watchers, by psychotherapy, by diuretics, by thyroid preparations, or by anorectic agents such as amphetamines, the lost pounds are usually regained together with a few extra ones as soon as the intense weight-reducing regimen has ceased. In fact, weight loss is usually disappointingly low. In a classic study of 100 patients subjected to an intensive weight-reducing regimen by four dietitians, 77% lost less than 10 lb., and only one patient lost more than 20 lb.

Although the use of *drugs* for the treatment of obesity has been disappointing in the past, advances are being made in the development of new agents and in the application of multiagent protocols. The appetite suppressant drug amphetamine has been in clinical use for over 50 years, but it has a long history of abuse. Safer new agents are now being introduced, including fenfluramine, phenylpropanolamine, and mazindol. Hopefully these new drugs also will prove useful in the morbidly obese. Until they do, however, surgery remains the therapy of choice.

Exercise may be useful in maintaining the physical ability of the morbidly obese but in this group of patients has not been shown to produce significant weight loss. Similarly, *psychological measures* with behavior modification also have proven useless in these massive individuals.

SURGERY FOR MORBID OBESITY

Because diets are ineffective in the management of morbid and malignant obesity, most authorities now agree with the recommendation of the NIH National Consensus Conference on Surgery for Obesity that surgery has become the treatment of choice of that small percentage of persons who suffer from severe obesity. The first effective bariatric operation, that is, a procedure designed to cause weight loss, was the *intestinal bypass*, which excluded the majority of the small bowel from alimentary flow. The operation is no longer done because it failed to produce permanent weight loss in most patients and was associated with a large number of metabolic complications, including liver failure.

The most important advance in bariatric surgery occurred in 1966, when Mason, concerned by the frequency and seriousness of the complications from intestinal bypass, devised the gastric bypass, which was designed to interfere with food intake rather than with digestion and absorption. The procedure and various modifications were adopted rapidly when others confirmed that the gastric bypass was not only safer than but also as effective as the intestinal bypass in producing weight loss in the morbidly obese.

Two operations are commonly performed today: the gastric bypass (GB) and the vertical banded gastroplasty (VBG). A third, gastric banding, is gaining increasing application; a fourth, the biliopancreatic bypass or Scopinaro procedure, may have application in the superobese.

The *gastric bypass* partitions the stomach with several rows of staples to form a proximal pouch with a volume of 15 to 30 ml. Instead of draining the pouch into the distal stomach as in the VBG, however, the narrow gastric outlet (0.8 to 1.5 cm.) is developed with a Roux-en-Y gastrojejunostomy, with the alimentary segment measuring about 40 to 60 cm.

The operation can be performed with a mortality rate of about 1% to 2%, depending on the health of the patient population. The most common perioperative complications include sepsis due to subphrenic abscesses or anastomotic leaks, pulmonary emboli, and wound infections. The gastric bypass operation produces significant and durable weight loss. In a series of 608 primary gastric bypasses in the last 14 years, patients lost about 30 lb. in 1 month, 60 lb. within 6 months, and 100 lb. by 1 year. An average maximum weight loss of 70% of excess body weight occurred approximately 2 years after surgery. At the end of 5 years, mean weight loss was 58% of excess body weight, 55% after 10 years, and 49% after 14 years.

Even more striking is the *control of adult-onset diabetes*. Before surgery, 164 of the 608 patients (27%) had non-insulin-dependent diabetes mellitus (NIDDM), and another 166 of 608 (27.3%) proved to have impaired glucose metabolism (IGT). Currently, 91% of these patients continue to be euglycemic. No other therapy for diabetes, medical or surgical, has ever reported such a high rate of success in controlling the hyperglycemia and the hyperinsulinemia associated with that disease.

Before surgery, 353 (58.1%) of the patients had *hypertension.* After surgery, this rate has been reduced to 14%. In addition to these improvements, patients generally demonstrated *improvement of cardiopulmonary function, in their disabilities from arthritis, and in fertility.* The gastric bypass produced long-term improvement in the *health and physical functioning* of the morbidly obese, but the *emotional and social changes* for the better proved to be temporary.

The primary problem with the gastric bypass is a failure rate of about 15% with regain of weight, primarily due to disruption of the staple line used to partition the stomach. Newer approaches for partitioning the stomach, such as triple staple lines for division of the stomach, are promising solutions now under evaluation.

The *vertical banded gastroplasty* consists of a stapled partition of the stomach with a proximal pouch volume of about 15 ml. to limit intake and a small gastric outlet of about 1 cm. in its inner diameter. The outlet is buttressed either with a strip of Marlex mesh or a circle of Silastic tubing to prevent stretching. The operation is somewhat less challenging than the gastric bypass but carries a similar mortality and morbidity rate. The procedure produces about 10% to 15% less weight loss than the GB, suffers also from disruption of the staple lines, but is associated with fewer nutritional deficiencies. The popularity of this procedure is waning because of problems with the plastic mesh and its failure to produce as much weight loss as the GB.

The *gastric banding operation* partitions the stomach with a 1-cm. external silicone band that is wrapped about the proximal stomach like a belt. The proximal pouch in this procedure is also about 15 to 30 ml., and the gastric outlet size is adjustable with a small saline reservoir in the band that can be inflated through an implanted port in the rectus muscle. The operation can be done safely with a mortality of less than 1%, does not enter a viscus, and produces weight loss similar to that of the VBG. The recent demonstration that the operation can be done with the laparoscope has enhanced its popularity.

The *biliopancreatic bypass* of Scopinaro is a radical procedure that includes a gastric bypass with marked shortening of the intestine, resection of the distal stomach, and cholecystectomy. The procedure is certainly effective in producing weight loss even in the superobese, but the safety of the operation remains in doubt. Some groups report few problems; others compare the rate and severity of complications to the intestinal bypass. Deaths from liver failure after the operation have been reported.

CONCLUSION

Morbid obesity is a serious and increasingly common disease for which the only successful therapy to date is surgery.

Surgery not only controls weight but also controls and may even reverse many of the co-morbidities of the disease, such as diabetes, hypertension, cardiopulmonary failure, arthritis, and endocrine abnormalities. Even more important, surgery can rehabilitate these unfortunate individuals and allow them to return to a high quality of life. The gastric bypass operation is currently the procedure of choice because it produces durable weight loss with a mortality rate of about 1% and reasonable postoperative and long-term morbidity, but gastric banding and the biliopancreatic bypass will probably also be adopted widely because "one size does not fit all patients," and different challenges require different solutions.

VI

Meckel's Diverticulum
Bryan M. Clary, M.D., and H. Kim Lyerly, M.D.

Meckel's diverticulum is the most commonly encountered congenital anomaly of the small intestine. Reported initially in 1598 by Hildanus, this abnormality was described in detail by Johann Meckel in 1809. Autopsy studies have estimated the incidence of Meckel's diverticulum to be 1% to 2%, with men being more commonly affected than women by a ratio of 2:1. Although most commonly presenting as an incidental finding on laparotomy (and now laparoscopy), this entity can be associated with several life-threatening disease states.

EMBRYOLOGY

Meckel's diverticulum is an embryologic derivative of the vitelline duct. The midgut loop remains in open connection with the yolk sac by way of the vitelline duct (omphalomesenteric duct) until the eighth to tenth week of gestation, at which time the vitelline duct becomes obliterated. Persistence of the vitelline duct may lead to (1) a fistula between the umbilicus and the ileum when the entire duct remains patent, (2) Meckel's diverticulum due to failure of closure of the intestinal end of the duct, (3) an umbilical sinus when the umbilical side of the duct is not obliterated, (4) a fibrous cord between the umbilicus and the ileum representing an obliterated duct and its vessels, or (5) any combination of these four entities, the most frequent being Meckel's diverticulum. Up to 25% of Meckel's diverticula are connected to the umbilicus by a fibrous strand. Meckel's diverticulum is a

See the corresponding chapter or part in the *Textbook of Surgery*, 15th edition, pp. 946–950, for a more detailed discussion of this topic, including a comprehensive list of references.

true diverticulum containing all layers of the intestinal wall, usually arising from the antimesenteric border of the ileum 45 to 90 cm. proximal to the ileocecal valve. The blood supply to a Meckel's diverticulum is provided by persistent vitelline vessels present within a distinct mesentery. It varies in length and diameter, ranging from 1 to 12 cm. Since the cells lining the vitelline duct are pluripotent, it is not uncommon to find heterotopic tissue within a Meckel's diverticulum. Gastric mucosa is present in 50% of all Meckel's diverticula but in over 75% of symptomatic individuals. Pancreatic mucosa is encountered in approximately 5% of diverticula. Less commonly, these diverticula may harbor colonic mucosa. Tumors are an uncommon finding in a Meckel's diverticulum and include lipoma, leiomyoma, neurofibroma, angioma, leiomyosarcoma, carcinoid, and less commonly, adenocarcinoma.

CLINICAL PRESENTATIONS

It is estimated that only 4% of patients who possess a Meckel's diverticulum will become symptomatic during their lifetimes. The most common clinical presentation is incidental identification during abdominal exploration. Symptomatic presentations are secondary to hemorrhage, small bowel obstruction, diverticulitis, perforation, associated umbilical abnormalities, and tumors. Over half of patients presenting with symptoms are under the age of 2. The average mortality in patients developing symptoms is 6%, with an excessive proportion of deaths occurring in the elderly. The most common clinical problem associated with Meckel's diverticulum is gastrointestinal bleeding presenting as bright red blood per rectum. The usual source of the bleeding is a chronic acid-induced ileal ulcer in the ileum adjacent to a Meckel's diverticulum that contains gastric mucosa. Diagnosis of a Meckel's diverticulum possessing gastric mucosa can be made utilizing ^{99m}Tc-pertechnetate radioisotope scanning which is readily taken up by gastric mucosa. Another common symptom associated with a Meckel's diverticulum is intestinal obstruction. The cause of this obstruction may be volvulus of the small bowel around a diverticulum associated with a fibrotic band attached to the abdominal wall, intussusception, or rarely, incarceration of the diverticulum in an inguinal hernia (Littre's hernia). Volvulus is usually an acute event and, if allowed to progress, may result in strangulation of the involved bowel. In intussusception, a broad-based diverticulum invaginates and then is carried forward by peristalsis. This may be ileoileal or ileocolic and presents as acute obstruction associated with an urge to defecate, early vomiting, and occasionally, the passage of the classic "currant jelly" stool. Barium enema reduction of an intussusception secondary to a Meckel's diverticulum can be performed, although with a decreased level of success in comparison with non-Meckel's-associated intussusception. Resection of the diverticulum is indicated even if hydrostatic reduction is successful.

Diverticulitis

Diverticulitis accounts for approximately 10% to 20% of symptomatic presentations. This complication is more frequent in older patients than in children under 2 years of age. Infection of a Meckel's diverticulum often presents as indistinguishable from appendicitis, although the peritoneal signs may vary in location. As with appendicitis, failure to promptly diagnose the diverticulitis may lead to perforation, peritonitis, and death. During exploration for suspected appendicitis where the appendix is found to be normal, it is critical to inspect the distal ileum for a Meckel's diverticulum. The indications for resection of the diverticulum in this clinical setting parallel those of appendectomy. Inflamed diverticula and diverticula incidentally found when other causes of the acute abdomen are not evident and that do not preclude safe diverticulectomy should undergo resection.

Umbilical Anomalies

Umbilical abnormalities occur in approximately 8% to 10% of patients with a Meckel's diverticulum. These include fistulas, cysts, sinuses, and fibrous bands between the diverticulum and the umbilicus (filum enterale). A fibrous band, if found on laparotomy, should be removed because of the risk of internal herniation and volvulus. It is generally recommended to resect the diverticulum when a fibrous band is found, although in situations where this is not safe, simple resection of the fibrous band is sufficient. The identification of external umbilical abnormalities is usually not a difficult endeavor. The presence of intestinal mucosa at the skin level or persistent drainage from the umbilicus is the most common form of presentation. To delineate the nature of the enterocutaneous fistula draining at the umbilicus, cannulation and dye injection are useful. Elective surgical exploration of the umbilicus is indicated in the management of these external umbilical abnormalities.

Surgical Management of Asymptomatic and Symptomatic Meckel's Diverticulum

The management of a Meckel's diverticulum found incidentally on laparotomy is controversial. It is clear that diverticulectomy under these circumstances has an extremely low morbidity and mortality. There is general agreement that diverticula which on physical inspection appear to have heterotopic mucosa should be resected given their higher risk of subsequent complication. Age less than 40 years, diverticula longer than 2 cm. and fibrous bands to the umbilicus or mesentery are also risk factors for the development of complications and thus relative indications for resection. Resection of asymptomatic diverticula in children discovered on laparotomy is generally recommended.

Because of the decreasing likelihood of complications associated with a Meckel's diverticulum with increasing age, the management of incidentally discovered diverticula in adults that are not found to have fibrous bands or thought to possess heterotopic mucosa is the subject of much controversy. Although the standard of care in recent decades has been the selective resection of incidentally discovered diverticula based on estimated risks of future complication, recent studies have demonstrated that the performance of prophylactic diverticulectomy under appropriate operative conditions is safe and may be beneficial. Symptomatic Meckel's diverticula should undergo resection. Resection in this setting is associated with a 5% to 10% mortality.

Controversy exists over whether diverticulectomy or segmental resection should be performed. In patients with hemorrhage from adjacent ileal ulcers, simple diverticulectomy will not remove the ulcer, and postoperative bleeding may recur. Segmental resection is also advocated in small children with broad-based diverticula, in whom the risk of ileal stenosis is greater if diverticulectomy is performed. In other clinical scenarios, segmental resection of the diverticulum with careful attention to divide the associated blood supply is sufficient. This can be performed either by a handsewn technique or by stapling across the base of the diverticulum in a diagonal or transverse line so as to minimize the risk of subsequent ileal stenosis. Recent reports have demonstrated the feasibility of laparoscopic techniques in the performance of diverticulectomy. Although long-term results from these newer techniques are not available, the increasing frequency with which Meckel's diverticula are diagnosed via laparoscopic examination will lead to further controversy in the management of asymptomatic diverticula.

VII

Carcinoid Tumors and the Carcinoid Syndrome
Haile T. Debas, M.D., and Susan L. Orloff, M.D.

Carcinoid tumors arise from cells with APUD characteristics and represent 55% of all gut endocrine tumors. The incidence is 1 to 5 per 100,000 of the general population.

CARCINOID TUMORS

SITE OF ORIGIN. These derive from the three portions of the embryonic gut. Carcinoids of the foregut develop primar-

See the corresponding chapter or part in the *Textbook of Surgery,* 15th edition, pp. 950–954, for a more detailed discussion of this topic, including a comprehensive list of references.

ily in the stomach, pancreas, and lungs and frequently produce atypical carcinoid syndrome. Midgut carcinoid tumors are most common and arise primarily in the appendix and terminal ileum. They produce multiple secretory products and are often associated with the typical carcinoid syndrome. Hindgut carcinoid tumors arise almost exclusively in the rectum. They do not produce secretory products and therefore do not cause carcinoid syndromes.

CLINICAL MANIFESTATIONS. Foregut Tumors. Gastric carcinoid tumors may be silent but may cause upper abdominal pain or bleeding. Bronchial carcinoid tumors have initial clinical manifestations of hemoptysis, recurrent pneumonitis, or localized wheezing or present as a "coin lesion" on chest film. Both gastric and bronchial carcinoid tumors may be associated with the carcinoid syndrome.

Midgut Carcinoid Tumors. Appendiceal and small intestinal tumors may be silent. Appendiceal carcinoid tumors may cause acute obstructive appendicitis. Small intestinal tumors may cause bowel obstruction due to fibrotic kinking or intussusception. They also may have initial clinical manifestations of diarrhea, bleeding, and weight loss and rarely may present as an abdominal mass.

Hindgut Tumors. These present as rectal lesions on endoscopy or may cause bleeding.

DIAGNOSIS. The most useful diagnostic finding is an elevated level of 5-hydroxyindoleacetic acid (5-HIAA). In foregut carcinoid tumors, the urine contains little (but above-normal) 5-HIAA but large amounts of 5-hydroxytryptophan (5-HTP) and serotonin (5-HT), because these tumors are deficient in dopa-decarboxylase and cannot convert 5-HTP into 5-HT. Plasma levels of neurotensin, substance P, motilin, somatostatin, and vasoactive intestinal polypeptide are sometimes elevated. The most promising new localizing technique takes advantage of the presence of somatostatin receptors in most carcinoid tumors. *In vivo* receptor scintigraphy using radioiodine- or radioindium-labeled octreotide, the eight-amino-acid analogue of somatostatin, can localize carcinoid tumors and their metastases both preoperatively and intraoperatively.

TREATMENT. Early resection, while the tumor is small, offers the patient the best likelihood for cure. Resection is often necessary regardless of the presence or absence of metastases. Appendiceal tumors smaller than 1.5 cm. in diameter may be treated by routine appendectomy. When they are larger than 1.5 cm. or are associated with invasion of the ileum or lymphatic spread, a right hemicolectomy is required. Rectal carcinoid tumors smaller than 1 cm. may be removed endoscopically. Tumors measuring 1 to 2 cm. should be excised operatively with margins. Those larger than 2 cm. require anterior resection.

CARCINOID SYNDROME

CAUSES. The carcinoid syndrome occurs in less than 10% of patients with carcinoid tumors. The syndrome occurs when venous drainage from the tumor gains access to the systemic circulation so that vasoactive secretory substances escape hepatic degradation. This occurs under the following conditions: when hepatic metastases are present, when venous blood from retroperitoneal metastases drains into paravertebral veins, and when the primary carcinoid tumor is outside the gastrointestinal tract—for example, bronchial, ovarian, or testicular tumors.

CLINICAL MANIFESTATIONS. The syndrome consists of flushing, diarrhea, wheezing, and tricuspid and/or pulmonic valve insufficiency. Other symptoms include sweating, abdominal pain and borborygmi, and pellagra dermatosis.

BIOCHEMICAL MEDIATORS. Serotonin is thought to be responsible for diarrhea and fibrosis, including that in cardiac valves. The vasomotor changes are thought to be mediated by kinins and such vasoactive peptides as substance P, neuropeptide K, neurokinin A, and neurotensin.

DIAGNOSIS. Elevated urinary 5-HIAA and elevated 5-HT in whole blood or platelet-poor plasma are the best confirmation of the diagnosis. Occasionally, the pentagastrin provocative test may be used to induce symptoms and to elevate circulating levels of 5-HT and peptides secreted by the tumor.

TREATMENT. Primary tumors should be resected. Debulking procedures of either primary or secondary tumors in the liver may provide significant palliation. Liver transplantation, when the primary has been eradicated and the tumor is confined to the liver, has been suggested, but this treatment is as yet unproved. Pharmacologic treatment with antisecretion agents or interferon is relatively ineffective. The best symptomatic treatment involves the use of long-acting somatostatin analogue. The best cancer chemotherapeutic regimen is a combination of streptozotocin and 5-fluorouracil.

VIII

Malabsorption Syndromes
John P. Grant, M.D.

Impaired absorption of fats, carbohydrates, proteins, vitamins, electrolytes, minerals, and/or water can occur following surgery.

ESOPHAGECTOMY. Mild steatorrhea usually occurs, likely related to the vagotomy performed as a part of esophageal resection.

TOTAL GASTRECTOMY. Malabsorption of fat and protein occurs as a result of truncal vagotomy and inefficient mixing

---

See the corresponding chapter or part in the *Textbook of Surgery,* 15th edition, pp. 955–960, for a more detailed discussion of this topic, including a comprehensive list of references.

of food with digestive enzymes. Pernicious anemia occurs rarely. Loss of the stomach reduces dietary intake. Although creation of a jejunal pouch improves storage capacity and a Roux-en-Y esophagojejunostomy decreases reflux alkaline esophagitis, anorexia often persists, and poor dietary intake remains a major cause of nutritional depletion.

PARTIAL GASTRECTOMY. A reduction in the gastric reservoir reduces dietary intake. In addition, malabsorption is often present due to decreased gastric digestion, more rapid and less regulated gastric emptying, and decreased intestinal transit time. A Billroth II reconstruction may aggravate malabsorption for these reasons: less stimulation of biliary and pancreatic secretions with bypass of the duodenum, inadequate mixing with pancreatic enzymes and bile salts, stasis in the afferent loop with bacterial overgrowth and abnormal metabolism of bile salts, and loss of the duodenum as the principal surface for iron, calcium, fat, and carotene absorption. Up to 50% of patients following a Billroth II procedure demonstrate steatorrhea greater than 8 gm. per 24 hours, but less than 20% develop clinically significant malabsorption. Only 25% demonstrate steatorrhea following a Billroth I procedure, and less than 10% show clinically significant malabsorption.

Anemia occurs in up to 30% of patients within 15 years following subtotal gastrectomy due to malabsorption of iron, folate, and occasionally vitamin B_{12}. A metabolic bone disease occurs in up to 33% of patients after 10 to 20 years.

FOLLOWING VAGOTOMY. Malabsorption follows truncal vagotomy due to diarrhea, poor mixing of pancreatic secretions and bile salts with food, and diminished release of secretin and cholecystokinin. The reported incidence varies from 28% to 68%, but significant diarrhea occurs in only about 5%. The diarrhea may be caused by rapid small bowel transit due to vagal denervation or stasis of food with bacterial overgrowth and dumping. In addition, truncal vagotomy reduces the time that food remains in the terminal ileum, leading to malabsorption and depletion of bile salts with steatorrhea. Steatorrhea also may be caused by abnormalities of gastric grinding and sieving of food particles. The incidence of malabsorption following selective vagotomy is less than 10%.

Vagotomy with drainage reduces glucose absorption up to 30%. Plasma glucose and insulin peaks, however, are two to four times higher than normal, reflecting rapid gastric emptying and initial absorption of glucose. The relatively short period of absorption with normal clearance of glucose may lead to "reactive" hypoglycemia.

ENTEROCUTANEOUS FISTULAS. Distal fistulas produce little malabsorption. Significant loss of ingested food may occur, however, if the fistula is proximal. Low-output fistulas (<200 ml. per day) are rarely clinically significant, but high-output fistulas (>800 ml. per day) can cause marked nutrient losses. Leakage of bile and pancreatic enzymes may produce malabsorption of fat, protein, and starch.

PANCREATIC INSUFFICIENCY. Resection of a major portion or all of the pancreas or ligation or obstruction of its duct can cause malabsorption and diabetes. Lack of lipase and protease accounts for the malabsorption of fat and protein.

BILIARY TRACT DISEASE. Reduction or absence of bile salts in the duodenum causes steatorrhea. Loss of vitamin D and calcium can lead to osteoporosis and osteomalacia. Loss of vitamin K can prolong the prothrombin time and produce bleeding.

SMALL BOWEL RESECTION. Malabsorption becomes significant with resection of more than 50% of the small bowel. Loss of the ileocecal valve causes rapid transit. Resection of the distal ileum leads to vitamin B_{12} deficiency and bile salt diarrhea. Depletion of bile salts leads to steatorrhea and increased stool calcium. Resection of the proximal small bowel removes sites of calcium, iron, and lactose absorption.

Intestinal resection leads to gastric hypersecretion and hyperacidity proportional to the amount resected. High solute load and acid injury to the mucosa may impair absorption, increase secretions, and inactivate lipase and trypsin.

BLIND LOOP SYNDROME. This syndrome occurs when there is stasis of intestinal contents. It is seen most commonly when a blind loop is created, as with a Billroth II procedure or intestinal bypass. The syndrome is characterized by diarrhea, steatorrhea, anemia, weight loss, abdominal pain, and multiple vitamin deficiencies.

Vitamin B_{12} deficiency can occur due to use of vitamin B_{12} by bacteria in the stagnant intestine or bacterial production of a toxin inhibiting enzymatic transfer of vitamin B_{12} across the small intestinal mucosa.

IX

Radiation Injury to the Intestine

Jerome J. DeCosse, M.D.

The aim of both surgical and radiation therapy is regional control of tumor. Combined treatment may permit a less extensive procedure. With widespread application of radiation therapy to abdominal and pelvic viscera for both cure and palliation, an occasional patient sustains intestinal injury. Energy transferred by ionizing radiation generates a series of biochemical events within injured tissues; DNA appears to be the most vulnerable target. Rapidly proliferating cells are particularly sensitive. Therapeutic levels of irradiation to the abdomen or pelvis lead to an acute disruption of cell kinetics in intestinal stem cells. Thus an early and self-limited effect

---

See the corresponding chapter or part in the *Textbook of Surgery,* 15th edition, pp. 960–964, for a more detailed discussion of this topic, including a comprehensive list of references.

of radiation therapy is transient diarrhea, painful bowel movements, and occasionally, rectal bleeding. These changes are readily managed by simple supportive measures.

Irradiation also may lead to a progressive vasculitis, diffuse collagen deposition, fibrosis, and a depleted blood supply in irradiated tissues. Visceral injury from irradiation may become apparent many years after treatment. Low-flow states such as congestive heart failure or atherosclerosis may aggravate subclinical injury. Some chemotherapeutic agents, called *radiomimetic*, enhance the biologic effect of irradiation. The visceral tissues affected are those within the radiation portals. Adhesions from prior operation may fix small intestine within the radiation field and increase risk. Injury to the small or large intestine may lead to partial or complete obstruction. Damage to the rectum results in rectal bleeding from proctitis, a radiation-induced ulcer, stenosis, and rarely, cancer. Injury at either site may be associated with damage to other viscera, particularly the genitourinary system; damage to the latter can be more life-threatening. Injury at either site can lead to progressive necrosis, abscess formation, perforation, and fistulization.

In addition to basic supportive measures, oral and rectal sucralfate and oral sulfasalazine and rectal steroids have shown benefit in reducing symptoms.

When an operation is warranted for intestinal obstruction, resection is favored, but a bypass may be necessary. The anastomosis should be performed outside the radiation portal, ordinarily to the transverse colon. When an abscess or perforation is present, the bowel must be excluded from the peritoneal cavity, and a stoma is necessary.

Injury of the rectum can lead to massive bleeding or to fistula formation. A colostomy is usually necessary and may be permanent. Occasionally, the diseased area in the rectum can be removed operatively and intestinal continuity restored.

Appendicitis
David C. Sabiston, Jr., M.D.

While the majority of patients with acute appendicitis can be diagnosed with ease, there remain a number in whom the signs and symptoms are quite variable, making a firm diagnosis difficult. For this reason, diagnostic criteria should remain rather liberal with the expectation that some patients will be operated on and found to have a normal appendix (10% to

---

See the corresponding chapter or part in the *Textbook of Surgery*, 15th edition, pp. 964–970, for a more detailed discussion of this topic, including a comprehensive list of references.

15%). This is far preferable to missing the diagnosis and having some patients perforate the appendix and develop generalized peritonitis, with its considerable morbidity and even mortality.

While descriptions of acute appendicitis had been made earlier, Reginald Fitz deserves much credit for his classic clinical and pathologic description of the disease published in 1886. After this paper, appendicitis became rapidly recognized, and the diagnosis was made frequently, with the saving of many lives.

The vermiform appendix lies in the right lower quadrant and is largely free to move in a 360-degree circle around the base of the cecum. The symptoms and signs of appendicitis depend on its anatomic location. Appendicitis most often follows *obstruction* of the appendiceal lumen, where bacteria multiply and produce exotoxins and endotoxins and ulcerate the mucosa. The bacteria in the lumen can then penetrate the wall of the appendix and establish an inflammatory process, which may penetrate the serosa and cause generalized peritonitis or a localized abscess.

The clinical diagnosis of acute appendicitis is made primarily on the basis of the history and physical findings, with additional support from laboratory examinations. The typical history is that of generalized abdominal pain beginning in the epigastrium, with anorexia and nausea and later vomiting. The pain gradually moves toward the umbilicus and finally into the right lower quadrant. Tenderness and spasm are present in the right lower quadrant and may become more extensive with the passage of time as the pathologic process spreads. The temperature is usually mildly elevated. Rovsing's sign may be elicited by applying pressure in the left lower quadrant, which is reflected by pain in the right lower quadrant. The psoas sign may be positive as well as the obturator sign, indicating an inflammatory process on the surface of these muscles. If perforation occurs, the temperature rises to 38 to 40° C., with accompanying tachycardia.

The leukocyte count is usually elevated (10,000 to 20,000), and for those for whom the count is normal, there is usually a shift to the left, indicating acute inflammation. In the elderly, the leukocyte count may be normal or only minimally elevated. Urinalysis may reveal a few red cells but is otherwise negative. Radiographic studies are seldom indicated. In patients in whom the diagnosis is not clear, plain films of the abdomen may show a dilated cecum with a fluid level (cecal ileus) and occasionally a calcified fecalith. The barium enema may fail to fill the appendix in more than three-quarters of patients with acute appendicitis. An ultrasound examination may be helpful in demonstrating signs of an enlarged appendix or an abscess. Computed tomography (CT) scans also may be helpful in establishing the presence of an abscess.

The differential diagnosis of acute appendicitis includes acute gastroenteritis, cholecystitis, pyelitis, salpingitis, tubalovarian abscess, and ruptured ovarian cysts. Ectopic pregnancy also may simulate acute appendicitis, as may regional enteritis, especially in the first attack. Testicular torsion and epididymitis also should be considered in the differential diagnosis. Most agree that antibiotics should be administered shortly before operation. Both cefoxitin and cefotetan have been used widely, and for patients with a perforated appendix, additional antibiotics may be necessary, especially if *Bacteroides fragilis* is involved, which responds to metronidazole. The treatment of acute appendicitis is appendectomy. This can be done by an open approach or by a laparoscopic technique. Both these operations have their advocates, although there appears to be increasing use of the laparoscopic approach. Those who advocate laparoscopic appendectomy emphasize that it provides additional information concerning the differential diagnosis and can be utilized simultaneously to remove the appendix. Moreover, the hospital course is associated with less pain and more rapid return to normal activity.

If an appendiceal abscess is palpated and the process appears to be subsiding, the patient may be managed with antibiotics, intravenous fluids, and careful observation until recovery. An elective appendectomy should be performed 3 months or so later, since more than half these patients have recurrence of acute appendicitis.

32

THE COLON AND RECTUM

I

Surgical Anatomy and Operative Procedures

Rolando H. Rolandelli, M.D., and Joel J. Roslyn, M.D.

The colon contains the same inner circular muscular layer as does the small bowel, but its outer longitudinal muscle layer is concentrated into three separate longitudinal strips named *taeniae coli*. The state of contraction of the taeniae coli creates *haustra*. These sacculations only partially encircle the colonic wall and give the colon a typical radiographic appearance. Coursing upward from the cecum to the transverse colon is the ascending colon, covering the right ureter and duodenum. The transverse colon is the most mobile portion of the colon and may be found in the upper abdomen or as far down as the pelvis and is completely intraperitoneal. The descending colon courses from the splenic flexure down into the pelvic brim and is only partially peritonealized and in intimate association with the left ureter. The sigmoid colon is S-shaped and extends from the pelvic brim to the peritoneal reflection, where it joins the rectum. The sigmoid colon is frequently redundant, and its mesentery may become elongated to produce a sigmoid volvulus. The rectum projects posteriorly and downward to conform to the curve of the sacrum, and as it descends into the pelvis, it loses the peritoneal investment. The cecum, ascending colon, and proximal portion of the transverse colon (right colon) derive arterial blood supply from the ileocolic, right colic, and middle colic branches of the superior mesenteric artery. The inferior mesenteric artery supplies blood to the distal transverse colon and descending and sigmoid colon (left colon) via the left colic artery and branches of the sigmoid and superior hemorrhoidal vessels. The rectum is supplied by a rich network of vessels from the middle hemorrhoidal and inferior hemorrhoidal arteries. As these vessels course through the mesentery toward the bowel wall, they bifurcate and form arcades at 1 to 2 cm. from the mesenteric border that define the marginal artery of Drummond. The anastomosis of arcades between the superior and inferior mesenteric vessels is known as the *long anastomosis of Riolan*. The colon is drained by a rich and vast network of lymphatics that follows the course of the major vessels.

Surgical treatment of colon cancer is based on the principle of excising all the segment containing the tumor and any other adjacent structures involved, as well as the lymphatic

See the corresponding chapter or part in the *Textbook of Surgery*, 15th edition, pp. 971–974, for a more detailed discussion of this topic, including a comprehensive list of references.

channels draining such segment. Tumors of the cecum and ascending colon require a right hemicolectomy with resection of the right colon to the level of the middle colic vessels. In tumors involving the hepatic flexure, the resection of the transverse colon is extended beyond the middle colic vessels. For tumors involving the descending colon, the left colon is removed. Sigmoid resections are frequently performed for diverticulitis. Tumors involving the rectum that preclude low anterior resection and restoration of gastrointestinal continuity are best managed by a combined abdominoperineal resection of the rectum (APR). Until recently, APR also was performed for patients with ulcerative colitis. Newer operations, however, maintain transanal fecal flow while removing all diseased mucosa and creating an ileal pouch–anal anastomosis (IPAA).

Colostomy refers to opening of the colon onto the surface of the abdomen, which may be necessary (1) as the outlet of feces when the distal colon or rectum has been removed, (2) to protect a distal anastomosis, (3) to serve as a "vent" of a more distal colonic obstruction, and (4) to divert the fecal stream from a pathologic process.

II

Physiology
Rolando H. Rolandelli, M.D., and Joel J. Roslyn, M.D.

The colon serves two major functions: the recycling of nutrients and stool formation and elimination. The recycling of nutrients involves the metabolic activity of the colonic flora and active absorption. Stool formation also involves absorption of solutes and water and depends on dehydration of colonic contents.

During the digestive process, food is diluted within the gut lumen by mixing with gastrointestinal, hepatobiliary, and pancreatic secretions. The small intestine absorbs most of the nutrients ingested and some of the secreted fluid. However, the ileal effluent is still rich in water, electrolytes, and nutrients such as proteins (enzymes) and resistant carbohydrates. In the colon, bacteria ferment carbohydrates and proteins, transforming their caloric content into short-chain fatty acids (SCFA), which are then absorbed by the colon and can account for as much as 10% of the daily energy expenditure of a normal subject.

For many years, urea was thought to be the end product of

See the corresponding chapter or part in the *Textbook of Surgery,* 15th edition, pp. 975–977, for a more detailed discussion of this topic, including a comprehensive list of references.

nitrogen metabolism in humans. Tracer studies have demonstrated that 10% of urea being synthesized is split by bacterial ureases, yielding ammonia, which is then absorbed by the colonic mucosa.

The total absorptive area of the colon is estimated to be approximately 900 sq. cm. Daily, 1000 to 1500 ml. of water is delivered from the ileum into the cecum. The daily volume of stool water is estimated to be only 100 to 150 ml., with a sodium concentration of 25 to 50 mEq. per liter. The mechanism of sodium absorption by the colonic epithelium is an active transport process directed against a combined transepithelial chemical, concentration, and electropotential difference. The net effect of active sodium transport is the return of water from the lumen, and therefore, absorption of water is a passive process. The colon is also the site of bile acid absorption, which is a process of non-ionic or passive diffusion.

The preferred fuel for the colonic epithelium is *n*-butyrate, which is only produced by bacterial fermentation. The lack of *n*-butyrate, such as that resulting from inhibition of fermentation by broad-spectrum antibiotics, leads to less sodium and water absorption and thus diarrhea. Mineralocorticoids stimulate potassium secretion by colonic epithelium. Bicarbonate is also secreted by an active process directed against a difference in both chemical concentration and electrical potential.

In the right colon, *antiperistalsis* waves produce retrograde flow to maintain some degree of stasis and allow for fermentation. In the left colon, contents are propelled caudad by *tonic contractions*, separating them into a series of globular masses. A third type of contraction, referred to as *mass peristalsis*, is interspersed with these contractions and occurs at varying intervals but typically more frequently after meals. Each mass peristaltic contraction advances a column of colonic contents through one third of the colonic length. The rectum undergoes receptive relaxation to accommodate stool until defecation takes place.

Fecal continence implies deferment of stool and gas elimination until socially acceptable. Two sphincter muscles surround the anorectum: the internal and external anal sphincters. The internal sphincter consists of circular smooth muscle, and it is tonically contracted, maintaining the anal canal closed. As the rectum becomes distended, the internal sphincter relaxes and the external sphincter contracts until a voluntary increase in intra-abdominal pressure, in conjunction with a contraction of the levator muscle, produces the passage of stool through the anus.

III

Diagnostic Studies

Joel J. Roslyn, M.D., and Rolando H. Rolandelli, M.D.

Symptoms of colonic diseases include change in the caliber of the stool, diarrhea, constipation or obstipation, hematochezia, or rectal tenesmus or urgency. All patients in whom a diagnosis of colonic disease is being considered should undergo a complete physical examination including pelvic and rectal examinations. In patients with diarrhea, a stool sample should be examined for enteropathogens and for *Clostridium difficile* toxin. The differentiation between malabsorptive and secretory diarrhea can be done by calculating the osmolar gap from the measurement of electrolytes and osmolality in stool. The diagnosis of malabsorptive diarrhea can be further investigated by measurement of fecal fat. Blood assays for gastrin, vasoactive intestinal polypeptide (VIP), and other enterohormones should be obtained when the history and stool analysis suggest secretory diarrhea of endocrine origin. Liver function tests are obtained when liver metastases are suspected. Serial measurements of the carcinoembryonic antigen (CEA) are used to detect recurrences of colonic carcinoma following curative resections.

Plain radiographs and contrast studies of the colon continue to be invaluable diagnostic methods in the assessment of patients with suspected obstruction or mucosal lesions. A colonic transit time can be calculated by obtaining plain films of the abdomen 4 and 6 days following the ingestion of radiopaque markers. This study also assesses severity and locates segmental defects versus global inertia. Cinedefecography involves instilling contrast media into the rectum and recording the act of defecation with static radiographs and videofluoroscopy. The static radiographs demonstrate the relationships of the anorectum to bony landmarks during defecation. Videofluoroscopy may disclose very subtle and transient abnormalities such as rectal intussusception that can be missed in static radiographs. Computed tomographic (CT) scans and magnetic resonance imaging (MRI) are helpful in assessing the resectability of rectal tumors and the involvement of contiguous organs and the liver in malignant processes.

Endoscopic evaluation of the colon remains the most important technique in the accurate diagnosis of colonic disease, especially carcinoma. The anoscope or proctoscope is invaluable for the assessment of internal hemorrhoids and rectal tumors that are within 8 to 10 cm. of the anal verge. Anoscopy is usually painless unless the patient has an anal fissure,

---

See the corresponding chapter or part in the *Textbook of Surgery*, 15th edition, pp. 977–979, for a more detailed discussion of this topic, including a comprehensive list of references.

thrombosed external hemorrhoids, or the anoscope is introduced forcefully. Rigid sigmoidoscopy allows visualization of the distal 20 to 25 cm. of the colon. Flexible sigmoidoscopy can reach as far as the splenic flexure or 45 cm. Colonoscopy provides an examination of the entire colon and even the terminal ileum. Endoscopies are not only diagnostic but also can be therapeutic by producing hemostasis of bleeding sites, removing foreign bodies, and excising polyps.

Anorectal manometry registers internal and external sphincter pressures and the presence of the anorectal inhibitory reflex, which is particularly useful in assessing patients with fecal incontinence. Electromyography records the action potentials derived from the different muscles involved in defecation through endoscopically placed mucosal electrodes along the colon. In patients with paradoxical pelvic floor contraction, the pubis rectalis muscle remains contracted during defecation.

IV

Intestinal Antisepsis

Rolando H. Rolandelli, M.D., and Joel J. Roslyn, M.D.

The human colon is the site of more than 400 bacterial species in concentrations that approach 10^{12} colony-forming units per ml. The typical microorganisms found in the colon are *Bacteroides*, *Bifidobacterium*, and *Eubacterium*. While the colonic microflora are an integral part of the colonic physiology, luminal bacteria become a threat during colonic surgery. The rate of wound infection in patients undergoing colonic procedures who have not received appropriate preparation may be as high as 75%.

To reduce the bulk of feces and bacteria within the colon, patients undergo mechanical cleansing and intestinal antisepsis prior to surgery. Mechanical cleansing is presently accomplished by drinking of 1 gal. of a polyethylene glycol solution that also contains electrolytes to compensate for the ensuing losses. Intestinal antisepsis is performed by the administration of antibiotics.

In 1973, Nichols and associates demonstrated the benefit of orally administered nonabsorbable antibiotics in combination with mechanical cleansing. The findings of this study were confirmed several years later in a prospective, randomized, multi-institutional trial. In a study of over 1000 patients undergoing colonic surgery, there was no significant benefit from the

See the corresponding chapter or part in the *Textbook of Surgery*, 15th edition, pp. 979–982, for a more detailed discussion of this topic, including a comprehensive list of references.

addition of parenteral antibiotic prophylaxis to an appropriate mechanical preparation with oral nonabsorbed antimicrobial agents. A large number of studies have subsequently attempted to identify the ideal agents for either oral antimicrobial therapy or parenteral administration. There are certain characteristics that any ideal prophylactic antibiotic regimen, whether oral or parenteral, should include. The regimen selected should provide broad suppression of fecal flora with high activity against aerobic and anaerobic organisms. Toxicity should be minimal, and there should be no emergence of resistant organisms. Additionally, a single agent is preferable to multiple drugs, there should be a short term of administration, and the drugs should be cost-effective. Orally administered neomycin and erythromycin base or metronidazole have become the most common agents used for oral antibiotic preparation. These agents are generally administered at 1:00 P.M., 2:00 P.M., and 11:00 P.M. the day before operation. It was thought initially that absorption of these drugs was not desirable. It is now thought that increased tissue levels of the drug at sites distant from the colon aid the normal host resistance mechanisms when contamination of the wound occurs.

Appropriate regimens for parenteral antibiotics should include agents that have considerable activity against aerobes and anaerobes. Several investigators have reviewed multiple-drug regimens, including aminoglycosides and metronidazole or clindamycin, rather than single-agent regimens. In recent years, the second-generation cephalosporins have gained considerable popularity as useful agents for antimicrobial prophylaxis. However, these combinations or single agents are not effective against group D streptococci (enterococci). More recent studies have compared the third-generation cephalosporins used as a single dose compared with multiple-dose administration of the second-generation cephalosporins.

V

Diverticular Disease of the Colon
Anthony L. Imbembo, M.D.

The prevalence of diverticular disease of the colon is estimated to be less than 5% at age 40, increasing to as high as 65% by age 85. Males and females appear to be affected equally. Diverticular disease is much more common in the United States and western Europe than in less industrialized regions such as Africa, South America, and Asia.

See the corresponding chapter or part in the *Textbook of Surgery*, 15th edition, pp. 982–993, for a more detailed discussion of this topic, including a comprehensive list of references.

Clinical studies have implicated low-fiber diets as a prominent etiologic factor. Diets lacking vegetable fiber are presumed to predispose to the development of diverticula by altering colonic motility. There is evidence that patients with diverticular disease manifest exaggerated contractile responses to feeding and hormonal stimuli. These abnormal muscular contractions are believed to result in increases in intraluminal pressures with resultant smooth muscle hypertrophy and the formation of diverticula. Decreased tensile strength of the colonic wall may be a contributing factor.

ANATOMIC FEATURES

Diverticula form at so-called weak points where the nutrient blood vessels (vasa recta) penetrate the circular muscle layer en route to the mucosa. These "perforating" vessels tend to penetrate the colonic wall along the mesenteric border of the two antimesenteric taeniae. It is estimated that 90% to 95% of patients with diverticulosis will have involvement of the sigmoid colon and 65% of patients will have disease limited to the sigmoid colon alone. Conversely, only 2% to 10% of patients will have disease confined to the ascending or transverse colon.

NATURAL HISTORY

Only 10% to 25% of patients will ever develop symptoms of diverticulitis. An overall mortality of less than 5% follows an initial attack of diverticulitis. Almost one third of patients may experience recurrence of diverticulitis within 3 to 5 years. Another 30% to 40% will suffer from intermittent abdominal pain, while the remainder can be expected to remain symptom-free. Only 30% of patients will demonstrate radiologic evidence of progression of their disease, in the form of either an increased number of diverticula or involvement of other segments of the colon. Progression of disease following resection also is unusual, occurring in less than 10% to 15% of patients.

COMPLICATIONS OF DIVERTICULOSIS

Hemorrhage

Bleeding can be expected to develop in 15% of patients with diverticulosis, and diverticular disease accounts for 30% to 50% of massive colonic bleeding. Diverticular hemorrhage arises from the right colon in 70% to 90% of patients, and 70% of patients with diverticular hemorrhage stop bleeding spontaneously. The risk of rebleeding is only 30% but increases to 50% in patients who have suffered a second episode of hemorrhage. Diverticular hemorrhage is thought to result from injury and subsequent rupture of blood vessels lying adjacent to a diverticulum. Most patients with diverticular hemorrhage present with self-limited, relatively minor bleeding. One third of patients with diverticular hemorrhage present with massive, exsanguinating hemorrhage. Abdominal pain secondary to active diverticulitis is extremely uncommon during a bleeding episode. A 10% to 20% morbidity and mortality is associated with massive diverticular hemorrhage.

DIAGNOSIS. The first step in the management of any patient with massive gastrointestinal hemorrhage is resuscitation. All patients should then undergo proctoscopy to exclude the rectum as the bleeding source. Patients who stop bleeding spontaneously should undergo elective evaluation, whereas continued massive bleeding is an indication for emergent operation. In actively bleeding patients who maintain relative hemodynamic stability, attempts at localization, either by selective mesenteric arteriography, radioisotope scanning, or colonoscopy, should be made. Emergent selective mesenteric arteriography will identify the site of hemorrhage successfully in 40% to 60% of patients. In order for arteriography to be diagnostic, bleeding must be taking place at a minimal rate of 0.5 ml. per minute.

TREATMENT. About 15% of all patients presenting with massive diverticular hemorrhage will require emergency surgery before further diagnostic information can be obtained. Their mortality approaches 30% to 50%. In patients with an identifiable site of bleeding, selective intra-arterial infusion of vasopressin may control hemorrhage in over 90% of cases. Vasopressin treatment is associated with a 50% rate of rebleeding. Diverticular hemorrhage is usually not amenable to endoscopic therapy.

Indications for emergent operation include persistent hemodynamic instability, a large transfusion requirement, and recurrent hemorrhage. If the bleeding site has been identified, a segmental resection can be performed with control in 90% of patients. Segmental resection should not be performed when the site of hemorrhage has not been identified, since the rebleed rate is 35% to 50% and the resultant mortality is about 30%. Total abdominal colectomy with ileoproctostomy is the preferred treatment when preoperative localization has been unsuccessful.

Diverticulitis

The term *diverticulitis* refers to inflammation of one or more diverticula and represents, at an anatomic level, perforation of a diverticulum into the pericolic space. Unfortunately, a clear distinction between diverticulitis and painful colonic spasm is often difficult. Diverticulitis ultimately will develop in 15% to 20% of patients with diverticulosis. Inflammation is limited to the sigmoid colon in over 90% of cases. Isolated right-sided diverticular inflammation occurs in only 5% of patients with diverticulitis. The inflammatory process is usually walled off by pericolic fat and mesentery. Involvement of other abdominal organs in this walling-off process may lead to intestinal obstruction or fistulization. A contained perforation may result in intra-abdominal abscess formation, while generalized peritonitis may occur if a perforation is not well contained.

CLINICAL FEATURES. Patients with diverticulitis usually manifest signs and symptoms of ongoing inflammation, such as progressive left lower quadrant pain (70%), anorexia, nausea and vomiting (20%), diarrhea (30%), low-grade fever, and urinary tract symptoms (15%). The pain is usually present for several days prior to presentation, unlike other acute surgical conditions, such as appendicitis or perforated peptic ulcer, which typically are more rapidly progressive. A tender abdominal mass is found in 20% of patients, and its presence portends a worse prognosis. Physical findings are consistent with localized peritonitis.

DIAGNOSIS. Most patients can be diagnosed on the basis of their clinical presentation. However, confirmation of the diagnosis is of importance. Routine abdominal x-rays are helpful in excluding other acute surgical problems such as intestinal obstruction or a perforated viscus. Contrast radiography or colonoscopy may lead to free rupture of a previously well-localized peridiverticular abscess and therefore should be undertaken with extreme caution in patients with suspected acute diverticulitis. Computed tomography (CT) has been shown to be as accurate as barium enema in diagnosing diverticulitis and therefore has substantially reduced the use of contrast studies. CT will demonstrate pericolic inflammation, bowel wall edema, abscess formation, and even fistulization, in 63% to 95% of patients. Elective evaluation of a patient following resolution of diverticulitis should include colonoscopy, barium enema, or both.

TREATMENT. Most patients require hospitalization. Therapy consists of bowel rest, intravenous antibiotics, and fluid resuscitation. The antibiotic regimen should provide coverage of normal colonic flora. Therefore, cefoxitin or the combination of an aminoglycoside with either clindamycin or metronidazole often is prescribed. With resolution, patients should be placed on a high-fiber diet. Barium enema or colonoscopy should be scheduled within several weeks of the acute episode to confirm and define the extent of disease.

Patients who fail to respond or deteriorate within the first 24 to 48 hours usually require urgent surgical treatment. Occasionally, patients who are known to have a diverticular abscess can be stabilized temporarily by percutaneous CT-guided drainage. This may permit adequate resuscitation of a critically ill patient. Such drainage should never be construed as definitive treatment. Approximately 20% of patients who develop acute diverticulitis will eventually require surgery. Following a second attack, the incidence of complications approaches 50% to 60%, with a mortality rate that is twice that associated with an initial attack. Recurrence of acute diverticulitis warrants surgical resection once active inflammation has subsided.

SURGICAL OPTIONS. Patients undergoing elective surgery are best served by resection of the involved segment and primary anastomosis. Bowel preparation usually has been possible, and antibiotics (both systemic and oral) can be administered safely and easily. The mortality for elective colon resection after the resolution of inflammatory diverticular disease should be less than 2%.

In patients with fulminant disease, bowel preparation is not usually possible. Therefore, a two-stage procedure consisting of colonic resection with colostomy initially, followed by colostomy closure 3 months later, is required.

Sequelae of Diverticulitis

The distribution of the various complications of diverticulitis in patients requiring surgery is abscess formation (40% to 50%), intestinal obstruction (10% to 30%), free perforation (10% to 15%), and fistulization (4% to 10%). Each of these conditions may coexist in any given patient. Complications develop in up to 25% of patients with active diverticulitis, and surgical intervention is necessary in almost all such instances.

VI

Benign Neoplasms of the Colon, Including Vascular Malformations
Anthony L. Imbembo, M.D., and Alan T. Lefor, M.D.

A polyp is a discrete tissue mass that protrudes into the bowel lumen. They are generally acquired lesions and are defined by their size, shape, number, and histology. Polyps may be responsible for gastrointestinal bleeding and can cause obstruction by a variety of mechanisms. Recent data support the contention that most carcinomas of the colon and rectum begin as neoplastic adenomatous polyps.

SUBMUCOSAL LESIONS. The various submucosal lesions include carcinoid tumors, lymphoid polyps, lipomas, metastatic lesions, and pneumatosis cystoides intestinalis. Endoscopic biopsy usually reveals normal mucosa; excision is usually required if a specific diagnosis is indicated.

NONNEOPLASTIC MUCOSAL LESIONS. These include hyperplastic polyps, juvenile polyps, and inflammatory polyps. Hyperplastic polyps are small lesions in the distal colon, most common in older patients. They do not have malignant potential. Inflammatory polyps are a response to colonic injury and are commonly associated with ulcerative colitis. Juvenile polyps are hamartomas that have no malignant potential and vary greatly in size, some being as large as 20 mm. They commonly present with hematochezia.

NEOPLASTIC MUCOSAL LESIONS. There are three major types, classified by histologic appearance: tubular ade-

---

See the corresponding chapter or part in the *Textbook of Surgery*, 15th edition, pp. 993–1001, for a more detailed discussion of this topic, including a comprehensive list of references.

nomas, tubulovillous adenomas, and villous adenomas. Tubular adenomas are the most common type, comprising 60% to 80% of benign neoplasms of the colon. They may be pedunculated (on a stalk) or sessile (broad-based). The likelihood of any neoplastic polyp containing malignancy is related to its size and histologic type. Of tubular adenomas, only 5% are malignant. Villous adenoma is the most common type seen in polyps greater than 20 mm. in size and is the most likely to be malignant. The tubulovillous adenomas have an intermediate malignant risk.

MOLECULAR BIOLOGY. There is excellent evidence that most carcinomas of the colon begin as neoplastic benign polyps. The changes leading to malignancy are believed to be multiple, no one of which alone results in malignancy. Several of the specific genetic defects have been identified. An early event is the loss of tumor suppressor gene function at the familial adenomatous polyposis locus on chromosome 5q, called the *APC* gene. The *K-ras* oncogene is activated as an intermediate step, and later steps include mutations of the *DCC* (deleted in colon cancer) and *p53* genes. A recent study demonstrated that colonoscopic polypectomy does in fact reduce the incidence of malignancy, thus justifying an aggressive approach to excision. Patients in whom the polyp cannot be resected completely endoscopically usually require surgical resection.

FAMILIAL POLYPOSIS SYNDROMES. There are a number of inherited adenomatous polyposis syndromes, including familial adenomatous polyposis (FAP), Gardner's syndrome, and Turcot's syndrome. Patients with FAP invariably develop malignancies and therefore require resection, usually at the time of diagnosis. While total proctocolectomy with ileostomy is curative, the ileostomy is not well accepted by some patients. Therefore, total colectomy with ileorectal anastomosis and ileoanal pull-through with rectal mucosectomy are more desirable alternatives. Patients undergoing ileorectal anastomoses require intensive follow-up, since tumors can develop in the residual rectal mucosa.

The Cronkhite-Canada syndrome is a noninherited hamartomatous polyposis syndrome, which is characterized by diffuse polyposis, dystrophy of the fingernails, alopecia, cutaneous hyperpigmentation, diarrhea, weight loss, abdominal pain, and complications of malnutrition. There is a progressive malabsorption syndrome. Inherited familial hamartomatous polyposis syndromes include neurofibromatosis, Peutz-Jeghers syndrome (mucocutaneous pigmentation and gastrointestinal polyposis), and juvenile polyposis. Unlike FAP, patients with juvenile polyposis have symptoms in childhood and generally bleed or obstruct, necessitating resection.

VASCULAR MALFORMATIONS. Angiodysplasia is due to the formation of small arteriovenous shunts, most commonly presenting as hematochezia. Angiodysplasia is responsible for about 6% of all lower gastrointestinal hemorrhages. It is most common in the right colon. Hemangiomas are much less common than angiodysplasia, occurring most commonly in the rectum. Kaposi's sarcoma lesions are considered hemangiomas. Mesenteric varices secondary to portal hypertension and telangiectasias are other types of vascular malformations in the large intestine.

VII

Ulcerative Colitis

James M. Becker, M.D., and Frank G. Moody, M.D.

Chronic ulcerative colitis is a diffuse inflammatory disease of the mucosal lining of the colon and rectum. The disease is characterized by bloody diarrhea that exacerbates and abates without apparent cause and without a clearly identified etiologic agent or specific medical therapy. Total removal of the colon and rectum provides a complete cure. Surgical alternatives developed over the last 15 years have eliminated the need for a permanent ileostomy following definitive resection of the involved colon and rectum.

The cause of ulcerative colitis remains unknown despite intensive work by many investigators. The examination of bacterial and viral agents continues to be an area of considerable activity, although there is uncertainty as to the fundamental role that infectious agents have in the primary pathogenesis of ulcerative colitis. Genetic factors appear to have an important role, since most studies have demonstrated that ulcerative colitis is two to four times more common in Jewish than in non-Jewish white populations and is approximately 50% less frequent in nonwhite than in white populations. In addition, there is a 10% to 15% greater frequency of ulcerative colitis in family members of patients with confirmed ulcerative colitis. Psychological factors may have a role in exacerbations of the disease but are not of primary importance in the pathogenesis of the disorder.

There has been considerable speculation that ulcerative colitis is an autoimmune disease. A number of immunologic studies have supported this concept, and there is currently much interest in the role of cytokines and immunoregulatory molecules in control of the immune response in patients with inflammatory bowel disease. Other studies have suggested that ulcerative colitis represents an energy-deficient disease of the colonic epithelium. It also has been suggested that there might be alterations in colonic mucosal glycoprotein composition in patients with ulcerative colitis. Over the last decade, animal models of intestinal inflammation have substantially augmented our understanding of the pathogenesis of ulcerative colitis, particularly in the areas of inflammatory mediators

See the corresponding chapter or part in the *Textbook of Surgery,* 15th edition, pp. 1001–1015, for a more detailed discussion of this topic, including a comprehensive list of references.

and cytokine regulation, genetic susceptibility, and the influence of ubiquitous luminal bacterial constituents.

Ulcerative colitis, for the most part, is a disease confined to the mucosal and submucosal layers of the colonic wall. It is a continuous colonic disease with the rectum essentially always involved. This is in contradistinction to the transmural inflammatory changes found in Crohn's disease of the colon, in which all layers of the colonic wall may be involved in a granulomatous inflammatory process.

CLINICAL MANIFESTATIONS. Bloody diarrhea is the most common early symptom of ulcerative colitis. Occasionally, arthritis, iritis, hepatic dysfunction, skin lesions, or other systemic manifestations may be paramount. The disease presents as a chronic, relatively low-grade illness in most patients. In a small number of patients (15%), it has an acute and catastrophic fulminating course. Such patients present with frequent bloody bowel movements, high fever, and abdominal pain. Onset of the disease occurs in patients less than 15 years of age in approximately 15% of cases, and presentations over 40 years of age are not uncommon. The incidence of ulcerative colitis is 3.5 to 6.5 per 10^5 population, and the prevalence is 60 per 10^5.

Physical findings are directly related to the duration and presentation of the disease. Weight loss and pallor are usually present. In the active phase, the abdomen in the region of the colon is usually tender to palpation. During acute episodes or in the fulminant form of the disease, there may be signs of an acute abdomen accompanied by fever and decreased bowel sounds. It is also in these patients with toxic megacolon that abdominal distention may be identified.

Sigmoidoscopy is the first step in diagnosis, since ulcerative colitis involves the distal colon and rectum in 90% to 95% of patients. The mucosa of the rectum and sigmoid colon is erythematous and friable. Normal colonic vascular markings may be lost or the mucosa may be hyperemic, and the intracolonic haustra are thick and blunted. Superficial mucosal ulcerations are seen. In advanced disease, the areas of ulceration may surround areas of accumulated granulation tissue and edematous mucosa, which are termed *pseudopolyps*. The use of flexible sigmoidoscopy has improved diagnostic accuracy and patient acceptability. Colonoscopy may be useful in determining the extent and activity of the disease, particularly in patients in whom the diagnosis is unclear or if cancer is suspected.

A plain abdominal film shows colonic dilatation, which has been termed *toxic megacolon*, in approximately 3% to 5% of patients. Most frequently seen is dilatation of the transverse colon, although there may be free air within the peritoneal cavity from perforation of the diseased colon. Barium enema examination of the colon is useful in most patients, although potentially dangerous in those with toxic megacolon. Radiographic signs suggesting ulcerative colitis on barium enema include loss of haustral markings and irregularities of the colon wall, which represent small ulcerations. Later in the course of the disease, pseudopolyps may be identified. In long-standing chronic ulcerative colitis, the colon assumes the appearance of a rigid, contracted tube, the "lead pipe" appearance.

In all patients presenting for the first time, it is necessary to exclude infectious causes of the enterocolitis. Therefore, stool specimens must be obtained for smears and cultures to exclude colitis due to viruses, *Chlamydia,* bacterial pathogens, and parasites. It has become increasingly important to differentiate ulcerative colitis from Crohn's colitis. Crohn's disease of the colon, compared with ulcerative colitis, would be suggested by the findings of small bowel involvement, rectal sparing, absence or infrequency of gross bleeding, perianal disease, focal lesions, segmental distribution (skip lesions), asymmetric involvement, fistulization, granulomas or transmural involvement on biopsy, and the distinct endoscopic appearance.

MEDICAL MANAGEMENT. Patients who present with advanced signs of acute illness require hospitalization and supportive as well as specific therapy for associated metabolic and hematologic derangements. Because of the massive fluid and electrolyte loss per rectum, such patients usually present with metabolic acidosis, contracted extravascular volume, and prerenal azotemia. Intravenous potassium and blood transfusion are often needed. Symptoms of toxicity are treated by nasogastric suction, intravenous corticosteroids, antibiotics, and total parenteral nutrition.

Corticosteroids and immunosuppressive agents have both been demonstrated to be effective in the management of ulcerative colitis. These agents, however, are capable of producing significant side effects. Corticosteroids remain the mainstay of therapy during acute episodes. Between 40 and 60 mg. of prednisolone in a single daily dose is effective in most cases in inducing remission. Patients with more active disease or toxicity may require parenteral steroids in the form of hydrocortisone or methylprednisolone. Although steroids may be useful in controlling symptoms of patients with continuing activity, maintenance therapy with small-dose corticosteroids for patients with inactive disease have not been demonstrated to prevent relapse. Sulfasalazine has not been of significant value in treating patients with severe ulcerative colitis but may have a role in controlling acute exacerbations in patients with chronic disease. In an effort to eliminate the side effects associated with the sulfa carrier, newer forms of the drug, such as 5-ASA, have been developed and are available for clinical use either in topical or oral form. A number of immunosuppressive agents have been utilized for the management of ulcerative colitis, including azathioprine and 6-mercaptopurine. Cyclosporine, which has a more rapid onset of action, has been advocated for the treatment of severe, refractory acute ulcerative colitis. There is, however, significant theoretical risk of irreversible cyclosporine-associated nephropathy following treatment of ulcerative colitis with high doses of the drug, and severe infectious complications also may occur. Before immunosuppressive agents are prescribed, familiarity with the dosing, monitoring, toxicity, and possible induction of lymphoma or other malignancies associated with these drugs is mandatory. Although widely prescribed for both ulcerative colitis and Crohn's disease, metronidazole and other antibiotics are of no proven value in the treatment of inflammatory bowel disease.

INDICATIONS FOR SURGICAL TREATMENT. Common indications for surgical intervention include (1) massive unrelenting hemorrhage, (2) toxic megacolon with impending or frank perforation, (3) fulminating acute ulcerative colitis that is unresponsive to maximal medical therapy, (4) obstruction from strictures, and (5) suspicion or demonstration of colonic cancer. Surgical therapy is also recommended in children who fail to mature at an acceptable rate. For most patients with ulcerative colitis, a colectomy is performed when the disease enters an intractable, chronic phase and becomes a physical and social burden to the patient.

Acute perforation occurs infrequently, with the incidence directly related to both the severity of the initial episode and the extent of the bowel disease. Specifically, although the overall incidence of perforation during the first attack is less than 4%, if the attack is severe, the incidence rises to approximately 10%. If there is pancolitis, the perforation rate is approximately 15%, and if the attack is both severe and involves the entire colon, it increases to almost 20%. The site of perforation is most often in the sigmoid colon or splenic flexure. Perforation occurs usually in patients with toxic megacolon. This complication causes more deaths than does any other complication of ulcerative colitis.

Obstruction due to benign stricture formation occurs in approximately 10% of patients with ulcerative colitis, with one third of these occurring in the rectum. It is important that the obstructive lesions be differentiated from carcinoma by biopsy or excision and particular attention given to excluding Crohn's disease.

Massive hemorrhage is a rare complication of acute ulcerative colitis that occurs in fewer than 1% of patients. Prompt surgical intervention is indicated if transfusion of more than 3000 ml. of blood is required within 24 hours. It must be remembered that 50% of patients with acute colonic bleeding have toxic megacolon. Uncontrollable hemorrhage from the entire colorectal mucosa may be the one clear indication for an emergency total proctocolectomy. In selected cases, the rectum can be spared for a later sphincter-saving operation, with the realization that this may be a continued source of bleeding.

Toxic megacolon occurs in approximately 10% of patients with ulcerative colitis. If toxic colitis, with or without megacolon, does not improve within 48 hours, an emergency operation is indicated. The operation of choice in this setting is abdominal colectomy with Brooke ileostomy and Hartmann closure of the rectum. Emergency operation for acute toxic megacolon has a high operative morbidity and a mortality of 3% to 30%. The mortality appears to be higher following a total proctocolectomy than following abdominal (subtotal) colectomy. Subtotal colectomy also preserves the rectum, thus allowing subsequent mucosal proctectomy and ileoanal anastomosis.

Although recent studies have suggested that previous reports may have overestimated the risk of cancer in the adult population with ulcerative colitis, patients with this disease remain at a 10% to 20% risk of developing carcinoma within 20 years of the diagnosis of ulcerative colitis. Adenocarcinoma, in association with ulcerative colitis, is multicentric in 50% of cases. In addition, the cancers tend to be more infiltrated and more difficult to identify colonoscopically. These tumors are evenly distributed throughout the colon, with approximately 50% found proximal to the splenic flexure. The likelihood of carcinoma in patients with ulcerative colitis appears to relate to both the extent of colonic involvement and the duration of disease. Although it was held for some time that the carcinoma associated with ulcerative colitis was more aggressive than that of the general population, recent studies have demonstrated that the natural evolution of the cancer is probably the same in both groups. The question of timing of surgical therapy for cancer prophylaxis remains controversial. After 10 years of follow-up, prophylactic colectomy needs to be considered because of the accelerating risk of cancer. The role of colon or rectal biopsy in directing the timing of colectomy remains controversial. Patients followed more than 5 to 7 years should undergo an annual colonoscopy and multiple biopsies for detection of epithelial dysplasia. The end-point of endoscopic surveillance, however, remains controversial. Severe dysplasia on several biopsies is associated with cancer of the colon in up to half the patients and is a clear indication for colectomy. Recent studies also have suggested that even low-grade dysplasia, if unequivocal and unassociated with severe inflammation, should prompt colectomy. A number of studies have demonstrated that surveillance programs are associated with high false-negative and false-positive rates. In addition, to date no study has clearly documented that surveillance lowers the mortality from colorectal cancer associated with ulcerative colitis.

The relationship between systemic extracolonic manifestations of ulcerative colitis and colectomy is not entirely clear. Although arthritis and skin lesions respond to colectomy, ankylosing spondylitis and liver dysfunction or failure may not respond.

The most common indication for operation remains intractability. Elective operations for medically intractable ulcerative colitis include total proctocolectomy and Brooke ileostomy or continent ileostomy (Kock pouch), subtotal colectomy with ileostomy or ileorectal anastomosis, and colectomy with mucosal proctectomy and ileal pouch–anal anastomosis. Because of the availability of the sphincter-sparing operations, patients and their physicians are now electing surgical therapy for intractability earlier in the course of the disease. Criteria regarding timing of operation and indications for operation are therefore undergoing considerable revision.

SURGICAL MANAGEMENT. Since chronic ulcerative colitis is cured when the colon and rectum are removed, single-stage total proctocolectomy has until recently been the operation of choice for elective surgical treatment. Despite the fact that proctocolectomy eliminates the diseased mucosa and the risk of malignant transformation, it has remained controversial and poorly accepted by patients and their physicians. This is due primarily to the fact that a permanent abdominal ileostomy is required after standard proctocolectomy. Although most patients adjust to their ileostomy, a significant percentage have chronic appliance-related problems, and there are significant psychological and social implications of an ileostomy for young and active patients. Fortunately, a number of other surgical alternatives to total proctocolectomy and ileostomy are currently available.

Subtotal colectomy with ileorectal anastomosis has been employed as a compromise operation for ulcerative colitis for decades. The operation eliminates an abdominal stoma, and since the pelvic autonomic nerves are not disturbed, impotence and bladder dysfunction are not risks. The operation, however, does not eliminate the proctitis, and thus patients may have persistent, severe rectal disease and a poor functional result. In addition, there is a 15% to 20% risk of developing cancer in the rectal stump after many decades. Kock first proposed the concept of a continent ileostomy in 1969. In constructing the continent ileostomy, the colon and rectum are removed just as in proctocolectomy with a standard ileostomy. However, the creation of the ileostomy incorporates the concepts of an intestinal pouch or reservoir and a one-way valve at the abdominal wall. Patients can then empty the pouch by passing a tube through the valve into the pouch via the stoma. The pouch has the advantage that a definitive or curative procedure may be performed, and the majority of patients are continent. Nevertheless, at least 15% of patients are incontinent owing to failure of the nipple valve, and ultimately, 40% to 50% of patients may require reoperation for technical or anatomic complications. With the success of ileoanal anastomosis, the Kock pouch is being performed much less frequently. Continent ileostomy is currently most useful in patients who have already undergone total proctocolectomy and ileostomy and who strongly desire a continence-restoring operation or in patients who have failed ileoanal anastomosis.

In 1947, Ravitch and Sabiston proposed an anal sphincter–sparing operation that consisted of abdominal colectomy, mucosal proctectomy, and endorectal ileoanal pull-through and anastomosis. As initially proposed, the operation was performed by first resecting the abdominal colon in a standard manner. Rather than removing the entire rectum and anus, the disease-bearing mucosa of the rectum was dissected free and resected, preserving an intact rectal muscular cuff and anal sphincter mechanism. Continuity of the intestinal tract was re-established by extending the terminal ileum into the pelvis within the muscular tube and circumferentially suturing it to the anus. Potential advantages of this approach are elimination of all diseased mucosa; preservation of parasympathetic innervation to the bladder and genitalia, thus avoiding impotence; avoiding a permanent abdominal ileostomy; and preservation of the anorectal sphincter apparatus that is responsible for fecal continence. Despite these theoretical advantages, the operation was associated initially with a high complication rate and an unpredictable functional result and was performed on very few patients until the early 1980s.

Improved successes with the operation were noted, in part, because of a generalized advancement in perioperative and intraoperative surgical care but more specifically because of a number of technical improvements in the operation. Perhaps the most important modification of the operation was the creation of an ileal pouch or reservoir proximal to the ileoanal anastomosis. Several pouch configurations exist: J, S, and W. Studies comparing the functional results following ileoanal anastomosis, with and without an ileal reservoir, have found that 24-hour stool frequency was significantly reduced in patients with ileal pouches, particularly in the early postoperative period.

The selection of patients for this operation is key to a good result. Crohn's disease contraindicates the operation, although patients with indeterminant colitis do well after this operation. The patient must have a good anal sphincter for control of the semisolid stool, and this can be tested using anorectal manometric techniques. Anorectal sepsis precludes this operation. Obesity is a relative contraindication. Chronologic age of the patient may be a relative contraindication, but more important is the physiologic age and pre-existing continence. The functional results in most large series of patients undergoing ileoanal anastomosis have been encouraging. By providing an adequate intestinal reservoir and preserving nearly normal anal sphincter function, the operation provides anal continence and acceptable stool frequency. The number of bowel movements is four to nine daily, with an average of six. Nocturnal bowel movements occur one to two times nightly, with a mean of slightly more than one. Of greater importance are control and urgency of bowel movements, which are variable, depending on the time after operation. Daytime incontinence is extremely uncommon, although nocturnal leakage occurs in 10% to 50% of patients. Improvement of these factors continues for more than 2 years after operation. In an effort to control stool output, patients are placed on loperamide hydrochloride, a synthetic opioid antidiarrheal agent, a high-fiber diet, and supplementary fiber in the form of psyllium or methylcellulose.

Although results with mucosal proctectomy and ileal pouch–anal anastomosis have been excellent, divergent points of view have arisen regarding the operative technique and its effect on anal physiology and functional result. Some surgeons have advocated an alternative approach to conventional endoanal rectal mucosal resection that eliminates distal mucosal proctectomy altogether. Instead, the distal rectum is divided near the pelvic floor, leaving the anal canal largely intact. The ileal pouch is then stapled to the top of the anal canal. The rationale for this approach is that by preserving the mucosa of the anal transition zone, the anatomic integrity of the anal canal would be preserved and the rate of fecal incontinence improved. While several studies have suggested that patients have improved sensation and better functional results following preservation of the anal transition zone, this has not been documented by prospective study. The obvious concern is that by leaving disease-bearing mucosa in the anal canal, the patients are exposed to a lifelong risk of persistent or recurrent inflammatory disease as well the potential for malignant transformation. Until this technique is further evaluated, patients will require careful lifetime surveillance. Mucosectomy must be recommended in patients with rectal dysplasia, proximal rectal cancer, diffuse colonic dysplasia, and familial polyposis.

Mortality for elective surgical therapy for ulcerative colitis is 0% to 2%; for emergency operation, it is about 4% to 5%; and for toxic megacolon, it rises to 17%. A major complication in all reported series is sepsis, either in the wound or in the intra-abdominal cavity. The most common late complication of proctocolectomy with a Brooke or continent ileostomy or an ileoanal anastomosis is intestinal obstruction, which occurs in about 10% of patients. Other complications following proctocolectomy include delay in perineal closure, sexual dysfunction, and renal stones. The most frequent late complication in patients undergoing ileal pouch–anal anastomosis is ileal pouch dysfunction or pouchitis, which has been reported to occur in 10% to 50% of patients undergoing this procedure for ulcerative colitis. Pouchitis is an incompletely defined and poorly understood clinical syndrome consisting of increased stool frequency, watery stools, cramping, urgency, malaise, and fever. The etiology of this condition is unknown; speculations have included Crohn's disease, bacterial overgrowth or dysbiosis, either primary or secondary malabsorption, stasis, ischemia, and nutritional or immune deficiency. Fortunately, treatment with a short course of metronidazole is successful in most patients. All patients undergoing surgical therapy for ulcerative colitis benefit from support through ileostomy clubs, enterostomal therapists, and patient-oriented support groups.

Thus ulcerative colitis is a chronic inflammatory disease of the mucosa of the colon and rectum. It can be controlled effectively in most patients with diet, salicylates, steroids, and immunosuppressant agents. Eventually, a significant proportion of patients require operation, particularly if the inflammatory process involves the entire colon and rectum. Ulcerative colitis is cured if the colon and rectum are removed. In the past, definitive treatment required total proctocolectomy and permanent ileostomy. Currently, surgical alternatives that preserve continence but may be associated with distinct morbidity are available.

VIII

Volvulus of the Colon

Anthony L. Imbembo, M.D., and Karl A. Zucker, M.D.

Volvulus is the abnormal twisting or rotation of a portion of the bowel about its mesentery. This may result in occlusion of the lumen at each end of the segment with resultant obstruction and/or vascular compromise. The sigmoid colon, cecum or right colon, transverse colon, or splenic flexure may be involved. Colonic volvulus generally occurs in the setting of a dilated redundant colonic segment with a narrow mesenteric base. The redundant segment is freely mobile while the points of fixation are quite close, serving as a fulcrum for development of volvulus or twisting of that segment of bowel. These features may be acquired, as in sigmoid volvulus, or congenital in origin, as is likely with cecal volvulus. Left untreated, volvulus generally progresses rapidly from colonic obstruction to strangulation and gangrene.

Volvulus is an uncommon cause of obstruction in English-speaking countries, accounting for only 1% to 3% of all admissions for bowel obstruction. It remains, however, a major health problem in parts of eastern Europe, Iran, India, and Africa, where volvulus may constitute the most common cause of intestinal obstruction.

SIGMOID VOLVULUS

Approximately three quarters of all cases of large bowel volvulus involve the sigmoid colon. The age and sex distributions of patients with sigmoid volvulus appear to have two distinct patterns. Patients in Iran, Africa, and eastern Europe are predominantly middle-aged males (mean age 40 to 50 years), where the pathogenesis has been ascribed to an acquired redundancy of sigmoid colon secondary to high-residue diets. In the United States, Australia, the United Kingdom, and Canada, sigmoid volvulus occurs in elderly individuals (mean age 60 to 70 years) of either sex, with almost all patients reporting a long history of disordered bowel habits. Many patients are referred from chronic care facilities with disorders such as Parkinson's disease, Alzheimer's disease, multiple sclerosis, paralysis, chronic schizophrenia, pseudobulbar palsy, and senility. The usual bedridden state of these patients and the use of various neuropsychotropic drugs are both known to alter bowel motility. Acute sigmoid volvulus generally presents with the sudden onset of severe, colicky abdominal pain, obstipation, and ab-

---

See the corresponding chapter or part in the *Textbook of Surgery*, 15th edition, pp. 1015–1020, for a more detailed discussion of this topic, including a comprehensive list of references.

dominal distention. Generalized abdominal pain, tenderness, fever, and hypovolemia suggest that strangulation has already occurred. Occasionally, patients present with a history of intermittent pain and distention consistent with chronic recurrent volvulus.

Plain abdominal radiographs often reveal a dilated colon forming the so-called bent inner tube or omega-loop sign. The convexity of the loop points toward the right upper quadrant, or away from the point of obstruction. Barium enema is usually not required for diagnosis and is contraindicated whenever strangulation is suspected.

Initial treatment of sigmoid volvulus consists of attempted nonoperative reduction, which is successful in 70% to 80% of patients. Successful detorsion permits deferral of surgery in acutely ill patients with unprepared bowel. The most widely used nonoperative procedure for reduction of sigmoid volvulus is the combination of proctoscopy and rectal tube placement. Following successful nonoperative reduction of a sigmoid volvulus, delayed sigmoid colonic resection with appropriate bowel preparation is recommended for most patients. In such a setting, primary anastomosis may be performed safely. In patients who fail nonoperative reduction, the appropriate surgical approach is less clear. Proximal colostomy alone is contraindicated, since this procedure will not prevent strangulation of the segment or recurrent volvulus. Operative detorsion alone is associated with up to a 40% recurrence. Other procedures that have been used include tube sigmoidostomy, extraperitonealization of the sigmoid colon, sigmoidopexy, and resection with end-colostomy (with or without mucous fistula). Unfortunately, there is insufficient experience reported to evaluate the efficacy of these procedures. If gangrene is present at the time of laparotomy, immediate resection is indicated, with end-colostomy and mucous fistula or Hartmann's pouch.

CECAL VOLVULUS

Cecal volvulus accounts for 20% to 40% of all cases of colonic volvulus. Approximately 90% of patients with cecal volvulus have an axial twist of a segment of the proximal colon or even the entire right colon, while in the remainder there is a cephalad fold of the cecum across the ascending colon (cecal bascule). A mobile cecum is a prerequisite for the development of a cecal volvulus. As many as one half to two thirds of these patients have undergone previous abdominal surgical procedures. Colonic distention resulting from distal obstruction also has been implicated in the development of cecal volvulus and should be excluded.

Cecal volvulus presents with the acute onset of severe, colicky pain, nausea, vomiting, and obstipation along with a compressible mass extending from the right lower quadrant to the midabdominal region. Abdominal x-rays reveal marked distention of the cecum, while barium enema may show the narrowing of bowel lumen accompanying the twisting of the colon ("bird's neck" deformity). Nonoperative techniques for the reduction of cecal volvulus have been much less successful than for sigmoid volvulus. Approximately 25% of patients are found to have gangrenous changes at the time of laparotomy, and the mortality in this setting approaches 40%. Therefore, once the diagnosis of cecal volvulus has been made, prompt surgical intervention is advised. When the cecum is gangrenous, resection is mandatory, usually with ileotransverse colostomy. However, in the setting of viable bowel, the procedure of choice is again less clear. Right hemicolectomy is recommended in many institutions. Perhaps the best of the other options is detorsion with cecopexy.

IX

Carcinoma of the Colon, Rectum, and Anus
H. Kim Lyerly, M.D.

NONNEOPLASTIC POLYPS

An intestinal *hamartoma* is a localized overgrowth of normal mature intestinal epithelial cells, which is usually pedunculated, the stalk being lined with normal mucosa. *Peutz-Jeghers syndrome* is an autosomal dominant condition in which numerous hamartomatous polyps are present throughout the gastrointestinal tract, including the small intestine, large intestine, and stomach. Over 95% of patients with Peutz-Jeghers syndrome also have a brownish pigmentation of their lips, buccal surfaces, periocular skin, and perianal regions. *Cowden's disease* is an autosomal dominant condition consisting of multiple intestinal hamartomas. *Juvenile or retention polyps* occur mainly in children and are hamartomatous epithelial retentions composed of cystically dilated glands filled with mucous and inflammatory debris. *Inflammatory polyps* are usually multiple and are associated with ulcerative colitis and Crohn's disease. *Hyperplastic polyps* are the most common small benign tumors of the colon. They are the product of excessive replication of the mucosal epithelium resulting in small sessile mucosal elevations.

NEOPLASTIC POLYPS

Neoplastic or adenomatous polyps are relatively common in patients in the United States and may be either sporadic or

---

See the corresponding chapter or part in the *Textbook of Surgery*, 15th edition, pp. 1020–1032, for a more detailed discussion of this topic, including a comprehensive list of references.

associated with an inherited polyposis syndrome. Although the inherited forms of polyps occur in young patients, there is an increase in incidence of the sporadic type with advancing age, with adenomatous polyps being most common in patients older than 60 years of age. These polyps may be classified histologically as tubular or villous depending on the glandular pattern. Patients with the inherited forms of adenomatous polyps or polyposis have an extremely high rate of colorectal carcinoma. Adenomatous polyps are therefore considered premalignant, and the majority, if not all, of colorectal carcinomas are thought to arise from these polyps, in a succession of events termed the *adenoma carcinoma sequence.*

Colorectal adenomas tend to grow slowly and continuously, and a polyp may take 10 years to double in size. Adenomas may be sessile (flat) or pedunculated (long stalked). Although polyps may cause symptoms related to blood loss from an ulcerated surface, they are most frequently occult and are detected by barium enema or proctosigmoidoscopy or colonoscopy. Adenomas rarely may result in hemorrhage or diarrhea, although villous adenomas sometimes may produce a mucoid diarrhea with resultant hypokalemic alkalosis. Villous adenomas also may produce an excessive secretion of mucus with loss of protein, which rarely causes hypoalbuminemia. Very large polyps may cause abdominal pain from partial intestinal obstruction or may be the lead point in colonic intussusception in an adult.

Removal of all colorectal adenomatous polyps is recommended. Pedunculated polyps may be excised by endoscopic snare cautery. With large polyps with a high risk of malignant change, such as a large villous adenoma, a segmental colectomy often is indicated. Following endoscopic polypectomy, the patient should have routine colonoscopic surveillance to detect new or additional lesions, since about 40% of patients will have another adenoma at follow-up.

COLORECTAL MALIGNANCIES

Several factors are associated with an increase in the incidence of colorectal malignancies and include familial polyposis and ulcerative colitis. Screening tools of asymptomatic patients involve digital rectal examination, routine stool guaiac testing, proctosigmoidoscopy or pancolonoscopy, and barium enema with air contrast studies.

The clinical features of colorectal carcinomas are related to the tumor size and location. Some 70% to 80% of these lesions are located below the middle descending colon. Tumors in this location are often infiltrating or annular and may cause obstructive symptoms, changes in bowel habits, or bleeding. Due to the semisolid or solid contents and the small diameter in this location, gas pains, a decrease in caliber of the stool, and the use of laxatives are common symptoms. In the right colon, large, bulky tumors are more common, due perhaps to the wide diameter of the colon and its liquid contents, which allow growth into the lumen without symptoms of obstruction. Patients may complain of abdominal pain that may be confused with gallbladder or peptic ulcer disease or may have bleeding, weight loss, or anemia.

The diagnosis of colorectal carcinomas requires a high index of suspicion. Proctosigmoidoscopy is an important diagnostic tool in the symptomatic patient, and colonoscopy is used frequently to evaluate all patients with symptoms or occult fecal blood. Barium enema with air contrast usually detects all colonic lesions that are at least 5 mm. in diameter.

Carcinoma of the colon and rectum extends by six routes: intramucosal extension, direct invasion of adjacent structures, lymphatic spread, hematogenous spread, intraperitoneal spread, and anastomotic implantation. The modes and routes of spread must be considered in deciding on the appropriate surgical extirpation to provide the highest cure rate and to appropriately stage the patient. Excision of the primary lesion must be accompanied by adequate margins of normal tissue and the draining lymphatics. Almost 90% of patients have tumors that can be resected completely, and the mortality ranges from 2% to 10%. The critical determinant of success is the degree to which the tumor has spread at the time of operation. The principles of surgical resection include excision of the primary lesion with adequate margins, restoration of continuity of the intestine, and maintenance of function whenever possible with minimal morbidity and mortality. Inadequate resection close to the macroscopic tumor border, tumor inoculation into the anastamotic region, and spread of tumor cells within the operative field are examples of common technical maneuvers that result in suboptimal outcomes.

The exact surgical procedure depends on location of the tumor in the colon. Preoperatively, the patient undergoes bowel preparation. Wide margins surrounding the primary tumor must be removed with an *en bloc* resection of the draining lymphatics. This need to remove the draining lymphatics necessitates interruption of blood supply to a region of the colon, since the lymphatic drainage parallels the blood supply.

The standard treatment of neoplasms of the cecum and ascending colon is right colectomy, which includes a segment of the terminal ileum, the cecum, and the right half of the transverse colon. The ileocolic vessels, right colic artery, and right branch of the midcolic artery, with mesentery including regional lymphatics, are resected. Carcinomas of the splenic flexure or descending colon are treated by excision of the distal transverse, descending, and sigmoid colon, together with the associated mesocolon excised to the aorta. For tumors of the sigmoid colon, the proximal resection can be limited, and the transverse colon need not necessarily be removed. For carcinomas in the upper rectum, an anterior resection and reanastomosis can be performed; however, preservation of the distal rectum to provide continence is extremely important, and a detailed discussion follows regarding the preservation of the rectum for mid and low rectal carcinomas.

In tumors involving the upper rectum, a low anterior colon resection (LAR) may be performed with a distal margin of 2 in. or 5 cm. In general, tumors within 7 to 8 cm. of the anal verge are treated by abdominal perineal resection (APR) with a permanent colostomy, whereas those greater than 12 cm. from the anal verge are adequately managed by LAR. Lesions lying between 7 and 11 cm. from the anal verge may be managed by either procedure, depending on the size of the lesion, the size of the pelvis, and the differentiation of the tumor. The use of circumferential stapling devices greatly facilitates the construction of the LAR. New combined-treatment modalities have allowed some surgeons to perform sphincter-sparing operations for rectal carcinomas that would have been managed previously by APR. These modalities include preoperative radiotherapy combined with chemotherapy. Several recent reports about the feasibility and safety of laparoscopic and laparoscopically assisted colectomy for malignant disease have appeared; however, issues such as compromised cancer control and complications have emerged when discussing the role of laparoscopic surgery in curative resections.

Both radiation therapy and chemotherapy have been used in the adjuvant setting following resection of colon cancer with high risks of recurrence. Radiation therapy has been used to minimize local regional recurrence.

Current recommendations for adjuvant therapy include adjuvant 5-FU and levamisole for Dukes C patients. However, ongoing and further trials are apt to modify these recommendations.

X

Disorders of the Anal Canal
Roger R. Dozois, M.D.

The anal canal extends from the anorectal ring to the hairy skin of the anal verge and can be the site of common benign disorders and rare malignant disease. The columnar epithelium of the proximal anal canal and of the mixed lining of the transition zone area is separated from the squamous epithelium of the distal anal canal by the corrugated dentate line. Its lining and musculature together with the pelvic floor structures contribute significantly to the regulation of defecation and maintenance of continence.

Complete prolapse of the rectum, which is of obscure etiology and is characterized by full-thickness extrusion of the rectum, is seen predominantly in women, in those with excessive straining, and in those with chronic mental disorders. It is likely due to the intussusception of the rectum and rectosig-

---

See the corresponding chapter or part in the *Textbook of Surgery,* 15th edition, pp. 1032–1044, for a more detailed discussion of this topic, including a comprehensive list of references.

moid. Surgical treatment includes transabdominal rectal fixation with or without sigmoidectomy in healthy patients and transperineal excision of intussusceptum in elderly, debilitated patients. Impaired continence may improve spontaneously in at least 50% of patients. If not, a postanal repair can be attempted 12 months later in incapacitated patients.

Hemorrhoids are specialized "cushions" in the left lateral, right anterior, and right posterior anal canal that normally aid in continence. Downward sliding of these cushions with straining and irregular bowel habits may lead to bright red bleeding with defecation and protrusion and even incarceration. Treatment may be conservative (diet, stool softener, rubber band ligation) for painless bleeding with or without reducible protrusion or surgical if protrusion requires manual reduction or the hemorrhoids are permanently prolapsed.

Fissure-in-ano is a linear ulcer, usually located in the posterior midline and quite painful on defecation. An external tag or sentinel pile and an enlarged anal papilla frequently are associated with the ulcer. If avoidance of constipation and local measures fail, a lateral internal sphincterotomy relieves the pain in most patients.

Anorectal suppurative disorders most often originate in the intersphincteric plane from infection of cryptoglandular structures. An intersphincteric abscess may cause severe pain. Vertical, downward extension results in a perineal abscess, while upward extension leads to an intermuscular abscess within the rectal wall or a supralevator abscess. If the intersphincteric suppurative process spreads horizontally across the external sphincter, an ischiorectal fossa abscess results in a red, tender, fluctuant mass. Finally, if the infectious process spreads circumferentially from one side to the other of the intersphincteric space, the supralevator space, or the ischiorectal fossa, a horseshoe abscess forms. Abscesses should be drained surgically. An intersphincteric abscess is drained by dividing the internal sphincter, while perianal and ischiorectal abscesses are drained through a skin incision. Horseshoe abscesses are drained through a posterior midline incision into the deep postanal space together with para-anal counterincisions.

Fistula-in-ano derives from sepsis originating in the anal canal glands at the dentate line. Most commonly, they track from the intersphincteric space into the ischiorectal fossa, directly to the perineal skin. In some instances, the process may track circumferentially from one fossa to the contralateral one to constitute a horseshoe fistula. Rarely, the track may extend in the intersphincteric plane over the puborectalis before taking a downward course through the ischiorectal fossa to the perineal skin (suprasphincteric). Finally, the track may be totally extrasphincteric, extending from the rectal wall, the levator ani, down to the perineal skin.

Treatment requires (1) accurate definition of the abnormal anatomy by gentle probing and fistulotomy, (2) drainage of the primary intersphincteric infection as well as primary and secondary tracts, and (3) close follow-up and local measures including sitz baths, irrigation, and packing to ensure healing from the depth of the wound to the surface. Suprasphincteric and extrasphincteric fistulas may require referral to colorectal specialists.

Crohn's disease of the anal area is characterized by large, edematous, purplish tags, skin ulcerations and excoriations, off-midline fissures, and complex abscesses/fistulas. Incontinence may result from the local disease or aggressive surgical procedures and loss of rectal compliance. While conservatism is paramount to avoid unwarranted complications, under-treating patients, especially those with pain due to abscess, should be avoided. Sphincterotomy and fissurectomy should be avoided.

Neoplasms of the anal area are rare and require a high degree of suspicion to diagnose. *Bowen's disease* is an *in situ* intraepithelial squamous cell carcinoma that appears as thickened, erythematous skin that can be confirmed by punch biopsies. Wide local excision with primary closure or advancement flaps is the treatment of choice. *Extramammary Paget's disease* of the anus is a rare intraepithelial adenocarcinoma with an underlying carcinoma in 50% to 85% of patients. The typical appearance is that of well-demarcated eczematoid plaques. Treatment consists of wide local excision for limited disease, abdominoperineal resection for those with underlying rectal adenocarcinoma, or combined chemoradiotherapy for associated epidermoid cancer of the anal canal. *Basal cell carcinoma* is very rare and may be difficult to differentiate from cloacogenic cancers arising in the transitional zone area. Most often, basal cell cancer can be treated by wide local excision. *Squamous cell carcinomas* that resemble other skin cancer in their behavior are treated by wide local excision if early and by abdominoperineal resection if locally advanced. *Verrucous carcinomas,* also referred to as *giant condyloma acuminatum,* are intermediate lesions between condyloma acuminatum and invasive squamous cell carcinomas and are large, soft, warty-like lesions caused by papillovirus. Their treatment includes wide local excision or abdominoperineal resection. *Epidermoid carcinoma* arising in the anal canal or in the transitional zone with squamous, basaloid, cloagenic, or mucoepidermoid epithelium has a similar behavior and is treated successfully in most instances by chemoradiation. *Melanoma* has a poor prognosis whether treated locally or radically. Other rare lesions include adenocarcinoma, leiomyosarcoma, and lymphoma.

Hidradenitis suppurativa is an inflammatory process affecting the apocrine sweat glands of the region that can follow multiple fistulas that communicate with the dentate line and is characterized by a purplish discoloration of the skin and drainage of watery pus. Treatment consists of unroofing sinuses in more limited disease and wide excision in more advanced disease.

Condyloma acuminatum or perianal warts that may involve the anus, perineum, and anal canal are caused by a papillomavirus. Their prevalence in the anorectal and anogenital regions points toward a sexual mode of transmission. If few lesions are present, podophyllin may suffice; when the lesions are extensive, electrocoagulation or laser therapy is effective for small lesions, and wide excision is necessary for larger lesions. Sexually transmitted diseases may involve the alimentary canal from mouth to anus and include colitis, proctitis, and ulcerations of the genital, perianal skin or anorectum. The offending agents may comprise amebiasis, giardiasis, shigellosis, *Neisseria gonorrhoeae, Chlamydia trachomatis, Treponema pallidum,* and herpes simplex virus type 2. Any mass should be biopsied to exclude Kaposi's sarcoma or other anal carcinoma. Disorders of the anorectum are common in AIDS, and treatment should focus on drainage, biopsy, fistulotomy, and local excision.

33

THE LIVER

I

Anatomy and Physiology
William C. Meyers, M.D., and Ravi S. Chari, M.D.

ANATOMY

The liver is the largest gland in the body, weighing approximately 1500 gm. in the adult and representing about one-fiftieth of the body weight. The liver conforms to the undersurface of the diaphragm, and its inferior surface is in contact with the duodenum, colon, kidney, adrenal gland, esophagus, and stomach. It is under the protection of the ribs.

Lobar Anatomy

The topographic lobes do not correspond to the true lobar anatomy. Distribution of the major branches of the veins, arteries, and bile ducts divides the liver into two relatively equal masses by a plane (the portal fissure) passing from the left side of the gallbladder fossa to the left side of the inferior vena cava, creating the right and left lobes. The left lobe consists of a medial segment lying to the right of the falciform ligament and a lateral segment to the left of the falciform ligament. The right lobe consists of an anterior and posterior segment, for which there is no visible superficial demarcation.

French Segmental System

Another nomenclature takes into greater consideration the hepatic venous drainage but also applies to the portal biliary and arterial anatomy. Instead of four, there are eight segments: four on the right, three on the left, and one corresponding to the caudate lobe. The three hepatic veins divide the liver into four sectors. The planes contain the right, middle, and left hepatic veins and are termed *portal scissurae*; the planes containing portal pedicles are termed *hepatic scissurae*. Segments, according to the French system, correspond generally to the subsegments described in the lobar anatomic classification.

Biliary System

The biliary ductal pattern becomes more variable distally. Basically, one duct drains each segment and joins into two

---

See the corresponding chapter or part in the *Textbook of Surgery*, 15th edition, pp. 1045–1046, for a more detailed discussion of this topic, including a comprehensive list of references.

main trunks. However, it is not uncommon to have three or even four relatively equally converging ducts into one confluence. The left hepatic duct joins the right at a much more anterior and acute angle, an anatomic consistency that becomes important during common duct exploration or cholangiography. The upper limit of the normal diameter of the common duct is controversial, although most references list 6 to 8 mm. except after cholecystectomy, when it may dilate. The gallbladder is a pear-shaped distensible appendage of the extrahepatic biliary system containing 30 to 50 ml. of bile. The valves of the cystic duct are extremely tortuous, sometimes making cholangiography difficult. The sphincter of Oddi has three principal parts: the sphincter of the choledochus, the pancreatic sphincter, and the ampullary sphincter. Knowledge concerning possible biliary variations is extremely important in avoidance of injury even in seemingly simple procedures such as cholecystectomy.

The liver acinar unit is a concept of microscopic masses of liver cells functionally situated around terminal portal venules. Blood flow is from the venules into the sinusoids coming into contact with hepatocytes until it drains into the terminal hepatic venules. Zones of hepatocytes have been divided arbitrarily into three sections, with Zone 1 being the area immediately adjacent to the portal venule and Zones 2 and 3 being farther away. Certain functions are readily explained by this concept, such as Zone 1 cells being the first to receive blood and oxygen and therefore the last to undergo necrosis.

PHYSIOLOGY

The liver is an amazingly dynamic organ, active in the uptake, storage, distribution, and disposition of various nutrients from the intestine or blood and responsible for the synthesis, transformation, and metabolism of many endogenous and exogenous subtrates.

The liver expends approximately 20% of the body's energy and consumes 20% to 25% of the total oxygen utilized despite constituting only 4% to 5% of the body weight. About 70% to 75% of the total hepatic blood flow is derived from the portal vein, and the remaining 25% to 30%, from the hepatic artery. There is a reciprocal increase in hepatic arterial flow in response to reduction in portal venous flow, but the converse does not occur. Approximately 1000 ml. of blood can be made available to the body by the liver in periods of stress. The portal and arterial systems converge in the sinusoidal bed, where the pressure remains remarkably constant and low. Deprivation of portal flow causes deterioration in hepatic structure and function marked pathologically by Zone 3 centrilobular hepatocyte atrophy and fatty infiltration.

Bile Formation

Bile formation is an active process relatively independent of total hepatic blood flow except during conditions simulating shock. There appears to be both a transcellular and a paracellular route for canalicular and ductular bile formation. The paracellular route is of lesser importance under physiologic conditions. Intraluminal receptors also likely play a role in bile formation.

The principal organic compounds in bile are the conjugated bile acids, cholesterol, phospholipid, bile pigments, and protein. Total unstimulated bile flow in a 70-kg. man has been estimated to be between 0.41 and 0.43 ml. per minute. Of this, 0.15 to 0.16 ml. per minute is bile acid–dependent flow, another 0.16 to 0.17 ml. per minute is bile acid–independent canalicular flow, and approximately 0.11 ml. per minute is from ductular secretion. Under physiologic conditions, total bile flow in 1 day is estimated to be 600 to 1000 ml. The total flow varies considerably depending on the presence or absence of various physiologic stimulants or inhibitors. The two most important factors in this variability in the surgical setting are the presence or absence of a fistula and fasting versus feeding.

Lymph Formation

Hepatic lymph collection transports large and small molecules, plasma protein, débris, bacteria, other foreign substances, and fluid. Lymph is 3% to 5% protein, mainly albumin, and its electrolyte composition estimates that of plasma. Greatly increased numbers of lymph channels are present in cirrhosis.

Enterohepatic Circulation

Bile salts are secreted into the biliary system and empty into the intestine, where they are efficiently reabsorbed into the portal circulation. The liver extracts the bile acids and transports them to the canalicular membrane, where they are resected into the biliary system. This process is referred to as the *enterohepatic circulation*. Total bile salt pool size in humans is 2 to 5 gm. and undergoes this circulation 2 to 3 times per meal and 6 to 10 times daily, depending on dietary habits. In addition, 0.2 to 0.6 gm. is lost per day in the stool, and this quantity is replaced by newly synthesized bile acids.

Bilirubin Metabolism

The primary breakdown product of heme, bilirubin, is excreted almost entirely in the bile. With hepatocellular disease or extrahepatic biliary obstruction, free bilirubin may accumulate in blood and tissues and cause toxic effects. A number of disorders of bilirubin metabolism have been described that vary from kernicterus, which is an extreme example of bilirubin toxicity occurring in children, to Gilbert's syndrome, which is benign.

Other Hepatocyte Functions

Hepatic protein synthesis and catabolism are vitally important, and measurement of these functions often provides a useful indication of the degree of liver impairment. Albumin is the most studied of the various proteins synthesized in the liver. Synthesis of this protein is influenced by nutrition, various hormones, and oncotic pressure. Much information is presently being accumulated on the genes expressed by the liver. A large number appear to be expressed primarily in the liver compared with other organs, such as albumin and tyrosine aminotransferase. The expression of various proteins has led to an appreciation of the heterogeneous functions of portions of the liver.

II

Pyogenic and Amebic Liver Abscess

Gene D. Branum, M.D., and William C. Meyers, M.D.

Abscess of the liver remains a challenging diagnostic and therapeutic problem for the clinician despite modern imaging techniques for diagnosis of the disorder, effective antibiotics, and a range of effective methods for drainage. Pyogenic (bacterial) and amebic organisms are the most common pathogens encountered, with bacteria the cause in 80% to 90% of the cases in the United States. Early diagnosis and treatment are critical in successful management of liver abscess.

PYOGENIC LIVER ABSCESS

INCIDENCE AND PATHOGENESIS. The incidence of pyogenic liver abscess is probably increasing, owing to the aggressive treatment of malignant disorders. The current estimate of prevalence is 13 to 22 patients per 10,000 hospital admissions. The pathophysiologic mechanism of liver abscess in general, or pyogenic abscess in particular, involves two basic elements: (1) the presence of the organism and (2) vulnerability of the liver. The spread of bacterial or other organisms to the hepatic parenchyma may occur via (1) the portal system, (2) ascension from the biliary tree, (3) the hepatic artery during generalized septicemia, (4) direct extension from subhepatic or subdiaphragmatic infection, or (5) a direct route

---

See the corresponding chapter or part in the *Textbook of Surgery,* 15th edition, pp. 1061–1068, for a more detailed discussion of this topic, including a comprehensive list of references.

as a result of trauma. Most organisms arise in the liver via the portal route, and hepatic clearance of portal bacteria is probably a common event in healthy individuals. Bacterial organisms superimposed on necrotic tissue, hepatic injury, malignant tumors, or acquired biliary or vascular obstruction, however, may cause multiplication, tissue invasion, and abscess formation.

Appendicitis was formerly the most common source of bacterial organisms, but it has been replaced in recent series by benign and malignant biliary obstruction as the most common source. Other significant sources include diverticulitis, regional enteritis, trauma, generalized sepsis, and pelvic inflammatory disease. Patients receiving chemotherapy for hematologic or solid malignancies are at increased risk. Despite great advances in diagnostic techniques and aggressive searches for a source, no probable cause of hepatic abscess was identified in 13% to 35% of cases since 1984.

PATHOLOGY AND MICROBIOLOGY. Pyogenic hepatic abscesses have some characteristic gross and microscopic pathologic features. Right lobe involvement predominates by a 3:1 ratio. Bilobar metastases occur in approximately 10% of patients. Most series indicate a nearly equal distribution between solitary and multiple liver abscesses. Hepatic abscesses appear yellow, compared with the normal deep maroon hepatic parenchyma that surrounds them. The organ is usually enlarged, and palpation may reveal a fluctuant area corresponding to the pus-filled cavity. On microscopic examination, acute inflammatory reaction is seen in necrosis and hepatocyte cords in the portal triad regions. Cholestasis may be evident in adjacent tissue.

Organisms recovered from liver abscesses vary greatly in reported series but generally reflect biliary or enteric flora. Solitary abscesses are more likely than multiple ones to grow multiple organisms. Presently, the most common aerobic organisms cultured are *Escherichia coli, Klebsiella*, and enterococcus. The most common anaerobes are *Bacteroides*, anaerobic streptococci, and *Fusobacterium* species. Streptococcal species (aerobic, anaerobic, or microaerophilic) are found in 25% to 30% of cultured abscesses and are believed to be of increasing importance in the pathogenesis of pyogenic abscess.

AMEBIC ABSCESS

INCIDENCE. Recent epidemiologic data in the United States are lacking concerning the incidence of amebic infestation. In general, the prevalence is higher in (1) countries in tropical or subtropical zones, (2) locations with poor sanitation, (3) mental institutions, and (4) cities in the United States with large immigrant populations. American tourists to tropical areas are more likely to develop invasive amebiasis than are permanent residents, presumably owing to a partial immunity of local inhabitants. Amebic abscess affects males more than females in a 9 to 10:1 ratio. In general, the patients are younger than their counterparts with pyogenic abscess, with the peak incidence in the fourth decade. There does not appear to be any particular racial susceptibility except for that related to living conditions.

PATHOLOGY. Amebic liver abscess follows intestinal infestation by *Entamoeba histolytica*. *Entamoeba* infestation occurs via contaminated drinking water, food, or person-to-person contact. *Entamoeba* cysts are ingested and resist digestion in the gastrointestinal tract. Trophozoites then colonize the colon and are transported via the portal circulation to the liver area, where they either degenerate in the portal venous radicles or migrate to an adjacent area, causing necrosis and liquefaction. Areas of destruction then coalesce to form, most commonly, a single large cavity in the right lobe. The contents are a mixture of necrotic hepatic parenchyma and blood, which yields the classic "anchovy paste" appearance. Bacterial superinfection occurs in approximately 10% of cases, which may change the color and odor of the contents. Greater than 90% of the abscesses are in the right lobe, and older abscesses have a well-formed fibrous capsule. The lesions may grow to an extremely large size and rupture intraperitoneally, intrathoracically, or into the pericardial space.

Diagnosis

The diagnosis of hepatic abscess is challenging because clinical signs are usually not specific. Early differentiation between pyogenic and amebic liver abscess may be difficult but is important because the treatments are radically different. Hepatic abscess is apparent at the time of admission in a minority of patients but if suspected is readily diagnosed by ultrasonography or computed tomography (CT) in over 95% of patients.

The majority of patients with hepatic abscess have an illness of less than 2 weeks' duration, although one-third have been ill for a month or longer. The primary symptoms are fever, malaise, chills, anorexia, weight loss, abdominal pain, or nausea. With amebic abscess, a recent diarrheal syndrome is present only in a minority of patients. Physical findings include right upper quadrant tenderness, pleural dullness to percussion, fever, hepatomegaly, and jaundice. Most patients have leukocytosis and some liver enzyme abnormality. The most common findings on plain abdominal or chest radiographs are right-sided atelectasis, an elevated hemidiaphragm, pleural effusion, or pneumonia. Occasionally, a subdiaphragmatic air-fluid collection is seen with pyogenic abscess or superinfected amebic abscess.

Ultrasonography has become the most useful screening test when the suspicion of hepatic abscess arises. The test is highly sensitive, is more accurate than CT in imaging the biliary tree, and allows diagnostic or therapeutic drainage or biopsy at the time of performance. CT scanning is the most sensitive of the imaging procedures (95% to 100%) and allows diagnostic or therapeutic intervention to be performed. Technetium-99m–sulfur colloid scanning has been useful in diagnosis of abscesses for four decades. Although very sensitive, the test has significant limitations of (1) being unable to detect lesions smaller than 2 cm. and (2) not allowing diagnostic or therapeutic procedures at the time of performance.

DIFFERENTIAL DIAGNOSIS. When an abscess has been demonstrated, a distinction must be made between pyogenic and more unusual types. Serum antibody titer for *E. histolytica* or counterimmunoelectrophoresis is highly specific and of great benefit when positive. Percutaneous aspiration may help in the identification of a bacterial organism; however, such aspiration is usually not helpful in the diagnosis of amebae. If amebic serologic study is not available or the results are delayed, the best method of early distinction between pyogenic and amebic abscess is a trial of an amebicidal agent. If the patient has not responded clinically in a 24- to 36-hour trial, pyogenic abscess should be the primary diagnosis. Clinical response is determined by relief of pain, fever, and leukocytosis.

MANAGEMENT

Untreated pyogenic abscesses are 95% to 100% fatal, with death following rupture, sepsis, or both. Prognostic factors include the patient's age, multiplicity of abscesses, multiplicity of organisms, and the presence of associated malignant or other immunosuppressive disease. Survival has improved in recent years, and mortality should be less than 20% with current therapy.

Effective management involves elimination of the abscess and the underlying source. Treatment of the abscess usually requires both intravenous antibiotics and effective drainage. Drainage may be accomplished by either *percutaneous* or *open* surgical methods. Recent series have documented the ease, effectiveness, and safety of percutaneous drainage of most hepatic abscesses. Solitary abscesses in the peripheral posterior of the right lobe are particularly amenable to percutaneous treatment. However, a combination of appendiceal or diverticular abscess and hepatic abscess is usually best treated by open drainage. Multiple abscesses remain difficult management problems by percutaneous, open, or even a combination of the two approaches. Laparoscopy has an increasing role in the management of pyogenic abscess.

Adjunctive antibiotic therapy is critical to effective treatment of hepatic abscesses. Directed therapy is based on the results of Gram stain and culture of diagnostic abscess aspirates. The most common isolates are gram-negative aerobes, colonic anaerobes, and microaerophilic streptococcal species. An appropriate regimen might include an aminoglycoside, an antibiotic directed primarily against anaerobes (such as clindamycin or metronidazole), and a penicillin. This regimen is adjusted appropriately after definitive culture results become known.

Surgical approaches available for use include the transpleural, extraperitoneal, and transperitoneal approaches. Most surgeons presently prefer the transperitoneal route because it allows inspection of the entire abdominal cavity for an underlying source as well as the best mobilization for appropriate drainage. The transpleural route is occasionally useful for high posterior lesions.

AMEBIC ABSCESS. Except where there is rupture or secondary infection, amebicidal agents are the treatment of choice for hepatic amebiasis. The drug of choice is metronidazole, and the usual dosage is 750 mg. orally three times daily for 7 to 14 days. If the patient is too ill to receive oral agents, intravenous administration is effective.

If clinical symptoms do not resolve within 48 hours of treatment, an incorrect diagnosis or secondary bacterial infection should be suspected. At that time, percutaneous aspiration or surgical drainage may be considered. Surgical therapy also has a role in suspected rupture, erosion, or perforation of an adjacent viscus or extrahepatic problems such as colonic obstruction. Mortality from amebic liver abscess should be less than 5% in the absence of secondary bacterial infection.

III

Neoplasms of the Liver
William C. Meyers, M.D.

PRIMARY MALIGNANT TUMORS
Hepatocellular Carcinoma

The most prevalent malignant disease worldwide today is hepatocellular carcinoma. The tumor is much more common in Africa and Asia than in the United States, where it may be increasing in incidence. Epidemiologic and laboratory studies have now firmly established a strong and specific association between both hepatitis B and hepatitis C virus and hepatocellular carcinoma. Other etiologic factors include cirrhosis from other causes, aflatoxin, oral contraceptives, and Thorotrast. Symptoms of hepatocellular carcinoma are extremely variable, but over half the patients have metastatic disease at the time of initial presentation. A large number of paraneoplastic manifestations are associated with hepatocellular carcinoma, including protein abnormalities, the most important of which is elevation of alpha-fetoprotein level.

Alpha-fetoprotein is of particular diagnostic significance because over half the patients with tumor exhibit the antigen. During the past several years in the Orient, the combination of alpha-fetoprotein level and real-time ultrasonography has been used as a screening method for hepatocellular carcinoma. Other radiologic investigations of importance in the diagnosis

See the corresponding chapter or part in the *Textbook of Surgery*, 15th edition, pp. 1140–1145, for a more detailed discussion of this topic, including a comprehensive list of references.

of hepatocellular and other tumors of the liver include computed tomography (CT), magnetic resonance imaging (MRI), endoscopic or percutaneous cholangiography, and radionuclide scanning. Recently, laparoscopy with ultrasound has an increasing role in the diagnosis and staging of these tumors. Primary treatment of hepatocellular carcinoma is resection whenever possible. Liver transplantation sometimes achieves resectability, but the long-term survival is relatively poor. Five-year survival for patients with hepatocellular carcinoma is generally considered to be about 20%.

Bile Duct Cancer (Cholangiocarcinoma)

Bile duct cancers represent 5% to 30% of all hepatobiliary neoplasms and may occur anywhere within the biliary system. Both intra- and extrahepatic bile duct cancers have been associated with ulcerative colitis and may be confused with sclerosing cholangitis. The tumor is often a markedly sclerotic adenocarcinoma. Approximately 20% to 25% of the tumors are resectable, which is usually advised if possible. Biliary intubation without resection may provide excellent palliation. With more aggressive invasive treatment, survival often has been extended from several weeks to many months or even years. Although patients with bile duct cancer might be expected to be a favorable group for hepatic transplantation, this has not been substantiated. Overall survival may be enhanced by more aggressive hepatic resections, which include Segment 1.

Other Primary Malignant Tumors

These tumors represent approximately 5% of cases and include *combined hepatocellular-cholangiocarcinoma, bile duct cystadenocarcinoma, squamous cell carcinoma*, and the incurable *angiosarcoma*. Sarcomas, carcinoid, and other mixed malignant tumors occur more rarely. *Epithelioid hemangioendothelioma* is considered a malignant neoplasm because of the diffuse involvement within the liver and the metastatic characteristics.

METASTATIC TUMORS

Metastatic cancer comprises the largest group of malignant tumors in the liver. Most occur in the liver probably as a result of primary tumor cells shedding into the vascular system. According to one autopsy study, bronchogenic carcinoma was the most common primary lesion causing hepatic metastases. Next in frequency were colonic, pancreatic, breast, and stomach tumors. CT portography has emerged as the most sensitive preoperative imaging test for these lesions.

The liver is the most common site of metastatic colorectal cancer. Approximately one-fourth of metastatic colorectal cancers to the liver are resectable. Several studies have documented the unfavorable prognosis of untreated hepatic metastases from colorectal cancer. Three-year survival in recent reports of resection for metastatic colorectal cancer is approximately 35% to 40%. Five-year survival appears to be 20% to 30%. Although there is little question that aggressive surgical therapy benefits selected patients, the precise numbers of and methods for selecting such patients preoperatively are still lacking. The probable significant prognostic factors include size and number of metastatic lesions. Undoubtedly, the most important predictor is the presence or absence of extrahepatic or residual local disease.

BENIGN HEPATIC NEOPLASMS

A number of primary benign lesions may occur in the liver. Some require resection, whereas others do not. Therefore, it is important to be familiar with the types of lesions that affect the liver and the methods of diagnosis. Liver cell *adenoma* and *focal nodular hyperplasia* are frequently difficult to differentiate, although each has distinct pathologic and clinical features. Both affect women and are associated with the use of oral contraceptives. Hepatic adenomas are usually solitary but vary in size up to 38 cm. in diameter. Occasionally, they are multiple and cluster in families. The lesions are prone to rupture, and malignant change is possible. In contrast, focal nodular hyperplasia typically does not produce symptoms, and bleeding, rupture, and malignant changes do not occur. Probably the most common benign tumor to come to the attention of surgeons is *cavernous hemangioma*, which is found in approximately 2% of livers at autopsy. Spontaneous rupture is unusual but can be dramatic. Complications include congestive heart failure, arteriovenous shunting, and consumptive coagulopathy. Resection is usually determined by the presence of symptoms, danger of rupture, and the amount of liver tissue involved. *Hemangioendotheliomas* are rare vasoformative cellular tumors usually occurring in the first 2 years of life. Resection may be indicated when there is no response to prednisone. A number of other benign solid tumors that may occur in the liver include *lipoma, leiomyoma, myxoma, teratoma, carcinoid tumor,* and *mesenchymal hamartoma*.

CYSTS

Cysts of the liver can be divided into those which are parasitic and those which are nonparasitic. Large solitary *parenchymal (developmental) cysts* are rare; they occur most commonly in the right lobe of the liver, probably representing an arrest of development. By definition, a cyst contains epithelium, often resembling biliary epithelium. Most small cysts require no treatment, although they may be difficult to differentiate from cystadenoma or cystadenocarcinoma. Preferred treatment of large cysts that are causing symptoms is resection, although other surgical treatments may be attempted. One consideration in the surgical treatment of large hepatic cysts is whether there is communication with the biliary system. Polycystic liver disease often accompanies polycystic kidneys. A surgical procedure of choice for a symptomatic dominant cyst in polycystic disease is the fenestration operation, in which the symptomatic cyst is made to communicate with the peritoneal cavity. A cyst (*pseudocyst*) also may form as a consequence of trauma or inflammation; however, these are not true cysts, since they have a fibrous rather than an epithelial lining.

Choledochal cysts are more common in the Orient than elsewhere and may be associated with supraduodenal entry of the pancreatic duct. There is a premalignant potential of choledochal cysts. The extreme form of choledochal cysts consists of multiple cystic dilatations in the intrahepatic ducts, termed *Caroli's disease.*

Echinococcus is the most frequent cause of parasitic liver cysts. The problem is endemic in Greece and other parts of eastern Europe, South America, Australia, and South Africa. It is rare in the United States. The most common form is due to *E. granulosus*. The other primary form is *E. multilocularis* and is endemic to Alaska. The eggs of *E. granulosus* are passed in the stool and ingested by cows, sheep, moose, caribou, or humans. The primary treatment of *Echinococcus* (hydatid) cysts is surgical resection without peritoneal contamination.

MAJOR HEPATIC RESECTION

Because of reduction of operative mortality in elective hepatic resection to less than 1% in several centers, it has become the primary therapy for resectable primary or metastatic tumors as well as selected benign conditions. Segmental resection has become increasingly popular.

IV

Hemobilia
Ravi S. Chari, M.D., and William C. Meyers, M.D.

Bleeding into the biliary tract is a common, usually inconsequential problem but also may be life-threatening. By far the most common cause of hemobilia is trauma. Some degree of hemobilia often accompanies hepatobiliary diagnostic and therapeutic techniques, such as liver biopsy, transhepatic or endoscopic cholangiography, and lithotripsy.

The bleeding can occur anywhere within the biliary system: liver parenchyma, intra- or extrahepatic bile ducts, gallbladder, pancreas, or ampullary region. In an early review (1972), trauma comprised 48% of the cases, infection 28%, and gall-

See the corresponding chapter or part in the *Textbook of Surgery*, 15th edition, pp. 1145–1148, for a more detailed discussion of this topic, including a comprehensive list of references.

stones 10%. The classic cause of dramatic hemobilia is blunt trauma causing injury deep within the liver without disruption of Glisson's capsule. As the resultant hematoma expands, rupture occurs into the biliary system or a false aneurysm forms that creates the same problem in a more delayed manner. An important cause of hemobilia in the Far East is parasites, most notably *Clonorchis* or *Ascaris*, which may cause hemobilia associated with cholangitis or pericholangitic abscesses. Other relatively common causes of hemobilia include pancreatic disease, various types of aneurysms, hepatoma, other tumors, and sickle cell anemia.

The classic triad of hemobilia is gastrointestinal bleeding, right upper quadrant pain, and jaundice. These symptoms also suggest other diseases such as terminal cancer, but in the setting of trauma, general good health, or biliary tract manipulation, the triad should suggest the possibility of hemobilia. Other findings may include a palpable mass in the right upper quadrant or right upper quadrant bruit.

Arteriography remains the single most accurate and helpful diagnostic test in the evaluation of patients in whom bleeding into the biliary ducts is suspected. Cholangiography also may be helpful. However, these procedures also may confuse the diagnosis because manipulation may create a new source of bleeding. Technetium-labeled red blood cell scans occasionally may be an efficient way of establishing the diagnosis. An external biliary drainage catheter also may, of course, demonstrate the bleeding.

Management of hemobilia can be divided into two phases. The first phase is general evaluation and resuscitation with blood transfusions as needed. The second phase is treatment, for which there are several options. The majority of cases of severe hemobilia are best treated by arteriographic embolization. Generally, operation should be considered a last resort.

V

Surgical Complications Of Cirrhosis and Portal Hypertension
Layton F. Rikkers, M.D.

Cirrhosis is the end result of a variety of mechanisms that cause the combination of hepatocellular injury, fibrosis, and regeneration. Even though only 15% of heavy drinkers are afflicted, alcoholic cirrhosis is the most common type of

---

See the corresponding chapter or part in the *Textbook of Surgery*, 15th edition, pp. 1355–1361, for a more detailed discussion of this topic, including a comprehensive list of references.

chronic liver disease in the United States, making cirrhosis the sixth leading cause of death between the ages of 35 and 54. Cirrhosis results in two major phenomena, hepatic failure and portal hypertension. Complications of portal hypertension include variceal hemorrhage, portal systemic encephalopathy, ascites, and hypersplenism. The most life-threatening complication is variceal hemorrhage, which ranks second to hepatic failure as a cause of death in patients with cirrhosis.

PATHOGENESIS OF PORTAL HYPERTENSION AND VARICEAL RUPTURE

Since increased portal venous resistance is usually the initiator of portal hypertension, classifications are generally based on the site of elevated resistance. However, increased portal venous inflow secondary to a hyperdynamic systemic circulation and splanchnic hyperemia is often a significant contributor to the maintenance of portal hypertension. Prehepatic, presinusoidal portal hypertension is usually due to extrahepatic portal vein thrombosis and is most common in the pediatric age group. Hepatic function remains normal because portal flow is restored through collaterals. The most common cause of intrahepatic, presinusoidal portal hypertension is schistosomiasis. Again, liver function is generally well preserved. Depending on the etiology of cirrhosis, the site(s) of increased resistance within the liver may vary. Alcoholic cirrhosis usually involves sinusoidal and postsinusoidal levels, while some types of nonalcoholic cirrhosis have a presinusoidal component as well. Elevated portal vein pressure stimulates portal systemic collateralization. The most important pathway clinically is through the esophagogastric venous network to the azygous system.

Esophagogastric varices do not develop until portal pressure exceeds 12 mm. Hg and, once present, bleed in only one-third to one-half of patients. In 90% of patients, variceal rupture occurs within 2 to 3 cm. of the esophagogastric junction. The remaining 10% of patients bleed from gastric varices. Gastritis secondary to portal hypertension (portal hypertensive gastropathy) usually involves the proximal stomach and may also be a cause of hemorrhage.

PATIENT EVALUATION

Patient evaluation begins with a detailed history and physical examination. Stigmata of chronic liver disease include spider angiomata, palmar erythema, gynecomastia, testicular atrophy, and altered mental status. Splenomegaly, ascites, and visible abdominal wall veins each indicate the presence of portal hypertension.

Child's classification, composed of three clinical variables (ascites, encephalopathy, and nutritional status) and two biochemical tests (serum bilirubin and albumin) are an indirect, but useful, estimate of hepatic functional reserve. This classification scheme is particularly valuable in predicting outcome after surgical intervention. Operative mortality rates for

Child's A, B, and C Class patients are in the ranges of 0% to 5%, 10% to 15%, and greater than 25%, respectively.

In patients with alcoholic cirrhosis and many varieties of nonalcoholic cirrhosis, portal pressure can be estimated indirectly by measurement of hepatic venous wedge pressure. This variable is normal in patients with presinusoidal hypertension. Selective visceral angiography has been the most frequently used method for definition of portal venous anatomy, qualitative estimation of hepatic portal perfusion, and determination of postoperative shunt patency. Duplex ultrasonography is a less accurate but noninvasive alternative to angiography for assessment of these same parameters.

Endoscopy is the key procedure for diagnosing the site of upper gastrointestinal hemorrhage in a patient with portal hypertension. In approximately 90% of instances, bleeding will be secondary to portal hypertension (esophageal varices, gastric varices, or portal hypertensive gastropathy). The remaining 10% of bleeding episodes in portal hypertensive patients usually are due to duodenal ulcer, gastric ulcer, or Mallory-Weiss tear.

MANAGEMENT OF ACUTE VARICEAL HEMORRHAGE

Since the greatest risk of death from variceal bleeding is within the first few days after the onset of hemorrhage, prompt and effective therapy is essential for maximal patient salvage. Many patients have decompensated hepatic function secondary to either recent alcoholism or hypotension and are high risks for surgery. Therefore, emergency treatment should be nonoperative whenever possible. However, failure of nonoperative therapy should be recognized promptly so that the appropriate operation can be performed before the patient is moribund.

Presently, endoscopic therapy is the most commonly used treatment for management of the acute bleeding episode. This technique offers the opportunity to control hemorrhage at the same time the diagnosis is made. Sclerotherapy results in cessation of acute hemorrhage in over 80% of patients. Failure of acute sclerotherapy can be defined as persistent bleeding after two sclerotherapy sessions. Sclerotherapy is generally ineffective for bleeding gastric varices.

Since the reintroduction of endoscopic therapy, pharmacotherapy and balloon tamponade have been used less frequently. The mainstay of pharmacotherapy has been intravenous infusion of vasopressin, a potent splanchnic vasoconstrictor, but recent trials have shown that somatostatin and its analog, octreotide, are as effective as endoscopic therapy. Pharmacotherapy is an important component of treatment for patients awaiting endoscopy, for sclerotherapy failures, and for individuals bleeding from gastric varices or portal hypertensive gastropathy.

The advantage of variceal tamponade with the Sengstaken-Blakemore tube is immediate control of hemorrhage in over 85% of patients. To avoid complications, this device needs to be used according to a strict protocol. It may be lifesaving for individuals with exsanguinating hemorrhage and for sclerotherapy failures who do not respond to pharmacotherapy. Because rebleeding is common after balloon deflation, either surgery or endoscopic sclerotherapy should be planned.

Transjugular intrahepatic portosystemic shunt (TIPS) is the newest option for control of acute bleeding. Its advantage is immediate and usually effective portal decompression. Disadvantages include a high long-term shunt failure rate and a fairly high frequency of encephalopathy.

Although routine emergency surgery has been advocated by some, there is no evidence that this approach is superior to acute endoscopic therapy followed by elective surgery or by chronic endoscopic treatment. The major disadvantage of emergency surgery is that operative mortality rates exceed 25% in most series. The most frequently used emergency operations are stapled esophageal transection and the portacaval shunt.

PREVENTION OF RECURRENT VARICEAL HEMORRHAGE

Although only one-third to one-half of patients with varices bleed, once hemorrhage has occurred it recurs in over 70% of untreated individuals. Available definitive therapies include pharmacotherapy, chronic endoscopic therapy, TIPS, three types of portal systemic shunts (nonselective, selective, and partial), a variety of nonshunt procedures, and hepatic transplantation.

Long-term drug therapy for prevention of recurrent variceal bleeding decreases the likelihood of rebleeding by about 20%. Most trials have evaluated propranolol and other beta blockers given in a titrated dose to reduce heart rate by 25%.

During the past 15 years, chronic endoscopic therapy has become the most frequently used treatment for prevention of recurrent variceal hemorrhage. Varices can be eradicated completely in approximately two-thirds of patients. Although rebleeding rates after endoscopic treatment approach 50% in most trials, many episodes of recurrent hemorrhage can be treated successfully by further sclerotherapy or variceal ligation. However, this therapeutic approach eventually fails in approximately one-third of patients, most of whom require surgery. Nevertheless, chronic endoscopic therapy is a reasonable initial approach for many patients as long as surgical rescue is readily available.

TIPS has been used in the elective setting more often than as an emergency. Because of the high shunt stenosis or thrombosis rate (up to 50% by 1 year), patients should be selected carefully. Ideal candidates for TIPS are patients who require only short-term portal decompression (transplant candidates and nontransplant candidates with advanced hepatic disease who are unlikely to survive for long). TIPS is a nonselective shunt and has been followed by a high incidence of encephalopathy in some series.

Portal systemic shunts are the most effective means of preventing recurrent variceal hemorrhage. In addition to providing adequate variceal decompression, nonselective shunts (end-to-side and side-to-side portacaval, interpositional, and conventional splenorenal shunts) divert the entire portal venous flow away from the liver. Since portal blood contains hepatotrophic hormones and cerebral toxins, adverse consequences of these procedures are accelerated hepatic failure and frequent postshunt encephalopathy (20% to 50% of patients). Because of these side effects, controlled trials have failed to show a survival advantage of nonselective shunts over conventional medical management. All nonselective shunts, except the end-to-side portacaval shunt, decompress the hepatic sinusoidal network in addition to the portal venous system. Therefore, these procedures effectively relieve ascites in addition to preventing recurrent variceal bleeding.

The distal splenorenal shunt is a selective shunt that compartmentalizes the portal venous circulation into a decompressed gastrosplenic component and a high-pressure mesenteric component. Because hepatic portal perfusion is maintained into the late postoperative interval in approximately 40% to 50% of patients (greater in nonalcoholic and less in alcoholic cirrhotics) undergoing this procedure, the majority of series have reported less frequent encephalopathy (10% to 15% of patients) following the distal splenorenal shunt than after nonselective shunts (20% to 50%). No controlled trial has shown a survival advantage of selective over nonselective shunts. Contraindications to the distal splenorenal shunt are medically intractable ascites and incompatible anatomy (prior splenectomy or splenic vein diameter less than 7 mm.).

The small-diameter (8 to 10 mm.) portacaval H-graft is a partial shunt that also preserves hepatic portal perfusion in some patients. Initial experience with this procedure suggests that the frequency of postoperative encephalopathy is low when portal flow is maintained.

Nonshunt operations range from simple stapled transection and reanastomosis of the distal esophagus to extensive esophagogastric devascularization (Sugiura procedure). The advantage of these operations is minimal alteration of hepatic portal perfusion and liver function. A significant disadvantage is a high rebleeding rate (20% to 40%) in Western series. Nonshunt procedures are the only applicable operations for patients with diffuse splanchnic venous thrombosis.

Hepatic transplantation is the only definitive therapy for variceal hemorrhage that addresses the underlying liver disease. Variceal bleeders who are transplant candidates include nonalcoholic cirrhotics and abstinent alcoholic cirrhotics with either limited functional hepatic reserve (Child's Class C) or a poor quality of life secondary to their disease. Future transplant candidates (Child's Classes A and B), who receive another therapy initially (chronic endoscopic therapy, TIPS, or shunt), should be monitored carefully so that transplantation is accomplished before they become high operative risks for this procedure.

In selecting an appropriate definitive therapy for variceal bleeding, patients are first grouped according to their transplant candidacy. Immediate transplant candidates should undergo this procedure as soon as a donor liver is available. Most future transplant and nontransplant candidates should receive initial sclerotherapy unless they bleed from gastric varices or have limited access to emergency surgical care. These latter individuals and those who fail sclerotherapy should receive the appropriate shunt or nonshunt operation depending on their clinical circumstances and portal venous anatomy.

VI

Peritoneovenous Shunts for Intractable Ascites

Paul D. Greig, M.D.,
and Bernard Langer, M.D.

PATHOGENESIS OF ASCITES IN CIRRHOSIS

Ascites in the cirrhotic patient results from renal sodium and water retention. With portal hypertension, the increased splanchnic hydrostatic pressure and reduced oncotic pressure (from hypoalbuminemia) cause an imbalance of Starling forces and movement of fluid into the peritoneal cavity. Reduced glomerular filtration and increased renin and aldosterone contribute further to sodium retention, which aggravates the ascites. This may progress to uremia and oliguria (*hepatorenal syndrome*), an uncommon form of functional renal failure.

CLINICAL MANIFESTATIONS OF ASCITES IN CHRONIC LIVER DISEASE

Cirrhotic ascites usually is chronic and progressive and indicates advanced liver dysfunction. Transient ascites may develop in cirrhotic patients following laparotomy or from resuscitation following variceal bleeding. Resistant ascites occurs in 10% of patients and indicates less than 50% 1-year survival. Severe ascites may be associated with pleural effusions, leg edema, abdominal wall hernias, and spontaneous bacterial peritonitis.

TREATMENT OF ASCITES

Treatment includes dietary restriction of sodium (400 mg. per day) and fluid (1 liter per day) plus diuretics, usually an

---

See the corresponding chapter or part in the *Textbook of Surgery*, 15th edition, pp. 1104–1110, for a more detailed discussion of this topic, including a comprehensive list of references.

aldosterone antagonist (spironolactone or amiloride) with a thiazide or furosemide when necessary, aiming to mobilize up to 1 liter per day. Complications include hypokalemia, metabolic alkalosis and hyponatremia, acute tubular necrosis, or hepatorenal syndrome. Therapeutic paracentesis with albumin infusions may be effective in patients with tense or refractory ascites. Physiologic side-to-side portosystemic shunts and transjugular intrahepatic portosystemic shunt with stent (TIPSS) lower portal pressure and decrease ascites, but these have a high risk and incidence of encephalopathy.

PERITONEOVENOUS SHUNTING

The peritoneovenous shunt (PVS) is a prosthesis with a one-way valve between the peritoneal cavity and the superior vena cava (SVC). The LeVeen shunt has a pressure-activated valve with Silastic peritoneal and venous catheters. Others (e.g., Denver shunt) have a pumpable valve.

Indications for PVS include (1) cirrhosis with chronic refractory ascites, (2) hepatorenal syndrome, and (3) acute ascites following a portosystemic shunt. The PVS is contraindicated in infected ascites or other sepsis, acute viral or alcoholic hepatitis, or end-stage liver disease. Relative contraindications are recent GI bleeding or peritonitis, hepatic encephalopathy, complications of alcoholism, malnutrition, a serum bilirubin more than 3 times normal, a prothrombin time greater than 4 seconds prolonged, or a creatinine more than 2.3 times normal.

Preoperative diagnostic paracentesis, liver biopsy, liver biochemical tests, and coagulation studies are performed, and prophylactic antibiotics are administered. Local or general anesthetic may be used. The LeVeen valve is placed in the abdominal wall deep to the rectus muscle. A pumpable valve is placed over the chest wall. The peritoneal end lies freely in the ascites. The venous limb is tunneled subcutaneously and inserted into the SVC via the internal jugular or subclavian vein. The tip is placed just inside the right atrium under radiologic control. Postoperative coagulopathy is reduced by replacing the ascitic fluid with Ringer's lactate. Furosemide is used to maintain the urinary output over 60 ml. per hour. Weight, girth, hematocrit, electrolytes, renal function, and coagulation are monitored. Ultimately, there is reduction of ascites.

Complications occur in up to 80% of patients. Most develop a coagulopathy, and up to 20% develop disseminated intravascular coagulation requiring temporary ligation of the shunt and provision of fresh frozen plasma, cryoprecipitate, and platelets. Epsilon-aminocaproic acid also may be useful. Shunt infection is a serious complication requiring systemic antibiotics and removal of the shunt. Shunt blockage may be diagnosed by a direct injection of radiopaque contrast material into the shunt (*shuntogram*). The operative mortality ranges up to 30%.

The renal and hemodynamic improvements persist in the late postoperative period. Even with a blocked shunt, most patients become and remain ascites-free with an improvement in nutrition. Late complications include shunt blockage, infection, SVC thrombosis, and bowel obstruction. The patency rate of 5-year survivors has been only 40%. Most late deaths are due to bleeding esophageal varices and hepatic failure.

The peritoneovenous shunt is a palliative procedure that may control ascites but does not prolong life. It should be avoided in potential liver transplant patients.

VII

Viral Hepatitis and the Surgeon

John D. Hamilton, M.D.

Although viral hepatitis has been recognized clinically for centuries, its causes have been established only in the last three to four decades. As of now, there are certainly five and likely six distinct groups of viruses that cause hepatitis, namely, hepatitis A, B, C, D, E, and possibly F.

VIRUS CHARACTERIZATION

Each of these classes of virus is distinct and separate from the others, with no common antigens or cross-reactive antibodies. Identification of each class is dependent on specific serologic studies because other methods such as tissue culture, electron microscopy, and animal infectivity are either not possible or impractical for clinical use. Sensitive and specific serologic tests are available commercially for hepatitis A to D.

EPIDEMIOLOGY

The Centers for Disease Control and Prevention reported over 24,000 cases of HAV, over 3000 cases of HBV, and almost 5000 cases of non-A, non-B hepatitis in 1993. Each of the first two are generally decreasing in number with successive years. Nonetheless, the CDC projects that up to 300,000 cases of HBV occur yearly in the United States and that 5000 deaths yearly are due to viral-induced cirrhosis or hepatocellular carcinoma.

TRANSMISSION

Parenterally transmitted viruses constitute the greatest concern for the practicing surgeon. Of the hepatitis viruses, HBV,

See the corresponding chapter or part in the *Textbook of Surgery*, 15th edition, pp. 1110–1116, for a more detailed discussion of this topic, including a comprehensive list of references.

HCV, and HDV are blood-borne and therefore capable of being transmitted by the parenteral route. In addition, because each of these viruses may exist in an infectious form in asymptomatic individuals, the potential for transmission from the asymptomatic patient to the practicing surgeon is quite real. In addition, transmission from surgeon to a patient has been documented but is considered to be remote.

For the surgical patient who on occasion requires transfusion, the risk of hepatitis exists but has been reduced dramatically by routine testing for HBV and HCV. Hepatitis C is presently the major cause of postransfusion hepatitis.

CLINICAL DISEASE

Typically, viral hepatitis is asymptomatic, but if symptomatic, the disease persists for several weeks to several months and is characterized by some combination of fever, anorexia, fatigue, nausea, dark urine, and yellow sclera. Laboratory studies generally reflect liver cell necrosis, including primarily elevations of aminotransferase.

Fortunately, 90% of individuals with a clinical illness recover with supportive but not specific therapy. Around 5% become chronic carriers, and another 5% develop a chronic form of hepatitis that may lead to cirrhosis or contribute to the development of hepatocellular carcinoma. A small number (less than 1%) develop an acute, fulminant, and usually fatal form of hepatitis.

PREVENTION

The mainstays of preventing viral hepatitis are the correct diagnosis and reporting of new cases, the attention to standard principles of cleanliness and hygiene, specific measures to eliminate the sources of infection, and in the case of the surgeon, scrupulous surgical technique. Additional measures available include the administration of immune or hyperimmune globulin after or in anticipation of an exposure to HAV, HBV, or HCV. More definitively and reliably protective, however, are vaccines, which are routinely recommended for individuals at risk of exposure. HBV vaccines are especially relevant for the practicing surgeon and should be considered as essential in the preparation for a surgical career.

TREATMENT

Therapy for viral hepatitis is nonspecific and supportive, with particular attention to hydration, nutrition, and metabolic balance. Under certain circumstances, treatment of chronic hepatitis with prednisone and interferon may be considered, but there is no role for these drugs in the acute illness.

34

THE BILIARY SYSTEM

David L. Nahrwold, M.D.

Knowledge of the anatomy of the biliary duct system and its associated blood vessels is essential for safe surgery of the biliary tract. Surgically important anomalies include a very long or very short cystic duct, a cystic duct that courses behind the common bile duct to enter it on the left or posteriorly, and fusion of a long cystic duct to the common duct, with which it may share a common wall. The most important is an abnormal entrance of the anterior or posterior right segmental duct of the liver into the cystic duct, leading the unwary surgeon to excise a portion of the common bile duct. Anomalies of the cystic and hepatic arteries are frequent.

CONGENITAL ANOMALIES OF THE GALLBLADDER

Gallbladder agenesis is very rare. Some adults have biliary tract symptoms and may have bile duct dilatation or choledocholithiasis. Ultrasonography may be interpreted as showing a small, contracted gallbladder. When the gallbladder is not found at operation, a cholangiogram should be performed to exclude choledocholithiasis.

Ectopic gallbladders are found in the falciform ligament or within the liver. Torsion may occur when the organ is suspended by a long mesentery.

CHOLEDOCHAL CYSTS

The most common type of choledochal cyst is the fusiform-shaped extrahepatic cyst, thought to be caused by a distal stricture and destruction of the proximal duct epithelium by pancreatic juice. The entire duct system may resemble a fusiform cyst. Another type is a diverticulum from the common duct. Cholangitis is frequent. Cysts are imaged by ultrasonography, but cholangiography is the definitive test. Patients have an increased incidence of pancreatitis and cancer within the cyst. The treatment of extrahepatic cysts is excision and Roux-en-Y hepaticojejunostomy.

CHOLEDOCHOLITHIASIS

Bile duct stones may migrate from the gallbladder (secondary stones) or form within the duct system (primary stones).

See the corresponding chapter or part in the *Textbook of Surgery*, 15th edition, pp. 1117–1125, for a more detailed discussion of this topic, including a comprehensive list of references.

Arbitrarily, stones discovered more than 2 years after chole-cystectomy are designated as primary stones.

CLINICAL MANIFESTATIONS AND DIAGNOSIS. Bile duct calculi may be asymptomatic or cause biliary colic, bile duct obstruction, cholangitis, or pancreatitis. Central nervous system symptoms and hemodynamic instability signify acute toxic cholangitis, caused by complete obstruction and infected bile under pressure.

The physical examination is usually normal, but jaundice and abdominal tenderness may be present. The white blood cell count and the serum bilirubin, alkaline phosphatase, and amylase may be elevated. The definitive diagnosis is made by cholangiography.

TREATMENT. The initial treatment is antibiotic administration. Emergency decompression of the duct system is essential in acute toxic cholangitis; this may be performed by endoscopic sphincterotomy and stone extraction, percutaneous transhepatic drainage, or laparotomy and insertion of a T-tube in the common duct.

CHOLEDOCHOLITHOTOMY. The laparoscopic procedure entails an incision in the cystic duct and removal of stones utilizing choledochoscopy, a stone basket, and fluoro-cholangiography. Antegrade sphincterotomy is also used. Because not all stones are amenable to these techniques, preoperative and postoperative endoscopic sphincterotomy and stone extraction are utilized. When these are unsuccessful, open choledochotomy is necessary.

BILE DUCT INJURIES

EARLY MANAGEMENT OF INJURIES. Injuries may be manifested in the immediate postoperative period by leakage of bile through the wound, biliary ascites, or biloma. Endoscopic cholangiography is indicated and demonstrates the leak, which should be treated by stenting if the duct system is intact. When the duct system is not intact, percutaneous transhepatic cholangiography and insertion of proximal catheters are indicated prior to reconstruction by a biliary-enteric anastomosis.

LATE STRICTURES. Reconstruction by Roux-en-Y hepaticojejunostomy is the conventional therapy. Excellent results are achieved in 75% of patients. The early experience with plastic stents, changed every 3 months and removed after 6 to 8 months, suggests that results equivalent to surgery are obtained in selected patients. Balloon dilation is successful in 75% of carefully selected patients after 2 years.

BILE DUCT CANCERS

A majority of bile duct cancers are proximal to the entrance of the cystic duct and often involve one or both hepatic ducts. Risk factors include congenital cystic disease of the biliary tract, primary sclerosing cholangitis, and infestation with *Clonorchis sinensis*. Cholangiocarcinoma usually presents with jaundice. The diagnosis is made by cholangiography and brushings or fine-needle aspiration of the lesion. Computed tomography and angiography help to determine resectability.

TREATMENT. Lesions in the proximal two thirds of the extrahepatic duct system require excision and hepaticoje-junostomy. Those in the distal third are treated by the Whipple procedure. Percutaneous or endoscopic insertion of a stent and radiation therapy may provide palliation. Only about 10% of patients are cured.

SCLEROSING CHOLANGITIS

Sclerosing cholangitis is an inflammatory disease of the bile ducts that causes fibrosis and thickening of their walls and multiple short, concentric strictures. The disease is progressive and gradually causes cirrhosis, portal hypertension, and death from hepatic failure. Patients with sclerosing cholangitis have an increased incidence of cholangiocarcinoma.

Consideration of percutaneous balloon dilation or stenting arises when the patient is jaundiced and clearly has one or more points of obstruction within the biliary duct system. Some patients are improved by these procedures. In the very rare patient who has an isolated obstruction within the extra-hepatic duct system, a Roux-en-Y hepaticojejunostomy proxi-mal to the obstruction may be indicated. However, the defini-tive management of patients with sclerosing cholangitis is hepatic transplantation.

I
_____

Acute Cholecystitis
David L. Nahrwold, M.D.

Acute cholecystitis is a chemical or bacterial inflammation of the gallbladder. Acute calculous cholecystitis is associated with cholelithiasis, and acalculous cholecystitis, representing only 5% of cases, is not.

ACUTE CALCULOUS CHOLECYSTITIS

Obstruction of the outlet of the gallbladder by a stone is probably the fundamental cause of acute calculous cholecysti-tis, but other factors are involved. Toxic bile acids gain access to the wall of the gallbladder when the obstructing stone erodes the gallbladder mucosa. The role of bacteria, which

---

See the corresponding chapter or part in the *Textbook of Surgery*, 15th edition, pp. 1126–1132, for a more detailed discussion of this topic, including a comprehensive list of references.

colonize gallbladder bile or the gallbladder wall in most but not all cases, is not clear.

Sloughing of the mucosa, edema of the gallbladder wall, and an infiltration of neutrophils are typical in acute cholecystitis. As the inflammation progresses, the organ becomes gangrenous and may perforate, leading to a pericholecystic abscess, spreading peritonitis, or a cholecystoenteric fistula.

CLINICAL MANIFESTATIONS. The inflammatory process causes pain in the epigastrium or right upper quadrant. Some patients have nausea and vomiting, but moderate to severe pain is the cardinal symptom.

Physical examination reveals right upper quadrant and epigastric tenderness, often associated with muscle rigidity and rebound tenderness. Murphy's sign, inspiratory arrest during deep palpation of the right upper quadrant, is said to be pathognomonic. A mass can be palpated in the right upper quadrant in 40% of patients. It may be the distended gallbladder, omentum adherent to the organ, or a pericholecystic abscess. Absorption of bile pigments throughout the damaged mucosa may cause jaundice or signify choledocholithiasis.

A majority of patients have fever or an elevated white blood cell count, manifestations of the inflammation.

DIAGNOSTIC STUDIES. Gallbladder scintigraphy using a derivative of technetium-99m iminodiacetic acid (IDA scan) is the specific test for acute cholecystitis, providing a sensitivity of almost 100% and a specificity of 95%. The gallbladder is not visible on the scan because the outlet obstruction prevents entry of the nuclide into the lumen. Ultrasonography demonstrates gallstones and may show edema or pericholecystic fluid, but the test is not specific for acute cholecystitis.

TREATMENT. Initial management is hospitalization and administration of a combination of antimicrobial agents effective against both gram-positive and gram-negative aerobes and anaerobes. The most frequent organisms are *Escherichia coli, Klebsiella aerogenes, Streptococcus faecalis, Clostridium welchii, Proteus* species, *Enterobacter* species, and anaerobic streptococci.

The definitive treatment of acute cholecystitis is laparoscopic cholecystectomy with conversion to the open technique if the laparoscopic procedure cannot be completed safely or when bleeding or a bile leak cannot be stopped without risking injury to important structures. Conversion is carried out in patients who have the complications of acute cholecystitis. The mortality rate is less than 0.2%, and the major morbidity rate is less than 5%.

ACUTE ACALCULOUS CHOLECYSTITIS

This disease often occurs after or in association with other conditions such as trauma, burns, major operations, or chronic, debilitating conditions such as the collagen vascular diseases. Susceptible patients are frequently critically ill, requiring life-support measures and total parenteral nutrition.

The diagnosis is difficult because the typical signs and symptoms are masked by the concurrent condition. Cholescintigraphy is often falsely positive. Right upper quadrant pain and tenderness to palpation in the right upper quadrant are the most reliable clinical features.

UNUSUAL TYPES OF CHOLECYSTITIS

Acute emphysematous cholecystitis is a rare form characterized by gas in the lumen and the wall of the gallbladder caused by infection with one or more gas-forming organisms. *Clostridium perfringens* is cultured in 50% of cases. The disease has an abrupt onset and progresses rapidly, causing gangrene of the gallbladder and severe toxicity.

Typhoid fever occasionally gives rise to acute cholecystitis caused by *Salmonella typhi*. A typhoid carrier may harbor this organism in the gallbladder, a condition usually eradicated by quinoline antibiotics, but when gallstones are present, cholecystectomy may be necessary to eradicate the carrier state.

II

Chronic Cholecystitis and Cholelithiasis
David L. Nahrwold, M.D.

Chronic inflammatory changes are found in the gallbladders of many symptomatic patients with gallstones, but gallstones are also present in an otherwise normal gallbladder, and gallbladder symptoms may occur without inflammation.

INCIDENCE AND CLASSIFICATION. Approximately 500,000 cholecystectomies are performed annually. The prevalence of gallstones increases with increasing age, and the incidence in women of childbearing age is higher than in men of the same age. Approximately 70% of stones are composed predominantly of cholesterol, and 30% are pigment stones. The latter are classified as black pigment stones, which are associated with hemolysis and cirrhosis, and calcium bilirubinate stones, which are associated with infection in the biliary tract.

PATHOLOGY. Chronic cholecystitis occurs primarily (primary chronic cholecystitis) or follows an attack of acute cholecystitis (secondary chronic cholecystitis). In the secondary type, the entire organ is thickened, and there are granulomas containing cholesterol clefts, fibrosis of the muscular layer, and loss of the villous architecture of the mucosa. The gall-

---

See the corresponding chapter or part in the *Textbook of Surgery*, 15th edition, pp. 1132–1139, for a more detailed discussion of this topic, including a comprehensive list of references.

bladder retains its thin-walled appearance and villous architecture in the primary type, and the inflammatory infiltrate is
predominantly lymphocytes. Stones are almost always present
in both types.

CLINICAL MANIFESTATIONS AND DIAGNOSIS. Right
upper quadrant or epigastric pain, the cardinal symptom of
chronic cholelithiasis and cholecystitis, is caused by obstruction of the outlet of the gallbladder during its contraction. The
pain typically follows large meals and radiates around the
side to the tip of the right scapula. Nausea and vomiting are
frequent. Between attacks, patients often have bloating and a
sensation of fullness. Physical findings, present only during
an attack, include right upper quadrant and epigastric tenderness and voluntary muscle guarding, but no signs of peritonitis.

The diagnosis of cholelithiasis is confirmed by ultrasonography, which has an accuracy rate of over 95%. Oral cholecystography, which is less accurate, should be performed when
the symptoms are typical and ultrasonography is normal or
equivocal.

TREATMENT. Initial treatment is parenteral narcotic administration, which effectively relieves the pain. The definitive
therapy is elective laparoscopic cholecystectomy after co-morbid conditions have been treated appropriately. A preoperative prophylactic antibiotic is administered in patients over
age 60 and in those recovering from acute cholecystitis or
suspected of having bile duct stones.

Laparoscopic cholecystectomy is performed except when it
is impossible to safely establish pneumoperitoneum or when
adhesions or other anatomic abnormalities prevent safe access
to the gallbladder. Conversion to the open procedure is necessary in approximately 5% of patients when gallbladder and
bile duct anatomy is unclear or when bleeding or leakage of
bile cannot be controlled satisfactorily.

The mortality of laparoscopic cholecystectomy ranges from
0% to 0.3%, and the rate of complications ranges from 1.3%
to 11.2%. The bile duct injury rate is approximately 0.4%, but
this will probably fall with more experience. The advantages
over the open procedure are a reduced length of hospital stay,
earlier return to normal activity, and a better cosmetic result.

Oral dissolution therapy (ursodiol) is used in patients who
refuse operation or who have risk factors precluding operation, but the efficacy is low.

ASYMPTOMATIC STONES. Cholecystectomy is not indicated routinely in patients who have asymptomatic stones.
Some recommend operation in patients who are candidates
for heart or kidney transplantation, patients receiving total
parenteral nutrition, and during bariatric surgery for morbid
obesity.

CHRONIC ACALCULOUS CHOLECYSTITIS. Occasionally, patients present with typical gallbladder symptoms but
without gallstones. Reproduction of symptoms after cholecystokinin administration, poor contraction of the gallbladder,
and the presence of cholesterol crystals in bile collected from
the duodenum are taken by some to be indications for cholecystectomy.

III

Cholangitis
David L. Nahrwold, M.D.

Cholangitis is a bacterial, parasitic, or rarely, a chemical inflammation of the biliary duct system.

PATHOGENESIS. Bacteria and parasites may enter the bile duct system through the liver, having been delivered through the portal venous system from the intestine. Bacteria and parasites also may enter the duct system through the ampulla of Vater, usually after sphincterotomy or a biliary-enteric anastomosis. A characteristic feature of cholangitis is that it does not occur in the absence of partial or complete bile duct obstruction. Therefore, the biliary tract must be investigated for concomitant disease when cholangitis is diagnosed.

Cholangitis is life-threatening when bacteria or their toxic products enter the general circulation from hepatic sinusoids, which communicate with bile canaliculi. This cholangiovenous reflux occurs during episodes of increased pressure within the biliary duct system, an obvious consequence of complete or partial bile duct obstruction. In complete obstruction, the bile duct system may become filled with pus—in effect, a large abscess. The organisms most frequently found in the blood of patients with cholangitis are *Escherichia coli*, species of *Klebsiella*, *Proteus*, and *Pseudomonas*, and the gram-positive organisms *Streptococcus faecalis* and enterococcus species. The anaerobic species *Bacteroides* and *Clostridium* and the fungus *Candida* also have been isolated.

ASSOCIATED CONDITIONS. Bile duct calculi account for approximately 60% of cases. They may migrate from the gallbladder or form *de novo* in the bile ducts. The latter are usually predominantly calcium bilirubinate, the formation of which involves beta-glucuronidase produced by biliary bacteria. Malignant strictures involving the bile ducts, pancreas, or ampullary area may be associated with cholangitis. Benign strictures, resulting from previous surgery, choledocholithiasis, or chronic pancreatitis, may be heralded by cholangitis. Cases frequently follow instrumentation of the biliary system for cholangiography or the insertion of tubes or stents. Other causes include infestation with *Clonorchis sinensis* or *Ascaris lumbricoides* or chemical irritation from carbamazepine or sulindac.

CLINICAL MANIFESTATIONS. Charcot's triad—chills and fever, abdominal pain, and jaundice—occurs in 50% to 70% of patients who have cholangitis. Nevertheless, all patients will manifest at least one element of Charcot's triad. The pain is

---

See the corresponding chapter or part in the *Textbook of Surgery*, 15th edition, pp. 1140–1145, for a more detailed discussion of this topic, including a comprehensive list of references.

usually mild and in the right upper quadrant. Nausea and vomiting are the only other frequent symptoms.

In acute toxic cholangitis, a potentially fatal condition, patients may manifest hemodynamic instability and confusion or coma. In them, rapid diagnosis and emergency treatment are lifesaving.

Most patients have tenderness in the right upper quadrant or epigastrium, but signs of peritoneal irritation are not found commonly. Bowel sounds are normal. Abnormal laboratory tests include elevated white blood cell count, serum bilirubin, and alkaline phosphatase.

DIAGNOSIS. After controlling the infection, cholangiography is performed. The percutaneous transhepatic method is used less often because of the availability of endoscopic cholangiography and the ability to perform concomitant sphincterotomy and stone extraction, when indicated.

TREATMENT. Initial therapy in mild cholangitis is a second- or third-generation cephalosporin. Acute toxic cholangitis should be treated initially with a penicillin, an aminoglycoside, and either clindamycin or metronidazole.

Emergency decompression of the duct system is performed in patients with acute toxic cholangitis, usually by endoscopic sphincterotomy and nasobiliary drainage. When this is not available or possible, decompression is performed by percutaneous transhepatic catheterization. Laparotomy and insertion of a T-tube in the common duct are indicated if the noninvasive procedures fail or are not available.

IV

Gallstone Ileus and Fistula
Francis E. Rosato, M.D.

BILIARY FISTULAS

A biliary fistula is an abnormal communication between any portion of the biliary tree and some other area. External fistulas are most often due to trauma, especially operative trauma, and present as bile leaks to the outside. Internal fistulas to other structures are most often caused by inflammatory or neoplastic disease. Biliary-intestinal fistulas may allow gallstones to enter the intestinal tract, with resulting distal small bowel obstruction (see later); biliary-bronchial connections cause biloptysis (bile-stained sputum); biliary–urinary bladder connections produce bile-stained urine.

See the corresponding chapter or part in the *Textbook of Surgery*, 15th edition, pp. 1145–1148, for a more detailed discussion of this topic, including a comprehensive list of references.

COMPLICATIONS. There are four important complications of fistula: (1) hyponatremia due to the external loss of the sodium content of bile either externally or into other structures, (2) weight loss (the loss of bile to the gastrointestinal tract in all but biliary–high intestinal fistulas can cause malabsorption syndrome), (3) infection (all bile fistulas potentially allow bacterial contamination of bile, i.e., cholangitis; the classic presentation of such cholangitis is Charcot's triad of jaundice, pain, fever, and shaking chills, and (4) gallstone ileus (see following section on gallstone ileus).

TREATMENT. There are five major components to treatment.

1. *Define the fistula.* This is done most easily through an external fistulogram with the injection of contrast material into the external opening of the fistula. For internal fistulas, other studies, including a gastrointestinal series, barium enema, cholangiography, bronchoscopy, or cystography, may be necessary for delineation of the fistula.

2. *Discover the cause of the fistula.* The studies mentioned for delineating the extent of the fistula also may provide evidence as to the cause. Cytologic studies help to establish neoplasm when it is the cause of the fistula. Presently, 85% of all internal fistulas are due to gallstone disease, with inflammation establishing a cholecystoenteric fistula, whereas 8% are due to peptic ulcer disease. Operative trauma is responsible for most external fistulas.

3. *Control infection.* Cholangitis is a prominent part of the problem. Bile cultures can be useful in choosing the most appropriate antibiotic, usually one with a spectrum against gram-negative aerobic and anaerobic organisms.

4. *Correct electrolyte abnormalities,* particularly sodium depletion.

5. *Surgical therapy.* The initial approach is usually percutaneous drainage of any bile collections. This measure alone suffices to allow the resolution of most external biliary fistulas. Where indicated, the relief of distal common ductal obstruction through papillotomy by endoscopic retrograde cholangiopancreatography may allow normal flow of bile with resolution of many external and internal fistulas. When jaundice, sepsis, electrolyte abnormalities, or worsening nutrition continue despite such measures, surgical therapy is indicated. At operation, an attempt is made to establish the cause of the fistula. For external fistulas, relief of obstruction may suffice. At times, formal biliary-enteric anastomoses must be constructed and bile duct repairs done in conjunction with attempts at relieving obstruction. For internal fistulas, separation of the partner structures is done with surgical closure of each. When neoplasia is the underlying cause, separation is often not possible, but relief of obstruction to bile flow is the objective. For fistulas secondary to gallstone disease, a simple cholecystectomy with repair of the biliary partner structure is sufficient. When peptic ulcer disease is the underlying cause, separation of the communicating structures, repair of both, and definitive acid-reducing procedures are combined for definitive treatment.

GALLSTONE ILEUS

When an antecedent cholecystointestinal or choledochointestinal fistula occurs, the potential exists for the migration of gallstones into the intestine. They cause obstruction when they can no longer negotiate the more narrow reaches of the small intestine. They are most common (4:1) in women, and 80% occur in those over the age of 70 years. The diagnosis is based on a recognition of the following diagnostic features: air in the biliary tree of dilated small bowel loops, the finding of an opaque stone in the intestinal tract by radiography, and more recently, the finding of nonopaque stones in the distal small bowel with the use of ultrasound.

TREATMENT. The first priority in gallstone ileus is removal of the obstructing stone, usually located in the distal small bowel. If the patient is at high risk, or if there has been instability of vital signs in the course of the operation, this suffices. If definitive "takedown" of the underlying biliary-enteric fistula (usually cholecystoenteric) is not performed, there is a 10% likelihood of recurrence of the phenomenon. Where possible, therefore, definitive correction of the underlying fistula should be performed either as a part of the initial procedure or as a planned second operation when the patient is judged to be well enough.

V

Carcinoma of the Gallbladder
David Fromm, M.D.

Carcinoma of the gallbladder is the most common malignant lesion of the biliary tract and is more frequent in those at least 50 years old and female. There is a well-established association with gallstones, which are present in at least 70% of cases. Cancer of the gallbladder associated with cholelithiasis occurs in about 0.5% of autopsies and from about 1% to 2% in patients undergoing cholecystectomy. There is no predilection for carcinoma developing in a gallbladder containing single as opposed to multiple stones. Other conditions believed to be associated with the development of carcinoma include cholecystoenteric fistula, porcelain gallbladder, congenital biliary dilatation, a long common biliary channel distal to entry of the pancreatic duct, xanthogranulomatous cholecystitis, and ulcerative colitis. The reported association with adenomyomatosis may be coincidental. Adenomas are prema-

See the corresponding chapter or part in the *Textbook of Surgery*, 15th edition, pp. 1148–1151, for a more detailed discussion of this topic, including a comprehensive list of references.

lignant and present as a polypoid lesion, which is best detected by ultrasonography. Surgical treatment of a polypoid lesion is recommended if the lesion exceeds 1 cm. in diameter, or is single or associated with stones, or if the patient is older than 50 years. These features are associated more often with a malignant polyp.

Adenocarcinoma constitutes 82% of cases; undifferentiated carcinoma occurs in 7%, and squamous cell occurs in 3%. Unusual tumors include adenoacanthoma, lymphosarcoma, rhabdomyosarcoma, reticulum cell sarcoma, fibrosarcoma, melanoma, carcinoid, and carcinosarcoma. The tumor spreads by several routes: lymphatic, vascular, intraperitoneal seeding, neural, intraductal, and direct extension. The various forms of liver involvement include spread along the bile ductules, veins, and lymphatics and spread by direct extension.

The symptoms of carcinoma of the gallbladder are not specific. Pain occurs in 66%, weight loss in 59%, jaundice in 51%, anorexia in 40%, and right upper quadrant mass in 40% of patients. Malignancy in patients with pre-existing biliary symptoms generally produces a noticeable change in symptoms. A right upper quadrant mass may be apparent and is usually tender. Jaundice most often is due to invasion of the common duct or compression from involved pericholedochal lymph nodes and, less frequently, involvement of the liver; rarely, it is due to concurrent stones in the biliary tract. The diagnosis is infrequently made by radiographic studies or even preoperatively. Those with early, resectable lesions tend to have symptoms of benign biliary disease.

Malignancy of the gallbladder usually is associated with a dismal prognosis. About 88% die within a year of diagnosis, and only about 4% are alive after 5 years. Most of the long-term survivors are those in whom the surgeon was unaware of the presence of the tumor at the time of cholecystectomy (approximately 12% of cases), the diagnosis being made by the pathologist. Practically all patients with invasion confined to the mucosa and muscularis and who survive operation are alive at 5 years, whereas only about 7% with serosal (or adventitial) involvement are alive at 5 years. It is a rare patient who is symptomatic from the tumor and who enjoys prolonged survival following operative treatment.

There continues to be debate about the utility of radical resection of the tumor. Proponents of a radical approach optimistically maintain that up to 30% of patients present with tumors that could be treated by radical cholecystectomy, which includes in-continuity resection of its hepatic bed or right hepatic lobectomy (or even trisegmentectomy) and regional lymph node dissection. Yet only a handful of long-term survivors have been reported following radical surgery. Data are inconclusive to support the proposition that the patient with unexpected carcinoma found histologically should undergo reoperation with intent for radical excision. There are indirect suggestions that the prognosis of gallbladder carcinoma may be improving, but it is not clear if this is spontaneous or due either to earlier diagnosis or surgical management.

Moderate palliation is occasionally achieved by operation, even though its benefits are usually of short duration. Palliation is directed chiefly at relieving common duct obstruction or bypassing an obstructed portion of the gastrointestinal tract. Some palliation also may be achieved by removing the gallbladder, when feasible, in the hope of delaying obstruction of surrounding structures. Chemotherapy and/or radiation therapy have questionable benefit.

Obstructive jaundice occurring some time after cholecystectomy can be difficult to treat by operation because of tumor encroachment in the porta hepatis. Placement of a prosthesis endoscopically or percutaneously through a malignant stricture in the common duct or hepatic bifurcation can reduce symptoms relating to biliary obstruction successfully. However, long-term palliation appears more related to tumor extent than to resolution of jaundice.

35

THE PANCREAS

Charles J. Yeo, M.D., and John L. Cameron, M.D.

ANATOMY. The pancreas is a retroperitoneal organ that extends obliquely from the duodenal C loop to the hilum of the spleen. It is divided into four portions: head, neck, body, and tail. The head is intimately associated with the second portion of the duodenum, and these two structures are jointly supplied by the pancreaticoduodenal arteries. Blood is supplied to the body and tail of the pancreas through a variable complex of arteries. The venous drainage of the pancreas corresponds with the segmental arterial supply and terminates in the portal vein. Multiple lymph node groups drain the pancreas, largely corresponding to the venous drainage patterns.

HISTOLOGY. The pancreas incorporates both an endocrine and exocrine organ system. The endocrine portion resides in nearly spherical collections of cells scattered throughout the pancreatic parenchyma, the islets of Langerhans. Each islet is composed of several distinctive cell types. Beta cells produce insulin and make up the majority of the islet cell population. Alpha cells produce glucagon and constitute approximately one quarter of the total islet cell number. Other cells found within the islets include somatostatin-producing delta cells, as well as cells that produce pancreatic polypeptide. The acinus is composed of a single layer of acinar cells, which contain zymogen granules in their narrow, centrally located apical portion. The pancreatic ductal system originates in the centroacinar cells of each individual acinus and includes intercalated duct cells and cells of the main excretory duct.

PHYSIOLOGY. Exocrine. The final product of the exocrine pancreas is a clear isotonic solution with a pH $\cong$ 8. There are two distinct components of pancreatic exocrine secretion: enzymes originating from acinar cells and water and electrolytes originating from the centroacinar and intercalated duct cells. Cholecystokinin is the most potent endogenous stimulant of pancreatic enzyme secretion, while secretin is the most potent endogenous stimulant of pancreatic water and electrolyte secretion.

Endocrine. The release of *insulin* into the portal blood is controlled by the concentration of blood glucose, vagal interactions, and local concentrations of somatostatin. The major stimulus for *glucagon* release is a fall in serum glucose. *Somatostatin* has a broad inhibitory spectrum of gastrointestinal activity.

ACUTE PANCREATITIS. Acute pancreatitis can vary from mild parenchymal edema to severe hemorrhagic destruction associated with loss of pancreatic viability, gangrene, and

---

See the corresponding chapter or part in the *Textbook of Surgery,* 15th edition, pp. 1152–1186, for a more detailed discussion of this topic, including a comprehensive list of references.

TABLE 1. Etiologies of Acute Pancreatitis

Alcohol	Pancreatic duct obstruction
Biliary tract disease (gallstones)	Tumor
Hyperlipidemia	Pancreas divisum
Hypercalcemia	Ampullary stenosis
Familial	Ascaris infestation
Trauma	Duodenal obstruction
External	Viral infection
Operative	Scorpion venom
Retrograde pancreatography	Drugs
Ischemia	Idiopathic
Hypotension	
Cardiopulmonary bypass	
Atheroembolism	
Vasculitis	

subsequent necrosis. Nine of 10 patients experience mild to moderate symptoms and improve with supportive care alone, while 10% of patients develop a severe life-threatening form of acute pancreatitis.

Etiology. There are many causes of acute pancreatitis (Table 1). In 90% of cases, the cause is related to excessive alcohol intake or biliary tract disease.

Clinical Presentation. The predominant clinical features of acute pancreatitis are midepigastric abdominal pain, nausea, and vomiting. Typical findings on examination include fever, tachycardia, epigastric tenderness, and abdominal distention. Patients with severe pancreatitis may manifest hypotension, hypovolemia, and obtundation.

Diagnosis. The diagnosis of acute pancreatitis is supported by appropriate laboratory determinations and radiographic findings. Serum amylase is the most widely used laboratory test. Persistent hyperamylasemia beyond the first week of illness may indicate the development of a pancreatic pseudocyst, abscess, or infected necrosis. Other laboratory and radiographic tests may be used for the diagnosis of acute pancreatitis (Table 2). Currently, the most widely accepted and sensitive radiographic method used to confirm the diagnosis of acute pancreatitis is computed tomography (CT). A correlation exists between the degree of CT abnormality and the clinical course and severity of acute pancreatitis.

Clinical Course. The severity and prognosis of acute pan-

TABLE 2. Diagnosis of Acute Pancreatitis

Laboratory Tests	Radiographic Procedures
Serum amylase	Plain chest roentgenogram
Serum amylase isoenzymes	Plain abdominal roentgenogram
Urinary amylase	Upper GI contrast series
Amylase-creatinine clearance ratio	Ultrasonography
Serum lipase	Computed tomography
Serum methemalbumin	Magnetic resonance imaging
Peritoneal fluid analysis	

TABLE 3. Ranson's Early Prognostic Signs of Acute Pancreatitis (Used in Patients with Pancreatitis Not Caused by Gallstones)

At Admission	During Initial 48 Hours
Age over 55 years	Hematocrit falls > 10%
WBC > 16,000 cells / cu. mm.	BUN elevation > 5 mg. / 100 ml.
Blood glucose > 200 mg. / 100 ml.	Serum calcium falls to < 8 mg. / 100 ml.
Serum lactate dehydrogenase > 250 I.U./L.	Arterial P_{O_2} < 60 torr
AST > 250 units / 100 ml.	Base deficit > 4 mEq. / L.
	Estimated fluid sequestration > 6 L.

creatitis can be predicted using routinely available clinical and laboratory determinations (Table 3). Patients with two or fewer prognostic signs generally require simple supportive care and usually incur no major morbidity or mortality. In contrast, patients with three or more prognostic signs have a stepwise increase in morbidity and mortality rates.

Nonoperative Management. The initial management of patients with acute pancreatitis is nonoperative. Therapy includes intravenous fluid and electrolyte replacement using crystalloid solutions. Nasogastric decompression is used in patients with significant ileus in an effort to prevent emesis and aspiration. Abdominal pain is treated with careful administration of meperidine. Oral intake, initially prohibited, is resumed when abdominal pain and tenderness have improved and ileus has resolved. Antibiotics are not indicated in the routine treatment of mild to moderate pancreatitis but reduce the risk of septic complications in patients with severe pancreatitis (three or more Ranson prognostic signs). Respiratory complications require appropriate supportive care.

Operative Management. Operative intervention is indicated in four specific circumstances:

1. *Uncertainty of clinical diagnosis.* In this uncommon situation, exploratory laparotomy may be indicated to exclude a surgically correctable disease with potentially fatal outcome in the unoperated state. With the widespread availability of abdominal CT scanning, these situations are becoming less frequent.

2. *Treatment of secondary pancreatic infection.* Pancreatic abscess, infected pseudocyst, or infected necrosis develops in up to 5% of all patients with pancreatitis. These often life-threatening complications occur with increasing frequency, in direct proportion to the severity of acute pancreatitis. The treatment of secondary pancreatic infections combines antibiotic therapy with prompt drainage.

3. *Correction of associated biliary tract disease.* Definitive biliary tract operations during the index admission (usually laparoscopic cholecystectomy) are now favored for the majority of patients with gallstone-associated pancreatitis. In patients with severe pancreatitis and a deteriorating clinical course, the use of early endoscopic retrograde cholangiopancreatography

(ERCP) to document choledocholithiasis and subsequent endoscopic sphincterotomy to retrieve stones should be considered.

4. *Deterioration of clinical status.* The most controversial
indication for surgical therapy involves patients with a deteriorating clinical condition. In such cases, proponents of early
operative intervention recommend procedures ranging from
local débridement of necrotic tissue to formal total pancreatectomy. To date, no controlled, randomized clinical trials allow
realistic evaluation of the efficacy of such early resectional
therapy.

CHRONIC PANCREATITIS. Chronic pancreatitis encompasses recurrent or persistent abdominal pain of pancreatic
origin combined with evidence of exocrine and endocrine
insufficiency and is marked pathologically by irreversible parenchymal destruction.

Etiology. Chronic pancreatitis is associated with alcohol
abuse, hyperparathyroidism, congenital anomalies of the pancreatic duct, cystic fibrosis, and pancreatic trauma. It also may
be idiopathic.

Clinical Presentation. Patients typically present in the
fourth or fifth decade of life with a history of alcohol abuse
and with epigastric and back pain. Up to a third of patients
have insulin-dependent diabetes, and up to one quarter have
steatorrhea. Narcotic abuse is common.

Diagnosis. Chronic pancreatitis is usually suspected based
on the clinical setting. Plain abdominal films may reveal pancreatic calcifications. An abdominal CT scan is used to evaluate the size and texture of the gland, to inspect for pancreatic
parenchymal calcifications and nodularity, and to assess the
pancreatic ductal system. Pancreatography can document ductal abnormalities not seen by CT.

Nonoperative Management. Nonoperative management
encompasses control of abdominal pain and treatment of endocrine and exocrine insufficiency. In some patients, pain
relief may be obtained by abstinence from alcohol. Pain control begins with nonnarcotic analgesics, followed later by narcotic analgesics. Diabetes may require cautious insulin therapy. Exocrine insufficiency is treated with exogenous pancreatic
enzyme supplementation.

Operative Management. Surgical treatment is categorized
into three groups of procedures: ampullary, ductal drainage,
and ablative. Prior to considering surgical intervention, mandatory evaluation involves pancreatic imaging by CT as well
as assessment of pancreatic ductal anatomy by ERCP. *Ampullary procedures* currently have limited application. The most
common *ductal drainage procedure* involves a side-to-side
pancreaticojejunostomy. Ductal drainage does not improve
established pancreatic exocrine or endocrine dysfunction, although it may delay the rate of progressive impairment. *Ablative procedures* are generally reserved for patients who are not
candidates for or who have failed ductal drainage procedures.
In carefully selected patients with parenchymal disease localized to the body and tail of the pancreas, distal pancreatectomy (40% to 80% pancreatectomy) has success. Subtotal distal
pancreatectomy (95% pancreatectomy) has been applied to

patients with severe diffuse parenchymal disease. Pylorus-preserving pancreaticoduodenectomy is an option in patients without ductal dilatation, in whom parenchymal disease primarily affects the head of the gland. Newer duodenum-sparing procedures have been applied in selected populations. Total pancreatectomy, combined with the necessary duodenal resection, is a last-resort measure in carefully selected patients who have lesser procedures.

DISRUPTIONS OF THE PANCREATIC DUCT. Disruptions of the pancreatic duct occur most commonly in the setting of alcoholic pancreatitis or following pancreatic trauma. Disruptions of the pancreatic duct can cause internal or external pancreatic fistulas.

Internal Pancreatic Fistula. *Pancreatic pseudocysts* are localized collections of pancreatic secretions that lack an epithelial lining, and they occur when surrounding tissues wall off a pancreatic duct disruption. Pancreatic pseudocysts may develop in up to 10% of patients after acute alcoholic pancreatitis. Patients with pseudocysts most often present with upper abdominal pain, nausea, and vomiting. The majority of patients have elevations of serum amylase. Definitive diagnosis is made by CT scan or ultrasound. Recent evidence suggests that up to 50% of pseudocysts can be managed nonoperatively without complication. Strict size criteria alone are not sufficient to determine the need for operative versus nonoperative management. For pseudocysts that require operative intervention, preoperative endoscopic retrograde pancreatography may be useful. Options for the management of pseudocysts include *internal drainage* via cystojejunostomy, cystogastrostomy, or cystoduodenostomy; *excision; external drainage*; and *percutaneous* or *endoscopic drainage* techniques.

Pancreatic ascites occurs when exocrine secretions extravasate anteriorly from the pancreatic duct and drain freely into the peritoneal cavity. *Pancreatic pleural effusion* can result when exocrine secretions extravasate into the retroperitoneum and track cephalad through the diaphragm into the thorax. Both entities occur most commonly as the result of alcohol abuse. Patients with pancreatic ascites typically present with painless massive ascites. Patients with pancreatic pleural effusion generally present with primary pulmonary symptoms such as dyspnea, chest pain, and cough. Nonoperative treatment is indicated initially and may resolve the clinical entity in 50% of patients. In patients not cured by nonoperative management, operative intervention follows delineation of pancreatic duct anatomy by ERCP.

An *external pancreatic fistula* is defined as drainage of exocrine secretions through a drain site or a wound that persists for more than 7 days. Complications of such fistulas include sepsis, fluid and electrolyte abnormalities, and skin excoriation. Sinography and CT are used to delineate the anatomy of the fistulous tract. Total parenteral nutrition is often utilized to avoid pancreatic stimulation by oral intake and to maximize tissue anabolism.

NEOPLASMS OF THE PANCREAS. Exocrine Tumors. Approximately 28,000 new cases of *cancer of the exocrine pancreas* are diagnosed each year in the United States. Cancer of the pancreas is more common in blacks, cigarette smokers, and males, and it appears to be linked to the presence of diabetes mellitus and chronic pancreatitis. More than 90% of these tumors are duct cell adenocarcinomas, with two thirds arising in the pancreatic head.

Periampullary Carcinoma. Four malignant neoplasms are classified as periampullary neoplasms: cancer of the head of the pancreas (85%), ampullary carcinomas (10%), and duodenal and distal common bile duct carcinomas (<5% each). The most common clinical features are jaundice, weight loss, and abdominal pain. The majority of patients have elevated serum bilirubin and alkaline phosphatase. Currently available serologic tests (such as CEA and CA 19-9) are not accurate enough for diagnosis or screening. CT scans determine the size of the primary neoplasm and detect hepatic metastases. The site of the biliary obstruction can be defined by cholangiography, using either the percutaneous transhepatic or the endoscopic retrograde route. In patients with potentially resectable tumors, selective celiac and mesenteric angiography or laparoscopy can be used to stage for resectability.

Nonoperative therapy is an option in patients with documented distant metastases, unresectable local disease, or acute or chronic debilitating illnesses. Efforts should be made to acquire a tissue diagnosis and to palliate abdominal pain and biliary obstruction.

Many patients with periampullary carcinoma are candidates for *operative therapy.* Hepatic metastases, serosal implants, and lymph node metastases outside the resection area indicate unresectable disease. Standard resection for periampullary carcinoma involves a pancreaticoduodenectomy, or Whipple resection. A modification of the standard Whipple resection, the pylorus-preserving pancreaticoduodenectomy, has gained popularity. Accumulated data indicate no compromise in survival in patients undergoing pylorus preservation. The major determinant of survival is the site of origin of the tumor, with resectable cancers of the duodenum, distal bile duct, and ampulla being associated with 5-year survival rates of 40% to 60%, whereas resectable carcinoma of the head of the pancreas is associated with a 5-year survival rate of up to 20%.

Palliative surgery for periampullary carcinoma is performed in patients with unresectable disease discovered at the time of laparotomy. Palliative surgery seeks to alleviate biliary obstruction, duodenal obstruction, and tumor-associated pain.

The combination of radiation and chemotherapy has been shown to prolong survival in patients with resected pancreatic adenocarcinoma.

Carcinoma of the body and tail of the pancreas accounts for up to 30% of all cases of pancreatic cancer. Patients generally present with weight loss and abdominal pain. Abdominal CT is the best initial radiographic study. ERCP commonly documents a pancreatic duct cutoff. Prior to laparotomy, visceral arteriography may be helpful. Good-risk patients without evidence of metastatic disease and with favorable arteriographic findings are best served by abdominal exploration with curative intent. The resectability rate for carcinoma of the body and tail of the pancreas is less than 7%, and the prognosis is generally poor (mean survival 5 to 6 months).

ENDOCRINE TUMORS. Pancreatic islet cell endocrine tumors are rare and are presumed to originate from neural crest cells. Functional endocrine tumors are conventionally named according to the major hormone produced by the tumor (Table 4). Malignancy is determined by the presence of local invasion, spread to regional lymph nodes, or the existence of hepatic or distant metastases. The general principles applicable to the management of patients with suspected functional pancreatic endocrine tumors involve (1) recognition of the abnormal physiology or characteristic syndrome, (2) detection of serum hormone elevations by radioimmunoassay, and (3) localization and staging of the tumor in preparation for operative therapy. Standard radiographic techniques used for tumor localization include CT with intravenous and oral contrast material, endoscopic ultrasonography, visceral angiography, transhepatic portal venous sampling, and intraoperative ultrasonography. The goals of surgical therapy include control of symptoms due to hormone excess, excision of maximal neoplastic tissue, and prevention of tumor recurrence.

Insulinoma is the most common endocrine tumor of the pancreas. Symptoms can be categorized into two groups: hypoglycemia-induced catecholamine-surge symptoms and neuroglycopenic symptoms. The most reliable method for diagnosing insulinomas involves a monitored 72-hour fast. Following biochemical diagnosis and appropriate localization studies, the treatment of insulinoma is surgical. Up to 90% of patients have benign solitary pancreatic adenomas amenable to surgical cure, often by simple enucleation techniques. Malignant insulinomas occur in 10% to 15% of cases.

Gastrinoma is the second most common functional pancreatic endocrine tumor. Clinical manifestations include peptic ulcer disease, abdominal pain, diarrhea, and reflux esophagitis. The fasting serum gastrin is almost always elevated above normal (100 to 200 pg. per ml.) and may be over 1000 pg. per ml. Gastric acid analysis differentiates ulcerogenic from nonulcerogenic states. Provocative testing using the intravenous secretin stimulation test should be employed in patients with fasting serum gastrin levels in the range of 200 to 1000 pg. per ml. After confirming the diagnosis, patient management involves (1) control of gastric acid hypersecretion (using omeprazole) and (2) alteration of the natural history of the gastrinoma (surgical resection). All patients undergo radiographic study to localize the primary tumor and to assess for metastatic disease. In the absence of documented unresectable disease, all patients should undergo exploration with curative intent. Improvements in preoperative localization and intraoperative assessment have yielded surgical cure rates approaching 35%.

PANCREATIC TRAUMA. Less than 2% of patients with abdominal trauma have pancreatic injuries. No laboratory test is sufficiently accurate for the specific diagnosis of pancreatic injury. CT has gained importance in the serial evaluation of pancreatic trauma. Patients who undergo laparotomy for abdominal trauma require complete assessment of the pan-

TABLE 4. Classification of Functional Pancreatic Endocrine Tumors

Tumor Name	Major Hormone(s)	Cell Type	Syndrome	Malignancy Rate	Extrapancreatic Location
Insulinoma	Insulin	Beta	Hypoglycemia	<15%	Rare
Gastrinoma (Zollinger-Ellison syndrome)	Gastrin	Non-beta	Peptic ulcer Diarrhea	50%	Frequent
Vipoma (Verner-Morrison syndrome)	VIP Prostaglandins	Non-beta	Watery diarrhea Hypokalemia Achlorhydria	Most	Occasional
Glucagonoma	Glucagon	Alpha	Hyperglycemia Dermatitis	Most	Rare
Somatostatinoma	Somatostatin	Delta	Hyperglycemia Steatorrhea Gallstones	Most	Rare

creas. The four classes of pancreatic injury include: *Class I injury,* pancreatic contusion without capsular rupture; *Class II injury,* pancreatic capsular or parenchymal rupture without injury to the main pancreatic duct; *Class III injury,* parenchymal injury associated with rupture or destruction of the main pancreatic duct; and *Class IV injury,* combined severe injuries to the pancreas and duodenum. Class I and Class II injuries are treated by drainage alone. Class III injuries to the body and tail are treated by distal pancreatectomy encompassing the site of the injury. Class III injuries to the head may be débrided and externally drained or drained via Roux-en-Y pancreaticojejunostomy. Surgical options for treatment of Class IV injuries include serosal patch technique, duodenal decompression with triple ostomy, duodenal diverticularization, or pancreaticoduodenectomy.

PANCREATIC TRANSPLANTATION. There are approximately 1 million Type I diabetics in the United States. Until recently, their primary therapy involved intermittent administration of subcutaneous insulin. Newer treatment methods include (1) sophisticated insulin delivery systems, (2) pancreatic islet cell transplantation, and (3) vascularized segmental or whole-pancreas transplantation. The transplantation of pancreatic islet cells alone is theoretically attractive because it avoids vascular and ductular anastomoses. Unfortunately, islet allotransplantation remains largely experimental. Segmental or whole-organ pancreas transplantation has been popularized at several centers. Whole-organ grafts are generally performed, providing exocrine drainage via a duodenal segment to the urinary bladder. Bladder-drained grafts allow the serial measurement of urinary amylase excretion as a measure of graft function. Immunosuppressive regimens usually involve quadruple-drug therapy. Patients with functioning pancreatic grafts demonstrate nearly normal glucose tolerance. Successful grafting appears to be protective against the development of diabetic nephropathy and can be associated with subjective improvement in peripheral neuropathy and diabetic retinopathy.

36

THE SPLEEN

George F. Sheldon, M.D., Robert D. Croom III, M.D., and Anthony A. Meyer, M.D., Ph.D.

An improved understanding of immune anemia, thrombocytopenia, and neutropenia has clarified the role of splenectomy in many hematologic diseases. Some diseases, such as immune thrombocytopenic purpura (ITP), appear to be increasing in incidence. Splenectomy as a means of staging Hodgkin's disease is no longer such an important diagnostic test in the overall approach to that disease, which now can be controlled in most patients using radiotherapy and chemotherapy. Splenectomy for splenomegaly associated with selected leukemias and non-Hodgkin's lymphomas is less commonly indicated as chemotherapy and radiation therapy have become more effective. The most frequent indications for splenectomy are now traumatic injury, ITP, and hypersplenism.

SPLENIC TRAUMA

If a splenic injury is suspected, admission to the hospital for monitoring is mandatory. A careful history should be obtained to include delineation of pain and a mechanism of injury consistent with splenic trauma. The signs and symptoms of splenic trauma are those of hemoperitoneum. Generalized and nonspecific abdominal pain in the left upper quadrant occurs in approximately one third of patients with splenic injury. Pain referred to the left shoulder (Kehr's sign) is inconsistent.

Diagnostic peritoneal lavage may reveal gross blood or an elevated red blood cell count indicating intraperitoneal hemorrhage. Computed tomography (CT) is the most accurate method available for diagnosing splenic injury. In selected splenic injuries, segmental resection of the spleen is practical and safe. In addition to partial splenectomy, splenorrhaphy, ligation of segmental vessels, and capsular repair are useful techniques for splenic salvage. Although technically more difficult than splenectomy, splenic repair can be performed with comparable transfusion requirements, reoperation rates, and morbidity. Conservatism in the management of splenic injury has extended beyond repairing and preserving an injured spleen when possible. Because bleeding from splenic trauma appears to be more self-limited in children than in adults, nonoperative therapy has proved to be safe in selected pediatric patients. However, 25% to 50% of adults with splenic injury can be treated nonoperatively.

See the corresponding chapter or part in the *Textbook of Surgery,* 15th edition, pp. 1187–1214, for a more detailed discussion of this topic, including a comprehensive list of references.

Nonoperative therapy requires a stable patient who is found by diagnostic tests to have an isolated splenic injury. One pitfall of nonoperative management of splenic trauma lies in the significant possibility of failing to diagnose and treat concomitant intra-abdominal injuries. An additional concern is that most reported series of nonoperative management of splenic injuries include patients with blood transfusion requirements substantial enough to expect an incidence of transfusion-related hepatitis greater than the statistical probability of postsplenectomy sepsis.

IMMUNE THROMBOCYTOPENIC PURPURA (ITP)

Immune thrombocytopenic purpura (previously idiopathic thrombocytopenic purpura) is a syndrome characterized by a persistently low platelet count. The thrombocytopenia is caused by a circulating antiplatelet factor that causes platelet destruction by the reticuloendothelial system. In most patients, the antiplatelet factor is an immunoglobulin (IgG) antibody directed toward a platelet-associated antigen. The majority of patients with ITP are young women. ITP is increasing in frequency, and the disease is now being diagnosed more often in men, caused in part by the association of immune thrombocytopenia with the acquired immunodeficiency syndrome (AIDS) and an increasing occurrence of ITP in homosexual men positive for human immunodeficiency virus (HIV), parenteral drug abusers, and hemophiliacs receiving multiple transfusions. The propensity for hemorrhage is reflected by the level of thrombocytopenia.

Diagnosis of ITP requires the exclusion of drug-dependent antibodies, isoantibodies, collagen vascular disease, lymphoproliferative disorders, thyroid disease, recent viral illness, and spurious thrombocytopenia. Patients with *classic* ITP rarely have a palpable spleen (<2%), whereas a palpable spleen that reflects mild to moderate enlargement and an associated high incidence of generalized lymphadenopathy have been found in ITP associated with AIDS. A peripheral blood smear shows thrombocytopenia, occasionally with an increased number of large platelets. A bone marrow aspirate reveals normal granulocytic and erythrocytic elements with an increased megakaryocyte count.

The goal of therapy in chronic ITP is to obtain a complete and sustained remission of the disease and to remove the patient from the risks of hemorrhage. This can be achieved in 80% to 90% of patients. Corticosteroid therapy (prednisone 1 mg. per kg. per day or the therapeutic equivalent) is instituted at the time of diagnosis. Most patients with ITP are improved with steroids, an increase in the platelet count occurring within 3 to 7 days and reaching a maximum in several weeks. Complete and sustained remission with steroids is rare. Splenectomy should be performed in patients with ITP that is refractory to corticosteroid therapy. In the majority of patients, splenectomy is performed electively. Emergency splenectomy is necessary in patients with ITP who have evidence of central nervous system bleeding.

ITP DURING CHILDHOOD

In children, particularly those under the age of 6, ITP often appears following a viral upper respiratory infection. In contrast to the adult form of the disease, childhood ITP usually undergoes spontaneous remission without specific therapy. Intracranial hemorrhage is a life-threatening complication of childhood ITP and is an indication for emergency splenectomy. Spontaneous and complete remission occurs in approximately 85% of children with ITP. Those in whom spontaneous remission does not occur within 1 year are considered to have chronic ITP and usually undergo elective splenectomy to avoid the risks of chronic thrombocytopenia.

High-dose intravenous gamma globulin is very effective in achieving an increase in the platelet count preoperatively in patients who do not respond to steroids or are not candidates for steroid therapy. It is postulated that intravenous gamma globulin therapy promotes a rise in the platelet count due to temporarily reducing platelet destruction by saturating macrophage Fc receptors, thus producing a transient blockage of the reticuloendothelial system. Immunizations with polyvalent pneumococcal vaccine (Pnu-Immune 23 or Pneumovax 23), *Hemophilus influenzae* vaccine, and *Neisseria meningitidis* vaccine should be administered as soon as it becomes likely that splenectomy will be performed. It is now being performed laparoscopically with good results. Over 80% of patients will have a normal platelet count in 3 months.

THROMBOTIC THROMBOCYTOPENIC PURPURA (TTP)

Thrombotic thrombocytopenic purpura (TTP) (Moschcowitz's syndrome) is a syndrome characterized by thrombocytopenia, microangiopathic hemolytic anemia, fluctuating neurologic abnormalities, progressive renal failure, and fever. TTP is produced by a widespread deposition of platelet microthrombi; clinical manifestations result from subendothelial and intraluminal deposits of hyaline material composed of aggregated platelets and fibrin in the capillaries. The etiology of TTP is unknown. TTP has a peak incidence in the third decade of life and occurs more frequently in females than in males.

Prognosis for untreated patients with TTP is very poor, with less than 10% surviving beyond 1 year. A combined therapeutic approach using plasma therapy, antiplatelet agents (aspirin and dipyridamole), and high-dose corticosteroid therapy is instituted immediately after the diagnosis is established. Plasma infusion or plasma exchange using plasmapheresis and replacement with fresh frozen plasma achieves response rates between 70% and 90%. If combined-modality therapy fails, splenectomy should be performed. Splenectomy occasionally results in spectacular improvement, particularly when combined with high-dose corticosteroid therapy and antiplatelet drugs.

HYPERSPLENISM

Hypersplenism is a concept, probably first used by Chauffard in 1907, that refers to a variety of ill effects resulting from increased splenic function which may be reversed by splenectomy. Hypersplenism is classified as *primary* when an underlying disease cannot be identified to account for the exaggerated splenic function. *Secondary hypersplenism* refers to those cases in which a specific or more or less well-defined disorder has been diagnosed. Primary hypersplenism is a diagnosis of exclusion and should be accepted only after an exhaustive search for a specific etiology of hypersplenism has been unrewarding. Secondary hypersplenism includes a number of diseases sharing the common feature of splenomegaly. Rather than listing these, it is more appropriate to consider the mechanisms producing splenic enlargement. Work hypertrophy from immune response and/or red blood cell destruction, venous congestion, myeloproliferation, infiltration, and neoplastic proliferation within the spleen produce variable degrees of splenomegaly. Diverse pathophysiologic mechanisms are involved in the resulting hypersplenism.

HODGKIN'S DISEASE

Hodgkin's disease is a malignant lymphoma characterized by the presence of typical multinucleate giant cells. The unique cell, described by Sternberg and later Reed around the turn of the century, is essential for diagnosis. The disease is slightly more common in men than in women. Most patients with Hodgkin's disease have asymptomatic lymphadenopathy at the time of diagnosis. The site of initial nodal involvement is the cervical area in most patients (65% to 80%), followed by the axillary (10% to 15%) and inguinal (6% to 12%) regions. Constitutional symptoms (B symptoms) such as fever, night sweats, weight loss, and pruritus usually are indicative of widespread involvement and are unfavorable prognostic signs. They may appear simultaneously with lymph node enlargement or may precede development of lymphadenopathy.

There are four histopathologic subtypes of Hodgkin's disease: lymphocyte predominance, nodular sclerosis, mixed cellularity, and lymphocyte depletion. Lymphocyte predominance and nodular sclerosis subtypes have a more favorable prognosis than mixed cellularity and lymphocyte depletion subtypes. Hodgkin's disease metastasizes initially in a predictable, nonrandom pattern via lymphatic channels to contiguous lymph node groups and organs with a prominent lymphatic tissue component. The predictable mode of spread of Hodgkin's disease provides the basis for irradiation of adjacent lymph node areas in patients with apparently localized disease. Treatment and ultimately survival of patients with Hodgkin's disease depend on the anatomic distribution of the disease and the presence or absence of specific symptoms, the stage of the disease, and the histopathologic subtype.

Since the concept of staging was introduced approximately 25 years ago, the staging process has undergone continued modification with the intent of accurately defining the anatomic sites of involvement and thus improving patient selection for the most appropriate type and amount of therapy. Stage I disease indicates nodal involvement in only one lymph node region. Stage II disease is limited to two or more lymph node regions on the same side of the diaphragm. Stage III refers to disease involving lymph node regions on both sides of the diaphragm (the spleen is considered a lymph node). Stage IV disease encompasses diffuse or disseminated involvement of one or more distant extranodal organs with or without associated lymph node involvement. The subscripts E and S are used to denote selected patients having localized extranodal disease (e.g., lung, bone, muscle, skin) contiguous with involved nodes and patients having splenic involvement, respectively. Stage is further classified as A (absence) or B (presence) with regard to fever, night sweats, weight loss, and pruritus. Staging laparotomy, which in the past was employed frequently for pathologic staging of Hodgkin's disease, now is being used less frequently.

Most patients with Hodgkin's disease present as Stage II or III, with 10% to 15% presenting as Stage I or Stage IV. Untreated Hodgkin's disease has a 5-year survival rate of 5%. Current survival rates for Hodgkin's, however, approximate 85% for all stages. The "gold standard" for management of Stage I and IIA Hodgkin's disease is external-beam radiation. The potential contribution of adjuvant radiation therapy to the management of advanced-stage Hodgkin's disease remains controversial. The cornerstone of therapy for advanced Hodgkin's disease is combination chemotherapy. Staging between IIA and IIIA can make some difference in treatment.

There are subsets of patients in whom the likelihood of any staging change that would alter therapy is remote. The risk of having abdominal involvement is less than 10% in clinical Stage I women, clinical Stage I men with lymphocyte predominance, and clinical Stage II women who are less than 27 years of age with three different sites.

Alternatively, the Stage I patient who has a large mediastinal mass now usually requires chemotherapy in addition to external-beam radiation because of recurrence outside the radiation ports and the fact of cardiac, especially pericardial, involvement with radiation. Stage IIIB patients require no staging, nor do ones with multiple E, IIA2.

Another contraindication or reason for the decline in staging has been the appearance of acute myeloid leukemia in significant numbers of patients who have had MOPP therapy and have received staging laparotomy with splenectomy.

The approximate results of different stages of Hodgkin's disease, then, are as follows: Stages I and IIA treated by external-beam radiation alone have an 80% FFP (free from progression) and a 90% regression-free survival; Stage IIIA has a 94% relapse-free survival at 10 years with MOPP; and

Stage IVA with alternating MOPP and ABD has 80% remission. The potential of bone marrow transplantation supplementing the treatment is an additional therapeutic maneuver.

The reason, then, that staging laparotomies are now less frequently done, is not entirely due to the ability to better stage the patient by noninvasive means, that is, CT, laparoscopic surgery, and so on. It speaks in part to the fact of the effectiveness of the various therapeutic modalities available. Salvage after recurrence is quite possible with most patients with Hodgkin's disease, making it less likely that the small differential changed by a staging process at the present time would make much difference in overall survival.

NON-HODGKIN'S LYMPHOMAS

Non-Hodgkin's lymphomas (NHL) constitute a diverse group of primary malignancies of lymphoreticular tissues. The clinical course and natural history of NHL are more variable than those of Hodgkin's disease, the pattern of spread is irregular, and more patients have leukemic features. In contrast to Hodgkin's disease, only about two thirds of patients with NHL initially have asymptomatic lymphadenopathy. In 20% to 35% of patients, the onset of NHL occurs in an extranodal site. In addition to peripheral and mediastinal lymphadenopathy, NHL commonly is found initially as an abdominal mass (retroperitoneal or mesenteric) or as hepatic and/or splenic enlargement. Constitutional symptoms such as fever, weight loss, and night sweats are frequently present. In NHLs the mode of spread generally is unpredictable, and most patients have disseminated disease at the time of presentation. As with Hodgkin's disease, chemotherapy and/or radiation therapy are the primary forms of treatment.

Splenectomy in NHL also is performed for hematologic depression secondary to hypersplenism or to relieve symptomatic splenomegaly or discomfort from recurrent splenic infarctions. Significant therapeutic benefit can be achieved by splenectomy in 80% to 90% of patients with advanced lymphomas (including Hodgkin's disease).

HAIRY CELL LEUKEMIA

Hairy cell leukemia (HCL, leukemic reticuloendotheliosis) is an uncommon form of leukemia characterized by pancytopenia, splenomegaly without significant lymphadenopathy, and characteristic mononuclear cells (hairy cells) in the blood and bone marrow. The disease is more common in males (ratio 4:1). The typical patient is a middle-aged man with moderate splenomegaly, absence of significant peripheral adenopathy, and variable hepatomegaly.

SPLENECTOMY FOR ANEMIA

Hemolytic anemia results from an increase in the rate of red cell destruction. Diagnostic evaluation should include a detailed family history, because many hemolytic anemias benefited by splenectomy have a hereditary basis. Congenital hemolytic anemias have a defect intrinsic to the red cell that may involve the cell membrane (hereditary spherocytosis), cellular metabolism (pyruvate kinase deficiency, G-6-PD deficiency), hemoglobin structure (sickle cell anemia), or hemoglobin chain synthesis rates (thalassemia). Acquired hemolytic anemias have an extracorpuscular factor that affects normal red cells.

Clinical features include variable pallor related to the degree of anemia, mild, fluctuating jaundice, and splenomegaly. Pigment gallstones are common after childhood and may produce biliary tract symptoms. Valuable laboratory studies include serum direct and total bilirubin and hepatoglobin levels. Jaundice associated with hyperbilirubinemia resulting from hemolysis is caused by an excess of unconjugated (free) bilirubin and is measured by an increase in the indirect reacting fraction of bilirubin. The unconjugated bilirubin bound to albumin does not enter the urine, and indirect hyperbilirubinemia is not associated with biliuria. Reticulocytosis and bone marrow erythroid hyperplasia reflect increased red cell production. Red cell morphology is often abnormal, as is osmotic fragility. Chromium-51 (^{51}Cr)–labeled red cell survival studies are sometimes useful to confirm hemolysis and a shortened red cell life span and to determine sites of red cell destruction.

HEREDITARY SPHEROCYTOSIS

Hereditary spherocytosis occurs primarily by autosomal dominant inheritance with variable expression. Between 20% and 25% of cases appear sporadically. The severity of the anemia and other clinical manifestations is variable. Aplastic crisis, which usually is precipitated by a viral illness such as human parvovirus, may produce a rapidly worsening anemia that may be life-threatening. Fluctuating jaundice due to hemolysis is common, and pigment gallstones are frequent, the incidence being directly related to the severity of the hemolysis and patient age. Cholelithiasis develops in 20% to 55% of patients with hereditary spherocytosis but is uncommon before age 10. Moderate splenomegaly is a characteristic physical finding. Diagnosis is established by the presence of spherocytes in the peripheral blood, reticulocytosis (usually 5% to 20%), an increased osmotic fragility, and a negative Coombs' test.

Splenectomy is indicated in virtually all patients. Following splenectomy, hemolysis is alleviated, and clinical cure of the anemia is achieved in most patients. The intrinsic red cell membrane defect is unaltered by splenectomy, but red cell survival becomes normal. With resolution of hemolysis, jaundice disappears, and the increased risk of calculous biliary tract disease is removed.

THALASSEMIA (THALASSEMIA SYNDROMES)

These hereditary hemolytic anemias result from a defect in hemoglobin synthesis in which one of the hemoglobin polypeptide chains is synthesized at a markedly reduced rate. Thalassemia is classified by the deficient peptide chain. Beta-thalassemia, in which there is a quantitative reduction in the rate of beta-chain synthesis, is the most common type of thalassemia. When the abnormal gene is inherited from both parents (homozygous), severe anemia, termed *thalassemia major*, results. Heterozygous patients have a mild anemia, termed *thalassemia minor*.

Thalassemia major results in a severe anemia and clinical manifestations usually within the first year of life. Pallor, retarded growth, and enlargement of the head with thalassemic facies are present, along with splenomegaly and hepatomegaly. The intense erythroid hyperplasia in the bone marrow results in expansion of the medullary cavities and attenuation of the cortex, producing bony abnormalities and a predisposition to fractures. Due to defective iron utilization coupled with increased iron absorption and frequent blood transfusions, iron overload is a common complication. Treatment consists of transfusion therapy and iron chelation, and splenectomy is effective in selected patients. Although the basic hematologic disease is not influenced, splenectomy will decrease blood transfusion requirements and relieve discomfort from splenomegaly.

AUTOIMMUNE HEMOLYTIC ANEMIA

Autoimmune hemolytic anemia (AIHA) is an acquired hemolytic anemia caused by antibodies produced by the body against its own red cells. Patients with AIHA have the usual manifestations of hemolysis with anemia, reticulocytosis, a shortened erythrocyte survival time, fluctuating jaundice, and splenomegaly. The blood smear in AIHA shows spherocytes and microspherocytes in numbers exceeded only in hereditary spherocytosis. The distinguishing feature of AIHA is a positive direct Coombs' test, which identifies antibody on the red cell surface.

The designation *autoimmune* in AIHA must not obscure the fact that in many cases the hemolytic process is associated with or related to a drug or a reversible disease that can be eliminated. When a drug exposure or an underlying disease is identified, AIHA is termed *secondary*. When no other etiologic association is demonstrable, AIHA is classified as *primary* or *idiopathic*. AIHA occurs at any age and in both sexes but is more common in women over age 50. Pallor and splenomegaly are the main physical findings in idiopathic AIHA, whereas in secondary AIHA additional clinical features of the underlying disease are present. Treatment is directed toward the hemolytic anemia and any underlying disease. Blood transfusions, corticosteroid therapy, and splenectomy are important aspects of treatment for the anemia. Splenectomy usually is performed in patients with AIHA in whom either steroids are ineffective or an excessive steroid dose is required or when complications preclude steroid use.

MYELOID METAPLASIA (AGNOGENIC MYELOID METAPLASIA, MYELOFIBROSIS, MYELOSCLEROSIS)

Myeloid metaplasia is an unusual illness resulting in gradual and progressive impairment of normal hematopoiesis due to continued fibroblastic proliferation, which ultimately produces sclerosis of the bone marrow and myelofibrosis. The panproliferative process causes increased connective tissue proliferation also in the liver, spleen, and lymph nodes and concomitant proliferation of hematopoietic elements in the spleen, liver, and long bones. Myeloid metaplasia is closely related to polycythemia vera, myelocytic (myelogenous) leukemia, and essential (idiopathic) thrombocytosis, and together these conditions constitute a disease spectrum termed *myeloproliferative disorders*. Characteristic features of myeloid metaplasia are (1) progressive fibrosis of the bone marrow, (2) extramedullary hematopoiesis, (3) presence in the peripheral blood of immature erythroid and granulocyte precursors (leukoerythroid response), and (4) massive splenomegaly. In some patients the enlarged spleen provides an expanded vascular space with an associated increase in plasma volume. By serving as a shunt, the enlarged spleen may result in a decreased peripheral vascular resistance and an increased cardiac workload. Portal hypertension with varices and ascites may develop in some patients from hepatic fibrosis, increased forward blood flow through the splenoportal system, or a combination of these factors.

Most patients are middle-aged or older and have symptoms related to anemia and splenomegaly. Malaise, dyspnea, and weight loss are common, and symptoms due to splenomegaly include abdominal fullness and discomfort, early satiety, and intermittent pain from splenic infarction. Splenomegaly due primarily to extramedullary hematopoiesis is invariably present, and myeloid metaplasia (myelofibrosis) has been responsible for some of the largest spleens we have encountered. Hepatomegaly is present in 50% to 75% of patients.

Treatment of patients with myeloid metaplasia is directed toward the anemia, thrombocytosis, and splenomegaly. Splenectomy is effective in controlling anemia and thrombocytopenia and relieving symptoms due to painful or massive splenomegaly. Splenectomy should be performed early rather than late in the course of the illness, since the risk of complications following splenectomy increases with progression of the disease. Indications for splenectomy are (1) an increasing transfusion requirement, (2) thrombocytopenic bleeding episodes, (3) symptomatic splenomegaly, (4) high-output cardiac failure, and (5) portal hypertension with bleeding varices.

Loss of the spleen as a major site of extramedullary hematopoiesis rarely has an adverse influence on the hematologic status of patients with myeloid metaplasia. Morbidity and mortality rates after splenectomy, however, are significantly higher for patients with myeloid metaplasia than for patients with other hematologic disorders. Additionally, following splenectomy, many of these patients have a marked thrombocytosis that is associated with an increased risk of thromboembolic complications, which include thrombosis of the portal vein and major mesenteric veins. Specific antiplatelet therapy may be needed in the preoperative preparation and postoperative care of patients undergoing splenectomy for myeloid metaplasia.

FELTY'S SYNDROME

Felty's syndrome consists of the triad of severe rheumatoid arthritis, granulocytopenia, and splenomegaly. It usually occurs in patients with a long history of rheumatoid arthritis. Patients with Felty's syndrome fail to show a substantial granulocytosis in response to infection, and severe, persistent, and recurrent infections are characteristic. Splenectomy is effective in most patients with Felty's syndrome and should be performed in those having significant recurrent infections. Controversy exists regarding the advisability of splenectomy for patients with Felty's syndrome who have severe granulocytopenia but have not yet developed severe or recurrent infections.

THE PROBLEM OF OVERWHELMING POSTSPLENECTOMY SEPSIS

Asplenic patients and those with deficient splenic function have an increased susceptibility to the development of overwhelming infection characterized by fulminant bacteremia, meningitis, or pneumonia. Singer's review of 2796 patients with splenectomy described a 4.2% incidence of sepsis and a 2.5% mortality rate. The risk of overwhelming sepsis is approximately 60 times greater than normal following splenectomy and may be as high as 0.5% to 1.0% per year. Although a lifetime risk of fulminant sepsis is incurred with splenectomy, the risk is greatest in children under 4 years of age and within 2 years of splenectomy (80% of patients). The risk for overwhelming postsplenectomy sepsis is highest in patients requiring splenectomy for thalassemia and reticuloendothelial system diseases such as Hodgkin's disease, histiocytosis X, or the Wiscott-Aldrich syndrome. It is lowest for patients with splenectomy for trauma, ITP, and hereditary spherocytosis.

The postsplenectomy sepsis syndrome typically occurs in a previously healthy individual following a mild upper respiratory infection associated with fever. Within hours, nausea, vomiting, headache, confusion, and shock, and coma occur, and death follows within 24 hours. Blood cultures reveal *Streptococcus pneumoniae, Neisseria meningitidis, Escherichia coli,* or *Haemophilus influenzae* in 75% of the cases with *S. pneumoniae* accounting for 50%. The fulminant nature of the syndrome makes it difficult to diagnose early enough for therapy to be effective. Adrenal hemorrhage is a common autopsy finding.

37

HERNIAS
Steve Eubanks, M.D.

Surgical management of the groin hernia has undergone extensive re-evaluation with renewed emphasis during the past 5 years. The rejuvenation of the surgeon's interest related to herniorrhaphy is partially attributable to the controversy regarding the application of laparoscopic techniques to this disease entity. Alterations in health care economics also have contributed to the renewed scrutiny the surgical treatment of hernia has received. The introduction of new techniques for the repair of hernia has highlighted the necessity for the surgeon to obtain a thorough understanding of the anatomy and pathophysiology of the hernia regardless of the repair technique applied.

A hernia is the abnormal protrusion of a peritoneal-lined sac through the musculoaponeurotic covering of the abdomen. The word *hernia* is a Latin term that means "rupture of a portion of a structure." Weakness of the abdominal wall, congenital or acquired in origin, results in the inability to contain the visceral contents of the abdominal cavity within their normal confines.

HISTORY

The earliest recorded mention of hernias appears in the Egyptian *Papyrus of Ebers* (1552 B.C.). Edoardo Bassini (1844–1924) reported the results of his new technique for the repair of the inguinal hernia in 1889. This was the first report that related consistently successful results with the surgical repair of inguinal hernias. Bassini described careful dissection with high ligation of the hernial sac and meticulous anatomic approximation of the conjoint fascia of the internal oblique and transversus abdominis muscles to the inguinal (Poupart's) ligament. The recurrence rate among his first 251 patients was only 3%. William S. Halsted (1852–1922) of the Johns Hopkins School of Medicine, working independently and unaware of Bassini's work, introduced a similar technique for the radical cure of inguinal hernia on November 4, 1889. Halsted's initial work differed slightly from that of Bassini in that the spermatic cord was transplanted above the closure of the external oblique fascia (Halsted I). The Halsted II procedure was a modification of the initial work in which the spermatic cord was allowed to remain in its normal position beneath the external oblique aponeurosis.

The popular Cooper ligament repair was first described in 1898 by Georg Lotheissen (1868–1935) of Vienna but was later

See the corresponding chapter or part in the *Textbook of Surgery*, 15th edition, pp. 1215–1233, for a more detailed discussion of this topic, including a comprehensive list of references.

popularized by Chester McVay (1911–1987) and subsequently came to be known as the McVay repair. The floor of the inguinal canal is repaired by suturing the conjoint tendon to Cooper's ligament.

The Shouldice (or Canadian) repair was described in the surgical literature in the 1960s. The Shouldice technique involves imbrication of the layers of the inguinal floor repaired under local anesthesia.

The preperitoneal approach for the repair of hernia was described by Cheatle in 1920. Cheatle's work received little attention until its rediscovery by Henry in 1936. Read described the preperitoneal approach and contributed significantly to our understanding of the development and history of the surgical treatment of hernias. Lloyd M. Nyhus, considered by many to be the leading authority on inguinal hernia, and his associates scientifically demonstrated the efficacy of the peritoneal approach for the repair of hernia.

Nyhus and colleagues popularized the use of prosthetic mesh for buttress repair of the groin hernia. The French surgeon Renée Stoppa described the repair of a groin hernia with a giant mesh prosthesis through the midline preperitoneal approach. The Stoppa procedure is more commonly known by the descriptive phrase *giant prosthetic reinforcement of the visceral sac* (GPRVS). The concept of tension-free repair was popularized by Lichtenstein and colleagues. The tension-free hernioplasty has received wide acceptance because of a low recurrence rate, rapid return to normal activities, minimal perioperative pain, and routine performance under local anesthesia.

The widespread acceptance of laparoscopic surgery and superb visualization of the groin hernia has led to the application of this technology to surgical repair of the groin hernia. The vast majority of laparoscopic interest today centers around the transabdominal preperitoneal approach (TAPP) and the totally extraperitoneal approach (TEPA) to the posterior inguinal wall with liberal use of mesh in essentially all patients. The surgical opinion regarding the appropriate technique for repair of the groin hernia is far from a consensus. Techniques for the repair of hernia continue to evolve, and the final chapter in the history of herniorrhaphy is yet to be written.

The complex anatomy of the inguinal region is often poorly understood by the student of surgery. The anatomy of the groin is frequently taught by describing layers of the abdominal wall, as are other regions of the human anatomy. The layers encountered at the level of the inguinal canal are skin, subcutaneous tissues (Camper's and Scarpa's fasciae), the external oblique aponeurosis, the inguinal canal (containing the spermatic cord structures, the ilioinguinal nerve, and the iliohypogastric nerve), the floor of the inguinal canal (transversalis fascia), preperitoneal fat, and peritoneum. The inguinal region also must be understood with regard to its three-dimensional configuration and relations. A knowledge of the convergence of tissue planes is the foundation upon which surgical cure can be effected.

The adult inguinal canal is approximately 4 cm. in length

and is located 2 to 4 cm. cephalad to the inguinal ligament. A canal extends between the internal (deep inguinal) ring and the external (superficial inguinal) ring opening. The inguinal canal contains either the spermatic cord or the round ligament of the uterus. The inguinal canal must be understood in the context of its three-dimensional anatomy. The canal courses from lateral to medial, deep to superficial, and cephalad to caudad. The inguinal canal is bounded superficially by the external oblique aponeurosis. The cephalad wall is composed of internal oblique muscle, tranversus abdominis muscle, and the aponeuroses of these muscles. The inferior wall of the inguinal canal is formed by the inguinal ligament and the lacunar ligament. The posterior wall (floor) of the inguinal canal is formed by the tranversalis fascia and the aponeurosis of the transversus abdominis muscle. The floor of the inguinal canal is the most important structure of the inguinal canal from an anatomic and surgical standpoint.

Hesselbach's triangle is bounded by the lateral edge of the rectus sheath, the inguinal ligament, and the inferior epigastric vessels. Hernias occurring within Hesselbach's triangle are considered to be direct hernias, whereas hernias occurring lateral to the triangle are thought to be indirect inguinal hernias.

The patient with a groin hernia usually presents with complaints of a bulge in the inguinal region. The patient may describe minor pain or vague discomfort associated with the groin bulge. However, extreme pain related to a hernia in the absence of incarceration and intestinal vascular compromise is very unusual and should raise the surgeon's suspicion of another etiology of the pain. Occasionally, patients will present with paresthesias related to irritation or compression of inguinal nerves by the hernia.

Around 75% of all hernias occur in the inguinal region. Approximately 50% of hernias are indirect inguinal hernias, and 24% are direct inguinal hernias. Incisional and ventral hernias comprise approximately 10% of all hernias, femoral hernias comprise 3%, and unusual hernias account for the remaining 5% to 10% of hernias. The vast majority of hernias occur in males. The most common hernia in males and females is the indirect inguinal hernia. Femoral hernias occur much more frequently in females than in males.

Around 25% of men will develop an inguinal hernia during their lifetime. Only 2% of females will develop an inguinal hernia during the span of a lifetime. Hernias occur more commonly on the right than on the left side.

Other types of hernias include the following:

UMBILICAL HERNIAS. Almost always congenital in origin, this hernia is usually diagnosed during childhood and repaired electively, since incarceration or strangulation is very unusual in umbilical hernias.

VENTRAL (INCISIONAL) HERNIA. This hernia occurs as a result of inadequate healing of a previous incision. Risk factors include obesity, steroid use, prior wound infection, diabetes mellitus, vascular disease, advanced age, malnutrition, ascites, pregnancy, peritoneal dialysis, and other conditions that place increased strain on the abdominal wall.

SLIDING HERNIA. One wall of the hernia sac in an inguinal hernia is composed of an abdominal viscus. The cecum is most commonly involved on the right side, and the sigmoid colon is most commonly involved on the left side.

RICHTER'S HERNIA. To satisfy the requirement of a Richter's hernia, the antimesenteric border of the intestine must protrude into the hernia sac, but never to the point of involvement of the entire circumference of the intestine.

LITTRE'S HERNIA. The presence of a Meckel's diverticulum as the sole component of the hernia sac defines Littre's hernia.

SPIGELIAN HERNIA. A hernia through the fascia along the lateral edge of the rectus muscle at the space between the semilunar line and the lateral edge of the rectus muscle is a Spigelian hernia. Most commonly, the Spigelian hernia occurs inferior to the semicircular line of Douglas.

OBTURATOR HERNIA. The obturator canal is covered by a membrane that is pierced by the obturator nerve and vessels. Weakening of the obturator membrane and enlargement of the canal may result in formation of a hernia sac, which can lead to intestinal incarceration and obstruction. The obturator canal, which is 2 to 3 cm. long, may contain a fat pad, which is considered by many surgeons to be pathologic. The patient may present with evidence of compression of the obturator nerve resulting in pain in the medial aspect of the thigh.

LUMBAR (DORSAL) HERNIAS. Lumbar or dorsal hernias can occur in the lumbar region through the posterior abdominal wall. Grynfelt's hernia appears through the superior lumbar triangle, whereas Petit's hernia occurs through the inferior lumbar triangle. Diffuse lumbar hernias are a third type and are most often iatrogenic. Most diffuse lumbar hernias occur following flank incisions for kidney operations.

38

PEDIATRIC SURGERY

Jay L. Grosfeld, M.D.

GENERAL CONSIDERATIONS

The newborn infant is a unique surgical patient who is physically and physiologically different from the adult. The cardiorespiratory dynamics in the newborn relate to conversion of a fetal circulation that bypasses the lungs to a postnatal state with elevated pulmonary artery pressure, patent ductus arteriosus, and patent foramen ovale producing a 15% to 20% shunt. Cardiac output in the neonate is rate-dependent, and stroke volume is limited when bradycardia occurs. The lung is not fully mature at birth. The more immature the infant, the fewer pulmonary units available and less surfactant produced, causing alveolar collapse, atelectasis, and hyaline membrane formation. Persistent pulmonary hypertension may cause significant extrapulmonary shunting and severe hypoxemia. The neonatal airway is quite small (tracheal diameter 2.5 to 4.0 mm.), and the tidal volume is 6 to 10 cc. per kg. Newborn infants are nasal and diaphragmatic breathers and have a relatively rapid respiratory rate (up to 60/min. is normal). Respiratory distress is heralded by tachypnea, nasal flaring, retractions, and cyanosis. The normal PaO_2 is 70 to 80 mm. Hg, $PaCO_2$ is 30 to 35 mm. Hg, and the pH is 7.3 to 7.4. The neonate has reasonably good renal function and handles a water lead quite well despite a reduced glomerular filtration rate and immature tubular function interfering with normal concentrating ability. Urine osmolality more than 400 mOsm. may reflect dehydration and less than 150 mOsm. overhydration. Normal urine output is 1 to 2 cc. per kg. per hour. The full-term infant is relatively immunodeficient, with decreased levels of IgG, opsonins, IgM, and the C3B component of complement and absent or severely diminished IgA. The more immature the infant, the less is the ability of his or her white blood cell leukocytes to phagocytize bacteria, leaving the baby at a greater risk for serious infection. The infant must be kept in a thermoneutral environment, and the body temperature is best monitored by a skin probe (36 to 36.5° C being normal). The baby's relatively large body surface area, lack of hair and subcutaneous tissue, and increased insensible losses make him or her vulnerable to hypothermia. Continued exposure to cold leads to metabolic acidosis despite nonshivering thermogenesis due to an increased metabolic rate caused by metabolizing brown fat. Maintenance of thermoneutrality may require overhead heaters, plastic body shields, extremity wraps, and metallic foil caps and wraps.

Liver function in the neonate is also immature, and physio-

See the corresponding chapter or part in the *Textbook of Surgery,* 15th edition, pp. 1234–1274, for a more detailed discussion of this topic, including a comprehensive list of references.

logic jaundice caused by relative deficiencies of glucuronyl-transferase is a common observation. Due to limited glycogen stores, the infant is prone to hypoglycemia (particularly small for gestational age infants), which may be manifested by seizures. Protracted hypoglycemia unresponsive to glucose infusions may signal the presence of hyperinsulinemia due to congenital pancreatic dysplasia. Hypocalcemia and hypomagnesemia are other causes of seizure activity.

The infant has a total body water space that represents 80% of body weight at birth and is mainly due to an increased extracellular fluid volume. Insensible losses are high (30 to 35 cc. per kg. per day) and are increased by fever, radiant warmers, overhead phototherapy for hyperbilirubinemia, and respiratory distress. Intravenous water requirements are 100 to 125 cc. per kg. per day in full-term infants and as high as 140 to 150 cc. per kg. per day in the premature. A solution of 10% glucose in 0.25% saline is used for maintenance fluids. The potassium and sodium requirements are 2 to 3 mEq. per kg. per day. Body weight, skin turgor, urine and serum osmolality, and urine output and specific gravity are good parameters to assess fluid requirements. Fluid losses from gastric drainage or stomal losses are replaced with lactated Ringer's solution. The infant's total blood volume can be estimated at 80 cc. per kg. Transfusion with packed red blood cells at 10 cc. per kg. is safe. Platelet and fresh frozen plasma infusions for thrombocytopenia or coagulation problems can be administered at a rate of 10 cc. per kg. as well.

The neonate has a metabolic rate 2.5 times that of the adult and a caloric requirement to grow of 120 cal. per kg. per day. Most formulas contain 20 cal. per oz., and 6 oz. per kg. therefore delivers an adequate caloric load. Caloric requirements are increased by fever, major illness, trauma, or sepsis. Most premature infants require gavage (oral-gastric or duodenal) feedings because of an immature suck reflex. A number of special infant formulas are available (soy, casein-derived, highly defined elemental diet with medium-chain fats, and so on). If the infant cannot tolerate an enteral diet, total parenteral nutrition is required. The calorie-nitrogen ratio is maintained at >150:1. A solution containing 18% to 25% glucose, 2.5 gm amino acids per kg. per day, and 3 to 4 gm fat per kg. per day delivers an adequate caloric intake. Adequate vitamins, trace minerals, iron, and folate are required additives. Total parenteral nutrition (TPN) is administered in neonates through a No. 4 French Silastic central venous catheter placed in the subclavian vein and passed into the superior vena cava at the entrance of the right atrium.

ALIMENTARY TRACT OBSTRUCTION

The cardinal signs of alimentary tract obstruction in the neonate are maternal polyhydramnios, bilious vomiting, abdominal distention, and failure to pass normal amounts of meconium in the first day of life.

Esophageal Atresia and Tracheoesophageal Fistula

Infants with variants of *esophageal atresia* may present with excess salivation, coughing, choking, and cyanosis. Aspiration of saliva and reflux of gastric juice through a *tracheoesophageal (TE) fistula* causes these symptoms. A high rate of associated anomalies may coexist in 40% to 60% of cases (especially cardiovascular defects). The most common defect type is Type C with a proximal esophageal atresia and distal TE fistula. These infants show a blind proximal pouch in the upper thorax and air in the stomach and intestine on chest radiograph. Infants with esophageal atresia without a TE fistula (Type A) present with maternal polyhydramnios and no air beneath the diaphragm on abdominal radiograph. Right thoracotomy and extrapleural division of the TE fistula and one-layer end-to-end esophageal anastomosis is the procedure of choice for Type C cases. If the atretic ends are too far apart, a proximal esophagomyotomy is a useful adjunct and often allows primary esophageal repair. Type A atresia (without a fistula) may be treated with prolonged dilatation to stretch the proximal pouch and insertion of a gastrostomy for feeding purposes. After 6 to 8 weeks, a single proximal myotomy or occasionally multiple myotomies often permit a primary anastomosis and avoid the need for esophageal replacement procedures. *H-type TE fistula without atresia* (Type E) is best detected by bronchoscopy and can be divided using a cervical approach. Type B proximal atresia and fistula and Type D proximal atresia with proximal and distal TE fistulas are less common anomalies. Complications include anastomotic leak (14% to 17%), stricture (18% to 30%), pneumonia, tracheomalacia (9% to 14%), and severe foregut motility disorders, including gastroesophageal reflux (50%). The overall survival is greater than 85% to 90%, with most deaths occurring in babies with severe associated anomalies (usually cardiac) or chromosomal syndromes.

Pyloric atresia presents with nonbilious vomiting, maternal polyhydramnios (66%), and a single gastric bubble on abdominal radiograph. The treatment program includes resection of a prepyloric web and pyloroplasty (Type I) or a pyloroduodenal anastomosis when a fibrous band or gap separates the tissues (Type II or III). *Duodenal atresia* can be diagnosed *in utero* by the appearance of a double bubble on prenatal ultrasonography. Maternal polyhydramnios is observed in 40% to 50% of cases, one third of the babies have Down syndrome, and one third are premature. Associated anomalies are observed in more than half the cases, with cardiovascular defects being most common. The diagnosis is confirmed following birth when a double bubble is noted on abdominal radiographs and bilious gastric aspirate is observed or bilious vomiting occurs. Annular pancreas and malrotation occur commonly (25% to 30%) in these cases, while an anterior portal vein is rarely seen. The operative procedure of choice is a duodenoduodenostomy. The distal segment should be checked for a second web (which occurs in 2% to 3%). Occasionally, a wind-sock web deformity is identified, and this can be managed by duodenotomy and web excision. Survival is currently 90%. Mortality is often due to serious cardiac anomalies. *Jejunoileal atresia* is due to a late intrauterine mesenteric vascular accident caused by volvulus, intussusception, or an internal hernia. Most cases present with a single atresia, but 10% to 15% may be multiple. The Type IIIa atresia with a mesenteric gap defect is the most common variant noted. These babies present with abdominal distention and bilious vomiting and often fail to pass meconium. Abdominal radiographs demonstrate dilated intestinal loops, often with air-fluid levels. A barium enema shows a microcolon, indicating that the colon is unused and that the site of obstruction is in the small intestine. At laparotomy, the dilated atretic bowel end is resected and bowel continuity restored with an end-to-oblique anastomosis. In babies with short bowel syndrome and a proximal jejunal atresia, bowel length can be preserved by the performance of a tapering jejunoplasty. Most babies with jejunoileal atresia have no other abnormalities and are more frequently full-term or small for gestational age patients. Approximately 35% require TPN, and 20% have short bowel syndrome. Survival is currently 87% to 90%. All babies with jejunoileal atresia require a sweat chloride determination prior to discharge to rule out cystic fibrosis.

Meconium ileus is a manifestation of cystic fibrosis and occurs in 10% to 15% of babies born with this hereditary disorder. This intraluminal form of obturator obstruction is characterized by bilious vomiting, abdominal distention, and failure to pass meconium. Abdominal radiographs show dilated loops of similar-sized bowel without air-fluid levels. A ground glass (soap bubble) appearance may be seen in the right lower quadrant due to admixture of inspissated meconium and air. Barium enema shows a microcolon, and in some cases the barium refluxes into the distal ileum and demonstrates obstructing meconium pellets. Treatment of choice for uncomplicated meconium ileus is nonoperative therapy using a hypertonic Gastrografin enema. Unsuccessful clearance of the inspissated meconium following Gastrografin enema requires surgical intervention. An enterotomy and irrigation are favored to clear the intraluminal obstruction; however, an enterostomy may be necessary occasionally. Complicated cases of meconium ileus include instances associated with atresia, perforation, volvulus, and giant cystic meconium peritonitis. Gastrografin enema is contraindicated in these cases. At operation, resection and enterostomy may be required. Cases of atresia usually can be managed by resection and anastomosis, as outlined above. The mortality has been significantly reduced in recent years, with more than 90% of patients surviving the neonatal period. The diagnosis should be confirmed with a sweat chloride determination and chromosomal studies showing an abnormality on the seventh chromosome (delta 508 position).

Other causes of neonatal small bowel obstruction include *internal hernia* due to volvulus around a *congenital band, mesenteric cyst,* or *Meckel's diverticulum;* an *incarcerated inguinal hernia;* or *duplication of the jejunum or ileum.*

Colon atresia is less common than either duodenal or jejunoileal atresia. The atresia usually occurs in the transverse or left colon and is probably related to intrauterine volvulus of these more floppy segments of the colon. Infants with colon atresia are usually big babies with no other serious anomalies. Preliminary colostomy and subsequent closure at 3 to 6 months of age have been a very successful method of management (100% survival). *Hirschsprung's disease* is a cause of neonatal colonic obstruction related to a lack of ganglion cells in the submucosal (Meissner's) and myenteric (Auerbach's) plexuses. Aganglionic megacolon occurs more frequently in boys (80%), most of the infants are full-term, and 3% to 5% have Down syndrome. Familial cases may have chromosomal aberrations on the tenth and thirteenth chromosomes. Presenting symptoms include bilious vomiting and abdominal distention, and 96% of cases will fail to pass meconium in the first 24 hours of life. Perforation and enterocolitis also may be presenting findings. The differential diagnosis includes meconium plug syndrome, small left colon syndrome, colonic neuronal dysplasia, maternal narcotic addiction, and hypothyroidism. Diagnosis is usually achieved with a barium enema, which may show a transition zone in the rectosigmoid or, in the newly born, a normal-sized colon with significant delays (>24 to 48 hours) in emptying the contrast material. Confirmation requires a suction rectal biopsy (submucosal), which shows an absence of ganglion cells. Full-thickness rectal biopsy may be necessary in some cases. Acetylcholinesterase staining of neurofibrils may be useful. Anal manometry may demonstrate an absent rectoanal reflex. The treatment of choice in the neonatal period is a preliminary sigmoid colostomy verifying the presence of ganglion cells at the stomal site. Aganglionosis is limited to the rectosigmoid in 80% of cases but can extend proximal to the splenic flexure in 10% and involve the entire colon and extend into the small bowel in 10%. In these latter instances, the preliminary stoma requires multiple frozen-section biopsies to determine the proper site of stomal formation in the small intestine. Definitive therapy is a pull-through operation at 6 to 12 months of age using the Soave endorectal pull-through, Duhamel retrorectal pull-through, or the Swenson procedure. In recent years, primary pull-through procedures in early infancy have been performed successfully. The modified Duhamel procedure is the most popular procedure for instances of total colonic aganglionosis, in which the ileum or even more proximal intestine is brought down to the anus at the time of the pull-through procedure. Survival is greater than 90%. Mortality is highest in patients with Down syndrome and those with extensive disease or cases complicated by enterocolitis.

Anorectal anomalies are classified as high, low, or intermediate lesions according to whether the rectal atresia is above, at, or below the level of the puborectalis sling. Between 85% and 90% of infants with variants of imperforate anus and rectal atresia have an associated fistula to the perineum, urethra, bladder, or vagina. Low lesions with imperforate anal membrane or rectoperineal fistula can be treated in the neonatal period with a perineal anoplasty, avoiding the need for colostomy. Intermediate- or high-level rectal atresia is treated initially with a high sigmoid colostomy and a formal posterior sagittal anorectoplasty (Peña procedure), with division of a rectourethral fistula (in boys), rectoforchette or vaginal fistula (in girls), or complete cloacal repair at 6 to 12 months of age. Many patients have associated anomalies, including cardiac defects, other gastrointestinal atresias (esophagus, duodenum), musculoskeletal disorders, urinary tract disorders, dysraphic spinal syndromes, other central nervous system abnormalities, and sacral abnormalities (hemivertebrae, sacral dysgenesis, and rarely, sacral agenesis), that may contribute to their ability to survive early and achieve continence at a later time. The lower the rectal atresia, the better is the prognosis. In intermediate and high lesions, the colostomy is kept in place until the new anoplasty site has been dilated adequately to avoid a stricture. Long-term success in achieving socially acceptable continence is possible in more than 90% with low lesions and 50% to 60% of infants with intermediate or high rectal atresia requiring posterior sagittal anorectoplasty.

ACUTE NEONATAL EMERGENCIES

Necrotizing Enterocolitis

Necrotizing enterocolitis (NEC) is a life-threatening intraabdominal condition affecting 1% to 2% of all neonatal intensive care unit (ICU) admissions. The vast majority of cases occur in premature or low birth weight infants. Predisposing factors include instances of shock, hypoxia, respiratory distress syndrome, apneic episodes, sepsis, polycythemia-hyperviscosity syndrome, exchange transfusion, patent ductus arteriosus, cyanotic heart disease with failure, hyperosmolar feedings, and treatment with indomethacin, xanthine derivatives (caffeine), and vitamin E. The pathophysiologic insult involves splanchnic vasoconstriction, hypoperfusion, and mucosal injury compounded by bacterial invasion. Symptoms and signs include increased gastric residuals, abdominal distention, lethargy, vomiting, occult or gross rectal bleeding, fever or hypothermia, an abdominal mass, abdominal wall erythema, oliguria, and instances of apnea/bradycardia. Abdominal radiographs may show pneumatosis intestinalis, portal vein air, pneumoperitoneum, fixed dilated loops, and ascites. Laboratory data usually show leukocytosis with a shift to the left on differential smear, anemia, hypoalbuminemia, acidosis, electrolyte disturbances, disseminated coagulopathy, and a progressively decreasing platelet count. Resuscitation includes cessation of feedings, insertion of an orogastric tube for gastric drainage, repletion of intravascular volume with crystalloid and colloid infusions, ventilator support (if not already in place), triple antibiotics, and administration of blood, platelets, and fresh frozen plasma as indicated.

Infants that show a prompt response to medical therapy often can be treated conservatively (nonoperatively). Babies with free air on abdominal radiographs, massive rectal bleeding, abdominal wall erythema, and abdominal mass and those who deteriorate on conservative therapy require operative intervention. Infants with portal vein air often have advanced disease and are candidates for early surgical intervention as well. In most cases, resection of infarcted bowel and a temporary enterostomy are the procedure of choice. On rare occasions, the process is so limited that a primary anastomosis may be reasonable. In colonic involvement a proximal stoma and distal Hartmann pouch procedure can be performed. Occasionally, insertion of a drain in the right lower quadrant is useful as a temporizing procedure in the very low birth weight micropremature infant with generalized peritonitis. If the baby improves, a formal delayed laparotomy is performed. The overall survival is 60% to 75% and varies with the severity of illness and the extent of bowel necrosis. Many babies have short bowel syndrome as a result of extensive enterectomy and require defined diets and TPN support. There is a 15% late mortality due to underlying disease factors that affected the premature infant prior to the development of NEC.

Malrotation and Midgut Volvulus

Anomalies of intestinal rotation and fixation cause the development of abnormal fixation bands across the duodenum and jejunum and make the infant vulnerable to a clockwise twist of the intestine and midgut volvulus (MGV). One-third of the cases of MGV occur in the first month of life. Infants with MGV present with the sudden onset of bilious vomiting and rapidly become seriously ill. If not recognized promptly, midgut infarction may occur, resulting in death or massive enterectomy and short bowel syndrome. The abdomen may be tender and distended. Bilious gastric returns are observed following passage of an orogastric tube. Occasionally, the infant passes blood and tissue (sloughed mucosa) per rectum. Abdominal radiographs may show distended bowel with air-fluid levels or a distended stomach and duodenum with a gasless abdomen beyond that point. Barium enema shows the cecum in an abnormal upper abdominal position, while barium swallow demonstrates a duodenal cutoff with a corkscrew appearance consistent with a twist. The infant is given triple antibiotics and fluid resuscitation and taken to the operating room promptly for laparotomy. At operation, the bowel is reduced in a counterclockwise fashion, and Ladd's bands (across the duodenum) or duodenojejunal bands are lysed to widen the base of the mesentery. The cecum is placed in the left lower quadrant next to the sigmoid colon, and an appendectomy is performed because of the atypical location of this appendage at the conclusion of the procedure. The Doppler probe or fluorescein dye and a Wood's lamp usually can predict bowel viability. If the entire small bowel and right colon appear necrotic, the bowel is detorsed, the abdomen closed, and the infant is treated supportively. If he or she survives more than 48 hours, a second-look laparotomy is performed to evaluate for bowel viability. The mortality for MGV remains high (18% to 25%). Most cases of incomplete or intermittent volvulus respond to a Ladd procedure and appendectomy as outlined above, and almost all of the latter group of patients survive.

Gastroschisis

Gastroschisis refers to an antenatal evisceration of the gastrointestinal tract *in utero*. The defect lies just to the right of an intact umbilical cord. The herniated bowel is exposed to the irritating effects of amniotic fluid (pH 7.0), causing an inflammatory reaction and foreshortening of the mesentery and intestine. The baby has malrotation and a small abdominal cavity. The diagnosis is often noted prior to birth on prenatal ultrasound study. At birth, the infant is prone to hypothermia and hypovolemia due to increased insensible losses and evaporative losses from the exposed viscera. Bowel atresia caused by volvulus or choking off of the blood supply to the herniated bowel in a very tight small defect may be seen in 10% to 15% of cases. Associated anomalies are otherwise uncommon. Aggressive parenteral fluid resuscitation is required, starting with a bolus of 20 cc. per kg. of lactated Ringer's solution or colloid. An orogastric tube is passed, and broad-spectrum antibiotic coverage is initiated. Extending the incision 2.0 cm. cephalad and caudad allows for a mechanical advantage to attempt reduction of the exposed viscera. The abdominal wall is stretched manually and the colon emptied of meconium (per rectum) to make more room within the small abdominal cavity for the herniated viscera. Primary closure is possible in 70% of cases. This is monitored by the ventilatory pressure and pulse oximeter. Excessive ventilatory pressure (>35 cm. H_2O) and hypoxemia are indications for application of a Dacron-reinforced temporary Silastic housing and a staged closure. Immediate postoperative care may require a short ventilator run and adequate fluid resuscitation. Due to a prolonged adynamic ileus, TPN is often necessary for a 2- to 4-week period. Most babies can tolerate full enteral feeds by 1 month of age. Hospital length of stay is approximately 3 to 5 weeks. Infants with associated atresia will require a temporary enterostomy and subsequent anastomosis. The length of hospitalization for complicated cases (e.g., atresias, perforations, etc.) is significantly longer than for uncomplicated cases. The current survival for infants with gastroschisis is 90%.

Omphalocele

An *omphalocele* is a covered defect of the umbilical ring into which abdominal contents herniate. The sac is composed of an outer layer of amnion and an inner layer of peritoneum. The incidence is 1 in 5000 births. More than 50% of patients have significant associated anomalies affecting the cardiovascular, gastrointestinal, musculoskeletal, urinary tract, and central nervous systems. Many of the infants are premature (25%), while others are affected by a number of chromosomal syndromes, including the Beckwith-Weidemann syndrome, trisomy 13–15 and 16–18, exstrophy of the bladder or cloaca, and the pentalogy of Cantrell, which includes epigastrically located omphalocele, anterior diaphragmatic defect, sternal cleft, ectopia cordis, intracardiac defects (usually a ventricular

septal defect), and occasionally a diverticulum of the left
ventricle. The size of the defect varies from a small herniation
of the umbilical cord to a 10.0-cm. defect containing the liver
and entire gastrointestinal tract. The abdominal cavity may be
quite small, and most patients have malrotation. The defect is
often recognized *in utero* on prenatal ultrasound studies. Due
to the size of the defect, a cesarean section may be necessary.
At birth, an orogastric tube is inserted to prevent gastric
distention, and the patient is placed feet first into a sterile
bowel bag, which is gently tied across the upper abdomen.
The infant is transferred to a tertiary neonatal care center in a
thermally neutral environment. Wet dressings should be
avoided because they macerate the sac and may cause hypothermia. The patient's general condition should be assessed
carefully for severe anomalies, chromosomal defects, prematurity, and so on. The covered sac gives the surgeon a number
of treatment options. Small defects can be managed by direct
primary closure of the abdominal wall. Medium to large defects may require a staged closure using a Dacron-reinforced
Silastic silo as a temporary housing for the herniated viscera.
The prosthetic material is sutured to the edge of the defect
with continuous 3-0 polypropylene suture. The silo can be
reduced gradually over a 3- to 7-day period on the newborn
unit, and the infant is then returned to the operating room for
removal of the prosthesis and abdominal wall repair. Infants
with giant (>10.0-cm.) defects, chromosomal syndromes, hyaline membrane disease, or severe cardiac defects producing
congestive heart failure or requiring ventilator support can be
treated initially nonoperatively with topical therapy using
0.25% mercurochrome, 0.5% silver nitrate solution, or silver
sulfadiazine as a topical agent. Higher concentrations of mercurochrome can result in mercury poisoning and should be
avoided. Continued nonoperative treatment with topical
agents is advised for infants with chromosomal syndromes
such as trisomy 13–15 or 16–18, where long-term survival is
not expected. The other patients can be treated definitively
when their underlying illness is brought under control and
their general condition stabilizes. The overall survival for infants with omphalocele depends on the size of the defect, sac
rupture and sepsis, complications of prematurity, and how
many and of what severity associated anomalies coexist. Infants with chromosomal syndromes and those with the pentalogy of Cantrell have a very high mortality. The overall mortality for omphalocele at the author's institution is 37%.

ACUTE RESPIRATORY EMERGENCIES

Congenital Diaphragmatic Hernia

Congenital posterolateral diaphragmatic hernia (CDH) of
Bochdalek is a defect of the developing pleuroperitoneal fold.
The fetal intestine usually ascends through the defect and
enters the chest in the eight to tenth week of gestation. The
herniated bowel acts as a space-occupying lesion and prevents
normal lung development and may result in pulmonary hypo-

plasia. The risk of occurrence is 1 in 2200 births, and CDH is more common in boys. The infants are usually full-term and weigh more than 3.0 kg. The defect can be detected by prenatal ultrasound and frequently is associated with maternal polyhydramnios, which is a poor prognostic marker. At birth, most of these infants develop symptoms of respiratory distress in the delivery room or shortly thereafter. The infant appears dyspneic, tachypneic, and cyanotic and has severe retractions with an increased chest diameter and a relatively scaphoid abdomen. Bowel sounds may be heard on auscultation of the affected chest. Chest radiograph demonstrates air-filled viscera in the thorax on the side of the hernia. The left side is affected in 88% of cases, the right side in 10%, and bilateral hernias are observed in 2%. In 10% of cases there is a peritoneal hernia sac. The infant develops extrapulmonary shunting accompanied by hypercarbia, severe hypoxemia, and a combined respiratory and metabolic acidosis. Treatment can be divided conveniently into three categories: (1) stabilization and preoperative preparation, (2) operative treatment, and (3) postoperative respiratory, circulatory, metabolic, and nutritional support. The infant with diaphragmatic hernia should have direct endotracheal intubation and ventilatory support with high oxygen concentration ($FIO_2 = 1.0$). The respiratory rate is set rapid intentionally to induce a respiratory alkalosis, which causes pulmonary vascular dilatation. Excessive ventilatory pressures are avoided to prevent barotrauma and contralateral pneumothorax. An arterial catheter is inserted, preferably in the right radial artery, to monitor preductal pH and blood gas tensions. An umbilical artery catheter is an alternative but measures postductal blood gas tensions. An orogastric tube is inserted to decompress the stomach and prevent air from entering the gastrointestinal tract and further compressing the lung. If the infant becomes stabilized and demonstrates an ApO_2 greater than 250 mm. Hg and $ApCO_2$ less than 40 mm. Hg on an FIO_2 of 1.0, delayed operative correction of the defect is attempted in the neonatal ICU. This is best accomplished with a transabdominal approach using a subcostal incision on the affected side. The bowel is reduced from the chest, carefully avoiding injury to the spleen on the left or the liver on the right, which may be displaced into the thorax. A chest tube is inserted under direct vision, and the defect is then repaired using 3-0 nonabsorbable interrupted mattress sutures. If the defect is too large or the diaphragm is absent, a prosthetic Gore-Tex patch is used to replace the diaphragm. The abdomen is closed in layers when possible; however, in some babies the abdominal cavity is too small to accommodate the viscera returning from the chest, and either a skin closure or temporary Dacron-reinforced Silastic housing may be necessary. Postoperatively, the infant remains in the neonatal ICU and is monitored closely. The endotracheal tube is left in place, and the infant is given ventilatory support with an FIO_2 of 1.0 to maintain the ApO_2 greater than 150 mm. Hg for 48 to 72 hours to avoid deterioration following this temporary period of stability referred to as the "honeymoon period." This set of circumstances may occur when the FIO_2 and ApO_2 are reduced too quickly. This type of deterioration is related to the sudden onset of pulmonary vascular vasoconstriction and persistent pulmonary hypertension. Surfactant to prevent alveolar collapse and pharmacologic agents such as tolazoline, prostaglandins, and acetylcholine to induce pulmonary vascular vasodilatation have been employed; however, the response to these medications has been disappointing. Recent treatments with inhaled nitric oxide have been disappointing. Dopamine and dobutamine may be necessary to maintain blood pressure, perfusion, and cardiac index. Infants older than 24 hours at diagnosis all survive; however, the survival for infants who are symptomatic shortly after birth has been less than 30% and is even lower (16%) if polyhydramnios is present. The mortality is directly related to the degree of pulmonary hypoplasia (especially if the contralateral lung is also hypoplastic) or whether associated congenital anomalies including congenital heart disease or chromosomal defects are present. The advent of extracorporeal membrane oxygenation (ECMO) has led to a number of innovative clinical programs. Infants who develop persistent pulmonary hypertension following repair of a diaphragmatic hernia can almost always be salvaged with ECMO. However, infants with pulmonary hypoplasia have not had the same postoperative benefits from treatment with ECMO and continue to have a significant mortality. In some instances, symptomatic babies with CDH are placed on ECMO preoperatively after failing conventional ventilator support, including use of the oscillating ventilator. When the infant's general condition improves (1 to 5 days), the baby can be weaned successfully from the ECMO circuit, and repair of the CDH defect can be performed. In some centers, CDH repair is performed while the infant is still on the ECMO circuit. The survival rate is approximately 65%. The outcomes have been similar whether the CDH is repaired on the ECMO circuit or after coming off this support. While ECMO has a significant role in the management of certain patients with CDH, it is not a panacea. Recent reports indicate survival rates of 70% to 90% using ECMO for all diaphragmatic hernia candidates who fail conventional treatment (including use of the oscillating ventilator and receiving NO_2) and have no other contraindications for extracorporeal life support therapy. An oxygenation index (O.I.) of greater than 40 has a mortality risk of greater than 80% and is an indication for ECMO. Oxygenation index is determined by O.I. = MAP (mean airway pressure) $\times$ FIO_2 $\times$ $100/APO_2$ based on three of five postductal APO_2 determinations. Gestational age less than 33 weeks, weight less than 2.0 kg., Grade III or IV intracranial hemorrhage, neurologic impairment, chromosomal disorders or anomalies incompatible with a meaningful life expectancy, and irreversible lung disease are contraindications for ECMO. Infants requiring ECMO who have a good cardiac output may be candidates for venovenous bypass, avoiding carotid artery cannulation.

Other Causes of Respiratory Distress

Other congenital abnormalities affecting the diaphragm include anterior *diaphragmatic hernia through the foramen of Mor-*

gagni (which is relatively uncommon in infants and children) and *eventration of the diaphragm*. The latter is most often related to birth injury following a breech delivery where the phrenic nerve is stretched and also may be associated with Erb's palsy and torticollis on the same side. The diaphragm is paralyzed and becomes attenuated, allowing the intra-abdominal contents to push up the thin muscle into the chest and compress the lung tissues, causing atelectasis and hypoxemia. Morgagni hernia can be repaired through the abdomen, while the author's institution favors a transthoracic diaphragmatic plication to correct instances of eventration.

Congenital cystic lung disease can cause respiratory distress in the neonate. These lesions are all derived from the primitive foregut, from which the lung bud originates. Lung cysts are categorized as *congenital lobar emphysema, cystic adenomatoid malformation, solitary lung cyst, pulmonary sequestrations (intra- and extralobar), bronchogenic cyst,* and *enteric duplication*. Each condition either traps air in the lung or compresses the tracheobronchial tree or pulmonary tissues, causing respiratory compromise due to obstruction or compression atelectasis. The treatment for each of these congenital cystic lesions is resection. Additional causes of respiratory distress in the newborn include *pulmonary interstitial emphysema, pneumothorax,* and *pneumomediastinum,* which are sequelae of the air-block syndrome in the neonate. *Micrognathia* associated with the Pierre-Robin syndrome and Sticker's syndrome, *choanal atresia or stenosis, hemangiomas, lymphangiomas,* and *teratomas* of the pharynx or tongue also can cause airway obstruction. The extent of the lesion can be defined by a CT examination. *Laryngomalacia, tracheomalacia, subglottic stenosis, laryngotracheal cleft,* and *congenital tracheal stenosis* are other conditions that must be considered when the neonate presents with noisy or obstructive stridorous breathing. The appropriate diagnosis usually can be arrived at with a careful physical examination, air tracheograms, indirect laryngoscopy, and bronchoscopy. Emergency intubation may be lifesaving, and in some cases, a temporary tracheostomy is required to secure the airway.

39

SURGICAL DISORDERS OF THE EARS, NOSE, PARANASAL SINUSES, PHARYNX, AND LARYNX

James B. Snow, Jr., M.D.

THE EARS

The external auditory canal makes a slightly S-shaped curve. The outer one third has a cartilaginous skeleton, and the inner two thirds has a bony skeleton. Cerumen glands and hair are borne in the outer third. The plane of the tympanic membrane makes an angle of 55 degrees with the long axis of the external auditory canal. The long process of the malleus is embedded in the fibrous layer of the tympanic membrane, and the head of the malleus articulates with the body of the incus. The lenticular process of the incus articulates with the head of the stapes. The footplate of the stapes articulates with the oval window.

The cochlea makes two and three quarter turns in the human. A cross section through the modiolus, or central bony framework, shows in each turn the scala vestibuli, the scala media, and the scala tympani. The scala vestibuli is separated from the scala media by Reissner's membrane. The scala media is separated from the scala tympani by the basilar membrane. The organ of Corti with its inner and outer hair cells rests on the basilar membrane. The hairs of the hair cells are in contact with the tectorial membrane. Dendrites of the neurons, the cell bodies of which are in the spiral canal of Rosenthal in the modiolus, arborize about the base of the hair cells.

The principal components of the vestibular labyrinth are the saccule, utricle, and semicircular canals. The saccule is spherical and is connected with the scala media through the canalis reuniens of Hensen. The saccular duct joins the utricular duct to form the endolymphatic duct. The utricle is larger than the saccule and is ovoid. The utricle has five openings for the three ampullated ends of the semicircular canals, the crus simplex of the horizontal semicircular canal, and the crus commune of the superior and posterior semicircular canals.

Sound waves impinging on the tympanic membrane set the tympanic membrane in motion. Movement of the tympanic membrane then causes movement of the malleus, incus, and stapes. Movement of the stapes causes pressure changes in the fluid in the inner ear. These pressure changes produce a traveling wave in the basilar membrane, from the base to the

---

See the corresponding chapter or part in the *Textbook of Surgery,* 15th edition, pp. 1275–1297, for a more detailed discussion of this topic, including a comprehensive list of references.

apex of the cochlea. Along the length of the basilar membrane, a point of maximal displacement occurs with each traveling wave. The location of the point of maximal displacement depends on the frequency of the stimulating tone. High-frequency tones cause maximal displacement near the base of the cochlea. As the frequency of the stimulating tone is decreased, the point of maximal displacement moves from the base to the apex.

Displacement of the basilar membrane causes movement of the organ of Corti and deformation of the hairs of the hair cells. In response to mechanical stimulation, the outer hair cells undergo alternating contraction and elongation. Mobility of the outer hair cells is thought to alter the physical properties of the organ of Corti to enhance the intensity, sensitivity, and frequency selectivity of the inner hair cells. A chemical transmitter is released in the region of the end boutons of the afferent eighth nerve fibers that attach to the hair cells. This chemical transmitter initiates depolarization of the dendritic terminals of the afferent nerve fibers.

Trauma and Foreign Bodies

Foreign bodies in the external auditory canal are a common problem. Beads, erasers, beans, and other objects may be inserted by children and their siblings into their ears. An insect may find its way into the ear canal and is particularly annoying to the patient until it is killed or removed. Foreign bodies are removed by passing a blunt hook deep to the foreign body and raking it out. A forceps is likely to push smooth foreign bodies ahead of it. If the foreign body is far medial, it is difficult to remove without injuring the tympanic membrane and ossicular chain. If a child is uncooperative or the mechanical problem is difficult, a general anesthetic is used for the removal of a foreign body. Metal and glass beads may be removed by irrigation, but care is used to be certain that the foreign body is not hygroscopic like a bean, because swelling with the addition of water complicates its removal. An insect is killed to give the patient immediate relief and facilitate its removal by filling the ear canal with mineral oil. The dead insect is removed with a forceps.

The tympanic membrane may be perforated with twigs of a tree, cotton applicators, and other objects placed in the ear canal, missiles such as hot slag in welding, and a sudden overpressure in an explosion (acoustic trauma). Perforations of the tympanic membrane may be associated with dislocations of the ossicular chain. Vertigo or a sensorineural hearing loss suggests that a portion of an ossicle or a missile has been driven into the inner ear or that there is a fistula between the perilymphatic space of the vestibule and the middle ear. These conditions require prompt exploration of the middle ear with an operative microscope and repair of the labyrinthine fistula. Most perforations of the tympanic membrane heal spontaneously in 6 weeks. For avoidance of infection during the healing period, the patient must be careful to avoid getting water in the ear. Prophylactic antibiotic therapy in the form of oral

penicillin for the first 7 days is recommended. If the perforation fails to heal or if there is a persisting conductive hearing
loss suggesting discontinuity of the ossicular chain, the middle
ear is explored and repaired.

FRACTURES OF THE TEMPORAL BONE. Basal skull
fractures follow blunt trauma to the head, particularly to the
occipital area. Basal skull fractures are in essence fractures of
the temporal bone, and they are a frequent cause of profound
sensorineural hearing loss. Bleeding from the ear following
an injury to the skull is pathognomonic of a fracture of the
temporal bone whether the bleeding is medial to an intact
tympanic membrane, from the middle ear through a rupture
of the tympanic membrane, or from a fracture line in the
ear canal. Hemotympanum gives the tympanic membrane a
blueblack color. Usually, there is a communication with the
subarachnoid space through the fracture line. Often there is
cerebrospinal fluid otorrhea. The immediate danger to the
patient is the development of meningitis. Therefore, prophylactic antibiotic therapy is initiated and continued for 7 to 10
days. More fractures of the temporal bone are longitudinal
(80%) than transverse (20%) to the long axis of the petrous
pyramid. Longitudinal fractures extend through the middle
ear into the ear canal and cause rupture of the tympanic
membrane. Transverse fractures extend across the cochlea and
fallopian canal to produce a profound, permanent sensorineural hearing loss and a facial paralysis. Approximately 35% of
longitudinal fractures produce a sensorineural hearing loss,
and approximately 15% produce facial paralysis. The fracture
extending through the middle ear may cause dislocation of
the ossicular chain that requires subsequent repair. Persistence
of a facial paralysis requires decompression of the facial nerve
under certain circumstances.

Infectious Diseases

ACUTE OTITIS MEDIA. Acute otitis media is an infectious
inflammatory process in the middle ear, usually secondary to
an upper respiratory tract infection. It is the most common
localized infection in children. Most children between 1 and 5
years of age have two or three episodes of acute otitis media
each winter. Acute otitis media may be viral or bacterial.

A myringotomy is indicated if bulging of the tympanic
membrane persists despite antibiotic therapy or if the pain
and systemic symptoms and signs such as fever, vomiting,
and diarrhea are severe. A large curvilinear incision is made
parallel to the annulus in the inferior quadrants midway between the umbo and the canal wall. The appearance and
movement of the tympanic membrane, tympanometry, and
the patient's hearing are followed until there is complete
resolution.

The infectious complications of acute otitis media are acute
mastoiditis, petrositis, labyrinthitis, facial paralysis, conductive and sensorineural hearing loss, epidural abscess, meningitis, brain abscess, lateral sinus thrombosis, subdural empyema, and otitic hydrocephalus. The most common intracranial
complication of acute otitis media is meningitis.

SEROUS AND SECRETORY OTITIS MEDIA. Serous and secretory otitis media are manifested as effusions in the middle ear. Such effusions are the result of incomplete resolution of acute otitis media or from eustachian tube obstruction due to inflammatory processes in the nasopharynx, allergic manifestations, hypertrophic adenoids, or benign or malignant nasopharyngeal neoplasms. Normally the middle ear is ventilated three to four times per minute as the eustachian tube opens during swallowing. If the patency of the eustachian tube is compromised, a relative negative pressure develops. At first there is mild retraction of the tympanic membrane. Soon a transudate of fluid occurs from the blood in the vessels in the mucous membrane of the middle ear. The presence of fluid in the middle ear may be recognized by an amber or dark gray color of the tympanic membrane, immobility of the tympanic membrane, a tympanogram indicating negative pressure in the middle ear, and conductive hearing loss.

Myringotomy for aspiration of the fluid and insertion of a tympanostomy tube for ventilation of the middle ear ameliorate the problem of eustachian tube obstruction regardless of the cause. In children, thorough adenoidectomy is frequently a necessary part of the treatment.

In children with middle ear effusions, initial treatment consists of antibiotic therapy appropriate for acute otitis media. Antibiotic therapy may sterilize the middle ear as well as ameliorate the eustachian tube obstruction secondary to purulent rhinitis, sinusitis, or adenoiditis and resolves the middle ear effusion in one third to one half of the patients.

CHRONIC OTITIS MEDIA. Chronic otitis media means a permanent perforation of the tympanic membrane. Perforations follow acute otitis media, mechanical trauma, thermal and chemical burns, and blast injuries. Chronic otitis media can be divided into two major categories depending on the type of perforation present. There is a benign tubotympanic type, with a central perforation of the tympanic membrane, and a dangerous type, with a pars flaccida or marginal perforation.

A central perforation is one in which there is some substance of the tympanic membrane between the rim of the perforation and the bony sulcus tympanicus. These perforations most commonly follow acute otitis media produced by relatively virulent microorganisms. Exacerbations of chronic otitis media produce painless, purulent otorrhea, which may be foul-smelling and occur secondary to upper respiratory infections and when water gains access to the middle ear in bathing and swimming.

The middle ear can generally be repaired in chronic otitis media with a central perforation. A tympanoplasty provides sound protection for the round window and restores sound pressure transformation to the oval window. Tympanoplastic procedures can be categorized into five types. The Type I tympanoplasty is applicable to the patient with a perforation of the tympanic membrane in which the ossicular chain is intact and mobile. The Type I tympanoplasty, sometimes termed a *myringoplasty*, restores the tympanic membrane by the use of a graft of soft tissue such as temporalis muscle fascia. A Type II tympanoplasty is required if there has been greater damage to the middle ear. Disruption of the ossicular chain, which often occurs as a result of necrosis of the long process of the incus, must be repaired in addition to grafting of the tympanic membrane. Often the remnant of the incus or the head of the malleus can be remodeled and repositioned to re-establish the continuity of the ossicular chain. Alloplastic materials are also used to restore the sound-conducting mechanism. A Type III tympanoplasty is required for a still more severely damaged middle ear in which the malleus and incus are not usable and only the stapes remains. Under these circumstances, the graft is placed in contact with the head of the stapes to produce a columellar effect similar to the single middle ear ossicle or columella found in birds. In more severe degrees of damage to the middle ear in which the superstructure of the stapes has been destroyed, only sound protection of the round window can be achieved by grafting from the promontory to the inferior remnant of the tympanic membrane. This Type IV tympanoplasty creates a small closed space that communicates with the eustachian tube and provides an air-filled cushion over the round window. A Type V tympanoplasty is utilized when the footplate of the stapes is fixed. It provides sound protection for the round window as in a Type IV tympanoplasty and fenestration of the horizontal semicircular canal for the admission of acoustic energy into the inner ear.

A cholesteatoma occurs when the middle ear is lined with stratified squamous epithelium. The stratified squamous epithelium desquamates in this closed space. The desquamated epithelial debris cannot be cleared and accumulates in ever-enlarging concentric layers. This debris serves as a culture medium for microorganisms. Cholesteatomas have the ability to destroy bone, including the tympanic ossicles. The presence of a cholesteatoma greatly increases the probability of the development of a serious complication such as a purulent labyrinthitis, facial paralysis, or intracranial suppurations.

Cholesteatomas are usually recognized by the small bits of white, amorphous debris in the middle ear and by the destruction of the external auditory canal bone superior to the perforation. Cholesteatomas are often associated with aural polyps, which may conceal the epithelial debris and bone destruction. Computed tomography of the temporal bone may demonstrate destruction of bone due to the cholesteatoma. Destruction of the scutum of Leidy (lateral wall of the epitympanum) and enlargement of the antrum greater than 1 cm. in diameter should be considered suspicious of cholesteatoma.

Cholesteatomas require surgical treatment. The objective of surgical therapy is to exteriorize the cholesteatoma and, if possible, remove it. In a radical mastoidectomy, the middle ear, including the attic and the antrum, and the mastoid air cell area are converted into one cavity that communicates with the exterior through the ear canal. If the cholesteatoma lies superficial to the remnants of the tympanic membrane and ossicles, a modified radical mastoidectomy can be performed. The modified radical mastoidectomy spares the tympanic membrane remnants and ossicles and preserves the remaining hearing. Under favorable circumstances, the cholesteatoma can be completely removed and the middle ear reconstructed. Exteriorization or removal of the cholesteatoma greatly reduces the likelihood of intracranial complications. The primary goal of surgical therapy for cholesteatoma is to make the ear safe, and the secondary goal is to maintain or improve the hearing.

Idiopathic Disease

OTOSCLEROSIS. Otosclerosis is the most common cause of a progressive conductive hearing loss in the adult with a normal ear drum. Otosclerosis is a disease of the bone of the inner ear with predilection for the anterior part of the oval window. On histologic examination, foci of otosclerosis show irregularly arranged, immature bone interspersed with numerous vascular channels. As the focus of the otosclerotic bone enlarges, it causes ankylosis of the footplate of the stapes and produces a conductive hearing loss. A second site of predilection is the posterior part to the oval window.

Otosclerosis tends to occur in families. It is more common in women than in men. Approximately 10% of the adult white population have foci of otosclerosis. Only 1 in 10 of these, or approximately 1% of the white population, has clinical otosclerosis as evidenced by conductive hearing loss. Otosclerosis is rare in blacks, Native Americans, and Japanese. It is common in Asiatic Indians. Otosclerosis also produces a sensorineural hearing loss if the focus is adjacent to the scala media. The conductive hearing loss becomes clinically evident in the late teenage and early adult years. The fixation of the stapes may progress rapidly during pregnancy. The conductive hearing loss can be corrected surgically in most instances. With microsurgical techniques, the superstructure (head, neck, and crura) of the stapes is removed and replaced with a prosthesis. A widely used prosthesis is one composed of a stainless steel wire and a Teflon piston. The wire, which is shaped like a shepherd's crook, is crimped around the long process of the incus, and the piston is placed through a hole created in the footplate of the stapes. The sound conduction characteristics of this arrangement are excellent. The complication of a profound sensorineural hearing loss occurs in 2% to 4% of patients. If a good initial hearing result is obtained, ordinarily a good result is maintained.

Neoplasms

Chemodectomas arise in the middle ear. These nonchromaffin paragangliomas are termed glomus jugulare or glomus tympanicus tumors, depending on their site of origin. The glomus tympanicus tumor arises from the area of Jacobson's nerve in the tympanic plexus on the promontory of the middle ear. The glomus jugulare tumor arises from the glomus jugulare body in the jugular bulb. Both tumors consist of rich networks of vascular spaces surrounded by epithelioid cells. Usually the neoplasms grow slowly, and symptoms may not be evident until the neoplasm is quite large. Pulsatile tinnitus, facial nerve paralysis, otorrhea, hemorrhage, vertigo, and paralysis of cranial nerves IX, X, XI, and XII are often the presenting symptoms and signs. Characteristically, a red mass that pulsates and blanches with compression with a pneumatic otoscope can be seen in the ear canal or middle ear. The pulsation also can be demonstrated with tympanometry. There may be evidence of bone erosion in the mastoid process, middle ear, or petrous pyramid on CT. Treatment consists of excision of the smaller neoplasms with or without a radical mastoidectomy. With large lesions, radiation therapy is the treatment of choice.

Acoustic neurinomas represent approximately 7% of all intracranial neoplasms. They arise twice as often from the vestibular division of the eighth nerve as from the auditory division. These neoplasms are derived from Schwann cells. Initially, they produce tinnitus and a neural hearing loss. The patient complains of unsteadiness or imbalance. True vertigo is not a common complaint. The hearing loss is predominantly a high-tone loss with greater impairment of the speech discrimination than would be expected with a cochlear lesion producing the same amount of pure-tone hearing loss. The structure of the five waves in brain stem response audiometry is disrupted, the interwave latency is increased, and the interaural latency difference of the fifth peak is increased. Initially, the tumor is confined to the internal auditory meatus. As it increases in size, it projects into the cerebellopontine angle and begins to compress the cerebellum and brain stem. Early diagnosis is based on auditory findings suggesting a neural loss of hearing. Auditory brain stem responses have become the most effective means of differentiating sensory from neural hearing losses. Acoustic neurinomas as small as 5 mm. in diameter can be visualized with magnetic resonance imaging (MRI) with enhancement with gadolinium. For the removal of small tumors, microsurgical approaches have been developed that utilize a translabyrinthine route if no useful hearing remains and a middle cranial fossa route for the preservation of the remaining hearing. Both routes allow preservation of the facial nerve. For very large neoplasms, the combined suboccipital and translabyrinthine approach offers the best likelihood of complete removal.

THE NOSE AND THE PARANASAL SINUSES

Trauma and Foreign Bodies

NASAL FRACTURE. Fractures of the nose are the most common fractures of the facial bones. Nasal fractures may involve the ascending processes of the maxillae and the nasal processes of the frontal bones as well as the nasal bones. A fracture of the nose is usually an open fracture. The skin of the dorsum of the nose may be lacerated, and the mucous membrane in the nasal cavity is usually torn. The most common deformity is a deviation of the nasal bones to the right with depression of the nasal bones on the left, characteristically occurring with a right hook. Fractures of the nose may be associated with septal fractures and hematomas.

Fractures of the nasal bones are generally associated with bleeding from the nose owing to the tear of the mucous membrane. A fracture should be suspected if blunt injury causes bleeding from the nose. Soft tissue swelling occurs fairly promptly and may tend to obscure the underlying bony deformity. The diagnosis can ordinarily be established by gentle palpation of the dorsum of the nose. Any deformity suggests a fracture. Radiographs of the nasal bones will tend to confirm the diagnosis.

Fractures of the nasal complex are often associated with fractures of other facial bones, and CT of the paranasal sinuses is obtained. Trauma to the facial bones is often associated with a cerebrospinal fluid rhinorrhea.

Nasal fractures in adults may be reduced under local anesthesia. General anesthesia is necessary for the reduction of nasal fractures in children. The fracture is manipulated into a good position by internal traction on the fracture fragments with a blunt periosteal elevator in association with external traction with the fingers. The need for internal and external splinting depends on the postreduction stability of the fracture.

Septal hematomas lie between the quadrangular cartilage and the perichondrium. If the perichondrium has been elevated from both sides of the septal cartilage, the cartilage will undergo avascular necrosis. Septal hematomas frequently become infected, and abscess formation produces avascular and septic necrosis of the septal cartilage, which causes a saddle deformity of the nose. Septal hematomas are incised and drained as soon as the diagnosis is made. The perichondrium is placed in contact with the septal cartilage by packing the nasal cavity with petrolatum gauze.

Septal abscesses are located between the cartilage and the perichondrium. They may involve both sides of the cartilage. Septal abscesses are incised and drained under general anesthesia as soon as the diagnosis is established. Incisions are made bilaterally if there is pus on both sides of the septum. A small rubber drain is sutured to a lip of the wound until the drainage subsides. Vigorous systemic antibiotic therapy is employed.

FOREIGN BODIES. Children put all manner of objects in their noses. Erasers, beans, buttons, pebbles, wool nap, paper, and sponge rubber are common foreign bodies. A foreign body in the nasal cavity produces a severe inflammatory reaction and causes a foul-smelling, bloody, unilateral discharge. Removal of the foreign body is facilitated by producing vasoconstriction anterior to it with a topical sympathomimetic amine such as phenylephrine. The foreign body is removed by placing a blunt hook posterior to it and raking it anteriorly. Attempts at grasping smooth, firm foreign bodies with forceps tend to push them farther posteriorly. General anesthesia is used if good cooperation from a child cannot be obtained by gentle reassurance.

If a foreign body dwells long in the nose, mineral salts are deposited on it and produce a rhinolith. The rhinolith tends

to conform to the contour of the nasal cavity, and its removal
is usually difficult.

Sinusitis

Acute rhinitis is the usual manifestation of a common cold.
Acute sinusitis is usually initiated by a viral upper respiratory
tract infection. Nearly all cases of acute sinusitis and most
cases of chronic sinusitis respond well to antibiotic therapy.
The complications of acute and chronic sinusitis often require
surgical therapy, as does unresponsive chronic sinusitis. Complications of maxillary sinusitis are rare. Ethmoid sinusitis is
frequently complicated in children by orbital cellulitis and
abscess. About 80% of all cases of orbital cellulitis are secondary to ethmoid sinusitis. In the patient who presents with
erythema and swelling of the eyelids, proptosis, and displacement of the globe laterally and inferiorly, the source of the
infection is sought by inspection of the nose for mucopus in
the middle meatus and by CT of the paranasal sinuses for
ethmoid sinusitis. CT of the orbits may allow differentiation
of orbital cellulitis from orbital abscess. Ethmoid sinusitis and
orbital cellulitis respond well to systemic antibiotic therapy. If
the proptosis fails to subside or progresses, incision and drainage of the abscess, which is between the lamina papyracea
and the orbital periosteum, is performed through a Killian
incision that extends from the lateral aspect of the nose to the
eyebrow. The orbital periosteum is elevated from the medial
wall of the orbit so that the abscess cavity can be reached.
The optic nerve tolerates 11 to 14 mm. of proptosis. The point
at which extraocular motion is lost is also the limit of stretch
of the optic nerve. Therefore, incision with drainage of an
orbital abscess is performed before complete loss of extraocular motion for prevention of blindness.

Frontal sinusitis may cause intracranial complications such
as meningitis, epidural abscess, subdural empyema, and brain
abscess. In severe acute frontal sinusitis that fails to respond
promptly to systemic antibiotic therapy, the floor of the frontal
sinus is trephined through an incision just inferior to the
medial part of the eyebrow. An opening of approximately 7
to 8 mm. is made, and a catheter is placed in the sinus for
maintaining drainage. Trephination is performed in an attempt to prevent the intracranial complications of frontal sinusitis.

Fractures of the frontal sinus cause development of mucoceles. Mucoceles are due to duplication of the mucous membrane. They gradually enlarge and destroy the floor of the
frontal sinus, and as they expand into the orbital cavity, they
produce proptosis and inferior and lateral displacement of the
eye. Mucoceles and other forms of chronic frontal sinusitis
that do not respond to medical management can be managed
surgically by an osteoplastic flap approach for obliteration of
the frontal sinus. The incision in the bone is made at the
periphery of the frontal sinus, and the anterior wall is rotated
inferiorly on the hinge of periosteum at the floor of the sinus.
Infected mucous membrane is removed with a gas-driven

burr under microscopic control, and the cavity of the frontal sinus is obliterated by the implantation of fat taken from the abdominal wall.

Approximately 25% of cases of chronic maxillary sinusitis are secondary to a dental infection. In chronic maxillary sinusitis, radiographs of the apices of the teeth should be obtained for excluding the possibility of a periapical abscess.

Infection and allergy can lead to hyperplastic tissue in the confluence of the ostia of the maxillary, anterior ethmoid, and frontal sinuses in the middle meatus, which produces obstruction of the ostia of these sinuses. Inflammation in the ostiomeatal complex is thought to account for a great deal of subacute and chronic sinusitis. Endoscopic excision of inflammatory tissue in the ostiomeatal complex is credited with resolution of chronic sinusitis without open operative procedures.

Chronic maxillary sinusitis that does not respond to medical management or endoscopic sinus surgery may be controlled with the Caldwell-Luc operation, which is a maxillary sinusotomy performed through an incision in the canine fossa. The bone of the anterior wall of the maxillary sinus is resected to permit access to the interior of the sinus for removal of infected mucous membrane, cysts, and epithelial debris. Drainage of the maxillary sinus is improved by creating a nasoantral window in the inferior meatus.

Chronic ethmoid sinusitis is often associated with allergic rhinitis and the formation of nasal polyps. In those individuals in whom the formation of nasal polyps and the symptoms of ethmoid sinusitis cannot be controlled adequately with medical management including topical corticosteroid therapy and immunotherapy, an ethmoidectomy is indicated. Ethmoidectomy is performed intranasally with endoscopic guidance or through an external approach by utilization of a Killian incision. In the external ethmoidectomy, the orbital periosteum is elevated, and the lamina papyracea is removed to give access to the ethmoid air cells. Infected mucous membrane, polypoid tissue, and epithelial debris are removed. The anterior half of the middle turbinate is excised to create a large opening between the ethmoid air cells and the nasal cavity. In essence, an ethmoidectomy incorporates the ethmoid air cell area into the nasal cavity.

Chronic sphenoid sinusitis that does not respond to medical management may be controlled by an operation in which the sphenoid sinus is approached with endoscopic guidance or through an external ethmoidectomy. After an ethmoidectomy has been accomplished, the anterior wall of the sphenoid sinus is resected to remove infected mucous membrane, polypoid tissue, and epithelial debris. The anterior and inferior walls of the sphenoid sinus are removed. In this way, the interior of the sphenoid sinus is incorporated in the posterior part of the nasal cavity and the nasopharynx, and in essence, the sphenoid sinus is eliminated as a separate entity.

Epistaxis

Bleeding from the nose is a common clinical problem. Around 90% of the time, epistaxis occurs from a plexus of vessels in the anteroinferior part of the septum. In the other 10% of cases, nasal bleeding occurs from the posterior part of the nose, particularly from far posterior in the inferior meatus at the junction of the inferior meatus and the nasopharynx. It is from this area that individuals with arteriosclerosis and hypertension are likely to bleed. This type of bleeding may be difficult to control and is associated with a 4% to 5% mortality. Mild epistaxis from the anterior part of the nasal septum is usually effectively controlled by steady pressure applied by squeezing the mobile portion of the nose between the index finger and thumb for 5 to 10 minutes. Treatment for epistaxis that is not controlled by this simple measure requires visualization of the bleeding point. The bleeding point can be controlled temporarily and anesthesia achieved with pressure applied over a cotton pledget impregnated with a vasoconstrictor and a topically active local anesthetic such as lidocaine. The bleeding point can be cauterized chemically or with electrocautery. Silver nitrate is preferred as the cauterizing agent, since it produces satisfactory intravascular coagulation without a severe burn of the mucous membrane. If the bleeding cannot be easily controlled with cautery or if the bleeding point cannot be visualized, strips of ½-in. petrolatum gauze are used to apply pressure to the bleeding point. Pressure is applied as atraumatically as possible. This method is preferred in a patient with a bleeding tendency because the periphery of a cauterized area may begin to bleed.

In order to pack the posterior part of the nasal cavity, the choana is obstructed with the balloon of a Foley catheter. If the bleeding point is in the inferior meatus, this area is packed tightly. The packing is left in place for 4 days. Prophylactic antibiotic therapy is indicated to prevent sinusitis and otitis media. Patients requiring postnasal packing generally have serious systemic vascular diseases. They have a low arterial PO_2 while the packing is in place and should be given supplemental humidified oxygen by mask.

An alternative method of treatment of patients with severe bleeding from the posterior part of the nose is ligation or embolization of the internal maxillary artery.

Severe epistaxis is often associated with pre-existing liver disease. Large amounts of blood may have been swallowed before the nasal packing. Blood is eliminated from the gastrointestinal tract as promptly as possible by the use of cathartics and enemas. Sterilization of the gastrointestinal tract to prevent the breakdown of blood by microorganisms and the absorption of ammonia is indicated by the presence of liver disease.

Replacement of blood that has been lost as a result of the epistaxis is accomplished as indicated by the hemoglobin and hematocrit determinations as well as by the patient's vital signs.

Neoplasms

BENIGN NEOPLASMS OF THE NOSE AND PARANASAL SINUSES. Exophytic squamous cell papillomas occur in the nasal cavity and are caused by the human papillomavirus. Exophytic papillomas occasionally recur after excision but have a benign course. Inverted papillomas are invasive and behave in a locally malignant manner. They arise from the lateral wall of the nasal cavity and invade bone. Inverted papillomas require removal of a margin of normal tissue through a lateral rhinotomy. Fibromas, hemangiomas, and neurofibromas occur occasionally in the nasal cavity. Fibromas, neurilemomas, and ossifying fibromas occur in the paranasal sinuses.

MALIGNANT NEOPLASMS OF THE NOSE AND PARANASAL SINUSES. The most common malignant neoplasm occurring in the nose and paranasal sinuses is squamous cell carcinoma. Adenoid cystic carcinomas, adenocarcinomas (particularly in the ethmoid sinuses), mucoepidermoid carcinomas, malignant mixed tumors, lymphomas, fibrosarcomas, osteosarcomas, chondrosarcomas, and melanomas also occur in the nose and paranasal sinuses. Metastatic tumors may involve the paranasal sinuses, and the most common neoplasm to metastasize to the paranasal sinuses is the hypernephroma.

A combination of radiation therapy and radical resection provides the best survival rates in carcinomas and sarcomas of the nasal cavities and paranasal sinuses.

THE PHARYNX

Nasopharynx

THE ADENOIDS. Adenoid hypertrophy in childhood often causes obstruction of the eustachian tubes and the choanae. Obstruction of the eustachian tubes produces serous or secretory otitis media, recurrent acute otitis media, and exacerbations of chronic otitis media. Obstruction of the choanae produces mouth breathing, a hyponasal voice, and rhinorrhea.

Recurrent serous or secretory otitis media is the most common indication for the removal of the adenoid tissue.

An adenoidectomy is performed under general anesthesia. The adenoid tissue is sheared from the posterior nasopharyngeal wall with a guillotine-type adenotome placed posterior to the soft palate.

BENIGN NEOPLASMS OF THE NASOPHARYNX. Juvenile angiofibromas are very vascular neoplasms that occur in pubescent males. Angiofibromas may extend into and obstruct the nasal cavity and encroach on the paranasal sinuses, the orbit, and the intracranial cavity. These neoplasms are composed of fibrous tissue and numerous thin-walled vessels without contractile elements.

Epistaxis is the major problem with angiofibromas, and the magnitude of the bleeding can be great. The extent of the neoplasm can be determined with CT and angiography. The main blood supply is usually from the branches of the internal maxillary artery, although the branches of the internal carotid artery and the middle meningeal artery also may contribute. Usually, angiofibromas are removed through a transpalatal approach. The blood loss during excision is often great, and rapid blood replacement is required. Treatment with estrogens and embolization of the internal maxillary artery at angiography have been used to reduce the operative blood loss. These neoplasms are responsive to radiation therapy. This is often the treatment of choice for the neoplasm that has invaded the orbit or the intracranial cavity or receives a large blood supply from intracranial vessels.

MALIGNANT NEOPLASMS OF THE NASOPHARYNX. Malignant neoplasms of the nasopharynx include squamous cell carcinomas, adenocarcinomas, adenoid cystic carcinomas, mucoepidermoid carcinomas, malignant mixed tumors, melanomas, chordomas, sarcomas including fibrosarcoma, rhabdomyosarcoma, liposarcoma and myxosarcoma, plasmacytomas, and lymphomas. Among children, lymphomas are the most common malignant neoplasms arising from and secondarily involving the nasopharynx. Among the carcinomas, lymphoepithelioma or squamous cell carcinoma is the most common type.

Carcinoma of the nasopharynx occurs at relatively young ages, and there is an unusually high incidence among the Chinese. The majority of patients with carcinoma of the nasopharynx present with nasal or eustachian tube obstruction. Obstruction of the eustachian tube may produce a middle ear effusion. The nasal obstruction may be associated with purulent, bloody rhinorrhea and frank epistaxis. The more dramatic symptoms following cranial nerve paralysis and cervical lymph node metastasis are, unfortunately, common presenting complaints.

The diagnosis is made by biopsy of the primary tumor. Adequate access to the nasopharynx ordinarily requires general anesthesia. General anesthesia also allows the opportunity to judge the extent of the primary lesion by palpation. Biopsy of the metastasis in the neck should be avoided until the nasopharynx has been inspected and palpated and any suspicious lesion has been biopsied. Biopsy of the cervical metastasis violates the integrity of the block of tissue that is removed in a radical neck dissection. It may cause implantation of the neoplasm in the skin and subcutaneous tissue. The necessity for demonstrating the neoplasm in the nasopharynx before treatment remains, even if a histologic diagnosis is obtained from biopsy of the cervical metastasis.

The treatment of choice for carcinoma of the nasopharynx is irradiation with a supervoltage source. The radiation should be delivered to the primary tumor-bearing area of the nasopharynx and to both sides of the neck whether there is clinically demonstrated metastasis or not. Those cervical metastases that remain clinically palpable following radiation therapy or that subsequently become apparent should be eradicated by radical neck dissection. The overall 5-year survival for carcinoma of the nasopharynx is approximately 35%.

Oropharynx

PERITONSILLAR ABSCESS. Peritonsillar cellulitis and abscess are complications of acute tonsillitis in which the infection has spread deep to the tonsillar capsule. Pus forms between the tonsillar capsule and the superior constrictor of the pharynx, and the tonsil is displaced medially. The uvula becomes tremendously edematous and is displaced to the opposite side. The soft palate is very red and displaced forward. There is marked trismus due to irritation of the pterygoid muscles, and the head is held tilted toward the side of the abscess. It is painful for the patient to talk and to swallow. Peritonsillar cellulitis or abscess is usually caused by a group A beta-hemolytic streptococcus or anaerobe. If a cellulitis without pus formation exists, it will respond in a matter of 24 to 48 hours to penicillin therapy. If pus is present, it may resolve or require incision and drainage. The incision need only split the mucous membrane, and the pus is obtained by spreading gently with a hemostat. No drain is required because the abscess cavity is emptied by each swallow.

These abscesses tend to recur and are an indication for tonsillectomy. Some advocate that the tonsillectomy be performed within a day or two after the antibiotic therapy is initiated.

PARAPHARYNGEAL ABSCESS. Parapharyngeal abscess may occur in infants and young children as well as in adults. The abscess is usually secondary to streptococcal pharyngitis or tonsillitis. Pus forms in the parapharyngeal space secondarily from the breakdown of lymphadenitis. The pus is located lateral to the superior constrictor of the pharynx and adjacent to the carotid sheath. There is marked swelling in the anterior cervical triangle. Penicillin is the antibiotic of choice. Pus formation can be demonstrated with CT or MRI before the abscess becomes fluctuant. When pus formation has been demonstrated, the abscess is incised and drained. The abscess is not drained through the lateral pharyngeal wall because of the proximity of the internal carotid artery and the internal jugular vein. An incision is made parallel to the skinfolds over the anterior border of the sternocleidomastoid muscle. The anterior border of the muscle is identified, and blunt dissection is carried toward the carotid sheath where the pus is encountered. A drain is sewn in place and removed when the drainage subsides.

RETROPHARYNGEAL ABSCESS. Retropharyngeal abscess occurs in infants and young children. These infections are located between the constrictors of the pharynx and the prevertebral fascia. They are secondary to pharyngitis and are due to the breakdown of retropharyngeal lymphadenitis. Infants with retropharyngeal abscesses usually present with stridor and hyperextension of the neck. A lumbar puncture is the appropriate diagnostic procedure in a febrile infant who presents in opisthotonos. If the cerebrospinal fluid is normal, the possibility of a retropharyngeal abscess must be excluded. The diagnosis is made by palpating the posterior pharyngeal wall. The infant is held in the prone position for the examination so that if the abscess is ruptured during the examination, the pus will flow out of the infant's mouth and not be aspirated. The abscess has a boggy fluctuant texture, and the bodies of the cervical vertebrae are not palpable. Inspection of the pharynx may not demonstrate the abscess because the whole posterior pharyngeal wall may be displaced forward and there may be no inflammatory reaction in the mucous membrane. The abscess also can be demonstrated by a radiograph of the lateral neck in which the posterior pharyngeal wall is displaced anteriorly, or by CT of the neck. For maintaining the airway, the child should be allowed to hyperextend the neck. A tracheotomy is rarely necessary. In addition to penicillin therapy, the posterior pharyngeal wall should be incised under general endotracheal anesthesia with the patient in the Rose position. The mucous membrane at the posterior wall of the pharynx is incised vertically. The incision need only split the mucous membrane. The pus is obtained by gently spreading a hemostat in the wound toward the retropharyngeal space. No drain is necessary because the abscess cavity tends to be emptied on swallowing.

TONSILLECTOMY. Recurrent acute bacterial tonsillitis caused by a group A beta-hemolytic streptococcus occurring three to four times during the year in children from 2 to 7 years of age can be adequately managed with penicillin or other appropriate antibiotics given for 12 days. The rationale for this length of treatment is that a shorter period may not eliminate a streptococcal infection. In addition to inappropriate selection of antibiotics and inadequate duration of therapy, passage of the streptococcus among family members is a cause of failure in the medical management of tonsillitis. This situation requires simultaneous cultures of the whole family and simultaneous treatment of all carriers. Despite these precautions, in some patients tonsillitis repeatedly develops within a few days after the completion of adequate treatment. When this pattern cannot be altered by medical management, tonsillectomy is indicated.

Chronic tonsillitis with persistent sore throat, either briefly relieved or not at all relieved by antibiotic therapy, constitutes an additional indication for tonsillectomy. Peritonsillar abscess is another indication for tonsillectomy

Tonsillar and adenoid hypertrophy frequently results in upper airway obstruction in children, causing sleep apnea. Tonsillectomy and adenoidectomy regularly solve this problem.

In adults, tonsillectomy is performed under local or general anesthesia. In children, general anesthesia is required. The technique involves an incision in the free edge of the tonsillar pillars. The dissection of the tonsil from the tonsillar fossa is performed in the plane between the tonsillar capsule and the superior constrictor muscle of the pharynx and is completed by closing a snare placed inferior to the lower pole of the tonsil. The objective is to remove the tonsil and its capsule intact and spare the musculature of the tonsillar fossa.

CARCINOMA OF THE TONSIL. Carcinoma of the tonsil represents 1.5% to 3% of all cancers and is second in frequency only to carcinoma of the larynx among malignant neoplasms of the upper respiratory tract. It is predominantly a disease of males, and smoking of cigarettes and consumption of more than 100 ml. of ethanol per day are etiologic factors. Squamous cell carcinoma is the predominant histologic type. Carcinoma of the tonsil usually remains asymptomatic until it has reached considerable size. Sore throat is the most common presenting complaint, and pain often radiates to the ear on the same side. Not infrequently the patient presents with a metastatic mass in the neck as the first symptom. The diagnosis is established by biopsy of the primary lesion. Treatment requires combined radiation therapy and operation. Radiation therapy may be given preoperatively or postoperatively. If preoperative irradiation is utilized, 5000 cGy is delivered to the primary lesion and both sides of the neck over a 5-week period. The patient is then given a 6-week rest. The operation consists of radical resection of the tonsillar fossa, hemimandibulectomy, and radical neck dissection if there are palpable metastases. If postoperative irradiation is utilized, 6000 cGy is delivered to the primary site and 5000 cGy to both sides of the neck. The 2-year disease-free survival approximates 50%.

LARYNX

Structural Changes in the True Vocal Cords Secondary to Misuse and Abuse of the Voice

Abuse and misuse of the voice can produce structural changes in the true vocal cords. Using the voice too loudly and too long produces acute and chronic changes in the true vocal cords. Prolonged use of intensity rather than frequency for emphasis, the employment of a monotone, the affectation of a frequency that is too low, and a very abrupt onset of high intensities (sharp glottal attack) produce structural changes in the true vocal cords.

POLYPS OF THE VOCAL CORDS. Polyps of the true vocal cords develop in response to use of the voice too loudly and too long. Chronic subepithelial edema develops in the lamina propria of the true vocal cords. Such polypoid swellings of the free edge of a true vocal cord interfere with the approximation of the true vocal cords and with the maintenance of periodicity and synchrony of the vibration of the vocal cords. They produce hoarseness and give a breathy quality to the voice. For restoration of the voice, polyps are removed by use of an operating microscope at direct laryngoscopy under general anesthesia.

VOCAL NODULES. Vocal nodules are caused by using a fundamental frequency that is unnaturally low and using the voice too loudly and too long. Vocal nodules occur in children as well as in adults and are likely to occur in robust, athletic boys 8 to 12 years of age who yell a great deal. Men affect an unnaturally low pitch to give an air of authority; women do it to give an impression of sexiness; and young boys probably do it to identify with older males in the family or community. Vocal nodules are condensations of hyaline connective tissue in the lamina propria at the junction of the anterior one third and the posterior two thirds of the true vocal cords. These nodules produce hoarseness and give the voice a breathy quality. In adults, these lesions are removed at direct laryngoscopy for restoration of the voice. However, it is necessary to begin voice therapy before the surgical therapy because if the underlying misuse of the voice is not corrected, the nodules will recur. In children, surgical removal is not usually necessary because the vocal nodules will regress with voice therapy.

Trauma

Trauma has replaced infectious diseases such as diphtheria, streptococcal croup, syphilis, tuberculosis, rhinoscleroma, and typhoid fever as the most common cause of laryngeal stenosis. Automobile accidents in which the patient is thrown forward and the larynx is crushed between the cervical vertebrae and the object against which it decelerates are the single most important cause of laryngeal stenosis. Children may fracture the larynx by falling against the handlebars of a bicycle or riding a horse or bicycle under a taut line. Another cause of laryngeal stenosis is the high tracheostomy in which a perichondritis of the cricoid cartilage follows pressure of the tube on the cartilage. Prolonged endotracheal intubation frequently produces subglottic stenosis, as do infectious processes.

Patients with crush injuries of the larynx complain of pain on swallowing. Hoarseness may progress to aphonia. Hemoptysis is usually present. Progressive dyspnea due to upper respiratory obstruction is to be anticipated. Subcutaneous emphysema is usually present in fractures of the larynx or trachea. The laryngeal cartilages cannot be distinctly palpated, nor can the trachea, owing to soft tissue swelling. On indirect laryngoscopy, the laryngeal lumen may appear disrupted or obliterated, and there may be exposed cartilage and lacerated mucous membrane. Vocal cord paralysis may be noted. Radiographs of the lateral neck and CT of the neck may indicate the type and degree of injury. Lateral neck radiographs may demonstrate associated fractures or dislocations of the cervical vertebrae.

In the initial management of the patient with a laryngeal fracture, a tracheostomy is performed and followed by direct laryngoscopy and tracheoscopy.

The repair of the fracture is done through a transverse incision in the neck. For gaining access to the interior of the larynx, a laryngofissure is performed by dividing the thyroid cartilage at its isthmus, or the fractures in the thyroid and cricoid cartilages are utilized. Mucous membrane lacerations are repaired, and the cartilages are returned to their normal alignment. Internal splinting is maintained with a solid-core mold for as long as 6 weeks.

In addition to external trauma, tracheal stenosis occurs secondary to pressure necrosis of the tracheal walls caused by the inflated cuff in prolonged endotracheal intubation. Tracheal stenosis also occurs secondary to tracheostomy, particularly when the wound becomes infected and there is cicatricial healing of large eroded tracheostomas. Tracheal stenosis may be managed by dilations, excision of the stenotic area with internal splinting for 6 weeks or more, or excision of the stenotic area with end-to-end anastomosis of the trachea. As much as 50% of the length of the trachea can be resected and end-to-end anastomosis performed.

Subglottic stenosis is a frequent complication of neonatal intubation, particularly in low-birth-weight infants. Subglottic stenosis in infants is repaired with an anterior or anterior and posterior cricoid cartilage split (vertical transection) with or without costal cartilage grafts.

Foreign Bodies of the Larynx, Tracheobronchial Tree, and Esophagus

Foreign bodies are retained in the larynx generally because they are sharp and stick into the mucous membrane or are irregular and soft and are caught between the two vocal cords in laryngospasm. A frequently fatal laryngeal foreign body is a bolus of meat. The resulting laryngospasm completely occludes the larynx and makes a choking individual mute. This "café coronary" may be distinguished from a myocardial infarction by the respiratory effort without exchange and the marked suprasternal, intercostal, and subxiphoid retraction. Death occurs rapidly unless an alternative airway is established or the foreign body is dislodged. As long as adequate respiratory exchange occurs, the individual should be allowed to employ protective reflexes to manage the problem. Maneuvers such as striking the choking individual on the back or turning a choking child upside down may make it more difficult for the individual to handle the problem successfully and may convert the situation into one that is less easily managed. If the individual is mute and makes no respiratory exchange, the Heimlich (abdominal thrust) maneuver should be attempted. In this maneuver, the operator places his arms around the choking individual from behind, grasps the fist of one hand in the other hand, and brings both hands up in the subxiphoid area briskly to apply pressure to the diaphragm. The pressure increases the intrathoracic pressure and may expel the foreign body. Should this maneuver fail, an alternative airway must be established by the prompt performance of a tracheostomy.

Smooth objects such as nuts, kernels of corn, watermelon seeds, beans, peas, and plastic toys pass through the larynx into the tracheobronchial tree. At the onset, there is severe spasmodic coughing that continues for approximately 30 minutes. During this period of time, the foreign body migrates from one portion of the tracheobronchial tree to another. It more frequently comes to rest in the right bronchus because the right bronchus is larger than the left and makes less of an angle with the long axis of the trachea, and the carina is to the left of the midline of the tracheal lumen. As it finally comes to rest, the coughing subsides, and a latent period begins during which the patient is free of symptoms. The mistaken inference is often made by the family and the physician in attendance that the foreign body has been expelled. However, careful auscultation of the chest may demonstrate an expiratory wheeze and the signs of obstructive emphysema. The most common mechanism of bronchial obstruction due to a foreign body is a one-way valve through which air may enter the bronchus distal to the foreign body during inspiration, but which affords limited egress on expiration. This type of obstruction produces emphysema distal to the foreign body. The obstructive emphysema may become apparent radiographically only on expiration. The mediastinum shifts away from the obstructed lung, and the obstructed portion of the lung becomes radiolucent compared with the normal lung.

A foreign body that completely obstructs the bronchus causes the rapid development of a more serious pathophysiologic state. Complete atelectasis of the obstructed lung occurs as a result of absorption of the remaining air in the lung. The mediastinum shifts toward the atelectatic lung, and the remaining lung undergoes compensatory emphysema. The atelectatic lung is useless as far as ventilatory exchange is concerned, and the efficiency of the emphysematous lung is greatly reduced. Rapid cardiorespiratory failure occurs unless the foreign body is removed. This type of complete bronchial obstruction is likely to occur with smooth hygroscopic foreign bodies, such as beans, that swell in the bronchus.

Vegetable foreign bodies are very poorly tolerated. Metallic and plastic foreign bodies that cause partial obstruction of the bronchus may be tolerated for long periods. Nuts, particularly peanuts, produce a severe tracheobronchitis. After a latent period of 24 hours, the patient develops a cough productive of purulent sputum, and a febrile course begins. A long-indwelling foreign body of the bronchus may produce bronchiectasis, recurrent pneumonitis, lung abscess, and empyema. Tracheobronchial foreign bodies are removed under general anesthesia through an open bronchoscope with forceps designed specifically for each type of foreign body.

Foreign bodies of the esophagus are likely to lodge just below the cricopharyngeus muscle. Around 95% of esophageal foreign bodies are found in this location. Other locations are the gastroesophageal junction and the indentations of the esophagus caused by the left bronchus and the arch of the aorta. The constrictors of the pharynx are very strong and can propel almost any irregular object through the cricopharyngeus muscle. When the foreign body has passed the cricopharyngeus, the muscular activity is very weak, and progress occurs mainly by gravity. Therefore, irregular objects are brought to an abrupt stop just below the cricopharyngeus muscle.

The symptoms of a foreign body of the esophagus are dysphagia and pain in the suprasternal area on swallowing. Bulky foreign bodies in the cervical esophagus may produce upper airway obstruction by extrinsic pressure through the membranous posterior wall of the trachea. Foreign bodies can be identified on a lateral neck radiograph if they are radiopaque. If they are radiolucent, evidence of a foreign body may still be obtained, because the foreign body tends to hold the esophageal walls apart and air may be seen in the cervical esophagus. If the foreign body cannot be located on a lateral neck film, posteroanterior and lateral chest films are taken.

If the foreign body cannot be located in this manner, an esophagogram may demonstrate it. A small pledget of cotton saturated with a solution of barium sulfate may hang on a sharp foreign body. A foreign body of the esophagus is removed under general anesthesia through an open esophagoscope. The foreign body is grasped, disengaged, and removed as a trailing foreign body or through the esophagoscope with a foreign body forceps appropriate to the object. The longer a foreign body remains in the esophagus, the greater the risk of perforation of the esophagus. Perforation of the esophagus produces air and soft tissue swelling in the paraesophageal tissue that may be demonstrated on physical examination and radiographically.

Infectious Diseases

CROUP. There are two forms of croup, epiglottitis (supraglottic laryngitis) and laryngotracheobronchitis. Croup occurs primarily in children over 1 year and under 5 years of age. It may be viral or bacterial. Parainfluenza type I is the most frequently isolated agent in viral croup. *Haemophilus influenzae* is the most frequently isolated agent in bacterial croup, but *Staphylococcus* and *Streptococcus* also may cause croup.

H. influenzae type b is the predominant microorganism in epiglottitis and frequently causes a bacteremia. Both epiglottitis and laryngotracheobronchitis may produce rapid onset of upper respiratory obstruction with inspiratory stridor and suprasternal, supraclavicular, intercostal, and subxiphoid retractions. The voice may be hoarse, and the cough has a brassy quality with subglottic edema.

Epiglottitis is more likely to cause abrupt and complete airway obstruction. When the diagnosis of epiglottitis is made, nasotracheal intubation is performed and maintained for 48 hours until the supraglottic swelling subsides. Fortunately, the *H. influenzae* type b (Hib) vaccine against meningitis also reduces the incidence of epiglottitis. In laryngotracheobronchitis, the airway obstruction results in part from edema, but there also are tenacious mucoid secretions. Humidification of the inspired atmosphere liquefies the material, and the patient may cough it out to reduce the degree of airway obstruction. Antibiotic therapy is initiated at the onset of both diseases; amoxicillin is the drug of choice because the infection is frequently caused by *H. influenzae*. Corticosteroid therapy is also initiated in an attempt to reduce the inflammatory swelling. Oxygen saturation is continuously monitored transcutaneously. With evidence of desaturation or fatigue, endotracheal intubation is accomplished. Prolonged endotracheal intubation increases the risk of laryngeal and subglottic stenosis in laryngotracheobronchitis. If tracheostomy is elected, it can be performed under general anesthesia in a relaxed patient and under unhurried and ideal circumstances. This approach reduces the incidence of pneumothorax and other complications.

Neoplasms

Benign neoplasms, including papillomas, fibromas, myxomas, chondromas, neurofibromas, hemangiomas, and so forth, may involve any part of the larynx including the true vocal cords. Such lesions can ordinarily be removed at direct laryngoscopy with restoration of the voice, the airway, and the functional integrity of the laryngeal sphincter.

MALIGNANT NEOPLASMS OF THE LARYNX. The majority of malignant neoplasms of the larynx are squamous cell carcinomas. Squamous cell carcinoma of the larynx represents approximately 2% of all cancer deaths. It is a disease mainly of males, with a sex ratio of 5:1. Twelve thousand new cases are expected each year in the United States. The peak incidence of carcinoma of the larynx is in the fifth and sixth decades of life. Laryngeal carcinoma occurs more commonly in individuals with a large ethanolic intake. It rarely develops in those who do not smoke.

Carcinoma may arise from the mucous membrane of any part of the larynx; however, there is a predilection for the true vocal cords, particularly the anterior portions of the true vocal cords. The epiglottis and pyriform sinus are common sites of origin of carcinoma. The natural history of the carcinoma varies considerably from one location to another. The early symptom of carcinoma of the true vocal cords is hoarseness. In any patient with hoarseness lasting 2 weeks, indirect laryngoscopy should be performed. Any discrete lesions of the mucous membrane of the larynx should be biopsied. Carcinomas of the true vocal cord limited to the middle third of the true vocal cord and not impairing the mobility of the cord are treated with radiation therapy or cordectomy with an overall 5-year survival rate of 85% to 95%. Because cordectomy causes permanent hoarseness and the use of irradiation usually returns the voice to normal, radiation therapy is the treatment of choice. Cordectomy is reserved for the 5% to 15% who have persistent carcinoma following radiation therapy. The likelihood of metastasis in early carcinoma of the true vocal cord is very slight.

The mobility of the vocal cord becomes impaired in more advanced carcinomas as a result of invasion of the intrinsic musculature and cartilage. With invasion of the intrinsic musculature, the rate of metastasis increases. With invasion of the thyroid cartilage, the rate of 5-year survival with radiation therapy decreases precipitously. Operation becomes the treatment of choice for lesions that involve the anterior commissure where cartilage is very early invaded and for larger glottic lesions in which the mobility of the true vocal cord is impaired. Often a vertical hemilaryngectomy can be performed for preservation of the phonatory and sphincteric functions of the larynx. In more advanced cases, total laryngectomy is required, and the laryngectomy may be combined with a radical neck dissection if palpable metastases are present.

Supraglottic carcinomas tend to be asymptomatic until they reach considerable size. They may produce hoarseness by secondary involvement of the vocal cords, or they may produce pain on swallowing as the first symptom. Often the pain radiates to the ears. Not infrequently, a patient with a supraglottic carcinoma presents with the chief complaint of a swelling in the neck that represents a metastasis. The likelihood of nonpalpable metastasis being present is 35%. Early supraglottic carcinoma is successfully treated with radiation therapy to the primary and both sides of the neck, but in advanced lesions, better survival rates are obtained with a combination of irradiation and surgical therapy. Better local and regional control is obtained with postoperative radiation therapy than with preoperative radiation therapy. The 2-year disease-free survival approximates 70%. In many patients with supraglottic carcinomas, the neoplasm can be completely removed by performing a supraglottic partial laryngectomy with preservation of the phonatory and sphincteric function of the larynx. If the glottis is involved, a total laryngectomy is usually required. These procedures are often combined with a radical neck dissection if there are palpable metastases.

Pyriform sinus carcinomas tend to remain asymptomatic for long periods of time. Often the patient presents with dysphagia and pain on swallowing that may radiate to the ear on the same side. Often the presenting complaint is a mass in the neck that represents a metastasis. A combination of preoperative or postoperative radiation therapy and operation yields better survival rates than does operation alone. Depending on the location of the lesion in the pyriform sinus, a partial laryngectomy can sometimes be accomplished with preservation of the phonatory and sphincteric functions of the larynx. More often, a total laryngectomy is required. Either of these procedures is combined with a radical neck dissection if there are palpable metastases. The 5-year survival rate for all stages is 30%.

A total laryngectomy requires the formation of a permanent tracheostomy in which the trachea is transected and anastomosed to the skin of the lower part of the neck. Rehabilitation of the postlaryngectomy patient requires the development of alaryngeal or esophageal speech. In this technique, the patient draws air into the esophagus during inspiration and gradually eructs the air through the cricopharyngeus muscle. The opening of the esophagus vibrates and serves as the sounding source. The sound is articulated by the pharynx, palate, tongue, teeth, and lips into speech. For those individuals who, because of age or other physical or emotional reasons, cannot develop alaryngeal speech, an electrolarynx can serve as the sounding source for modification by the articulators. The oscillator of the electrolarynx is placed in the submandibular area, and the sound is articulated into speech. Most patients who require a laryngectomy may return to their former occupation. With proper guidance in their rehabilitation, laryngectomees may resume all activities except swimming.

40

PLASTIC AND MAXILLOFACIAL SURGERY

Greg J. Mackay, M.D., Grant W. Carson, M.D.,
Robert J. Wood, M.D., and John T. Bostwick III, M.D.

Plastic surgery concentrates on restoring form and function to the human body. It is a specialty that is not confined to one system or anatomic region but concentrates on solving aesthetic and reconstructive problems throughout the body.

BASIC PRINCIPLES

Wound Closure

Optimal wound healing with a minimal scar that compromises neither appearance nor function is the desired result. This process is affected by both local and systemic factors. The following basic fundamental surgical techniques should be adhered to when managing any type of wound: (1) When placing incisions, design them to follow tension lines and natural folds in the skin, (2) handle all tissues gently and débride only devitalized areas, (3) eliminate tension at all skin edges, (4) evert wound edges, (5) ensure complete hemostasis, (6) use fine sutures and remove them early, and (7) allow time for scar maturation before revision is undertaken.

SKIN GRAFTS AND FLAPS

The technique used to close a wound is determined largely by the defect, its anatomic location, and the surgeon's preference. When minimal tissue loss is evident and the wound can be closed without undue tension, then direct closure is indicated. With significant tissue loss, or when direct closure of a wound might cause compromise of function or form, then a skin graft or flap may be indicated. Skin grafts are indicated primarily for covering wounds that have a suitable vascularized host bed to support them. Grafts do not "take" on bare cortical bone, denuded tendon, nerve, or cartilage. Flaps are generally reserved for deeper, more demanding reconstructive situations.

Split-thickness skin grafts, which are usually 0.012 to 0.018 in. in thickness, are used primarily for covering wounds with large skin defects. They can be meshed in ratios of 1:1.5 to 1:9. They are not as durable as full-thickness grafts, they undergo greater *secondary* contraction, and they may demon-

---

See the corresponding chapter or part in the *Textbook of Surgery*, 15th edition, pp. 1298–1329, for a more detailed discussion of this topic, including a comprehensive list of references.

strate abnormal pigmentation. They are harvested most often from the thighs, buttocks, or abdominal wall.

Full-thickness skin grafts include the entire epidermis and underlying dermis. They undergo greater *primary* contraction when harvested but maintain normal pigmentation and are quite durable. Full-thickness skin grafts are used primarily for covering wound defects in the face, where matching texture and skin color is of a greater cosmetic concern. Donor sites include the postauricular area, upper eyelid, supraclavicular region, groin crease, and antecubital fossa.

Flaps

Random flaps or *local flaps* are skin flaps that can be rotated, advanced, transposed, or transferred as an island to cover wound defects. These flaps are perfused by the dermal-subdermal plexus of multiple vessels but do not incorporate a specific cutaneous perforator.

Axial/arterial flaps are perfused by a specific cutaneous perforator. Their size and mobility are limited only by the length and territory supplied by the underlying vessel. These flaps consist of skin and subcutaneous tissue. Examples of these types of flaps include the groin flap, forehead flap, and radial forearm flap.

Musculocutaneous flaps are perfused by one or several dominant segmental vessels, which send perforators to the muscle and overlying skin and subcutaneous tissue. These large, robust flaps supply well-vascularized tissue for covering exposed bone and filling in dead space, or they can be shaped for such purposes as reconstructing a breast.

Free-tissue transfer involves the transfer of a wide variety of tissues, including bone, cartilage, muscle, skin, or any combination of the above for reconstructing a defect. The transferred tissue brings along its own blood supply, which is anastomosed to the local vessels using microvascular techniques. Free-tissue transfer is a useful procedure for reconstructing or closing complex wounds, particularly when local tissue is not available.

CRANIOFACIAL SURGERY
Congenital Deformities

Cleft lip and palate is the most common of the major congenital craniofacial deformities. The rate of clefting is 1 in 700 live births. *Cleft lips* present either as a unilateral or bilateral deformity and in all degrees of severity. A complete cleft of the primary palate extends through the lip and nostril floor, across the alveolus to the incisor foramen. Lip repair is generally undertaken between 3 and 4 months of age or according to the time-honored "rule of tens." The child should be at least 10 weeks of age, a weight of 10 pounds, and a hemoglobin of 10 gm. per 100 ml. There is often an associated cleft nasal deformity, which is repaired at some later stage in the child's development.

Cleft palate deformities develop from failure of fusion of the two lateral palatine processes that close anterior to posterior in the region of the incisor foramen during development. The incidence of isolated cleft palate is 1 in 2000 live births. A cleft palate deformity can affect speech and language development. The cleft palate is closed between 6 and 18 months by some form of palatoplasty.

FACIAL FRACTURES

Facial fractures are seen commonly following motor vehicle accidents, assaults, and other blunt trauma to the face. Assessment of the face should begin with examination of the scalp and calvarium for any laceration or bony irregularities. The eyes and orbits should be examined for any restrictions in gaze, enophthalmus, or irregularities. Nasal fractures present as a gross deformity, and the septum should be examined for the presence of a hematoma.

Radiographic assessment should include standard C-spine views and a facial series with posteroanterior, lateral, and Waters' views. If mandibular trauma is suspected, a mandible series with Panorex is indicated. Computed tomography (CT) remains the most sensitive technique for imaging facial fractures.

Orbital fractures are most commonly of the blowout type. This fracture involves the floor of the orbit. The mechanism of injury is usually a direct blow to the orbit. Orbital fat and often the inferior rectus muscle will herniate through the floor and become entrapped, causing a gaze restriction. Repair of this fracture involves exposure of the floor and often placement of a silicone sheet or bone graft to reconstruct the floor.

Maxillary fractures occur in a characteristic pattern described by Rene Le Fort. The *Le Fort I* is a transverse fracture across the maxilla separating the lower maxilla, hard palate, and pterygoid processes from the rest of the maxilla. The *Le Fort II* is a pyramidal fracture separation along the nasofrontal suture, floor of orbit, zygomaticomaxillary sutures, and the pterygoid processes. The *Le Fort III* fracture separates the entire facial skeleton from the cranium. This fracture extends from the pterygomaxillary fissure, through the zygomatical frontal suture, across the floor of the orbit to the nasofrontal junction. Maxillary fractures usually are reduced and secured with rigid fixation.

Mandibular fractures most often involve the condyle or angle of the mandible. Condyle fractures may be treated by a soft diet or intermaxillary fixation if minimally displaced. Angle fractures and those involving the body or symphysis are often displaced by the muscles of mastication and require open reduction and rigid fixation.

HEAD AND NECK CANCER

Epidemiology

The majority of head and neck cancers are squamous cell carcinomas (SCCs) of the upper aerodigestive tract. They are generally a disease of males in their fifth or sixth decade, accounting for roughly 8.5% of all malignancies in this age group. The male-to-female ratio is 4:1 but is decreasing because of an increase in female tobacco use. Ethanol consumption potentiates tobacco-related carcinogensis and is also an independent risk factor.

Diagnosis and Staging

The signs and symptoms of cancer of the upper aerodigestive tract vary with the location of the primary site and the stage of the cancer. Approximately 35% to 45% of patients present with early-stage disease and have vague symptoms and minimal physical findings. Many patients present with a mass in the neck. Chronology, patient's age, and mass location are important diagnostic factors. Inflammatory lesions generally have a brief duration and are common in the pediatric age group. A solitary mass in the neck of an adult that has been present for over 6 weeks should be presumed to be cancer until proven otherwise.

Physical examination identifies more than 90% of cancers of the upper aerodigestive tract. Examination under anesthesia is helpful to fully evaluate the primary cancer and to obtain biopsies. Triple endoscopy—direct laryngoscopy, bronchoscopy, and esophagoscopy—to evaluate for synchronous malignancies is not cost-effective and is not performed unless warranted by clinical suspicion. CT and magnetic resonance imaging (MRI) are the most useful radiographic studies for evaluating head and neck masses.

Natural History and Standard Therapy

The majority of head and neck cancer patients present with locally and regionally advanced disease. Stage I and II disease generally can be treated equally by surgery or radiation, with a control rate of 60% to 80%. Stage III and IV disease requires extensive surgery and postoperative radiation. Disease control is less than 30%, and the majority of patients die with locally or regionally persistent disease.

Management of the Neck

Management of the neck is not site-specific. The goals are to accurately stage the disease and decrease the likelihood of regional recurrence. Metastatic involvement of the cervical lymphatics reduces survival by 50% for all sites and is the single best prognostic factor in head and neck cancer.

Radical neck dissection is indicated in most N_2 nodal disease. A modified neck dissection is indicated in those patients with N_0 or N_1 disease. Adjuvant external-beam radiation therapy is generally used if greater than one node is found to be involved or there is evidence of extracapsular extension.

Head and Neck Reconstruction

Reconstruction after extirpation of head and neck cancer continues to be a surgical challenge. The majority of patients are debilitated and present with locally advanced disease. Poor long-term survival and the need for adjuvant radiotherapy demand that the reconstruction be immediate, single-stage, allow a rapid restoration of function, and have a low morbidity.

The pectoralis major muscle is a reliable, bulky flap with a favorable arc of rotation and is used successfully in many sites in the head and neck, including the oral cavity, oropharynx, and hypopharynx. Microvascular free-tissue transfer has supplanted the pectoralis major flap for the majority of head and neck reconstruction.

Salivary Gland Tumors

Neoplasms of the salivary glands are relatively uncommon, constituting 5% of hospital admissions for head and neck tumors. The major salivary glands include the parotid, submandibular, and sublingual glands. The minor salivary glands are scattered throughout the upper aerodigestive tract. Around 75% of salivary gland tumors involve the parotid. Nonneoplastic processes account for 25% of parotid masses.

Pleomorphic adenoma or benign mixed tumor is the most common parotid neoplasm, accounting for 50% of all parotid tumors. Surgical treatment is complete excision with negative margins. Tumors superficial to the facial nerve require a conservative total parotidectomy. The recurrence rate after complete resection is 1% to 5%.

Warthin's tumor or papillary cystadenoma lymphomatosum is the second most common benign parotid tumor. It can be bilateral in up to 10% of cases. Mucoepidermoid carcinoma is the most common malignancy of the parotid. Malignant mixed tumor or carcinoma ex pleomorphic adenoma is the second most common parotid malignancy. Adenoid cystic carcinoma constitutes less than 10% of parotid malignancy but is the most common cancer of the submandibular and minor salivary glands.

I

Pilonidal Cysts and Sinuses
Mark W. Sebastian, M.D.

Hodges introduced the term *pilonidal* (*pilus*, "hair," *nidus*, "nest") in 1880 and proposed a theory of congenital origin of

---

See the corresponding chapter or part in the *Textbook of Surgery*, 15th edition, pp. 1330–1334, for a more detailed discussion of this topic, including a comprehensive list of references.

the disease. Most commonly, it occurs in the sacrococcygeal area, about 3 to 5 cm. posterior and superior to the anal orifice; the evidence weighs heavily in favor of an acquired nature for all but the rare case of pilonidal disease. Stretching, particularly of the gluteal muscles, produces distention of hair follicles, sebaceous glands, and apocrine glands and sufficient spreading of their cutaneous orifices to allow insinuation of foreign substances. The tiny midline holes or pits (sinuses) that are seen in the cleft of almost all patients with sacrococcygeal pilonidal disease represent distorted hair follicles, which may ingest hair or become filled with keratin and other debris. In time, they become infected and rupture into the deeper fat. That hair may be ingested secondarily by some of these existing cavities was cleverly demonstrated by Page in 1969. Hair is present in the cyst in only half the patients.

Pilonidal disease has been reported in the umbilicus, the axilla, the clitoris, the interdigital webs of barbers' hands, the interdigital web of the foot of a worker in a hair mattress factory, the sole of the foot, and the anal canal. Pilonidal sinuses containing wool, grass, animal hair, and hair of a color different from that of the patient's have all been reported.

PRESENTATION. Patients with sacrococcygeal pilonidal disease may ask for advice about asymptomatic pits or pores in the natal cleft. Tenderness after physical activity or a long drive requiring the patient to sit for a prolonged duration is a common presentation. A tender or nontender nodule may be palpable. About 20% of such patients seek care for the severe pain and tenderness of an acute abscess. The diagnosis is usually readily apparent, although other conditions should be considered, including perianal abscess arising from the posterior midline crypt, hidradenitis suppurativa, and a simple carbuncle or furuncle. Some other focus of infection such as osteomyelitis rarely may give rise to a sinus in this area. The abscess enlarges rapidly, but since it may be located deep to relatively thick skin, it rarely ruptures spontaneously. In general, there is minimal cellulitis and induration surrounding the pilonidal abscess, and systemic reaction to the abscess is infrequent. Occasionally, fever, leukocytosis, and malaise are found.

The inflammatory process may subside early or progress until relief is obtained—usually by surgical means. After drainage has occurred, the purulent discharge may cease completely, but more commonly it recurs intermittently with drainage from one or more sinuses as the disease enters its chronic phase. In this setting, care must be taken to exclude a complicated anal fistula, which may angulate posteriorly before passing into a retrorectal abscess. Thorough examination of the anal cavity usually discloses the point of origin, and a probe inserted into a pilonidal sinus follows a course away from the anus.

About 80% of patients with pilonidal disease present with a chronic abscess and no history of a prior clinically apparent acute stage. Infection, particularly by anaerobic bacteria, has a central role in the extremely difficult problems of wound healing often associated with chronic pilonidal disease. *Staph-*

ylococcus aureus and *Bacteroides* species are the most important offending organisms.

TREATMENT. There is a growing consensus that pilonidal disease should be managed conservatively. Treatment in an outpatient setting has gained acceptance and is widely practiced. Simple incision and drainage of first-episode acute pilonidal abscess may effect healing *per primam* within 10 weeks of treatment, especially in patients with few pits and lateral tracts. Definitive treatment, which includes evacuation of hair and curetting of granulation tissue with wide exposure, is undertaken earlier than 10 weeks for those patients with pits and lateral tracts. With careful follow-up and local care, including shaving of hair, hot tub baths, and use of Water Pik irrigation, healing by secondary intention is generally completed in 2 weeks. Antibiotics are rarely indicated unless the patient has a medical condition such as rheumatic heart disease or is immunosuppressed.

However, because of the central role of bacterial infection in the perpetuation of chronic pilonidal disease, treatment of these patients is initiated with oral pain medication and an antibiotic regimen particularly directed against *S. aureus* and *Bacteroides* species. Under local or regional anesthesia, the chronic abscess is opened widely by a long incision that lies parallel to and 2 cm. to one side of the midline. Avoidance of the midline "ditch" containing the pits and sinuses is increasingly advocated. The abscess cavity is scrubbed free of hair with push gauze, with removal of portions of the cyst wall impregnated with hair and debris. A flap can be created and sutured to the sacrococcygeal fascia with skin closure and drainage. In the rare patient with long-standing disease, the abscess wall is covered with surface epithelium that has grown into the cavity. This is no longer a chronic abscess but an epithelial inclusion cyst, which is therefore excised. The lateral incision is left widely open to permit drainage; the small holes from the midline skin are excised, with minimal tissue loss, and closed with nonabsorbable suture material. The visible holes that represent enlarged follicles must be excised completely if recurrence is to be avoided. Multiple cavities may appear under insignificant-appearing follicles. Antibiotics are continued for 24 hours. Early ambulation is important. The patient is instructed in local care of the wound.

Pilonidal disease recurring after formal conservative primary treatment as outlined is usually limited to the caudal portion of the scar. A blind cavity or sinus is frequently encountered through a midline opening. Local exposure of the posterior wall of the tract, scraping of the granulation tissue, and débridement of the edges of the tract produce complete healing in 3 to 4 weeks. Hot baths and Water Pik irrigation at least once daily keep the healing wound clean.

COMPLICATIONS. Very rarely, malignant degeneration occurs in these lesions. Verrucous carcinoma (giant condyloma acuminatum) has been reported in an established pilonidal sinus.

41

NEUROSURGERY

I

Historical Aspects
Robert H. Wilkins, M.D.

The earliest cranial surgery was trepanation, which dates back to the Neolithic Period of the Stone Age. Skulls with "surgical" defects (many having evidence of healing) have been unearthed in widely separated geographic locations, indicating that the procedure was performed simultaneously among a variety of human cultures. Because there are no written records from that era, the rationale for trepanation remains unknown.

The oldest known writing concerning surgical topics, the Edwin Smith Papyrus, dates back to the seventeenth century B.C. It provided basic information about various types of head and neck injuries, with criteria relevant to prognosis and advice about management. Of note, trepanation was not mentioned.

Hippocrates revived the use of trepanation and also made important observations about common neurologic syndromes. He and his associates were astute observers but did not perform operations on the head or spine other than trepanation. The necessary prerequisites for successful surgical treatment of conditions affecting the nervous system, which were realized primarily during the second half of the nineteenth century, were the introduction and development of anesthesia, aseptic surgical technique, and the concept of the localization of function within the nervous system, especially the brain.

At the end of the nineteenth century, British surgeons took the lead in devising and conducting operations for the removal of brain tumors, spinal cord tumors, intracranial hematomas, and cerebral scars responsible for epileptic seizures. Rhizotomy of posterior spinal nerve roots and rhizotomy of the trigeminal nerve were developed to control pain.

Between 1900 and 1940, Drs. Harvey Cushing and Walter Dandy provided important leadership for the impressive growth and development of neurosurgery in the United States. During that period and subsequently, many technical advancements were made throughout the world that have expanded the scope of neurosurgery and have brightened the outlook of patients with diseases affecting the nervous system.

Computerized imaging techniques have revolutionized diagnosis and have permitted a degree of accuracy in neurosurgical operations not previously possible. Neurosurgery as a

See the corresponding chapter or part in the *Textbook of Surgery*, 15th edition, pp. 1335–1336, for a more detailed discussion of this topic, including a comprehensive list of references.

true medical discipline is only about 100 years old, but it is constantly changing at an ever-increasing pace so that current practice hardly resembles that of just a few decades ago.

II

Neuroradiology
Robert D. Tien, M.D.

Diagnostic neuroradiologic examinations available to the surgeon in the evaluation of neurologic diseases include plain films of the skull, sinuses, and spine, water-soluble myelography, cerebral angiography, computed tomography (CT), and magnetic resonance imaging (MRI).

PLAIN FILMS

At present, plain films are not very valuable in evaluation of intracerebral diseases. Plain films may still be useful in detecting facial fractures or diseases of paranasal sinuses.

MYELOGRAPHY

Noninvasive procedures such as CT and MRI have taken the place of myelography in evaluation of neurologic diseases. At present, myelography is necessary only for evaluating diffuse disease of the subarachnoid space that may be difficult to identify on MRI or CT, such as diffuse subarachnoid seeding of tumor. Another condition that may require a myelogram occurs when the clinician cannot determine the exact level of disease involvement, often because it is too time-consuming or difficult to use MRI for the whole spine.

CEREBRAL ANGIOGRAPHY

Cerebral angiography is an invasive procedure with a 0.5% to 2% complication rate. Actually, CT scanning and MRI have taken the place of cerebral angiography in many of its former functions. To date, cerebral angiography remains an important or definitive study in evaluation of the following situations: intracerebral aneurysms, arteriovenous malformations, vasculitis, vessel displacement or encasement by tumor when not readily apparent on CT or MRI, atherosclerotic disease of the carotid bifurcation, and intravascular neurointerventional

---

See the corresponding chapter or part in the *Textbook of Surgery*, 15th edition, pp. 1337–1344, for a more detailed discussion of this topic, including a comprehensive list of references.

procedures such as embolization of feeding vessels responsible for uncontrollable bleeding, hypervascular tumor, or cerebral arteriovenous malformations.

COMPUTED TOMOGRAPHY (CT)

CT is a method of x-ray evaluation in which a thin slice or planar volume of tissues is examined. Scans can be obtained at direct axial or coronal planes. Manipulation of controls on the computer console allows visualization of tissues on a soft tissue or bone window. By computer assistance, CT can differentiate various components of soft tissues in the brain such as gray matter, white matter, and cerebrospinal fluid (CSF).

Brain CT can be performed with or without iodinated contrast enhancement. A non-contrast-enhanced study is the best study in most acute situations; however, a contrast-enhanced study is usually the examination necessary in a chronic situation. In most acute situations, the clinical concern is either intracerebral hemorrhage or infarction. On the non-contrast-enhanced study, hemorrhage appears hyperdense (white) and is usually very obvious. Calcification also can be detected easily on a non-contrast-enhanced study as a hyperdense area. Contrast administration therefore is not necessary for visualization of hemorrhage or calcification. Most acute infarcts appear as a lucency (darker gray or black) and do not show any contrast enhancement for 1 to 2 weeks. In chronic neurologic disease, such as a tumor (primary tumor and metastasis) or an abscess, the definition of the lesion can be obtained only on the contrast-enhanced study. The abnormal enhancement exhibited by tumors and abscesses that are intra-axial is the result of breakdown of the blood-brain barrier, not abnormally increased vascularity. Metastases and abscesses frequently appear as sharply marginated, noncalcified nodules or ring-enhancing lesions with perifocal edema. Primary brain tumors tend to be less well marginated, irregularly enhancing lesions, with or without calcification and perifocal edema. To distinguish a primary brain tumor from metastasis or abscess is not always possible.

CT scans of the spine without contrast enhancement are useful in examining lumbar disc disease, degenerative spinal disease, and spinal trauma. However, in evaluation of cervical and thoracic disc disease or of involvement of the intraspinal contents by tumors, whether from metastatic disease or primary tumors of the spinal sac contents, opacification of the subarachnoid space on CT after intrathecal administration of water-soluble contrast material via lumbar puncture is often necessary (the CT-myelogram). The contrast-enhanced CT scans of the spine may aid in differentiating herniated disc from scar material.

In addition, CT scans can be applied in paranasal sinus diseases; lesions of the base of the skull (particularly tumors), temporal bone and inner ear lesions, and facial trauma; and laryngeal and other neck and upper airway tumors for location and staging.

ADVANCES IN COMPUTED TOMOGRAPHY (CT) TECHNOLOGY

Volume Scanning (Spiral CT, Helical CT)

A new advancement in the field of CT has been the development of volume scanning. The x-ray tube and detector within the CT gantry are moved continuously in a spiral or helical pattern as the patient is moved through the imaging zone. The benefits of this technology are the markedly reduced scanning time needed for acquisition of information and an elimination of motion-induced artifacts. The amount of contrast material needed is also decreased, resulting in increased patient safety and decreased cost. Because a volume of information is collected, re-formatting images or three-dimensional reconstructions will be smoother and more accurate.

Computed Tomographic Angiography (CTA)

The most accurate assessment of the carotid bifurcation remains carotid angiography. However, carotid angiography remains an expensive and invasive procedure. Noninvasive techniques such as duplex and color Doppler sonography are very operator-dependent and may underdiagnose distal plaque or may yield a false diagnosis of carotid occlusion. The magnetic resonance angiogram (MRA) also has been used to evaluate the carotid bifurcation, but it commonly overestimates the degree of carotid stenosis resulting from the turbulence dephasing at points of stenosis or irregularity. Recent advances in CT and in three-dimensional display have led to new vascular imaging methods that may overcome some of the limitations of sonography and MRI. The volume data obtained on spiral or helical CT can be reconstructed to produce a three-dimensional representation of the anatomic region scanned. Vascular structures can be imaged selectively by the use of a bolus intravenous infusion of contrast material. The potential utility of spiral CT with contrast enhancement is in imaging of the carotid bifurcation, aneurysm evaluation, and other vascular malformation of the brain.

MAGNETIC RESONANCE IMAGING (MRI)

MRI is a new development, with the information obtained as a result of magnetic properties of the tissues. Certain abnormalities that cannot be detected on CT scans are evident on MRI. Therefore, these two modalities have different sensitivities for detecting disease processes. Two types of images traditionally were included in an MRI examination. The T1-weighted images are used to obtain anatomic detail. On these images, CSF is dark (hypointense) and fat is very bright (hyperintense). Abnormal contrast enhancement is also clearly demonstrated on T1 contrast-enhanced images. T2-weighted images demonstrate the water-related contents (CSF) to be hyperintense and fat to be relatively hypointense. Anatomy on T2 sequences is less well demonstrated than that on T1 sequences, but T2 sequences are more sensitive than T1 sequences in detecting focal abnormality. The contrast material used with MRI is gadolinium chelating agent (Gd-DTPA), a paramagnetic substance administered intravenously that affects the magnetic properties of the tissues that accumulate the contrast material. Gadolinium is different from iodinated contrast material with very few of the systemic effects.

MRI has been proved to be a better modality than CT scanning in evaluation of disease of the central nervous system, such as diseases at the base of the skull, particularly the sellar and cerebellopontine angle cistern regions, and also for most tumors, white matter disease (e.g., multiple sclerosis), congenital abnormalities, vascular malformations, and spinal diseases. This is mostly due to the advantages of MRI with the absence of bone and dental artifacts that are commonly seen in CT, presence of multiplanar images (sagittal, coronal, axial, and oblique), and high sensitivity about the disease processes. However, CT is still better than MRI in evaluation of patients with acute intracerebral hemorrhage, acute head trauma, subarachnoid hemorrhage, or disease processes requiring analysis with fine bone detail such as facial or spinal fractures. Calcification is also poorly identified on all sequences of MRI. In addition, for patients who cannot cooperate sufficiently for the relatively long period of time required for MRI or have certain types of metal in their bodies (which may move because of the susceptibility to the magnetic field and cause injury to the patient or significant artifact), CT scanning remains the better option.

ADVANCES IN MAGNETIC RESONANCE IMAGING (MRI) PULSE-SEQUENCE DESIGN

Fast Spin Echo (FSE) MRI

FSE is a pulse-sequence technique with marked reduction in acquisition time needed for long repetition time (RT) images. This significant time saving may be extremely useful when imaging uncooperative patients (infants, ill patients, etc.).

Steady-State Free Precession (SSFP)

The MRI signal intensities of cystic masses of the brain on CSE MRI images can be similar to the signal intensities of the cerebrospinal fluid (CSF). With SSFP imaging, the signal intensities of all solid tissues are typically suppressed, leading to low signal of these tissues. However, the heavily T2-weighted SSFP images also show the high signal intensity fluid components of cystic masses, thereby differentiating solid from cystic. Similarly, SSFP MRI also can distinguish between epidermoid and arachnoid cysts, with the epidermoid cyst appearing with heterogeneous internal content and the arachnoid cyst with homogeneous CSF-like internal signal.

ADVANCES IN MAGNETIC RESONANCE IMAGING (MRI) APPLICATIONS

MRI of the Hippocampus

The most frequent type of seizure is the complex partial seizure (CPS). In patients with medically intractable CPS, mesial temporal sclerosis (MTS) is the most common pathologic abnormality. In cases of medically intractable CPS, surgical therapy (e.g., hippocampectomy) may be needed for seizure control. Before surgical therapy, accurate noninvasive evaluation of the seizure focus is essential. Recently developed FSE MRI has been shown to be extremely useful in detecting both the atrophy and signal abnormality associated with MTS.

MR Angiography in Hemifacial Spasm/ Trigeminal Neuralgia

Hemifacial spasm and trigeminal neuralgia are frequently due to vascular loop compression by either the vertebral-basilar arteries or their branches. These disorders may be relieved by vascular decompression procedures. A new MRI angiography (MRA) technique has been developed that can better delineate the branches of the vertebral-basilar system and the root entry zone of the seventh and eighth nerves and cisternal portions of the fifth nerves. With this technique, accurate demonstration of the compression is identified, and a roadmap for the surgeon is obtained preoperatively.

Diffusion-Weighted MRI

Diffusion-weighted MRI is a new development in MRI applications and sensitive to microscopic motion of water protons (brownian motion). Initial applications have involved imaging of early stroke, differentiation between edema and tumor, and identifying the nonenhancing part of the tumor. Other possible areas of use include white matter diseases and multiple sclerosis.

MR Angiography (MRA)

Conventional angiography remains the definitive technique for evaluation of cerebrovascular disease. New developments in MRI pulse sequences, however, have significantly improved the utility of MRA in noninvasive evaluation of vascular structures. The identification of vasculature by MRA is due to contrast material between the moving blood and stationary tissues. Both time of flight effects (TOF) and phase contrast (PC) effects can be exploited to generate an MRI angiogram. Currently, there are four established MRA techniques available: two-dimensional TOF, three-dimensional TOF, two-dimensional PC, and three-dimensional PC. Two-dimensional TOF is useful in the carotid bifurcation and cortical venous mapping. A frequent application of three-dimensional TOF is in the study of the circle of Willis for aneurysm evaluation.

When compared with TOF, the major advantage of two-dimensional and three-dimensional PC techniques is the extreme degree of stationary tissue suppression, including methemoglobin or fat, which could potentially confuse interpretation of TOF images. These techniques are extremely useful in the setting of venous thrombosis. Determination of velocity is also possible with PC techniques.

MR Spectroscopy

With MR spectroscopy, metabolites within a selected region of interest can be investigated, and spectral peaks that reflect the concentrations of the metabolite within the region of interest can be obtained. The metabolites, including lactate, amino acids [e.g., NAA (N-acetyl aspartate), a neuronal integrity marker], phosphorus metabolites (e.g., ATP), and so on, can be measured noninvasively. Reductions in the NAA level have been shown in multiple sclerosis plaques, mesial temporal sclerosis, ischemic brain lesions, and brain tumors.

MRI of the Spine

MRI has the ability to define normal age-related changes in the vertebral marrow of the axial skeleton and has emerged as the procedure of choice in evaluation of many bone marrow disorders, such as differentiation between a new compression fracture and a metastatic lesion in a patient with known primary carcinoma. The initial outcomes indicate that most malignant processes causing vertebral body pathologic compression show abnormal enhancement early during the sequence of images. This is opposed to the findings in benign, osteoporotic, compression fractures, which show no abnormal enhancement during the sequence of images. MRI also can provide kinematic studies of the spine. It is useful in patients with disease involving the craniovertebral junction and in evaluating the amount of canal compromise in these patients.

III

Intracranial Tumors
Robert H. Wilkins, M.D.

Primary intracranial tumors arise from tissues of the brain or pituitary gland or their coverings. Often, these lesions

---

See the corresponding chapter or part in the *Textbook of Surgery,* 15th edition, pp. 1344–1349, for a more detailed discussion of this topic, including a comprehensive list of references.

are not clearly separable into benign and malignant forms. Secondary intracranial tumors represent local extensions from regional tumors or metastases from a primary malignancy elsewhere in the body. The most common location of brain tumors in childhood is below the tentorium within the posterior cranial fossa; in adults, the most common location is above the tentorium. Within the various intracranial locations, certain types of tumors occur more commonly than others, both in childhood and in adulthood.

SYMPTOMS AND SIGNS. Intracranial tumors can present in several different ways. By their growth, they can cause an increase in intracranial pressure, either directly by the mass of the tumor or indirectly by obstructing the circulation of the cerebrospinal fluid and producing hydrocephalus. In addition, bleeding may occur into the tumor, with a sudden increase in its mass effect. The symptoms that may be produced by a generalized increase in intracranial pressure are headaches (especially prominent in the morning, with dependent head position, or during straining), nausea, vomiting, and a reduction in the level of consciousness. Such a patient may exhibit papilledema and unilateral or bilateral abducens paresis. A generalized increase in intracranial pressure may be tolerated for a period of time, but with further tumor growth, brain herniation may occur, with a rapid decline in the patient's neurologic function.

A second way in which an intracranial tumor may present is by the loss of function of the portion of the nervous system that is involved by the tumor. In contrast to the symptoms and signs caused by an increase in intracranial pressure, the symptoms and signs caused by the loss of function of a specific area of the nervous system often permit an accurate presumptive diagnosis based on the neurologic history and physical examination.

In addition, an intracranial tumor may be manifested by hyperactive function. The tumor can be the cause of this hyperfunction, such as a pituitary adenoma that overproduces one or more hormones or a choroid plexus papilloma that overproduces cerebrospinal fluid, or the tumor may stimulate seizures that arise from the adjacent or infiltrated brain.

DIAGNOSIS. The most common radiographic screening examination is computed tomographic (CT) scanning. Most intracranial tumors are demonstrated by such scanning, especially if scans made after the intravenous injection of an iodinated contrast agent (contrast-enhanced scans) are compared with analogous unenhanced scans. The bony structures forming the base of the skull are especially well demonstrated by CT scanning. However, these same bony structures are often the source of artifacts that degrade the images of adjacent portions of the brain. Magnetic resonance imaging (MRI) does not demonstrate bony detail but provides excellent visualization of the brain at the cranial base and at the craniocervical junction. MRI also offers much clearer and more easily obtained coronal and sagittal views. Among other types of radiologic studies are those done for specific purposes rather than for screening. For example, cerebral angiography may be useful for determining the vascularity of a tumor and its effect on the major adjacent vessels.

TREATMENT. The mainstay of the treatment of intracranial tumors is surgical removal. With CT- or MRI-guided stereotactic techniques, tumors within the nervous system can now be biopsied through a burr hole with low morbidity. The introduction of the operative microscope into neurosurgery and the development of neurosurgical microtechniques have permitted tumor exposure through a small cranial opening with the double aids of magnification and excellent illumination. The simultaneous evolution of bipolar electrical technology for tissue coagulation and cutting and the development of devices that employ laser energy, ultrasonic vibration, suction, or mechanical cutting for removal of tissue permits resection of intracranial tumors more easily and safely. These technological advances have improved the outlook for patients with certain types of intracranial tumors, such as meningiomas, pituitary adenomas, and schwannomas of the cranial nerves, but they have not had a large impact on the gliomas, which in most instances cannot be cured by surgical resection.

IV

Spontaneous Intracranial and Intraspinal Hemorrhage

Allan H. Friedman, M.D.

SUBARACHNOID HEMORRHAGE

Subarachnoid hemorrhage is characterized by the sudden onset of a severe headache. The headache is recalcitrant to minor analgesic medications and usually persists for days. Concomitant with the headache, the patient suffers a change in level of consciousness ranging from momentary confusion to persistent coma. Over the ensuing hours, the blood induces a sterile meningitis that produces a stiff neck, minor fever, and photophobia. Physical examination may reveal retinal hemorrhages. Approximately one-third of patients suffer a "warning leak" manifested as a severe headache before a life-threatening hemorrhage. Unfortunately, these warning events frequently go unrecognized. The clinical diagnosis of spontaneous subarachnoid hemorrhage is verified by brain computed tomographic (CT) scan or lumbar puncture. When the diagnosis of subarachnoid hemorrhage is made, a cerebral

---

See the corresponding chapter or part in the *Textbook of Surgery,* 15th edition, pp. 1349–1355, for a more detailed discussion of this topic, including a comprehensive list of references.

angiogram should be performed for localizing the source of the hemorrhage. While magnetic resonance imaging (MRI) and magnetic resonance angiography (MRA) will demonstrate many aneurysms, they are not sensitive enough to replace angiography.

Etiology

The most common cause of a nontraumatic subarachnoid hemorrhage is a ruptured intracranial aneurysm. The second most common cause is a ruptured arteriovenous malformation. In a smaller number of patients, the hemorrhage is caused by hypertensive cerebrovascular disease, primary or metastatic tumor, mycotic aneurysm, blood dyscrasia, anticoagulation therapy, eclampsia, intracranial infection, or spinal angiomatous malformation. In approximately 10% of cases, the etiologic factor is never discovered.

CEREBRAL ANEURYSMS

Intracranial berry aneurysms are thin-walled outpouchings that most often originate at the bifurcation of the large intracranial vessels that reside at the base of the brain. Berry aneurysms have been postulated to be due to congenital deficiencies coupled with degenerative changes in the vessel's wall. Some aneurysms are familial. As the aneurysm enlarges, its internal elastic lamina and muscularis fragment so that the dome of the aneurysm consists only of intimal and flimsy adventitial connective tissue.

Aneurysms usually present with a subarachnoid hemorrhage, but they may on occasion present as an intracranial mass. When presenting as a mass, berry aneurysms most frequently manifest as an optic or oculomotor nerve dysfunction. The median age of patients presenting with a subarachnoid hemorrhage from a berry aneurysm is 50 years. Patients who survive the first hemorrhage from a berry aneurysm are at risk for recurrent bleeding and vasospasm. One in five patients who have ruptured an intracranial aneurysm experience a second bleeding episode in the 2 weeks following the initial hemorrhage. Approximately 50% of patients experience a second hemorrhage within 6 months if the lesion remains untreated.

Cerebral vasospasm is an idiopathic narrowing of the intracranial vessels that occurs within 2 weeks of the subarachnoid hemorrhage. The phenomenon is encountered on the angiograms of approximately 60% of patients. Vasospasm is associated with decreased cerebral blood flow and becomes clinically manifest as cerebral ischemia or stroke in approximately one third of patients.

Therapy

The definitive treatment of an intracranial aneurysm is surgical. Most frequently the base of the aneurysm is ligated with a metal clip, with preservation of continuity of the parent vessel. In the few cases in which this is not possible, techniques have been devised for reducing the pressure within the aneurysm or for reinforcing its thin wall. The effects of vasospasm are prevented by treating the patient with nimodipine, a calcium channel blocking agent. Cerebral ischemia from vasospasm is treated by increasing the patient's intravascular volume and elevating the patient's systemic arterial blood pressure.

ARTERIOVENOUS MALFORMATIONS

Arteriovenous malformations are a collection of abnormal arteries and veins that shunt blood without an intervening capillary network. They may present as an intraparenchymal or sometimes subarachnoid hemorrhage. They also can come to clinical attention by precipitating seizures or headaches. Occasionally, the shunt within the malformation sumps blood from a critical portion of the brain, causing a progressive neurologic deficit. Arteriovenous malformations may bleed at any time during a patient's life, with the peak incidence in individuals between 30 and 39 years of age. The incidence of rehemorrhage from an arteriovenous malformation is much lower than that from an intracranial aneurysm. Treatment consists of surgical resection of the malformation when the lesion lies outside functionally important regions of the brain. Radiation therapy has proved effective in treating smaller, deeply placed lesions. The size of the malformation can be reduced by interventional radiologic techniques, although this is seldom curative.

HYPERTENSIVE HEMORRHAGE

Hypertensive hemorrhage within the parenchyma of the brain presents as a rapid loss of neurologic function. General physical examination reveals findings consistent with long-standing hypertension. The hemorrhage emanates from small, deep perforating arteries that have suffered degenerative changes secondary to long-standing hypertension. These hemorrhages most frequently begin in the putamen or external capsule. Patients with a hemorrhage in this location typically experience a rapidly progressive hemiparesis, hemisensory loss, and hemianopsia contralateral to the hemorrhage. Hypertensive hemorrhages within the cerebellum present with headache, nausea, and vomiting. As the brain stem is compressed by the cerebellar hemorrhage, the patient develops progressive difficulty with lateral gaze, sixth nerve dysfunction, and facial paralysis culminating in a loss of consciousness.

The best treatment for a hypertensive hemorrhage is prevention with medical control of blood pressure. Surgical evacuation of supratentorial hemorrhage is reserved for patients who manifest a deterioration in their level of consciousness. However, evacuation of a cerebellar hemorrhage may be life-saving and is performed on an emergency basis.

V

Craniocerebral Injuries
Allan H. Friedman, M.D.

Accidental injury is the fourth leading cause of death in the United States and the leading cause of death in individuals between the ages of 1 and 44 years. Head injuries are present in more than 50% of trauma-related deaths.

The final neurologic status of the patient who has sustained brain trauma is the sum of the irreversible damage acquired at the time of the initial injury and the damage that follows secondary insults. At the time of the initial head injury, the brain may suffer damage secondary to contusion, laceration, and shearing injuries. A portion of the brain sustains irreversible damage. Other areas of the brain sustain a lesser injury that has the potential to recover. Although several forms of intervention have been proposed for enhancement of the brain's normal repair processes, at this time the physician can do nothing to replace those cells which have suffered a fatal injury or to accelerate the restoration of recovering tissue. The physician's role is the prevention, recognition, and treatment of secondary brain insults.

SECONDARY BRAIN INSULTS

Secondary insults that further injure the already traumatized brain include metabolic abnormalities, expanding intracranial masses, cerebral ischemia, and sustained increased intracranial pressure. Systemic metabolic abnormalities are common after a head injury. The comatose patient is prone to oral airway obstruction and aspiration pneumonia. At the scene of the accident, an oral airway should be placed, and hypoventilation should be treated with positive-pressure ventilation. Concomitant injury to the chest or upper airway may produce hypoxia or hypercapnia, and abdominal or orthopedic injury may lead to hypotension.

Secondary injury may be due to an expanding intracranial mass such as a subdural, an epidural, or rarely, an intraparenchymal hematoma. Focal brain contusion with ensuing edema also can act as a focal mass. An expanding intracranial mass not only raises intracranial pressure but also can cause herniation of the brain through the tentorial notch or the foramen magnum. Transtentorial herniation follows downward movement of the supratentorial contents through the tentorial notch and secondary distortion of the midbrain, ocular motor nerve, and posterior cerebral artery. Clinically, this manifests as one of two syndromes outlined in Table 1. The treatment of a large

---

See the corresponding chapter or part in the *Textbook of Surgery*, 15th edition, pp. 1355–1361, for a more detailed discussion of this topic, including a comprehensive list of references.

TABLE 1. Signs of Transtentorial Herniation

	Level of Consciousness	Respiratory Pattern	Pupillary Size, Response to Light	Oculovestibular Reflex	Motor Response to Pain
Uncal herniation					
Early oculomotor nerve compression	Normal to obtunded	Normal	Unilaterally dilated, fixed	Full, conjugate	Appropriate
Late oculomotor nerve compression	Normal to obtunded	Normal	Unilaterally dilated, fixed	Unilateral third nerve palsy	Appropriate
Midbrain compression	Comatose	Hyperventilation	Bilaterally midposition, fixed	Dysconjugate gaze	Decerebrate posturing
Central herniation					
Early diencephalon compression	Obtunded	Deep sighs, yawns	Small, reactive	Conjugate	Appropriate
Late diencephalon compression	Barely arousable to comatose	Cheyne-Stokes respiration	Small, reactive	Conjugate without nystagmus	Cortical
Midbrain compression	Comatose	Hyperventilation	Midposition, fixed	Dysconjugate	Decerebrate

epidural or subdural hematoma is early recognition and rapid surgical evacuation. Intracranial pressure can be monitored by measuring pressure in the epidural space, subarachnoid space, parenchyma, or intraventricular fluid. Mortality is reduced without a concomitant increase in morbidity by aggressively lowering an increased intracranial pressure.

PATIENT EVALUATION

Following stabilization of the respiratory and cardiovascular systems, attention is turned to the central nervous system. The initial examination is recorded in detail so that it can be compared with subsequent examinations in order to detect a deterioration in the patient's condition. The head is inspected for scalp lacerations, compound skull fractures, or signs of a basilar skull fracture. In the awake patient, a detailed neurologic examination is performed with special attention to abnormalities in the patient's mentation, asymmetries in pupillary size, unilateral weakness, and asymmetries in deep tendon reflexes. In the comatose patient, the neurologic examination is confined to an observation of neurologic reflexes. Special attention is paid to the patient's respiratory pattern, pupillary size and response to light, oculocephalic reflexes, motor response to noxious stimuli, and deep tendon reflexes.

The patient's overall neurologic status is denoted by using the Glasgow Coma Scale (Table 2). This 15-point scale assesses the patient's neurologic responsiveness in three categories (eye opening, verbal response, and best motor response) and has a high concordance among different observers.

MANAGEMENT

Patients who sustained a transient loss of consciousness but are alert and awake upon arrival in the emergency room have

TABLE 2. Glasgow Coma Scale

Eye opening	
Spontaneous	E4
To speech	3
To pain	2
Nil	1
Best motor response	
Obeys	M6
Localizes	5
Withdraws	4
Abnormal flexion	3
Extension response	2
Nil	1
Verbal response	
Oriented	V5
Confused conversation	4
Inappropriate words	3
Incomprehensible sounds	2
Nil	1
Coma Score = E + M + V	

suffered a mild head injury. These patients are given a detailed neurologic examination for detection of early manifestations of an enlarging intracranial hematoma that could cause a delayed neurologic deterioration. Patients with a severe headache, lethargy, or restlessness should be admitted to the hospital for 24 hours of observation. Although these patients are expected to make an uneventful recovery, they frequently have postinjury disability in the form of persistent headaches, unsteadiness, memory deficits, and difficulties with activities of daily living that persist for weeks to months after the accident.

Patients who have sustained a moderate head injury are lethargic, stuporous, or combative when seen in the emergency room. Approximately 10% of patients entering the hospital with a moderate head injury are found to be harboring a focal intracranial lesion. Following assessment and stabilization of their cardiopulmonary systems and neurologic evaluation, these patients should have a brain computed tomographic (CT) scan. If no secondary insults occur, these patients become oriented and alert in the weeks following head injury. A high percentage of patients who have sustained a moderate head injury manifest some permanent alterations in mental acuity.

Patients who have a sustained loss of consciousness and have a Glasgow Coma Scale of less than 8 have sustained a severe head injury. These patients should undergo tracheal intubation for protection of the airway. Because 40% of patients who have sustained a severe head injury harbor an intracranial mass lesion, an immediate brain CT scan should be performed. Patients should be treated in an intensive care setting, with special attention given to changes in neurologic examination, respiratory care, and management of increased intracranial pressure. The potential for recovery is inversely proportional to the patient's age and proportional to the Glasgow Coma score. Poor prognostic factors include abnormal brain stem reflexes, focal intracranial lesions, concomitant abdominal or chest injury, systemic arterial hypotension, and elevated intracranial pressure.

VI

Intracranial Infections
Robert H. Wilkins, M.D.

CRANIAL OSTEOMYELITIS, EPIDURAL ABSCESS, SUBDURAL EMPYEMA

Cranial osteomyelitis is usually caused by adjacent spread from an infected paranasal sinus, by a penetrating wound, or

---

See the corresponding chapter or part in the *Textbook of Surgery*, 15th edition, pp. 1361–1363, for a more detailed discussion of this topic, including a comprehensive list of references.

by an operative infection involving a craniotomy flap. Treatment consists of surgical removal of the infected bone with simultaneous treatment of any coexisting sinusitis. Appropriate systemic antibiotics are administered as well.

An epidural infection is usually a well-confined bacterial abscess associated with one or more of the previously mentioned infections, and it is drained at the same time the coexisting osteomyelitis or sinusitis is treated. A subdural infection, however, is usually a more widespread empyema rather than a localized abscess, since the developing infection easily dissects open the subdural space to cover the surface of an entire cerebral hemisphere. Subdural empyema may begin by the extension of infection through the dura mater from without or through the arachnoid from within, or it may follow the operative infection of a subdural hematoma. In any event, a subdural empyema is usually treated by immediate evacuation through multiple trephine openings or a craniotomy flap in order to avert death or serious neurologic morbidity. Drains are usually left in the subdural space to be removed days later, after all drainage has ceased.

ENCEPHALITIS, CEREBRITIS, BRAIN ABSCESS

The neurosurgeon may be deceived into exploring and resecting an area of severe viral encephalitis, believing it is a malignant glioma. Herpes simplex, for example, may cause a necrotic and cystic mass in the temporal lobe that closely resembles a brain tumor. However, even if the correct diagnosis is suspected preoperatively, biopsy of the lesion may be of value for verification. In addition, resection of such a lesion or some type of decompressive operation also may be necessary if steroids and other medical measures are inadequate to control the severe elevations of intracranial pressure that frequently accompany encephalitis.

The term *cerebritis* is usually reserved for describing the focal area of cerebral inflammation that immediately precedes the development of a brain abscess. Such areas of cerebritis may arise from the following:

1. Extension of an infection through the meninges. In this way, mastoiditis may cause an abscess in the ipsilateral temporal lobe or cerebellar hemisphere, or frontal sinusitis may produce a frontal lobe abscess.

2. Hematogenous spread from some other site, especially from the lungs, pleura, or heart, or from other areas of the body via congenital heart defects that permit the paradoxical embolism of infected material. Brain abscesses that originate in this manner are distributed among the various areas of the brain in proportion to the vascular supply, so a large number occur in the distribution of the middle cerebral arteries.

3. Inoculation through the meninges, as by a compound depressed skull fracture or gunshot wound.

Typically, the patient with a brain abscess uncomplicated by meningitis has no systemic signs of infection, such as fever, tachycardia, or leukocytosis. The abscess presents clinically and by computed tomography (CT) and magnetic resonance imaging (MRI) as an intracranial mass that must be differentiated from a neoplasm, hematoma, or some other type of space-consuming lesion.

Formerly, the preferred treatment of a brain abscess was total surgical excision. Now that such abscesses can be followed closely by CT or MRI, stereotactic aspiration and drainage are frequently employed, at least initially, to reduce the mass effect, provide information about the causative organism(s), and lower the risk of intraventricular rupture while the abscess is treated by the systemic administration of antibiotics. A patient with a brain abscess also may require treatment with a steroid medication for reduction of reactive brain edema. There is a high incidence of seizures among survivors of abscesses of the cerebral hemispheres, which justifies the prophylactic administration of anticonvulsants in most of these patients.

VII

Intraspinal Tumors
Robert H. Wilkins, M.D.

Intraspinal tumors can be divided into three groups according to location: extradural, intradural extramedullary, and intramedullary.

EXTRADURAL NEOPLASMS

Extradural (epidural) tumors are usually malignant. The most common example is a metastasis to a vertebra from a primary carcinoma of the lung, breast, or prostate. Other examples of malignant extradural spinal tumors are lymphoma and myeloma. The most common location for an extradural neoplasm is in the thoracic area of the spine. The typical symptoms relate to the directions of tumor growth. The patient first develops back pain centered where the tumor involves the vertebral bone; then the patient experiences radicular pain and dysfunction (radiculopathy) extending around the trunk at the same level on one or both sides as the tumor involves the exiting spinal nerve roots; and finally, the patient develops a progressive interference with spinal cord function (myelopathy) with eventual paraplegia. If a patient presents with progressive back pain (and especially pain that is not

---

See the corresponding chapter or part in the *Textbook of Surgery*, 15th edition, pp. 1363–1365, for a more detailed discussion of this topic, including a comprehensive list of references.

improved by recumbency), radicular pain, and neurologic loss, the preliminary assessment should include plain roentgenograms, computed tomographic (CT) scanning, or magnetic resonance imaging (MRI) or all three. If such studies do not provide sufficient information, they can be supplemented by other studies such as radionuclide bone scanning and positive contrast myelography accompanied by postmyelographic CT scanning.

There are generally two treatment options, radiation therapy or surgical resection followed by radiation therapy. With either option, steroid administration is often advantageous; it can be given immediately and will reduce the bulk of the tumor (and the degree of neural compression) temporarily while the primary treatment modality is being accomplished. Depending on the nature of the tumor, hormonal therapy or chemotherapy also may be beneficial.

INTRADURAL EXTRAMEDULLARY NEOPLASMS

Tumors occurring in the spinal subarachnoid space are of two types. The first type consists of benign neoplasms that arise from the meninges (meningiomas) or the nerve roots (neurofibromas, schwannomas). The second type consists of malignant tumors that have spread through the spinal subarachnoid space from a primary intracranial location (e.g., medulloblastoma, ependymoma, certain pineal region tumors) or from a malignancy elsewhere in the body (meningeal carcinomatosis).

The treatment of intraspinal meningiomas, neurofibromas, and schwannomas is their surgical excision, which may include excision of the involved portion of the dura mater (meningioma) or the involved nerve rootlets or root (neurofibroma, schwannoma). If the gross total removal of a solitary intraspinal meningioma, neurofibroma, or schwannoma can be achieved, the patient is usually cured.

INTRAMEDULLARY NEOPLASMS

This type of tumor develops within the spinal cord, enlarging it in a fusiform manner. The patient experiences a progressive myelopathy, and the radiographic studies demonstrate evidence of spinal cord expansion. Intramedullary tumors are usually treated surgically through a laminectomy.

If an ependymoma is encountered, it may be possible to excise it completely with maintenance of the surrounding spinal cord; if only a partial resection can be achieved, radiotherapy can be given postoperatively. An intramedullary astrocytoma ordinarily cannot be completely removed surgically; the decision regarding postoperative radiotherapy is based on the exact histologic type of the tumor, the degree of surgical resection, and the age of the patient. The intramedullary hemangioblastoma is a benign tumor that can be cured by surgical excision without the need for radiotherapy. Intraspinal dermoid and epidermoid tumors and lipomas also are benign lesions; they can be found within the subarachnoid space or spinal cord or both. They are most common in the lumbosacral area and may be associated with spinal dysraphism. These various benign tumors can be resected surgically, with the risks and difficulties of such treatment being related to the degree of involvement of the tumor with critical areas of the spinal cord and to the extent of any associated dysraphic changes.

VIII

Ruptured Lumbar Intervertebral Disc
Robert H. Wilkins, M.D.

CLINICOPATHOLOGIC FEATURES. Degenerative changes in an intervertebral disc consist of two main forms: (1) the nucleus pulposus can herniate from its normally confined space (soft disc protrusion), or (2) the entire disc can lose substance, with loss of disc height and the formation of osteophytes that project outward from the adjacent rims of the vertebral body above and the vertebral body below the involved disc (hard disc protrusion).

Soft disc herniation begins with the development of a posterolateral or posterior fissure through the concentric rings of the annulus fibrosus. The nucleus pulposus may then begin to extend into this fissure. The patient at this stage may experience low back pain and perhaps some referred pain into the buttock or hip on the affected side. Further protrusion of the nucleus pulposus may then occur, causing bulging of the outer layers of the annulus and of the posterior longitudinal ligament sufficient to pinch the adjacent nerve root between the protruding disc and the lamina or the intervertebral facet. Finally, a fragment of the disc actually may be extruded completely through the remaining layers of the annulus fibrosus and become wedged anterior to the nerve root; this is referred to as a *free fragment*. When the nerve root is compressed by a protruding or extruded disc, the patient develops radiating pain along the distribution of the sciatic nerve (sciatica) on the involved side in addition to low back pain. The patient also may have neurologic deficits (hypesthesia, weakness, or reduction of the deep tendon reflex) in the distribution of the involved nerve root. This clinical pattern of radiating pain, perhaps with neurologic deficits, is referred to as a *radiculopathy.*

See the corresponding chapter or part in the *Textbook of Surgery*, 15th edition, pp. 1366–1368, for a more detailed discussion of this topic, including a comprehensive list of references.

Approximately 95% of lumbar disc herniations occur at the L5–S1 or L4–L5 level. About 4% occur at the L3–L4 level, and less than 1% occur at the L3–L3 or L1–L2 level.

SYMPTOMS AND SIGNS. The patient's pain is usually aggravated by back movement, by sitting or standing for long periods, by lifting an object from the bent position, and by coughing or straining. It usually is relieved temporarily by bed rest. The patient also may notice tingling paresthesias or numbness in certain aspects of the involved leg and foot, weakness in some muscle groups in that limb (less frequent), or rarely, urinary retention.

On physical examination, the patient may demonstrate one or more mechanical signs: lumbar scoliosis, paravertebral muscle spasm, limitation by pain of low back motion (especially forward flexion), limitation by pain of straight leg raising on one or both sides, or the initiation or intensification of sciatic and back pain by the popliteal compression test. Neurologic deficits, if present, have a typical pattern for each of the commonly involved lumbar discs: (1) L3–L4 disc lesions involve the L4 nerve root with reduced sensation along the anterior thigh and the anteromedial calf and motor loss of the quadriceps femoris with a reduction or loss of the knee jerk; (2) lesions of the L4–L5 disc involve the L5 nerve root with reduced sensation over the anterior calf and medial dorsum of the foot with motor loss of the foot dorsiflexors; and (3) L5–S1 lesions involve the S1 nerve root with sensory loss over the lateral calf, lateral dorsum of the foot, and small toe with motor loss of the plantar flexors of the foot and a reduction or loss of the ankle jerk.

MANAGEMENT. The initial treatment of the acute symptoms of lumbar disc disease consists of bed rest on a firm mattress with medication to combat pain and muscle spasm as needed. Locally applied heat, anti-inflammatory medication, pelvic traction, or the use of a lumbosacral corset may be helpful at times. If these maneuvers provide relief of the acute episode, recurrences may be minimized by a daily maintenance program of low back exercises and the avoidance of certain activities such as lifting heavy objects.

If conservative measures fail to relieve the patient's pain, or if the patient develops significant weakness or urinary retention, a more aggressive approach to treatment should be taken. The patient should have further diagnostic tests such as a magnetic resonance imaging (MRI) examination or a lumbar myelogram combined with a computed tomographic (CT) scan. If all available evidence indicates that a soft or hard lumbar disc protrusion is responsible for the symptoms and signs, it should be treated surgically.

IX

Cervical Disc Lesions
Robert H. Wilkins, M.D.

CLINICOPATHOLOGIC FEATURES. As with a lumbar disc, degenerative changes in a cervical intervertebral disc can assume two main forms: (1) the nucleus pulposus can herniate out of its normal confined space (soft disc protrusion), or (2) the entire disc can lose substance, with loss of disc height and the formation of osteophytes that project outward from the adjacent rims of the vertebral body above and the vertebral body below the involved disc. The second process is often combined with osteoarthritis of the apophyseal joints and the joints of Luschka. The combination of degenerative disc disease and osteophyte formation is called *spondylosis*.

Cervical disc herniations are most frequent at the C6–C7 level but also occur at C5–C6 and to a lesser extent at C4–C5 and other levels. With the usual posterolateral disc rupture, the patient experiences pain in the neck, and then as the nerve root is compressed, the patient develops pain radiating into the ipsilateral upper extremity and also may develop paresthesias, numbness, or weakness in an appropriate distribution. The pain and paresthesias may be intensified by neck movement, especially by extension or by lateral flexion to the side of the herniation, and by coughing or straining. They may be improved by bed rest.

On examination, the patient frequently exhibits restriction of neck movement, especially extension. Patterns of radiculopathy caused by cervical disc herniation or osteophyte formation for specific disc levels include (1) for C4–C5, the nerve root involved is C5 with reduced sensation over the deltoid area and weakness of the deltoid muscle; (2) for C5–C6, the nerve root involved is C6 with reduced sensory function of the thumb and index finger, biceps weakness, and a reduction or loss of the biceps reflex; (3) for C6–C7, the nerve root is C7 with reduced sensation of the index and long fingers, triceps weakness, and a reduction or loss of the triceps reflex; and (4) for C7–T1, the nerve root involved is C8 with reduced sensation in the ring and small fingers and weakness of grip.

If the disc herniation occurs more toward the midline (i.e., is a more direct posterior herniation), it compresses the spinal cord in addition to, or instead of, a nerve root. This produces cervical myelopathy, manifested by lower motor neuron dysfunction (muscle weakness and hypotonia, reduction or loss of appropriate deep tendon reflexes, dermatomal sensory impairment) at the level of the compression and upper motor neuron dysfunction (spasticity, clonus, increased deep tendon

---

See the corresponding chapter or part in the *Textbook of Surgery*, 15th edition, pp. 1369–1371, for a more detailed discussion of this topic, including a comprehensive list of references.

reflexes, Babinski's sign, reduction of sensation) below that level. Loss of voluntary control of bowel, bladder, and sexual function also may develop.

As in the lumbar area, spondylosis may cause compression of one or more cervical nerve roots or of the spinal cord at one or more levels. The resulting symptoms and signs are similar to those caused by disc herniation but tend to be more gradual in onset and more protracted in course.

MANAGEMENT. The initial treatment of the patient with acute radiculopathy consists of bed rest, with medication for pain and muscle spasm. Locally applied heat and cervical traction may provide additional comfort. Anti-inflammatory medication may be of value over a prolonged period for reducing the discomfort of cervical spondylosis.

If these measures do not provide adequate pain relief, or if the patient shows evidence of spinal cord compression, a more aggressive approach should be taken. Although electromyography and magnetic resonance imaging (MRI) may be useful, the best current study for assessing the presence and extent of cervical disc herniation or cervical spondylosis is the cervical myelogram combined with computed tomographic (CT) scanning.

Surgical treatment to provide nerve root decompression can be accomplished by a posterior approach through a hemilaminectomy or by an anterior approach through the intervertebral disc. The surgical treatment of spinal cord compression from spondylosis usually requires a larger operation, and the results are not as good. If the operation is done via a posterior approach, it necessitates a full laminectomy at multiple levels. If an anterior approach is chosen, it involves either a discectomy and osteophytectomy at one or more levels or the resection of the central aspects of one or more vertebral bodies, usually with the insertion of a bone graft to ensure the postoperative maintenance of vertebral alignment and stability.

X

Peripheral Nerve Injuries
Robert H. Wilkins, M.D.

ANATOMY AND PATHOPHYSIOLOGY. For correctly diagnosing and treating peripheral nerve injuries, the surgeon must understand the anatomy and pathophysiology of peripheral nerves. The "wiring diagram" of the human body is complex, in part because peripheral nerves contain varying

See the corresponding chapter or part in the *Textbook of Surgery,* 15th edition, pp. 1372–1373, for a more detailed discussion of this topic, including a comprehensive list of references.

proportions of motor, sensory, and sympathetic axons from diverse sources and in part because of the mixing that occurs not only in the cervical, brachial, lumbar, and sacral nerve plexuses but also within and between peripheral nerves.

In the Sunderland classification, there are five degrees of nerve injury. Seddon used only three terms to classify nerve injuries: *neurapraxia, axonotmesis,* and *neurotmesis.*

With neurapraxia, anatomic continuity is preserved, but there is selective demyelination of large nerve fibers that typically causes complete motor paralysis with little muscle atrophy and considerable sparing of sensory and autonomic function. Electrical conductivity of the nerve distal to the lesion is preserved. Surgical repair is not necessary, and recovery is rapid (within days or weeks). Recovery does not depend on regeneration, and there is no orderly sequence in the recovery of innervation. The quality of recovery is excellent.

With axonotmesis, anatomic continuity of the nerve and the Schwann sheaths is preserved, but the axons are interrupted and must recover by axonal regeneration. There is complete motor, sensory, and autonomic paralysis and progressive muscle atrophy. Surgical repair is not necessary. Recovery occurs at the rate of about 1 mm. per day (1 in. per month); it occurs according to the order of innervation, and the quality of recovery is excellent.

Neurotmesis is a more severe injury. There is significant disorganization within the nerve or actual disruption of its continuity, which precludes recovery without surgical repair. Wallerian degeneration occurs. At 10 to 20 days, fibrillations in the denervated muscles may first be detected by electromyography. From the time of the injury there is complete motor, sensory, and autonomic paralysis and progressive muscle atrophy.

At 10 to 20 days, axonal sprouting begins. If scar tissue blocks axonal entrance into the distal portion of the nerve, these sprouts coil into a disorganized, painful neuroma. In contrast, if the nerve has been repaired, axonal regrowth proceeds at approximately 1 mm. per day. The march of recovery occurs according to the order of innervation, and recovery is always imperfect.

SURGICAL THERAPY. Since surgeons first began to repair injured nerves, there has been controversy about the timing of such repair. For many years, delayed repair was favored; the rare exceptions involved clean lacerations made by sharp objects. With the development of microsurgery and replantation surgery, there has been increased interest in primary nerve repair at the time of injury.

If a clinically nonfunctioning nerve is in continuity when it is explored some weeks after the initial injury, the surgeon may find it helpful to electrically stimulate the nerve proximal to the injury and distally identify evidence of muscle contraction or transmission of nerve action potentials. If there is no evidence of transmission across the area of injury, the injured portion of the nerve should be excised, and the cut ends of the nerve should be sutured together. If there is transmission across the area of injury, surgical treatment should be limited to an external neurolysis.

If the nerve was divided initially in the accident or is divided by the surgeon, it should be reapproximated carefully and without tension after each end has been trimmed back to healthy fascicles. For regaining length so that the nerve can be sutured without tension, the nerve ends can be mobilized and rerouted and the adjacent joints can be flexed. If the ends cannot be brought together with these maneuvers, an interposed graft of an available cutaneous nerve, such as the sural nerve, can be used. Grafts of this type add another suture line that the regenerating axons must cross, and the results are not as favorable as with direct nerve reanastomosis.

XI

Congenital Abnormalities

Herbert E. Fuchs, M.D.

Congenital abnormalities of the central nervous system occur in 1% of live births and account for greater than 72% of fetal deaths prior to birth. Recent advances in diagnostic and therapeutic techniques have greatly improved the prognosis for children with these congenital malformations. The embryologic events responsible for these malformations are currently being elucidated and may in the future lead to improved therapies and even cures.

MYELOMENINGOCELE

Myelomeningocele is the most common defect of neurulation, the process by which the neural plate rolls up to form a tube. The open neural placode is not covered by skin but lies exposed on the dorsal surface of the infant above a cerebrospinal fluid (CSF)–containing sac, surrounded by dysplastic skin. Anomalies associated with the myelomeningocele are hydrocephalus and the Chiari II malformation, a complex anomaly involving hindbrain herniation into the cervical spinal canal. The child's neurologic examination, particularly spontaneous motor activity, will help to define the level of the lesion. Closure of the myelomeningocele should be accomplished within 24 hours of birth, and postoperatively, the child is monitored for the development of hydrocephalus, which is treated with a shunt. With vigilant care, the long-term outlook for these patients is actually quite good, since 90% will survive for 10 years, 62% will have an IQ of 80 or greater, and 85% will achieve social urinary continence with clean intermittent

See the corresponding chapter or part in the *Textbook of Surgery,* 15th edition, pp. 1374–1381, for a more detailed discussion of this topic, including a comprehensive list of references.

catheterization. Relentless neurologic deterioration is not the natural history of children with myelomeningocele, and any deterioration in neurologic function in these children must be investigated promptly and treated.

SPINA BIFIDA OCCULTA

Congenital spinal cord lesions with intact skin are termed *spina bifida occulta* and share a common clinical presentation due to tethering of the spinal cord. Cutaneous manifestations indicating underlying occult dysraphism include hemangioma, dermal sinus, subcutaneous lipoma, or hairy patch. Lesions in this category include lipomyelomeningocele, spinal lipoma, diastematomyelia (split cord malformation), fatty filum terminale/tethered cord, and dermal sinus. Pain, sensory loss, weakness, and bowel and bladder dysfunction are common presenting symptoms and signs of tethered cord. The surgical treatment of all these lesions is centered around release of the tethered cord, with restoration of more normal anatomic relationships of the spinal cord and surrounding structures.

HYDROCEPHALUS

Hydrocephalus is a condition in which there is a discrepancy between the rate of formation and absorption of CSF, causing the cerebral ventricles to dilate. A block in CSF flow results in noncommunicating hydrocephalus. A defect in absorption leads to communicating hydrocephalus. The young infant with hydrocephalus presents with increased head circumference, a full, bulging fontanelle, poor feeding, and vomiting. Cranial sutures may be diastatic, and the "sunsetting sign" of forced downgaze due to midbrain tectal compression may be seen. Older children may present more acutely with severe headache, vomiting, and lethargy. Radiologic imaging is critical for the diagnosis of hydrocephalus and to elucidate the cause. The development of valve-regulated CSF shunts has been the major advance in the treatment of hydrocephalus. The key feature of all shunt systems is that the drainage of CSF from the ventricle to a distant site (most commonly the peritoneal cavity or the right atrium of the heart) is controlled by a valve mechanism to prevent overdrainage of CSF. Complications of shunting include shunt malfunction, infection, abdominal viscus perforation (peritoneal shunts), pulmonary emboli, shunt nephritis, and cardiac arrhythmias (atrial shunts).

CRANIOSYNOSTOSIS

Craniosynostosis, or premature closure of the cranial sutures, may be sporadic or familial. When one or more sutures close prematurely, there is compensatory growth along the remaining open sutures, resulting in recognizable patterns of deformity. Sagittal synostosis is the most common and results in scaphocephaly. Coronal synostosis results in plagiocephaly if unilateral, brachycephaly if bilateral. Metopic synostosis results in trigonocephaly, and cloverleaf deformity (Kleeblatt-schädel) results from multiple-suture synostosis. Ridges along fused sutures may be palpable. Skull x-rays confirm the diagnosis. The therapy of craniosynostosis varies with the involved suture, but in general, early surgery provides the best cosmetic results.

XII

Neurosurgical Relief of Pain
John Gorecki, M.D.

The decision to treat chronic pain by surgical means is a major and sometimes difficult one, quite apart from choosing the appropriate procedure. Pain can be classified broadly into two categories. Patients with nociceptive pain referred to the neurosurgeon often suffer from cancer, although low back pain is probably the most common cause. Neural injury pain nearly always has a constant burning, dysaesthetic, or aching element, and this constant pain usually responds poorly to destructive procedures. Similarly, the surgical intervention for pain is classified into two broad groups: neuroablation and neuroaugmentation, which includes stimulation and delivery of pharmacologic agents to modulate the sensory pathways.

Pain in the head and neck should be considered separately, since the anatomic pathways are distinct, and these syndromes often respond to known therapy more favorably. Trigeminal neuralgia is an idiopathic condition that affects the elderly. The pain is intermittent, limited to the trigeminal distribution, and often is triggered. It responds well to pharmacologic treatment with carbamazepine, but when this fails, surgery is very successful. Pain limited to a single trigeminal branch can be relieved satisfactorily by avulsion or alcohol ablation. Pain in more than one division or recurrences respond in more than 95% of cases to percutaneous retrogasserian rhizotomy accomplished by radiofrequency lesion, glycerol injection, or compression. At least six centers report results from percutaneous, fluoroscopically guided procedures with no mortality in over 1000 cases each. For younger patients or those who wish to avoid sensory loss, microvascular decompression of cranial nerve V at the pons through a posterior fossa craniectomy (at times combined with open partial

---

See the corresponding chapter or part in the *Textbook of Surgery*, 15th edition, pp. 1381–1388, for a more detailed discussion of this topic, including a comprehensive list of references.

rhizotomy) is the procedure of choice, but it carries with it the added risk associated with craniotomy.

Reflex sympathetic dystrophy and causalgia are maintained by afferent conduction in the sympathetics, abnormal efferent activity in the sympathetics, or ephaptic connections between sympathetic and somatic fibers. These conditions, when treated early, respond favorably to systemic sympatholytics or a series of selected sympathetic blocks. When this management fails to establish a cure, surgical sympathectomy is indicated. Early aggressive treatment is justified by the poor results of delayed therapy.

For cancer pain, rhizotomy is an obvious solution for sufficiently localized lesions, and high percutaneous cordotomy is the treatment of choice for appropriately selected patients. There is limited experience with midline commissural myelotomy, and cordotomy can be performed bilaterally. Stereotactic mesencephalic tractotomy is the treatment of choice for pain extending above the C5 dermatome. Medial thalamotomy carries a lower risk and treats diffuse pain, but the beneficial effect is not always sustained. VCpc thalamotomy is promising for nociceptive pain, but experience is limited. Dorsomedial thalamic and anterior thalamic nucleus lesions as well as cingulumotomy reduce the complaint of suffering but do not affect the detection of a noxious stimulus. The success of the neuroaugmentation technique of chronic intraspinal narcotic analgesia has reduced the number of ablative procedures being performed. Intraspinal morphine acts directly on opioid receptors in the substantia gelatinosa to produce potent analgesia. Future experience should allow the introduction of other pharmacologic agents that act on the many sensory-modulating pathways located in the central nervous system.

Chronic low back pain is the most common syndrome referred for treatment. It consists of a variety of interrelated pain syndromes often complicated by psychogenic magnification, litigation, or compensation. Rare cases respond to facet rhizotomy or selective dorsal rhizotomy. If root deafferentation is prominent, dorsal column stimulation can be valuable. Of the more central procedures, chronic PVG stimulation would appear appropriate.

Neural injury pain in general has a 50% chance of amelioration by chronic stimulation. Destructive surgery in neural injury pain should be restricted largely to patients in whom stimulation has failed, particularly patients with prominent intermittent pain, allodynia, or hyperpathia. Stimulation occurs at the peripheral nerve, dorsal column, sensory thalamus, or periaqueductal gray. Periaqueductal gray stimulation is believed to exert its effect via the endogenous opioid system, is naloxone reversible, and also should affect nociceptive pain. When not relieved by stimulation, neuralgic pain may respond to medial thalamotomy or more focal destructive procedures for specific allodynia or hyperpathia. Dorsomedial thalamotomy, or cingulumotomy, with or without midbrain tractotomy, may reduce the associated depressive symptoms or suffering. Spinal cord injury is a common cause of neural injury pain and deserves special comment, since DREZ (dorsal root end zone) lesioning is often effective, particularly for end-zone pain. DREZ is most effective for the pain of brachial plexus avulsion, and also helps postherpetic neuralgia and phantom pain.

Chronic intrathecal narcotic infusion reduces nociceptive pain in nonmalignant disease, and it should relieve intermittent or evoked neural injury pain. However, its use for this indication is controversial, and long-term results remain to be proven.

XIII

Neurosurgical Relief of Epilepsy
Allan H. Friedman, M.D.

Epilepsy surgery is a prime example of laboratory research and clinical observation advancing clinical practice. Hughlings Jackson's clinical pathologic correlations laid the foundations for the localization of clinical function within the cerebral cortex and focal cortical resections for the treatment of epilepsy. The introduction of electroencephalography (EEG) by Jasper and Penfield allowed for the tracking down of the electrical origin of seizures. Advances in neuroimaging such as magnetic resonance imaging (MRI) demonstrate epileptic structural lesions that had not been visible to the surgeon.

CLASSIFICATION

The International League Against Epilepsy has developed the most widely used system to classify epileptic seizures for the purposes of the epilepsy surgeon (Table 1). The most important distinction is between partial seizures, which appear to begin with the activation of a limited portion of cerebral cortex, and generalized seizures, in which there is an early activation of neurons throughout both hemispheres. A complex seizure is one in which consciousness is lost, and in a simple seizure, consciousness is retained. Partial complex seizures, in which the patient first manifests focal seizure activity followed by a loss of consciousness, are the seizure types most commonly treated by focal resection of abnormal cerebral cortex.

PATIENT SELECTION FOR SURGERY

Surgical therapy for epilepsy is contemplated only when the patient's seizures are not adequately controlled by nontoxic

See the corresponding chapter or part in the *Textbook of Surgery,* 15th edition, pp. 1388–1392, for a more detailed discussion of this topic, including a comprehensive list of references.

TABLE 1. Classification of Seizures

I. Partial (focal, local) seizures
  A. Simple partial seizures (consciousness not impaired)
    1. With motor signs (focal motor, etc.)
    2. With somatosensory or special sensory symptoms (visual, auditory, etc.)
    3. With autonomic symptoms (pallor, sweating, etc.)
    4. With psychic symptoms (*déjà vu*, fear, anger, etc.)
  B. Complex partial seizures (impairment of consciousness)
    1. Simple partial onset followed by impairment of consciousness
    2. Impairment of consciousness at onset
  C. Partial seizures evolving to secondary generalized seizures (tonic-clonic, clonic or tonic)
II. Generalized seizures (may be convulsive, with motor movements, or nonconvulsive, without motor movements)
  A. Absence (sudden interruption of activity with blank stare)
  B. Myoclonic seizures (myoclonic jerks)
  C. Clonic seizures
  D. Tonic seizures
  E. Tonic-clonic seizures
  F. Atonic seizures (sudden loss of motor tone)

amounts of anticonvulsant medications, when the seizures limit the patient's activities, and when resection of the epileptogenic cortex will not produce a severe neurologic deficit. Most epilepsy surgical therapy is aimed at resection of the epileptogenic area of cerebral cortex responsible for initiating all the patient's seizures. The epileptogenic cortex is localized by the concordance of clinical manifestations of the seizures, abnormalities demonstrated by cerebral imaging studies, and epileptic electrical activity demonstrated by EEG. In the rare patient, the physical examination demonstrates a focal neurologic deficit or slight asymmetry in extremity size indicative of an abnormality in the contralateral cerebral hemisphere. The most pertinent clinical information comes from analyzing the physical manifestations of the patient's seizures. The initial symptoms of the seizures and the auras occurring prior to the loss of consciousness may reveal the site responsible for initiating the seizures. A wealth of brain imaging techniques including x-ray, computed tomography (CT), MRI, positron-emission tomography (PET), and single-photon-emission computed tomography (SPECT) help ferret out intracerebral abnormalities that potentially could be responsible for initiating the patient's seizures. MRI scans often can detect mesial temporal sclerosis, the most common pathology found in temporal lobe seizures. These scans can detect low-grade gliomas, areas of cortical dysgenesis, and epileptogenic lesions not detectable by older imaging modalities. PET and SPECT scans can demonstrate potentially epileptogenic areas of brain that have abnormal metabolism or receptor densities.

Empirically, EEG disturbances should be the hallmark of seizures. Unfortunately, EEG recordings collected by electrodes placed on the scalp are distorted by the intervening skull and scalp, and these electrodes do not record electrical activity from the medial and inferior surfaces of the brain. If the clinical data point to a locus of seizure inset that is not corroborated by scalp EEG recordings, electrodes may be placed in the brain or directly on a cortical surface. The risks and considerable costs of this invasive EEG monitoring limit its use to cases in which the patient's work-up strongly points to a specific seizure origin.

TEMPORAL LOBECTOMY

The most commonly performed surgical procedure for the treatment of intractable epilepsy is temporal lobe resection. The origin of the patient's seizures is localized to the temporal lobe by concordant clinical, imaging, and EEG data. Approximately 65% of selected patients become seizure-free following the operation, and an additional 25% significantly improve. Severe neurologic deficits are a complication of surgical intervention in approximately 2% of patients.

EXTRATEMPORAL CORTICAL RESECTIONS

The origin of seizures arising outside the temporal lobe is notoriously difficult to localize because of the rapid spread of electrical activity through the white matter pathways that interconnect areas of cerebral cortex. Clues to the seizure's origin can be garnered from observing the onset of the patient's clinical seizures. Cavernous angiomas, low-grade gliomas, cortical dysplasia, and cortical cicatrix, all of which can be imaged by MRI, are classic progenitors of epilepsy. Extratemporal cortical resections cause relief of seizures in 45% of patients and a reduction in seizure frequency in an additional 35% of patients.

HEMISPHERECTOMY

Hemispherectomy is performed to treat hemiplegic patients suffering from intractable seizures emanating from a single extensively damaged cerebral hemisphere. The disconnection frees the normal hemisphere from seizures emanating from the dysfunctioning hemisphere, allowing the normal hemisphere to function optimally. About 70% of selected patients undergoing a hemispherectomy are freed of generalized seizures, and an additional 20% are significantly improved.

CORPUS CALLOSUM SECTION

Sectioning the corpus callosum has been proposed as a method to stop the spread of the seizure when the initiating focus or foci cannot be resected directly. It has proven to be most effective in treating patients suffering from atonic seizures clinically manifested as a sudden drop attack.

XIV

Stereotactic Neurosurgery
Dennis A. Turner, M.D., M.A.

The goal of stereotactic procedures is to provide accurate navigation to a point or region in space. Stereotactic methods provide guidance techniques to access deep structures within the brain without the necessity of direct visualization. Initial stereotactic procedures were performed by defining radiographic landmarks close to the region of interest, such as the third ventricle for thalamic procedures. Further developments have included frame-based image-guided neurosurgical procedures for biopsy and treatment of lesions [using primarily computed tomography (CT) or magnetic resonance imaging (MRI)] and the advent of frameless stereotaxis, which provides accurate localization based on various forms of three-dimensional digitization of the skull and brain. Presently, there are two general indications for stereotactic procedures: (1) approaches to structural lesions (such as tumors and vascular malformations) and (2) treatment of functional abnormalities (such as movement disorders and pain conditions).

The concept of structural neurosurgery implies that a discrete abnormality can be detected on an imaging study, such as a tumor, vascular lesion, or abscess. This structural lesion can be approached for stereotactic biopsy using a stereotactic frame for guidance. The stereotactic frames developed for this purpose require a further set of images to orient the lesion with respect to the coordinates of the frame, following fixation of the frame directly to the skull, usually with sharp points. Thus the frame is applied; a repeat imaging study is performed to align the brain, lesion, and stereotactic frame; and then a biopsy is performed using an arc system attached to the frame. The arc holds constant both the twist drill to penetrate the skull and the biopsy needle. Sequential biopsies of structural lesions are checked with frozen section to enhance the likelihood of a positive diagnosis on permanent sections.

Additional treatment options are possible using a stereotactic frame. Radiobrachytherapy involves multiple catheters that are placed into the brain for local radioactive treatment of a malignancy to inhibit local recurrences. The Gamma knife involves the delivery of multiple point sources of radiation using a stereotactic head frame. The radiation is delivered to a region in a single fraction (1200 to 2400 rad.) for treatment of lesions (primarily AVMs and tumors) smaller than 25 to 30 mm. This single, focused radiation dose also may be delivered

---

See the corresponding chapter or part in the *Textbook of Surgery,* 15th edition, pp. 1393–1397, for a more detailed discussion of this topic, including a comprehensive list of references.

using a Linac radiotherapy machine, but giving continuous arcs rather than multiple, discrete delivery ports.

The stereotactic frame translates coordinates obtained from an imaging study into operating room coordinates with respect to the frame. Frameless stereotaxis relies on the rendering of scans (such as CT and MRI) into a three-dimensional image. The rendered view of the patient can then be aligned with the actual patient using a three-dimensional digitizer, performed by either a mechanical device (such as a robotic arm) or a line-of-sight device (such as a video camera or sound waves). The line-of-sight devices require a clear, unobstructed path from the digitizing device to the patient. The mechanical arms also may reach into the patient, around corners, and through sterile drapes but are limited in terms of flexibility. The digitizing device can be used as a simultaneous pointer both to brain structures and to the rendered image on the graphics workstation screen. Unfortunately, brain warping may occur following opening of the skull, CSF leakage, and partial tumor excision, affecting the accuracy of the device.

The concept of functional neurosurgery is to change the function of pathways in the brain by altering an intact aspect of the circuit. The target is usually anatomically defined and requires precise localization by brain atlases in coordination with the patient's own anatomy. For example, lesions in the globus pallidus may affect the overall function of the basal ganglia, thus improving the rigidity associated with Parkinson's syndrome. Other functional targets include the performance of lesions in the thalamus and midbrain to affect movement disorders and pain, placement of depth electrodes for localization of epileptic foci, stereotactic radiotherapy through the skull to lesion sites in the thalamus, and various anatomic methods of performing certain aspects of a frontal lobotomy. Lesioning methods have included radiofrequency heat lesions, mechanical lesions (with a small wire loop), freeze lesions (cryolesions using liquid N_2), balloon lesions to percuss the surrounding brain on inflation, and chemical lesions. The radiofrequency lesion can be graded the easiest, using direct temperature control of the electrode tip, and temporary lesions also can be produced prior to causing permanent damage to the area of the brain.

Other forms of stereotactic treatment include augmentative methods, such as cell or tissue transplants, which can in effect replace lost cells, as in Parkinson's disease or Huntington's disease. Gene transfer techniques involve transfection of host cells (either glia or neurons) with novel genes to produce either a missing enzyme or modify cells to create sensitivity to treating agents. These methods are highly novel and require further investigation to delineate their specific role in treatment of a number of CNS disorders.

42

FRACTURES AND DISLOCATIONS

I

General Principles

Michael E. Berend, M.D., John M. Harrelson, M.D., and John A. Feagin, M.D.

The treatment of fractures and dislocations requires a knowledge of anatomy, physiology, and biomechanics of the musculoskeletal system.

CLASSIFICATION OF FRACTURES

Sufficient force applied to a bone causes fracture. Fractures can be classified based on fracture pattern into *simple* and *comminuted* and status of the skin into *open* and *closed fractures*. The treatment and prognosis of open fractures are significantly different from those of closed fractures. Pathologic fractures occur through diseased bone caused by osteoporosis, metastatic carcinoma, and bone-wasting diseases.

FRACTURES IN CHILDREN

Fractures in children deserve special consideration. Fractures may occur through the physeal plates and cause future growth disturbance. The parents accordingly should be cautioned.

INITIAL EVALUATION

The initial evaluation of the fracture patient requires a careful history and physical examination. The examination should determine the motor function, sensory deficit, vascular status, and firmness of the associated fascial compartments. Radiographs of the fractured bone in at least two perpendicular planes should be performed. The films should visualize the entire fractured bone with its associated proximal and distal articulations.

FRACTURE REDUCTION

The goal of reduction is restoration of length of the extremity, correction of angulation and rotation, and apposition of

---

See the corresponding chapter or part in the *Textbook of Surgery*, 15th edition, pp. 1398–1401, for a more detailed discussion of this topic, including a comprehensive list of references.

the bone ends. The reduction of a fracture may be accomplished by *manipulative reduction, skeletal traction,* and/or *open reduction.*

IMMOBILIZATION

Immobilization may be accomplished in a number of ways. It is necessary to immobilize the joint above and below the fracture site. Plaster casts, splints, and traction may help immobilize fractures. Surgical options of internal fixation with plates and screws, intramedullary devices, and external fixators such as the Ilizarov device may be required in some fractures.

ACUTE COMPLICATIONS

Significantly increased *compartment pressure* due to bleeding may follow fractures and may cause muscular ischemia. The surgeon must be aware of these syndromes and be prepared to do a decompressive fasciotomy. *Adjacent organ injury* may occur with certain fractures.

OPEN FRACTURES

An open fracture should be treated as an emergency. Surgical débridement of the wound is required. Intravenous antibiotics should be administered, along with tetanus toxoid when appropriate. Cast immobilization with a window overlying the wound, delayed internal fixation, or external fixation may be appropriate initial stabilization methods in the care of open fractures. When extensive skin loss has occurred, split-thickness skin grafts or pedicled or free-flap grafting may be required.

FRACTURE HEALING

Osteogenic cells from the fracture hematoma and surrounding granulation tissue and their subsequent primitive bone formation constitute the *fracture callus.* As the bone matures, constant remodeling occurs, and trabeculae become oriented in the long axis of the bone.

LATE COMPLICATIONS

Complications following fractures include *loss of motion, nonunion/malunion,* and *traumatic arthritis.* These outcomes may require subsequent surgical intervention.

II

Fractures of the Spine

William T. Hardaker, Jr., M.D., and
William J. Richardson, M.D.

Trauma may subject the vertebral column to one or a combination of violent forces, including flexion, extension, axial compression, rotation, and shearing. If these forces produce motion greater than the physiologic range of the spine, a fracture or dislocation will occur.

The anatomic relationship for the vertebral supporting structures, the neural elements, and the types of forces producing the injury will determine the amount of displacement, stability, and neurologic involvement within a given spinal injury. Spine fractures are considered *stable* if the fragments are unlikely to move when the spine is physiologically loaded. Conversely, if movement and neural damage are likely, the injured spine is labeled *unstable*. The instability may be acute or chronic depending on whether the displacement is immediately threatening or if progressive deformity is likely to occur during the extended healing process.

A complete neurologic evaluation is essential in all individuals with suspected spine injuries. The intercostal and abdominal muscles should be examined as well as motor, sensory, and reflex testing of the extremities. The anal sphincter tone and bulbocavernosus reflexes must be included in the evaluation. Complete loss of motor and sensory function, including perianal sensation, during the first 24 hours after injury indicates complete cord injury. The bulbocavernosus reflex usually recovers within the first 24 hours. Recovery of this reflex and the presence of complete anesthesia and paralysis are compelling evidence that the patient will not recover functional motor power of the lower extremity muscle groups innervated below the level of fracture.

Anteroposterior and lateral roentgenographic views demonstrate most fractures involving the vertebral bodies. Computed tomography (CT) and magnetic resonance imaging (MRI) greatly improve the ability to evaluate thoroughly fractures and dislocations in the spinal canal.

THE CERVICAL SPINE

Fracture of the Atlas (Jefferson's Fracture)

This injury occurs from an axial load on the top of the head. The resultant forces are exerted laterally on the ring of C1,

---

See the corresponding chapter or part in the *Textbook of Surgery*, 15th edition, pp. 1401–1407, for a more detailed discussion of this topic, including a comprehensive list of references.

and the arches fracture at their thinnest and weakest points. Usually the spinal cord is not damaged, because the canal of the atlas is normally large, and with fracture, the fragments spread outward to further increase the dimensions of the neural canal. CT represents the best available roentgenographic study to evaluate the injury. When considerable instability is present, the halo vest is the preferred method of treatment.

Fractures of the Odontoid

Odontoid fractures often result from falls, blows to the head, and automobile accidents. If the injured patient complains of neck or occipital pain or headaches or has torticollis, the odontoid area should be examined thoroughly. Lateral views centered on the C2 vertebra and open-mouth views of the odontoid usually allow adequate visualization of the dens. However, CT scans may be necessary to demonstrate the fracture.

Anderson and D'Alonzo have described three basic types of fractures based on the anatomic level of the injury. Type I fractures are oblique and occur at the extreme upper level of the odontoid process. A hard cervical orthosis provides satisfactory stability of this fracture. Type II fractures occur through the junction of the odontoid process and the C2 vertebral body. Union will occur in most cases of Type II injuries with prompt diagnosis, satisfactory reduction, and rigid external fixation using the halo vest. Operative arthrodesis using autogenous iliac bone graft and wiring of C1–2 through a posterior approach are indicated if union is not achieved. Type III fractures extend through the cancellous bone of the C2 vertebral body. These injuries are rarely unstable and unite following 3 months of immobilization in an occipital-mandibular brace or halo vest.

Fractures of the Pedicles of the Atlas (Hangman's Fracture)

A fracture through the pedicles of C2 usually occurs from a severe extension injury such as an automobile accident or fall. Nonunion is uncommon in this fracture. If the injury is stable with little or no displacement, the four-poster brace is usually satisfactory treatment. In unstable circumstances, more rigid stabilization using the halo vest may be required.

Fractures and Dislocations of the C3 to C7 Vertebrae

Fractures and dislocations of the lower cervical spine are common. Dislocations of the cervical spine occur most commonly at the interspaces between C3 and C7. The injury is caused by a flexion-distraction force. These forces combine to dislocate the facet joints with concomitant fracture of the disc bond and varying degrees of failure of the longitudinal cervical ligaments. Dislocations of the cervical spine are managed by prompt realignment by means of serial traction under direct x-ray control and with concomitant serial neurologic examinations. If closed reduction cannot be achieved, operative reduction under direct vision followed by wire fixation and fusion using autogenous bone graft should be performed.

THE THORACOLUMBAR SPINE

Fractures or dislocations of the lumbar area require considerably more displacement to injure the neural elements than do fractures in the cervical or thoracic spine. A bursting fracture in the cervical or thoracic region may result in devastating neurologic loss, whereas a similar fracture in the lumbar area may produce no permanent neurologic deficit.

Flexion Injuries

Pure flexion injuries are the most common thoracolumbar fracture. These injuries usually involve only the anterior column and, therefore, are acutely stable. Neurologic loss is uncommon. If the compression is mild, a three-point brace will be satisfactory. When wedging is greater than 50% of the anterior body height, a modified polypropylene jacket may be necessary to prevent progressive angulation.

Axial Compression Injuries

Burst fractures result from axial compression of the spine frequently associated with varying degrees of flexion. These injuries, which occur most commonly at the thoracolumbar junction, are characterized by circumferential expansion of the entire involved vertebra with failure of the anterior, middle, and in some cases, posterior spinal columns. Middle-column failure in burst fractures results in retropulsion of the posterosuperior portion of the vertebral body into the spinal canal, compressing the dural tube, often with associated neurologic deficit.

Mild burst fractures with minimal anterior body deformation, minimal retropulsion of fragments into the spinal canal, no posterior element involvement, and minimal kyphotic angulation can be treated satisfactorily with a molded polypropylene body jacket. If there is incomplete neurologic involvement with bone fragments impinging on the neural elements, surgical management may be indicated. The goal of operation is to provide an optimal environment for potential spinal cord recovery. Fundamental to this goal are (1) decompression of the spinal canal to remove impinging bone and disc fragments, (2) restoration of the normal alignment of the spine at the thoracolumbar junction, (3) immediate stabilization of the fracture site with restoration of the normal vertebral body height, and (4) long-term stabilization by means of spinal arthrodesis using autogenous iliac bone graft.

Anterior exposure of the vertebral body for decompression

is gained by a transthoracic, transabdominal, or transpedicular approach. Spinal implants provide acute realignment and stabilization. Realignment of the spinal canal and restoration of the height will not always effectively decompress the spinal canal. The procedure should therefore be combined with definitive removal of bone fragments under direct observation.

Fracture-Dislocations

Fracture-dislocations usually involve translation of one spinal motion segment or a portion of one spinal segment in relationship to the remaining spine. A variety of failure modes including shear, compression, tension, and rotation can occur within the individual columns and produce characteristic radiographic fracture patterns. In the lumbar region, these injuries are usually grossly unstable, and great care must be exercised in handling patients with such injuries. Operative reduction and internal fixation are the most reliable means of creating a stable environment for potential maximum neurologic return.

Flexion-Distraction Injuries

Flexion-distraction forces classically occur in seatbelt injuries in which the individual is subjected to sudden deceleration and the torso is flexed forward over the restraining belt. Tension failure occurs in the posterior and middle columns. The failure mode of the anterior column depends on the location of the fulcrum of rotation. These injuries may be associated with marked displacement and usually are very unstable. Open reduction with realignment and internal fixation is usually required to regain stability.

III

Fractures and Dislocations of the Shoulder, Arm, and Forearm

Robert D. Fitch, M.D., and Kevin P. Speer, M.D.

TRAUMATIC ANTERIOR DISLOCATION OF THE SHOULDER

The shoulder demonstrates remarkable range of motion owing to the anatomic peculiarities of this unconstrained joint.

See the corresponding chapter or part in the *Textbook of Surgery*, 15th edition, pp. 1408–1415, for a more detailed discussion of this topic, including a comprehensive list of references.

However, these features also render it susceptible to dislocation. There is little contact between the shallow glenoid and the humeral head, and the capsular and ligament stability must be augmented by the surrounding rotator cuff musculature.

Following traumatic dislocation of the shoulder, the arm is held at the side. The acromion process is prominent, and the normal fullness of the shoulder is replaced by a concave contour just below the acromion. Evaluation must include complete neurologic and vascular examination because of the proximity of the brachial plexus and axillary artery to the site of injury. Anteroposterior and lateral views confirm the presence of dislocation and any associated fractures.

Treatment consists of prompt reduction of the dislocation. The longer the shoulder remains unreduced, the more muscle spasm there is to overcome. Reduction is accomplished by longitudinal traction on the arm, with countertraction applied in the axilla. An alternative method is the Stimson technique. The patient is placed prone with the arm allowed to drop off the table. Progressive weight is added to the extremity until a gradual gentle reduction is obtained. Following reduction, neurovascular status to the extremity is again reassessed. The arm is then immobilized in a sling held in internal rotation for approximately 3 weeks. Protected range-of-motion exercises are then begun, but excessive abduction and external rotation should be avoided for 3 months. Recurrence is a common complication in patients under 40 years of age.

FRACTURES OF THE PROXIMAL HUMERUS

Fractures of the proximal humerus occur more frequently with advancing age, and loss of normal trabecular bone with aging makes this area susceptible to injury. Minor trauma can cause fractures in the elderly; otherwise, fractures require considerable force. The major segments that can be involved include the anatomic neck, greater tuberosity, lesser tuberosity, and surgical neck. The fractures are described as nondisplaced or two-, three-, or four-part fractures depending on how many segments are involved and displaced. Most fractures occur as a result of a fall on the outstretched arm, which causes forced abduction, extension, and external rotation.

Clinically, some degree of ecchymosis and swelling about the shoulder should be present. The vascular supply to the limb must be assessed and a thorough neurologic examination performed for excluding associated arterial or nerve injury. Anteroposterior and lateral radiographs identify the extent of the injury and guide treatment.

Most proximal humeral fractures are minimally displaced, and treatment consists of temporary immobilization in a sling and swathe or commercially available shoulder immobilizer for 2 to 3 weeks followed by range-of-motion exercises. The prognosis for these fractures is quite good. Two-part fractures generally can be treated by closed reduction and immobilization. If significant displacement of the shaft or greater tuberosity persists following closed reduction, open reduction may be required. Three-part fractures generally require open reduction and internal fixation. In four-part fractures, prosthetic replacement of the humeral head has provided postoperative results superior to open reduction and internal fixation of all fracture fragments.

FRACTURES OF THE SHAFT OF THE HUMERUS

Humeral shaft fractures are caused by either direct trauma or a fall on the outstretched arm. Direct blow or bending movements usually cause a transverse fracture, whereas indirect torsional forces cause spiral fractures. The radial nerve is susceptible to injury because of its proximity to the bone at the junction of the middle and distal thirds of the shaft of the humerus. Clinical examination should include evaluation of the radial nerve function. Pain and swelling at the fracture site and crepitance are usually easily detectable. Radiographs identify the fracture location, pattern, and amount of commination.

Nondisplaced fractures can usually be treated by simple immobilization of the arm to the chest with a sling and swathe followed by early active range-of-motion exercises in 2 to 3 weeks. Displaced fractures are managed by a coaptation splint or a hanging-arm cast. Occasionally, open reduction and internal fixation are indicated if there is an associated vascular injury or if the radial nerve function is lost during manipulation of the fracture fragments. A radial nerve injury that occurs before any manipulation does not require surgical exploration, since most of these injuries are a result of stretching or contusion; function will return within several weeks. In the occasional case of nonunion, open reduction with internal fixation and bone grafting is indicated.

FRACTURES OF THE DISTAL HUMERUS AND ELBOW

Supracondylar and Intercondylar Fractures

Supracondylar fractures of the humerus represent 50% to 60% of all fractures about the elbow. There are two types: *flexion* and *extension*. The most common extension injury occurs as a result of a fall on the outstretched arm, which produces a compression and hyperextension force applied indirectly to the distal humerus. Clinically, pain and swelling are present. Neurovascular status must be carefully assessed because arterial or neurologic injury can occur by laceration and direct or indirect compression. Evaluation of the radiographs reveals the degree of displacement and amount of comminution. Subtle changes such as rotary malalignment and varus impaction must be identified.

In children, undisplaced fractures are treated by immobilization of the arm with the elbow flexed to 90 degrees. The period of immobilization is approximately 3 weeks. A varus impacted fracture may appear at first as a nondisplaced fracture, but if it is not recognized, a cubitus varus deformity will occur. Baumann's angle is a useful measurement for determining if varus position is present. If the fracture is significantly displaced, a reduction under anesthesia is warranted. If the fracture is unstable with the elbow flexed to 90 degrees, percutaneous pinning is recommended.

In the severely swollen, displaced supracondylar fracture without neurovascular compromise, preliminary sidearm traction or overhead traction may be useful. This can be provided by Dunlop skin traction or by olecranon pin traction. Attempts at obtaining and maintaining reduction while in traction are worthwhile. If the fracture cannot be aligned with traction after the swelling has subsided, a closed reduction with or without percutaneous pinning under general anesthesia is indicated.

Occasionally fractures cannot be reduced by traction or closed reduction because of soft tissue interposition. These fractures require open reduction and pinning. Similarly, in the case of neurologic deficit or vascular insufficiency, open reduction is required with exploration of the involved structures.

Supracondylar fractures in adults are often comminuted and have intra-articular extension; they are best managed by open reduction and internal fixation for allowing early range-of-motion exercises of the elbow.

The most serious complication is Volkmann's ischemia with subsequent contracture. Varus, valgus, and rotary malunion will not remodel and will persist. The most common malunion seen is that of cubitus varus (gunstock deformity), which may require corrective supracondylar valgus osteotomy.

Dislocations of the Elbow

Posterior dislocation by falling on an outstretched arm causes dislocation of the radius and ulna. Neurovascular structures are rarely affected, although arterial injury occurs occasionally. Anterior dislocations are caused by a blow on the flexed elbow. Dislocation of the radial head can occur as an isolated injury anteriorly or posteriorly. Dislocation of the ulna alone occurs rarely. Associated fractures of the coronoid process, medial epicondyle, or radial head can occur. Clinically, elbow motion is limited. There is deformity, and the neurovascular structures are usually intact. Median nerve injury occasionally occurs.

Gentle pull on the olecranon followed by flexion usually relocates the dislocation. After reduction, the elbow should be extended through a reasonable range of motion for testing stability. If the elbow is stable, temporary immobilization for comfort is recommended. Early range-of-motion exercises are instituted for avoidance of permanent stiffness. In simple dislocations, a functional range of motion usually results. Myositis ossificans, however, can produce mild or severe limitation of motion in a small percentage of patients.

FRACTURES OF THE SHAFT OF THE RADIUS AND ULNA

The two bones of the forearm, the radius and ulna, share an intricate relationship that allows pronation and supination. As the radius rotates around the ulna, a smooth articulation at the proximal radial-ulnar joint is required. The interosseous membrane serves as a hinge during forearm rotation, and the distal radial-ulnar articulation is stabilized by the triangular fibrocartilage complex. Distortion by fracture or dislocation alters the biomechanics of the forearm and therefore limits forearm rotation. One or both bones of the forearm may be fractured. The fracture of the proximal third of the ulna associated with a radial head dislocation is termed a *Monteggia fracture*. A fracture of the distal third of the radius in conjunction with dislocation of the distal ulna is termed a *Galeazzi* or *Piedmont fracture*.

Clinically, pain and deformity of the forearm are present. Evaluation of the neurovascular condition of the extremity must be made as well as of the presence or absence of increased pressure within the muscle compartments of the forearm. Swelling within the tight muscle compartments of the forearm can cause occlusion of venous and arterial circulation with resultant Volkmann's ischemic contracture. Significant swelling of the forearm compartments associated with pain on passive extension of the fingers should alert one to this possibility. Radiographs should include both the elbow and wrist joints for identifying the location of the fractures and any associated dislocations. In adults, displaced fractures of the shaft of the radius and ulna, the Monteggia or Piedmont fractures, should be treated by open reduction and internal fixation with plates and screws. Conversely, most forearm fractures in children can be managed by closed means. The thick periosteum allows stable reduction, and the osteogenic potential in children allows excellent remodeling of angular deformities.

The most serious complication of forearm fractures, neurovascular compromise and subsequent ischemic contracture, must be avoided. Nonunion of forearm shaft fractures occurs in 5% to 10% of cases in which closed treatment is used. Malunion is a frequent complication when open reduction with internal fixation is not utilized. Other complications include elbow stiffness, finger stiffness, and reflex sympathetic dystrophy.

IV

Fracture of the Carpal Scaphoid

Richard D. Goldner, M.D., and J. Leonard Goldner, M.D.

The initial physical examination consists of digital palpation, sensory assessment, and vascular patency. The response to digital pressure is the most important clue to the existence and location of a carpal injury. Tenderness to pressure in the anatomic snuffbox is present with a fracture.

If a scaphoid fracture is suspected, the radiographic examination should include anteroposterior, lateral, and supination and pronation oblique views. A projection in ulnar deviation and pronation (posteroanterior, palm down) may demonstrate an undisplaced fracture. The lateral view shows the linear relationship between the distal radius, lunate, and capitate.

If the films are negative at the initial injury but clinical findings suggest a fracture, the radiographs should be repeated 10 to 14 days after injury. Routine studies are done at that time, and if a fracture is not noted but suspected, then special techniques should be performed, including (1) magnification radiographs, (2) anteroposterior and lateral tomograms or direct sagittal and transverse computed tomographic (CT) scans, (3) stress radiographs in ulnar deviation, (4) fluoroscopic examination, and (5) technetium-99m bone scan.

TREATMENT. If a scaphoid fracture is suspected by the history and clinical examination but is not demonstrated on radiographs, a cast is applied with the hand in radial deviation and 10 degrees of flexion for immobilization of the thumb, including the proximal phalanx and the forearm. This cast is removed 10 to 14 days later, and the films are repeated. About 30% of the middle-third fractures and most proximal-third fractures develop aseptic necrosis of the proximal fragment because of the blood flow pattern. The distal location with limitation of major blood supply is the etiologic factor of nonunion and aseptic necrosis of the proximal fragment. The blood vessels passing from distal to proximal are interrupted when the fracture occurs.

The average healing time of a scaphoid fracture depends on the location and obliquity of the fracture line. Fractures of the distal third (10%) usually heal in about 8 weeks. For the middle third (70%), the healing time is generally 8 to 12 weeks or longer. Fractures of the proximal third (20%) heal more slowly (healing time 10 to 20 weeks). Most of the fractures of the proximal fifth of the scaphoid develop aseptic necrosis. Nondisplaced, stable fractures of the scaphoid are treated adequately by external immobilization in a cast. The cast may be a well-molded short-arm one that includes the thumb

---

See the corresponding chapter or part in the *Textbook of Surgery,* 15th edition, pp. 1415–1419, for a more detailed discussion of this topic, including a comprehensive list of references.

proximal phalanx and is changed every 10 to 14 days for the first 6 weeks, or it may be a long-arm cast that includes the thumb.

DIFFERENTIAL DIAGNOSIS OF CARPAL SCAPHOID FRACTURES. *Rotatory subluxation of the scaphoid* or scapholunate dissociation occurs after a tear of the complex ligaments between the radius, scaphoid, and lunate. The condition is not readily diagnosed unless suspected. Films showing the spread between the scaphoid and lunate are suggestive of this pathologic lesion.

Rupture of the flexor carpi radialis tendon may occur from a fall on the outstretched hand and can be in combination with ligamentous injury. This injury also may be spontaneous in older individuals.

Traumatic arthrosis occurs from cartilaginous damage during the original injury, incongruity of cartilage surfaces secondary to malposition or malunion, hypermobility from nonunion, or ligament injury.

In the management of nonunion, grafting of iliac crest bone to bridge both proximal and distal segments of the scaphoid on the palmar surface has been 90% successful. The Herbert screw has improved fixation of the fragments, diminishes the length of time of external immobilization, and may increase the union rate.

V

Fractures and Dislocations of the Hand

Richard D. Goldner, M.D., and J. Leonard Goldner, M.D.

Hands are exposed to many forces that may cause bone or joint trauma. Fractures of the metacarpals and phalanges are estimated at 10% of all fractures; of these, fractures of the distal phalanx are the most common, followed in order by fractures of the metacarpals, the proximal phalanges, and then the middle phalanges.

TERMINOLOGY

Terminology providing description of alignment is as follows. *Dislocation* means that the articular surfaces are not apposed or congruous. *Subluxation* means a partial displacement of one side of the joint on the other, but with less severe

---

See the corresponding chapter or part in the *Textbook of Surgery*, 15th edition, pp. 1419–1432, for a more detailed discussion of this topic, including a comprehensive list of references.

distortion than in a dislocation. The term *reduction* refers to the action required for obtaining anatomic alignment.

Fractures are described as stable, unstable, displaced, non-displaced, impacted, comminuted, intra-articular, extra-articular, transverse, oblique, or spiral. Angulation may occur in any direction: dorsal, volar, radial, ulnar, and combinations. Malrotation also may occur. If there is no wound, the fracture is referred to as *closed*, and if the skin is broken, the fracture is referred to as *open*.

RADIOGRAPHIC EXAMINATION

Films determine the exact location of the fracture: articular surface, epiphysis, neck, metaphysis, shaft, or base of the digit. They indicate the type of fracture: complete, incomplete, transverse, oblique, spiral, or comminuted; and they indicate the position of the fractured bones, the amount of displacement of one segment relative to the other, and the angulation of the segments compared with a straight line and with the apex of angulation either dorsal or volar. Correct rotation of the digit may be assessed radiographically by the relationship of the proximal to distal fractured segment but is best determined clinically by comparison with adjacent digits.

Multiple views of the involved hand or digit are essential for an accurate diagnosis. The usual views are posteroanterior, pronation and supination oblique, and true lateral. True lateral exposures must be obtained of the individual digits rather than of the entire hand, since in the latter case the digits are overlapping. A 10-degree supination film for the ulnar side of the hand and a 10-degree pronation film for the radial side of the hand provide additional information.

ANATOMIC REGIONS OF FRACTURES

Distal Phalanx and Distal Interphalangeal (DIP) Joint

DISTAL PHALANX FRACTURE. The fracture is splinted for 10 to 14 days to decrease discomfort and allow healing. The fingernail may be elevated by a hematoma trapped between the nail plate and nail bed, which is very painful. The hematoma is released by making a hole in the center of the nail plate with the round end of an open paper clip that has been heated in a flame or by a disposable ophthalmic cautery. If the nail bed has been lacerated, it should be removed and the laceration repaired with fine, absorbable sutures.

DORSAL AVULSION FRACTURE. A dorsal segment of bone is elevated when the extensor digitorum communis is avulsed. After extensor tendon continuity is lost at the distal joint, a "drop finger" or "mallet finger" occurs. If the fragment is small (less than 40%, displaced less than 2 mm.), slight hyperextension with a dorsal aluminum splint on the distal and middle phalanges produces sufficient apposition to allow healing. The splint is used for a total of 8 to 12 weeks. Similar treatment but longer protective splinting is used for the mallet finger of tendon origin in which no fracture or avulsion is noted.

AVULSION OF A FRAGMENT FROM THE FLEXOR SURFACE. This occurs when the flexor digitorum profundus is forcibly pulled from its distal phalangeal insertion, such as when the digit is hyperextended as a result of a forcible blow or fall or from catching the digit (usually the ring finger) in a football jersey. Physical findings are swelling, the patient's inability to flex the distal joint, and a palpable palmar mass at the base of the finger or in the palm. Radiographs may show the bone fragment in the digit. Operative treatment is required for reattaching the flexor tendon to the point of avulsion.

Middle Phalanx and Proximal Interphalangeal (PIP) Joint

The extrinsic muscles such as the extensor digitorum communis, flexor digitorum profundus, and flexor digitorum superficialis all affect the position of the fragments after phalangeal fractures. Active muscle contraction of the lumbricals and the interossei influences the position of the fragments and the deformity of the digit. Fractures through the distal portion (*neck*) of the middle phalanx are likely to have apex palmar angulation, because the proximal fragment is flexed by the superficialis tendon. A fracture through the proximal portion (*base*) of the middle phalanx is likely to have apex dorsal angulation caused by flexion of the distal fragment by the superficialis and extension of the proximal fragment by the central slip of the extensor. Fractures through the *middle* two-thirds may be angulated in either direction or not at all. Rotary deformities and radial and ulnar deviation also may depend on the intrinsic tendon pull as well as the force of the original injury.

Stable fractures of the middle phalanx can be immobilized initially in a splint followed by adjacent taping of the digit ("buddy" taping). Fractures that are stable after closed reduction are immobilized for approximately 3 weeks. Although the fracture may be protected for 6 to 8 weeks, gentle motion should be initiated at 3 to 4 weeks. Displaced, unstable fractures of the middle phalanx that cannot be reduced or maintained by external immobilization require fixation either by percutaneous pins or by open reduction, and the middle phalanx that cannot be reduced or maintained by external immobilization requires fixation either by percutaneous pins or by open reduction and internal fixation. Spiral and long oblique fractures are well suited for internal lag screw fixation.

A *chip fracture* at the PIP joint indicates either a collateral ligament tear or marginal capsular avulsion. This radiographic finding may be a subtle suggestion of more extensive instability, but as long as the phalanx can be placed in anatomic alignment, in the position that decreases tension and stress on the collateral ligaments, adequate healing usually occurs. Large, displaced avulsion fractures with collateral ligament attached are repaired surgically.

A nondisplaced *condylar fracture* should be splinted for 2 to 3 weeks. These fractures are followed frequently because displacement may occur after motion has been initiated. Displaced condylar fractures often cannot be reduced adequately and held by closed methods. Open reduction corrects incongruity of the articular surfaces that if uncorrected would cause traumatic arthrosis.

DORSAL DISLOCATION OF THE PIP JOINT. Dislocations of the PIP joint are classified by the location of the middle phalanx in relation to the proximal phalanx (palmar, dorsal, lateral).

Dorsal dislocation of the middle phalanx with avulsion of the volar plate from the middle phalanx is a common injury. The PIP joint is swollen and may be mistaken for a "sprained finger." The lateral radiograph demonstrates displacement and often a small volar fragment from the proximal end of the middle phalanx. After reduction, a splint is applied with the PIP joint flexed 20 to 30 degrees for 2 to 3 weeks. If the joint is completely stable, taping the involved digit to the adjacent one provides assistive motion and protects the joint.

DORSAL FRACTURE-DISLOCATION OF THE PIP JOINT. Dorsal dislocation of the middle phalanx with displaced fracture of its volar portion is a serious injury. Fractures of greater than 40% of the articular surface are usually unstable. If the fracture is reduced and is stable, it can be treated by a splint that blocks extension but allows flexion. If reduction is not maintained, and if the alignment of the joint cannot be re-established, an operative procedure is indicated.

PALMAR DISLOCATION OF THE PIP JOINT. Palmar dislocation of the middle phalanx may disrupt the central slip and dorsal capsule (palmar plate and one collateral ligament). This may produce a flexion deformity of the PIP joint and hyperextension of the distal interphalangeal joint (boutonnière deformity).

Proximal Phalanx

Fractures of the proximal phalanx are divided into oblique and transverse types.

TRANSVERSE FRACTURE OF THE PROXIMAL PHALANX. A fracture through the midportion of the proximal phalanx with volar angulation presses the long flexor tendons and causes a flexion deformity at the PIP joint. Internal fixation, by percutaneous pins or after open reduction, is required if the alignment cannot be maintained by plaster splint.

OBLIQUE FRACTURE OF THE PROXIMAL PHALANX. For treatment of the oblique fracture, the distal fragment is derotated and the joints on either side of the phalanx are flexed. The wrist is held in dorsiflexion, the metacarpophalangeal joints are flexed about 70 degrees, and the proximal and distal interphalangeal joints are flexed slightly. This portion of metacarpophalangeal flexion and interphalangeal extension is termed the *intrinsic-plus* portion.

INTERCONDYLAR FRACTURE OF THE PROXIMAL PHALANX. A condylar split fracture involving the distal end of the proximal phalanx is an intra-articular fracture. Collateral ligaments are attached to each of the condyles. If the condyles are malrotated and displaced greater than 2 mm., if adequate position cannot be obtained by manipulation, or if the reduction cannot be maintained, percutaneous pinning or open reduction and internal fixation of the condyles are performed.

METACARPOPHALANGEAL JOINT DISLOCATION. Metacarpophalangeal joint dislocation is due to a hyperextension force. The index is dislocated most frequently. If the palmar plate is avulsed from its origin and is trapped between the metacarpal head and the proximal phalanx, reduction is not possible by closed methods. Open reduction can be accomplished through either a palmar or dorsal approach.

THE METACARPALS

Metacarpal fractures are divided into (1) fractures of the metacarpal *head*, with intra-articular involvement and dorsal or palmar angulation of the fragments, (2) fractures of the metacarpal *neck*, with dorsal or palmar angulation and with a rotary element, (3) *transverse* fractures through the shaft of the metacarpal, (4) *oblique* fractures through the shaft of the metacarpal, and (5) *dislocation* at the base of the metacarpals. Metacarpal fractures that are nondisplaced are treated, closed, and immobilized for 3 weeks, followed by taping to the adjacent digit. Displaced fractures of the metacarpal head may require open reduction and internal fixation with small screws or wires. Severely comminuted fractures limited to the metacarpal head distal to the collateral ligament should be treated with early protective motion. Large articular fragments with collateral ligament avulsion may require open reduction and internal fixation.

A *fracture of the neck of the fifth metacarpal* is a common injury caused by a direct blow and is known as a "boxer's fracture" and occurs from a dorsal force applied directly to the metacarpal head. Films show the angulation on the oblique and lateral views. Up to 40 to 45 degrees of dorsal angulation is acceptable in the fifth metacarpal, approximately 30 degrees in the fourth metacarpal; in the index and long metacarpals, angulation greater than 15 degrees is unacceptable secondary to the lack of compensatory carpometacarpal motion. Rotation alignment should be restored in all fingers.

TRANSVERSE AND SHORT OBLIQUE METACARPAL SHAFT FRACTURES. *Transverse shaft fractures* are often caused by a direct blow with dorsal angulation secondary to exertion of palmar force by the interosseus muscles. The intermetacarpal ligaments prevent shortening, and the interossei stabilize the digits. If the fracture is minimally displaced, it can be controlled with a well-molded short-arm cast for 4 to 6 weeks with the metacarpophalangeal joints flexed 60 degrees.

Indications for internal fixation include any persistent rotational deformity, uncorrected dorsal angulation greater than 10 degrees in the second or third metacarpal, or uncorrected dorsal angulation greater than 20 degrees in the fourth or fifth metacarpals. Shortening more than 3 mm. or multiple displaced fractures usually require treatment. Internal fixation of long, oblique, or spiral fractures with interfragmentary screw fixation controls excessive shortening and angulation and allows early motion of the digits.

Long, oblique, or spiral metacarpal fractures, minimally displaced, are treated by splinting. Displaced fractures that are not able to be reduced adequately or that are unstable after reduction are best treated by lag screw fixation.

THUMB METACARPAL FRACTURES. Fractures at the base of the thumb are classified as follows: (1) *intra-articular fracture* through the proximal end of the metacarpal, leaving a fragment held by the intermetacarpal ligament, and the base of the metacarpal displaced laterally out of the joint by pull of the abductor pollicis longus (Bennett's fracture); simultaneously, the adductor pollicis pulls the proximal phalanx and distal metacarpal toward the palm and the proximal metacarpal away from its base; (2) a *comminuted intra-articular fracture* of the proximal end of the metacarpal (Rolando's fracture); (3) *fracture through the metaphysis,* extra-articular, with angulation dorsal or volar. Other variations may occur.

Treatment of the displaced thumb fracture depends on the type of injury. The *intra-articular fracture* with two segments (Bennett's) is managed by closed reduction and pinning.

The *comminuted fracture* at the base of the metacarpal (Rolando's) may be treated by either percutaneous pin fixation or traction obtained by placing a transfixation pin through the base of the proximal phalanx or neck of the metacarpal.

The fracture at the proximal metaphysis of the thumb metacarpal, which does not include the joint, is managed by manipulation, realignment, and plaster fixation, with the thumb in wide abduction and the metacarpophalangeal joint in flexion.

Injuries to the *metacarpophalangeal joint of the thumb* include chip fractures of the ulnar collateral ligament, the fragment being avulsed from the proximal phalanx or from the distal metacarpal. The ligament also can rupture in its central portion or pull from bone without a fracture. In addition to the collateral ligament injury, the palmar plate and the dorsal capsule are usually torn, causing the phalanx to displace palmarward and radially. In most instances, these injuries are detected by clinical examination (carpometacarpal flexion, metacarpophalangeal flexion with stress). The stress radiograph is not essential, but if there is any question about the extent of soft tissue injury, the stress radiograph under local or regional block is helpful.

If there is less than 30 degrees difference between the injured and uninjured thumb, incomplete tear is diagnosed. Treatment of an incomplete tear can be managed satisfactorily by application of a plaster or fiberglass cast that holds the phalanx in the neutral adducted position and realigns the metacarpal and the phalanx. If there is greater than 30 degrees difference, complete tear is diagnosed, and operative repair is usually indicated.

Displaced intra-articular fractures involving more than 15% to

20% of the articular surface and a small avulsion fracture displaced more than 5 mm. are relative indications for open reduction.

VI

Fractures of the Pelvis, Femur, and Knee

Thomas Parker Vail, M.D., and
Donald E. McCollum, M.D.

FRACTURES OF THE PELVIS

Because of the life-threatening nature of disruption to the pelvic ring, the mainstay of therapy is stabilization in the acute setting. This can include such maneuvers as placing the patient on his or her side to close an open book–type injury, application of MAST trousers, or application of external fixation to close an open pelvis and decrease the intrapelvic volume. These maneuvers are performed in an effort to stabilize the clot within the pelvis into a discrete and contained area and stop potentially life-threatening bleeding and should follow a standard algorithm for resuscitation of a severely traumatized patient. Retroperitoneal bleeding may mimic gastrointestinal trauma, and diagnostic peritoneal lavage is extremely helpful in distinguishing between them. Careful examination of the rectum and vagina may reveal blood—presumptive evidence of an open fracture of the pelvis via perforation of one of those structures.

The most common complication of the displaced pelvic fracture is massive hemorrhage. Bleeding may occur from laceration of the hypogastric or gluteal vessels from fractures extending into the sciatic notch. While a patient can appear stable initially, shock can rapidly ensue, as evidenced by changes in vital signs, urinary output, and central venous pressure. The patient must be massively transfused for correction of shock and maintenance of urinary output. Application of an external fixator on an emergent basis can decrease the pelvic volume by a factor of four and contribute to cessation of intrapelvic hemorrhage. If bleeding cannot be controlled, arteriography may be helpful to identify the source of the bleeding and allow embolization. In very rare circumstances, packing of the pelvis through a laparotomy can be helpful. Attempts at open ligation of vessels are extremely hazardous.

See the corresponding chapter or part in the *Textbook of Surgery*, 15th edition, pp. 1432–1444, for a more detailed discussion of this topic, including a comprehensive list of references.

Other injuries include those involving the intra-abdominal organs, neurologic structures, the lungs, and vascular structures. Internal injuries to the uterus, vagina, rectum, or abdominal viscera can create an open injury, which might require repair or intestinal bypass. In addition, intra-abdominal injury can be the source of bleeding. Diagnostic peritoneal lavage is therefore a helpful adjunct in evaluating intra-abdominal injury and remains a standard part of evaluation.

Displaced fractures through the roof of the acetabulum that fall within a 45-degree arc from a line drawn vertically through the center of rotation of the femoral head are generally treated by open reduction and internal fixation. Once the patient's condition allows, computed tomographic (CT) evaluation with three-dimensional reconstruction is helpful in recognizing all components of the fracture. The fracture may involve the posterior wall, the anterior wall, the posterior column, the anterior column, or any combination of these four elements of the acetabulum. The goal in treating fractures of the acetabulum is to achieve as near anatomic reduction as possible in order to prevent posttraumatic arthrosis.

FRACTURES OF THE HIP

Hip fractures are an extremely common problem in the elderly. According to Armstrong, fractures of the hips will affect one in four women by the age of 90 years and one in eight men. The rate of fractures of the hip in the United States appears to be highest in white women and least in black men. Review of mortality rates in Medicare patients sustaining hip fractures reveals that the lowest rates occur in white women, followed by black women, black men, and white men. Loss of bone density appears to be a risk factor for fracture of the proximal femur. In addition to the normal, steady 1% to 2% loss of bone density after age 35 to 40 years in both sexes, there is accelerated loss after menopause in women as well as in patients who smoke, use alcohol, and are steroid-dependent.

Fractures of the subcapital portion of the femur and the femoral neck generally have been classified by the Garden classification scheme. In this classification scheme, a Garden I fracture is an impacted valgus fracture, a Garden II fracture is a nondisplaced fracture, a Garden III is displaced less than 50% of the width of the neck, and a Garden IV is displaced greater than 50% of the width of the neck. Displacement increases the likelihood of disruption of the blood supply to the femoral head. The decision to treat an impacted valgus fracture with protected mobilization must be accompanied by close follow-up and frequent radiographs to rule out any internal displacement of the femoral head. An unstable or potentially unstable fracture of the subcapital region of the femur is best treated with application of internal fixation.

Treatment of displaced subcapital fractures and fractures of the neck of the femur is much more difficult to manage. Nonunion and avascular necrosis are much more frequent. These fractures should be treated as emergencies, with reduction being performed as quickly as possible with rigid internal fixation. One recent study has suggested that reduction within 6 hours can lead to a lower incidence of avascular necrosis. When moderate displacement is present, reduction can be accomplished by general abduction and internal rotation. In younger patients, if anatomic reduction cannot be obtained by manipulation, the capsule should be opened anteriorly and the fragments reduced under direct vision. In general, efforts at achieving an anatomic reduction with expeditious internal fixation are chosen for younger patients. For elderly patients or patients with pre-existing arthritic conditions, osteoporosis, or medical infirmity, arthroplasty may be preferred.

Intertrochanteric fractures occur below the inferior attachment of the hip capsule, outside the vascular ring supplying the femoral neck and head. Blood supply in this area is excellent, so avascular necrosis rarely develops. If adequate stability can be obtained, union in a functional position generally occurs. Thus the classification of intertrochanteric fractures is based on stability rather than blood supply.

FRACTURES OF THE FEMUR

Fractures of the femoral shaft have been classified by Winquist into five basic patterns. The type of fracture has direct relevance to surgical treatment, with the larger butterfly fragments and the comminuted fracture types requiring locked intramedullary nailing. Because fractures of the shaft of the femur can be associated with systemic complications such as respiratory distress syndrome, fat embolism, pulmonary embolism, and pneumonia, early stabilization and rapid mobilization of the patient have been recommended. The decision to perform either reamed or unreamed nailing will depend on the size of the patient, the pattern of the fracture, and whether the fracture is open or closed.

Displaced supracondylar fractures of the femur are best treated by open reduction, internal fixation, and early mobilization. Supracondylar fractures can extend into the knee joint. Displaced intra-articular fractures demand anatomic reduction. With an intra-articular fracture, reduction and early mobilization are imperative to avoid the complication of deformity and stiffness. Fixation is generally achieved through the use of lag-screw fixation in the case of condylar fragments. The supracondylar portion of the fracture can be treated with a supracondylar compression screw and side plate, a blade-plate configuration, or a buttress plate.

DISLOCATION OF THE KNEE

Most knee dislocations are easily reducible, sometimes spontaneously reducing prior to presentation in the emergency room. Unrecognized vascular injury can lead to ischemia and loss of the leg. Hyperextension of the knee or anterior displacement of the tibia may either completely tear the popliteal artery or produce intimal damage leading to thrombosis. Peripheral pulses must be assessed carefully on first examination and followed closely. If pulses are diminished, or if there is any question about the continuity of vessels, immediate exploration should be performed. Arteriography is time-consuming and unnecessary in a patient with a knee dislocation and an abnormal vascular examination after reduction. If a patient has a normal vascular examination after reduction, the surgeon in charge may elect to perform arteriography or careful and closely spaced repeated vascular examinations to rule out secondary thrombosis and ischemia from intimal damage. Delays in treatment while obtaining imaging studies in a patient with a documented knee dislocation and an abnormal vascular examination can negatively affect the salvage rate and success in obtaining adequate revascularization.

VII

Fractures of the Tibia, Fibula, Ankle, and Foot

L. Scott Levin, M.D., and
William G. Garrett, Jr., M.D., Ph.D.

FRACTURES OF THE TIBIA AND FIBULA

The tibia and fibula are two of the most frequently fractured long bones. High-speed motor vehicle accidents are responsible for a high proportion of these injuries. Open or compound fractures require treatment for the bone as well as soft tissue injury. The majority of the tibia is palpable along the medial lower leg as a subcutaneous structure. It bears the major portion of body weight. The lateral malleolus or distal fibula is also palpable through the subcutaneous tissue. The tibia and fibula are connected by a strong ligament, the interosseous ligament, which serves as an origin for muscles in the anterior and posterior compartment of the leg. The mechanism of injury is important in determining the prognosis of tibial fractures. The prognosis is directly related to the amount of energy absorption at the time of injury. Fractures of the fibula usually occur concomitantly with fractures of the tibia unless the fibula is struck by a direct blow. If the head of the fibula is fractured with an associated medial malleolus fracture, a Maisonneuve fracture results. Classification of tibial fractures is dependent on fracture location. Schatzker has classified the tibial plateau or tibial head fracture into six different types, Type VI being the most severe.

See the corresponding chapter or part in the *Textbook of Surgery*, 15th edition, pp. 1444–1452, for a more detailed discussion of this topic, including a comprehensive list of references.

The decision to treat tibial plateau fractures is based on the amount of articular surface depression (usually greater than 5 mm.) and the degree of joint incongruity or comminution. Fractures of the tibial shaft are classified into proximal, middle, and distal thirds. Delays in healing are seen commonly in the middle third. Open fractures have been classified by Gustilo and Anderson: Type I fractures have perforation of the skin, usually within wounds less than or equal to 1 cm.; Type II open fractures have lacerations of the soft tissue greater than 1 cm.; Type III injuries are divided into three subclasses depending on whether there is periosteal stripping (Type IIIb) or vascular injury (Type IIIc). The most important aspect of the physical examination for tibial fractures is to ascertain whether there is an impending compartment syndrome. Pain on passive stretch of muscle compartments in the alert patient is suggestive of compartment syndrome. In the unconscious patient with a closed tibial fracture, compartment pressure of greater than 30 mm. Hg for prolonged periods is an indication for fasciotomy. A number of radiographic techniques can be used for evaluation of tibial fractures. Tomography is helpful in the tibial plateau fracture.

Treatment is based on the fracture pattern and the presence of soft tissue injury. Cast immobilization can be used for closed diaphyseal fractures that can be maintained in adequate alignment. When soft tissue injuries accompany the tibial fracture, the external fixator is the standard method used for stabilizing the bone while soft tissues heal. Closed fractures that are amenable to intramedullary nailing can be treated with reamed or unreamed nails; locking the intramedullary device above and below the fracture creates more stability, which allows earlier weight-bearing. When there is a soft tissue defect of the tibia, the proximal third usually can be covered by a gastrocnemius rotational flap, the middle third by a soleus flap; the distal third usually requires free tissue transfer for healing of the soft tissue envelope. Complications of tibial fractures include delayed union, malunion, and nonunion. Methods such as electrical stimulation and bone grafting of various types have been used to achieve union. Despite major advances in bone and soft tissue care, there are patients whose wounds are so severe that primary amputation is still the treatment of choice. For Type III injuries, indications for this include comminution of bone greater than 20 cm., disruption of posterior tibial nerve, and ischemia greater than 6 hours.

FRACTURES AND DISLOCATIONS
OF THE ANKLE

Ankle injuries are among the most frequently treated conditions. Most ankle injuries involve external rotation of the foot in the ankle joint. The goal in treatment of ankle fractures is establishing and maintaining anatomic reduction. If this cannot be done by closed reduction and casting, then open reduction and internal fixation are performed. This is usually done with screws and plates.

FRACTURES OF THE FOOT

Fractures of the hindfoot are significant injuries in which functional disability often occurs. The talus has a delicate blood supply that may cause the bone to become avascular after injury. Fractures of the calcaneus are best defined by use of computed tomography. Open reduction and internal fixation of these fractures are difficult, and despite anatomic restoration, many patients develop hindfoot posttraumatic arthritis. Fractures of the midfoot include the Lisfranc fracture, which is a tarsometatarsal dislocation. This can be accompanied by severe soft tissue damage that may cause ischemia of the forefoot. Metatarsal fractures are usually treated with closed reduction and casting and usually do not produce any long-term ill effects. Stress fractures or fatigue fractures, which are not uncommon, should be suspected in anyone who presents with pain and puffiness in the foot following excessive activity. Fractures of the phalanges do not usually require reduction and can be treated by strapping the fractured toe to the adjacent toe or by the use of a cast shoe.

VIII

Amputations and Limb Substitutions

Sean P. Scully, M.D., Ph.D., and John M. Harrelson, M.D.

Amputations are commonly the result of congenital deformities, infection, trauma, or neoplasm. Current estimates suggest that between 20,000 and 30,000 amputations are performed in this country every year. Chronologically, the highest incidence of lower-extremity amputations is in the 50- to 75-year-old populations and is related to vascular disease and diabetes. This number is expected to increase as the population ages and the incidence of vascular disease and diabetic complications increase. Traumatic amputations and those involving the upper extremities tend to occur in a younger population. The combined etiologies produce approximately 350,000 to 1 million amputees to be cared for by the medical community.

SELECTION OF LEVEL

The determination of level of amputation should be based on physiologic, clinical, and anatomic considerations, with the

See the corresponding chapter or part in the *Textbook of Surgery,* 15th edition, pp. 1452–1458, for a more detailed discussion of this topic, including a comprehensive list of references.

aid of supporting laboratory data. Amputations for congenital deformities and neoplasm are determined by the existing anatomy, and prosthetic considerations have little, if any, role. In cases of infection and trauma, clinical judgment of what is viable tissue is of primary importance in determining the level of resection. In patients with dysvascular extremities and diabetes, clinical judgment can be augmented with noninvasive Doppler perfusion studies and transcutaneous oxygen tension.

SURGICAL PRINCIPLES

Basic principles of surgical procedures, especially with regard to soft tissue handling, are important in amputations because of the compromise of the local tissue by either ischemia, infection, or trauma. The tissue compromise is balanced by the desire to preserve length consistent with good surgical judgment. Attention to detail and gentle handling of tissue are important to creating a well-healed and functional stump.

SKIN, MUSCLES, NERVES, VESSELS, AND BONE

Soft tissue is frequently compromised, and to preserve existing tissue, skin flaps should be kept as thick as possible, avoiding unnecessary dissection between anatomic planes. In addition, myocutaneous flaps should be fashioned when possible, thereby preserving the deep circulation to the skin. The skin at the end of the residual limb should be mobile and sensate. Scar location has become less important with the development of total-contact sockets, but a scar adherent to underlying bone may break down over time. Stabilization of myotendinous structures by myodesis and myoplasty can improve residual limb function. Proponents believe that such treatment improves residual function, decreases the incidence of painful bursa formation, and perhaps decreases subsequent phantom pain. The transection of a nerve always causes the formation of a neuroma; however, neuromas placed in soft tissues and away from areas of pressure irritation are usually not problematic. Surgical technique to diminish clinically symptomatic neuromas includes a clean transection under tension, allowing the nerve to retract into the soft tissues away from the scar and prosthetic pressure points. Blood vessels should be isolated, clamped, transected, and ligated in a systematic fashion. Before the amputation wound is closed, the tourniquet should be deflated and hemostasis meticulously obtained with suture clips or electrocautery. Bone prominences such as in the distal anterior tibia during a below-knee amputation should be beveled and smoothed with a rasp. The bone prominences should be well padded with soft tissue when possible. Periosteum should be sectioned at the level of the bone.

POSTOPERATIVE MANAGEMENT

Immediately following amputation, the surgeon's efforts should be focused on establishing the optimal physical and metabolic circumstances for wound healing. Postoperative patients, in particular the elderly diabetic/dysvascular amputee, require great attention to detail to lower postoperative morbidity and mortality. Wounds can be managed by soft dressings, semirigid dressings, rigid dressings, and controlled environment gas systems (CET). There is no longer a perceived need to delay prosthetic fitting for residual limb maturation, and functional rehabilitation should proceed as soon as feasible. Temporary prosthetic fitting and limited weight bearing are begun early, but timing is based on individual patient factors. Young patients can be fitted immediately with a temporary prosthesis and begin weight bearing within the first few days following operation. In older patients with dysvascular extremities, early weight bearing can further compromise ischemic tissues, leading to wound separation. In these patients, weight bearing is delayed to accommodate slower wound healing.

COMPLICATIONS

Patients treated with amputation are at increased risk for postoperative complications because of many factors, including bone marrow suppression, radiation of soft tissue, ischemia of tissue in diabetic and dysvascular patients, and soft tissue compromise and wound contamination in trauma victims; these predispose patients to delayed wound healing and infection. Joint contracture tends to occur following operation but prior to prosthetic fitting. Long, rigid dressings, early prosthetic fitting, and stretching can prevent most contractures. Phantom sensation occurs in nearly all amputees and tends to decrease over time. It occurs in less than 10% of acquired amputations, and its incidence is decreased by perioperative epidural and intraneural anesthesia.

PROSTHETIC CONSIDERATIONS

Prosthetic use in patients who have sustained an amputation depends on a combination of proper prescription, manufacture, fitting, and training. Prescription entails identification of expected level of function, a means of weight bearing, suspension, and mechanical control. Manufacture and fitting are in the realm of prosthetists, and subsequent training involves skilled and experienced physical therapists. Together this group of professionals helps the surgeon in attaining the highest possible function for the amputee.

SUMMARY

In summary, amputation operations need to be viewed in a positive light, as a reconstructive procedure rather than as an objectionable chore that should be performed as rapidly as possible. Preoperative evaluation and planning should be as rigorous as they are for limb-salvage surgery and given fore-thought for rehabilitation. The surgical procedure should employ meticulous handling of usually compromised soft tissues. Postoperative rehabilitation should begin as soon as tissue healing permits and should involve a multidisciplinary group, including the surgeon, the prosthetist, the physical therapist, a vocational rehabilitation counselor, and not infrequently a clinical psychologist. Patients' efforts play a large role in rehabilitation, and patients should be given every opportunity to regain as optimal a functional level as possible following amputation.

IX

Infections and Neoplasms of Bone
Sean P. Scully, M.D., Ph.D., and John M. Harrelson, M.D.

Infection of bone (osteomyelitis) and many bone neoplasms share clinical and radiographic features, and both entities are discussed together. In any destructive lesion of bone one should be prepared to obtain cultures as well as histologic material for proper diagnosis.

PYOGENIC OSTEOMYELITIS

Suppurative infection of bone occurs either by hematogenous spread from a soft tissue focus or by introduction to the skeleton through penetrating wounds (trauma, surgery). Bloodborne infection (hematogenous osteomyelitis) is seen most commonly in childhood. *Staphylococcus aureus* is the most common offending organism. Hematogenous infection has a predilection for the metaphyseal ends of long bones, with the distal femur, proximal tibia, and proximal humerus being the most frequent sites in descending order. The physeal growth plate forms a barrier to the spread of infection into the adjacent joint, with the exception of the hip joint, where the physeal plate lies within the hip capsule.

The clinical symptoms of hematogenous osteomyelitis are fever, pain, swelling, and erythema. Loss of joint motion and inability to bear weight may be present. Laboratory findings include an elevated white blood cell count and elevated erythrocyte sedimentation rate and may include mild anemia. X-rays may be negative within the first 10 days of infection,

See the corresponding chapter or part in the *Textbook of Surgery*, 15th edition, pp. 1458–1470, for a more detailed discussion of this topic, including a comprehensive list of references.

although radionuclide scans and magnetic resonance imaging (MRI) may be diagnostic in the early stages. Late radiographic changes include lytic destruction of bone and reactive bone formation about the focus of infection.

Initial evaluation should include blood culture, which is positive in 50% of cases. Aspiration of the subperiosteal space or medullary cavity for culture may be indicated. Broad-spectrum antibiotics effective against *Staphylococcus* are initiated without awaiting the results of culture. In most circumstances, surgical drainage of the focus of bone infection is required in conjunction with appropriate antibiotic therapy.

Osteomyelitis arising from penetrating injury (exogenous osteomyelitis) is best treated by prevention. Patients presenting with open fractures or soft tissue wounds that extend to bone should be treated by vigorous surgical débridement of nonviable tissue, copious irrigation, antibiotic therapy, and redébridement if necessary. When osteomyelitis develops in an area of prior injury, wide débridement and irrigation are indicated. Wound management may be enhanced by the use of polymethylmethacrylate beads impregnated with antibiotics placed in the wound and sealed with plastic drape. These wounds frequently will require rotational or free-flap muscle coverage for closure because of the extensive tissue loss.

BACTERIAL PYARTHROSIS

Joint infection with pyogenic organisms is the result of either hematogenous seeding or penetrating joint injury. Hematogenous pyarthrosis is seen most commonly in children prior to age 5, with *S. aureus* the most common etiologic agent. *Haemophilus influenzae, Streptococcus,* gonococcus, and *Pneumococcus* also may be etiologic agents.

Patients with hematogenous pyarthrosis present with acute onset of pain, fever, irritability, loss of joint motion, and inability to bear weight. Examination reveals swelling, erythema, and exquisite tenderness to palpation of the affected joint. Laboratory studies demonstrate an elevated white blood cell count and elevated erythrocyte sedimentation rate. Aspiration of the joint with a large-bore needle is required for identification of the organism. Synovial fluid cell counts range from 50,000 to 200,000 polymorphonuclear neutrophils per ml. of blood. Treatment of acute pyarthrosis may be by repeated joint lavage with a large-bore needle, repeated lavage with an arthroscope, or open surgical incision and drainage. The latter is usually preferred for more advanced infections where the thick synovium and purulent material are not adequately removed by closed irrigation methods. The joint is immobilized until the infection is under control, at which point rehabilitation may be initiated.

Penetrating joint injuries need surgical incision and drainage and copious irrigation and coverage with prophylactic antibiotics in order to prevent the establishment of exogenous pyarthrosis. When joint infection develops from penetrating injury, the treatment is similar to that for acute hematogenous pyarthrosis.

SKELETAL TUBERCULOSIS

Skeletal tuberculosis results from hematogenous seeding with tubercle bacilli from either a pulmonary or gastrointestinal focus. Although the incidence of tuberculosis has steadily declined during the last half of the twentieth century, there has been a recent increase in this disease in patients with associated HIV infections. Resistant strains of tubercle bacilli have been encountered. Hematogenous seeding of tuberculosis affects the lower thoracic and upper lumbar intervertebral disc spaces in 30% of cases. The hip and knee joints are the next most frequently affected. Radiographs may demonstrate widening of the joint due to increased joint fluid pressure. Marginal erosions at the point of synovial attachment of bone are the first skeletal changes observed. As the disease progresses, joint narrowing occurs as a result of articular cartilage erosion.

Tuberculosis is most appropriately treated by antituberculous medications (isoniazid, rifampin, PAS, streptomycin, ethambutol). The affected joint is placed at rest either by splinting, bed rest, or thoracolumbar bracing. Failure of improvement on medical therapy is an indication for surgical débridement. Arthrodesis, frequently employed in past decades, is rarely indicated. Extensive joint destruction may require arthrodesis or prosthetic replacement in selected patients.

NEOPLASMS OF BONE

The most common neoplastic condition encountered in the skeleton is metastatic carcinoma from breast, prostate, lung, kidney, or thyroid. Primary benign and malignant skeletal neoplasms are much less common. Treatment decisions for benign and malignant skeletal neoplasms are based on staging information. Staging involves the radiographic imaging of lesions to determine their anatomic extent, relationship to adjacent structures, and presence or absence of metastatic disease. Another aspect of staging is the histologic grade of the lesion, as determined by biopsy. Biopsy is performed only after all imaging has been completed.

Benign lesions of bone can be staged by biplane radiographs in most instances. Stage I lesions are contained within the bone of origin and are well marginated by reactive bone. Stage II lesions may expand the overlying cortex but remain contained by bone and have a well-demarcated margin at the interface with medullary bone. Stage III lesions are aggressive with destruction of the overlying cortex or extension into adjacent soft tissues.

Malignant skeletal neoplasms are staged according to their anatomic locations (intracompartmental or extracompartmental) and their histologic grade (high-grade or low-grade) and the presence or absence of metastases. Low-grade lesions are designated by I and high-grade lesions by II. Intracompartmental lesions are designated by A and extracompartmental lesions by B. Thus one may have IA, IB, IIA, and IIB lesions in ascending order of severity. A Stage III lesion is any lesion in which metastases are present regardless of anatomic site or histologic grade.

The four surgical procedures for the treatment of skeletal neoplasms are intralesional curettage, local (marginal) excision, wide excision, and radical excision. Stage I benign lesions and some Stage II benign lesions are appropriately treated by intralesional curettage. Stage II and some Stage III lesions and Stage IA and IB lesions may be appropriately treated by wide excision. Stage IIA and IIB lesions may require radical margins unless the neoplasm can be modified by neoadjuvant chemotherapy.

X

The Hand: Compression Neuropathies of the Hand and Forearm

Richard D. Goldner, M.D., and J. Leonard Goldner, M.D.

The diagnosis of abnormal compression of the median, ulnar, or radial nerves may be easily overlooked, although these syndromes occur relatively frequently.

DIFFERENTIAL DIAGNOSIS

A focal compression lesion must be differentiated from a neuropathy associated with systemic disease such as diabetes, hypothyroidism, rheumatoid arthritis, acromegaly, heavy metal intoxication, or paresthesias due to certain medications. Other more proximal lesions such as cervical root irritation, brachial plexitis, or a lesion associated with cerebral cortex disease may cause distal paresthesias. Conditions such as spinal cord tumor or syringomyelia also may cause distal symptoms and signs suggestive of a nerve compression lesion.

COMPRESSION OF THE MEDIAN NERVE AT THE WRIST (CARPAL TUNNEL SYNDROME)

The median nerve is compressed within the carpal canal, which is formed by the transverse carpal ligament on the palmar surface and the carpal bones on the dorsal side. The

See the corresponding chapter or part in the *Textbook of Surgery*, 15th edition, pp. 1470–1486, for a more detailed discussion of this topic, including a comprehensive list of references.

flexor tendons travel in the carpal canal with the median nerve. Hypertrophic synovium, edema fluid, dislocated carpal bones, or space-occupying lesions can compress the median nerve within this confined area. Women are affected more frequently than are men and with a wide age range but in patients generally 40 years or older. The usual complaints are weakness, clumsiness, hypesthesia, or paresthesias often aggravated by use of the hand. This syndrome encompasses a wide range of characteristics, such as nocturnal or early morning numbness that is quickly relieved by moving the hand and finger tingling when a vibrating object such as an electric razor is held. Repetitive flexion and extension movements of the fingers and the hand may cause symptoms. Other conditions such as cold temperature, rapid weight gain, fluid retention associated with pregnancy, or compression from tight watchbands or rubber gloves may initiate or aggravate the original symptoms.

Physical examination commonly shows a positive percussion test of the median nerve at the wrist either proximal to, under, or distal to the ligament. Wrist flexion (Phalen's test) often causes paresthesias in the median nerve distribution. Light touch is frequently decreased. A venous tourniquet applied to the arm for 20 to 30 seconds may reproduce the symptoms.

TREATMENT. Initial treatment is nonoperative and consists of splinting at night, weight reduction, decreased repetitive activities of the hand, and use of anti-inflammatory medications. Occasionally a soluble corticosteroid mixed with 1% Xylocaine injected into the tendon sheaths of the flexor digitorum profundus, completely avoiding the ulnar and the median nerves, produces a remission of the medial nerve compression symptoms. If symptoms and signs persist despite nonoperative treatment, operative decompression is considered. This procedure is performed by incision of the transverse carpal ligament at the wrist just proximal to the ligament extending to the midpalmar extension of the ligament at the superficial palmar arch. The palmar cutaneous branch of the median nerve is avoided. The motor branch is protected; the nerve is isolated carefully proximally and protected as the transverse carpal ligament is incised.

COMPRESSION OF THE ANTERIOR INTEROSSEOUS BRANCH OF THE MEDIAN NERVE

The anterior interosseous nerve is a motor branch of the median nerve that is present in the proximal third of the forearm. It supplies the flexor pollicis longus, the flexor digitorum profundus of the index and long fingers, and the pronator quadratus.

Anterior interosseous nerve compression causes a vague pain in the proximal forearm that is aggravated by exercise and relieved by rest. The pinch between thumb and index finger is weak. Individual testing of the flexor pollicis longus and the flexor digitorum profundus of the index demonstrates these muscle bellies to be weak. There is no sensory deficit. This syndrome must be differentiated from a rupture of the flexor pollicis longus or the index profundus tendons.

If symptoms persist after a reasonable period of observation, and depending on the other diagnostic studies, surgical therapy is performed by isolating the median nerve proximal to the lacertus fibrosus and dissecting it distally through the pronator teres and distally to where the branches enter the flexor pollicis longus and flexor profundus of the index and long fingers. Electrical stimulation of the nerve during this decompression is very helpful.

ULNAR NERVE COMPRESSION AT THE ELBOW

Ulnar nerve compression occurs within the cubital tunnel or proximal or distal to it: (1) a dense fascia over the flexor carpi ulnaris distally or the firm ridge of the interosseous membrane proximally may cause nerve irritation with repetitive motion, (2) synovium or osteophytes within the cubital tunnel may irritate the nerve as a result of repetitive acute elbow flexion, (3) a synovial cyst arising from the elbow joint and extending into the canal may compress the nerve, (4) repeated subluxation of the nerve as it moves across the medial epicondyle may cause nerve compression, (5) positional stresses such as prolonged elbow flexion during sleep, external pressure on the elbow during general anesthesia, or repetitive use of the flexed elbow against the mattress by the patient's changing position while on bed rest can cause ulnar nerve compression, and (6) other anatomic structures such as a fibrous arcade (arcade of Struthers) proximally or a combination of proximal tethering and distal muscle hypertrophy may irritate the nerve.

SYMPTOMS AND SIGNS. The patient complains of deep aching along the ulnar aspect of the proximal and mid forearm and intermittent numbness, tingling, and combinations of these sensations in the ring and little fingers. The heel of the hand and the little finger "are asleep." Percussion of the nerve should be performed distally and advanced proximally for detecting the site of compression. Forced voluntary flexion of the elbow with the forearm held in that position for 2 minutes should produce tingling if the nerve is tethered or hypermobile at the elbow. Early compression shows no intrinsic atrophy or overt cutaneous sensory changes. Late and prolonged compression causes atrophy of the hypothenar and first dorsal interosseous muscles along with dryness and diminished sensibility of the little and the ulnar half of the ring fingers.

TREATMENT. Nonoperative treatment depends on an accurate diagnosis. The patient is advised to avoid resting the elbow on chair arms, table surfaces, and airplane arm-rests. If the elbow is acutely flexed during sleep, a splint is applied for prevention. An elbow pad worn during the day may diminish direct contusion of the nerve and limit repetitive elbow flexion. Anti-inflammatory medications diminish connective tissue irritation and lessen the intensity of the complaints.

Surgical treatment is considered if one or more of the following is present: (1) hypesthesia and paresthesias persist for several months and are constantly uncomfortable, (2) rest, splinting, and other forms of treatment have not improved the persistent or progressive symptoms after 3 months of observation, (3) atrophy of the intrinsic muscles of the hand is evident, and (4) electrophysiologic studies are positive in either motor or sensory conduction tests and abnormal action potentials are observed.

One method of surgical treatment is subcutaneous transfer of the ulnar nerve anteriorly. Alternative approaches of managing the compressed ulnar nerve are (1) excision of the medial epicondyle of the humerus without transferring the nerve anteriorly; this can be successful in some instances; (2) placement of the nerve anterior to the ulnar groove and within the forearm flexor muscles; this may be as successful as subcutaneous transfer, but the muscle tissue may eventually constrict or compress the nerve; and (3) placement of the nerve deep to the forearm muscles not only to warm the nerve as in the case of leprosy but also to protect the nerve during forceful exercise.

COMPRESSION NEUROPATHY OF THE RADIAL NERVE

Compression of the radial nerve high in the arm may cause total loss of function of the muscles extending the wrist, thumb, and fingers. A sensory defect also occurs along the course of the superficial radial nerve. The anatomic site of compression may be at the humeral midshaft near the radial groove or at the distal third of the humerus. A distal fracture may affect the nerve at this site.

Compression palsy (Saturday night palsy) or radial nerve injury after proximal or midshaft fracture of the humerus recovers spontaneously in 3 to 5 months in greater than 90% of the patients. A distal oblique fracture of the humerus, however, may entrap the nerve, and operative decompression may be required.

POSTERIOR INTEROSSEOUS NERVE COMPRESSION

After innervating the brachioradialis, extensor carpi radialis longus, and extensor carpi radialis brevis, the radial nerve divides into the posterior interosseous branch (motor) and the superficial radial branch (sensory). The posterior interosseous nerve supplies the thumb extensors and the finger metacarpophalangeal extensors. These muscles are weak if the posterior interosseous nerve is compressed significantly. The posterior interosseous nerve enters the radial tunnel between the superficial and the deep heads of the supinator muscle. This nerve may be compressed if the hands of the patient are performing repetitive pronation and supination several hundred times a day for months or years, or the lesion may occur between the radial head and the supinator after a fracture or dislocation of the proximal radius.

The clinical findings in an extremity with a *complete* posterior interosseous nerve lesion are active dorsiflexion of the hand in radial deviation but loss of thumb and finger extension at the metacarpophalangeal joints.

An *incomplete* posterior interosseous nerve lesion may show lack of extension of one or two digits and weakness of extension of the abductor pollicis and/or the extensor pollicis longus.

TREATMENT. If the compression lesion is localized proximal to the supinator and caused by the extensor carpi radialis brevis, a posterior interosseous neurolysis is performed if the distal extensor muscles are weak and then the common radial nerve is isolated anterolaterally. If the distal extensor muscles are weak, the common radial nerve is isolated anterolaterally at the elbow and the nerve is followed into the supinator and distally. The vascular leash (radial recurrent) is ligated, the proximal fascial bands in the supinator are incised, and the arcade of Frohse is released. Electrical stimulation is attempted proximally and distally on the nerve for determining whether epineurial splitting is necessary at any location on the nerve.

Results of treatment depend on the duration of compression and the severity of the nerve injury. If decompression is performed relatively early and repetitive physical activities are not resumed, then improvement follows. Reinnervation of the affected muscles may be determined electrically 3 months after decompression, and clinical examination shows evidence of early regeneration by 5 months. At least a year is required before maximal recovery is expected. If improvement of muscle function does not occur within a year after nerve decompression, tendon transfer should be considered.

COMPRESSION OF THE SENSORY BRANCH OF THE RADIAL NERVE

Hypesthesia or hyperesthesia on the dorsum of the thumb and/or the index finger may be related to compression of the cutaneous branch of the radial nerve at the point at which the nerve exits beneath the brachioradialis and the shaft of the radius or irritation occurs adjacent to an enlargement of the abductor pollicis longus annular ligament at the wrist. Direct trauma to the nerve at the wrist or at the base of the thumb may affect sensory conduction. The history is important in establishing diagnosis of proximal or distal irritation.

The clinical examination demonstrates an area of hyperesthesia or hypesthesia along the course of the nerve slightly proximal and always distal to the point of compression. The condition usually improves in time with elimination of the abnormal external compressive forces, such as avoidance of cutting with a blunt large scissors or removal of a tight elastic watchband.

If a sensory deficit persists, neurolysis is performed from the proximal point of compression under the brachioradialis tendon about 5 cm. proximal to the wrist joint to the distal area of compression as determined by skin sensitivity and percussion test.

43

REPLANTATION OF AMPUTATED LIMBS AND DIGITS

James R. Urbaniak, M.D.

Microvascular surgery implies repair of small blood vessels (3 mm or less in diameter) with use of an operating microscope, microsurgical instruments, and ultrafine suture material (usually about 20 μm. in diameter). *Replantation* is defined as reattachment of a part that has been completely severed; that is, there is no connection between the amputated part and the patient. *Revascularization* is the reattachment of a part of which some portion of the soft tissue (such as skin, nerves, or tendon) is still connected. Vascular repair is necessary to prevent necrosis of the partially severed distal limb. This may require repair of the arteries or the veins or both.

CARE OF THE AMPUTATED PART

Amputated or devascularized tissue will survive for about 6 hours if the part is not cooled. Because the digits essentially have no muscle tissue, they may be replanted successfully as long as 24 hours after amputation if they are cooled. The amputated part should be placed into a plastic bag containing Ringer's lactate or saline solution. The plastic bag is placed on ice. An alternative method of preserving the amputated part is to wrap it in a cloth or sponge moistened with Ringer's lactate or saline solution placed in a plastic bag, which is put on ice.

PATIENT SELECTION

Guillotine-type amputations are ideally suited for replanting. Organs for replantation are selected according to the following priorities: (1) thumb, (2) multiple digits, (3) partial hand (amputation through the palm), (4) almost any part of a child, (5) wrist or forearm, (6) above-elbow amputation (only sharp or moderately avulsed), and (7) isolated digit distal to the superficialis insertion (distal to the proximal interphalangeal joint). The prime parts for replantation are thumbs, multiple digits, and the complete hand. Replantation of these parts provides the best results. In children, an attempt should be made to replant almost any part; if the replanted extremity survives, excellent function can be expected.

Types of injuries that are not favorable for replantation are

---

See the corresponding chapter or part in the *Textbook of Surgery*, 15th edition, pp. 1487–1491, for a more detailed discussion of this topic, including a comprehensive list of references.

(1) severely crushed or mangled parts, (2) amputations at multiple levels, (3) amputations in patients with other serious injuries or diseases, (4) amputations in which the vessels are arteriosclerotic, (5) amputations in mentally unstable patients, (6) injuries with more than 6 hours of ischemia time, (7) severely contaminated parts, and (8) an individual finger in the adult with the amputation proximal to the superficialis insertions (proximal to the proximal interphalangeal joint). Replantation of isolated fingers at the base (proximal to the superficialis insertion) generally results in a finger that "gets in the way" because of diminished tendon excursion. Often the final decision cannot be made until the status of the damaged blood vessels is determined under the operating microscope.

SURGICAL TECHNIQUE

Microscopic evaluation determines the feasibility of restoration by revascularization.

The sequence of replantation of amputated digits or hands is as follows: (1) locate and tag the vessels and nerves, (2) shorten and fix the bone with an intramedullary pin, (3) repair the extensor tendons, (4) repair the flexor tendons, (5) repair the arteries, (6) repair the nerves, (7) repair the veins, and (8) obtain loose skin coverage (split-thickness graft if necessary).

The bone is shortened to facilitate the vascular anastomoses. *The most important factors in achieving permanent microvascular patency are easy coaptation of vessels with normal intima and the skill and expertise of the microsurgeon.*

MAJOR LIMB REPLANTATION

Major limb replantation implies replantation of limbs proximal to the wrist or of the lower extremity proximal to the ankle.

Whereas amputated digits may be replanted successfully 24 hours after amputation, an amputated arm at the elbow is in jeopardy if it has been ischemic for 10 to 12 hours, even if it has been cooled properly. Extensive muscle débridement both on the detached part and on the stump is essential for prevention of myonecrosis and subsequent infection, which is the major problem in major limb replantation but is uncommon in digital reattachment.

In replantations proximal to the metacarpal level, immediate arterial inflow is necessary for preventing or diminishing myonecrosis. If the amputated part and the patient arrive in the operating room more than 4 hours after injury, initiation of immediate blood flow to the detached part is desirable. This is best accomplished by using some form of shunt, such as a Sundt or ventriculoperitoneal shunt, to obtain rapid arterial inflow to the detached part. Shunting should be performed before bone fixation unless the bone can be stabilized rapidly and early blood flow obtained. After the establishment of temporary blood flow, further débridement can be continued, the bone stabilized, the shunt removed, and a direct arterial repair or interpositional vein graft of the vessels performed.

Stable bone fixation is necessary for major limb replantation; however, the method should be rapid. In major limb replantation, it is critical to perform the arterial anastomosis before the venous anastomosis. This sequence allows a physiologic washout of noxious agents such as lactic acid in the distal part. The administration of intravenous sodium bicarbonate before venous anastomosis is beneficial.

Extensive fasciotomies are always indicated in major limb replantations. *The two most common causes of failure in major limb replantation are myonecrosis with subsequent infection and failure to provide adequate decompression of the restored vessels.*

In replantations of major limbs, the patients should be returned to the operating room within 48 to 72 hours for evaluation of the state of muscle tissue. In major limb replantations, the best replantation results are obtained at the wrist, followed by the arm and distal forearm. The poorest results occur in the proximal third of the forearm, an area where the motor branches of the radial, median, and ulnar nerves enter the extrinsic musculature of the hand.

There are few indications for replantation of the lower extremity. Upper extremity prostheses poorly duplicate hand function; however, lower limb prostheses provide a stable stance and a functional gait. With the currently available lower extremity prostheses, considerable thought should be given before replantation of the lower extremities is attempted, even with rather cleanly severed limbs.

POSTOPERATIVE MANAGEMENT

Most patients receive some type of anticoagulation. Intravenous heparin at 1000 units per hour for about 7 days is usually administered. Low-molecular-weight dextran, aspirin, chlorpromazine, and dipyridamole have been used in difficult cases. Skin color, pulp turgor, capillary refill, and skin temperature are the most useful indicators for monitoring. Seldom is it necessary to return the patient to the operating room for a revision; however, if re-exploration is to be successful, it usually must be done within 24 to 48 hours after the primary procedure.

RESULTS OF REPLANTATION

Most major replantation centers are obtaining about an 80% viability rate in complete replantations. Cold intolerance is a problem in most patients, but this subsides in 1 to 2 years. Replanted thumbs provide the best functional results. Strong pinch, adequate motion, excellent sensation, and almost normal appearance are to be expected. Replantations of multiple digits, partial hands (through the palm), or complete hands provide good sensibility and useful function. Although amputations through the wrist or distal forearm provide good function of the hand, amputations at a more proximal level have varied results.

44

GYNECOLOGY:
The Female Reproductive Organs
Charles B. Hammond, M.D.

Gynecology is that branch of medicine concerning function and diseases of the female reproductive system. Increasingly, this specialty not only includes the pelvic reproductive organs themselves but other areas as well. These include the primary health care of women, the adjacent pelvic structures (urinary system and bowel), and even remote, hormonally reactive organs such as breast, bone, hypothalamus, and pituitary. It includes many other areas of interest, common to other surgical specialties.

CONGENITAL ANOMALIES

There are a number of abnormalities of the pelvic structures that are dictated by the developmental embryology of the systems. Awareness of the underlying embryology is necessary for understanding these deficits.

Imperforate Hymen

Imperforate hymen may cause retention of mucus or blood, with resulting hematocolpos, hematometrium, hematosalpinx, and even hematoperitoneum. Diagnosis is based on careful examination of the external genitalia, which shows a bulging hymen without communication with the vagina and a fluctuant pelvic mass that lies anterior to the rectum. Pelvic ultrasonography may be particularly useful for diagnosis. With adequate surgical drainage, the distended structures promptly return to normal.

Defects of Müllerian Fusion

Defects of müllerian fusion may exist, causing duplication of part or all of the reproductive structures. The classic abnormality is the uterus didelphis, with two vaginas, cervices, and uteri, each with a separate tube and ovary. Such patients can present with pelvic pain or a mass because of obstruction. Therapy, if indicated at all, is surgical excision or reconstruction.

Dysgenesis

There are a number of defects of the female genital tract due to hypoplasia or aplasia of the various components. Con-

---

See the corresponding chapter or part in the *Textbook of Surgery,* 15th edition, pp. 1492–1523, for a more detailed discussion of this topic, including a comprehensive list of references.

genital absence of both ovaries is rare, but absence of one tube or ovary at birth is not unusual. There are cases of complete absence of the vagina, usually associated with absence of the uterus and a number of other abnormalities. Whereas dysgenesis of the müllerian system with absence of the structures is the most common problem, a few patients present with androgen insensitivity, in which the gonads are testicular yet secondary sex characteristics are feminine, since the patient lacks the ability to respond to androgens. Usually, in patients with congenital absence of the pelvic structures, chromosomal studies are necessary for differentiation. If a testicular gonad is *in situ*, excision is necessary because of the risk of secondary malignancy. In all types of vaginal agenesis, a normally functioning vagina should be created surgically or by dilation. Other congenital anomalies of the urinary tract should be sought. There is a commonality of urologic and gynecologic anomalies, which approaches 50% in patients with more severe defects.

THE VULVA

A number of problems may occur in the area of the female external genitals. Trauma, allergy, inflammatory conditions, infections, degenerative changes, and neoplasia produce disorders ranging from minor annoyances to major hazards to life. An important precept in the evaluation and management of any noted abnormality of the vulva is to be absolutely sure to exclude neoplasia. Punch biopsy with local anesthesia should be done at any time a suspicious or unusual vulvar lesion is noted.

The vulva is rich in pigment, which increases in pregnancy. Vitiligo of the vulvar skin is the same as the lesion in other locations and does not require treatment. Vitiligo should not be confused with leukoplakia, in which the skin is whitish but thickened and leathery. Various skin eruptions involving the body as a whole may affect the vulva and appear, as do other lesions, elsewhere on the body. Varicose veins of the vulva are often found in association with varicosities of the lower extremities, and pregnancy may cause further hypertrophy. Therapy consists of lower extremity and vulvar support and ligation or injection in the nonpregnant patient. A severe direct blow to the vulva may be complicated by subcutaneous hematoma formation. Such a hematoma may dissect widely beneath the fascia of the vulva, and surgical evacuation is often necessary. It is frequently difficult to isolate bleeding points, and packing may be required. Vulvar lacerations should be cleansed and sutured as are lacerations elsewhere on the body.

Glandular Lesions

The vulvar glands are subject to a number of disorders. Skenitis usually occurs as a consequence of gonococcal infection. A Bartholin's abscess should be treated with heat until fluctuant and then sharply incised on the mucocutaneous junction between the vagina and vulva. Often, a small inflatable Worde catheter may be inserted. If the abscess is drained by incision, the margins of the incision are marsupialized. The vulva is also a common site of sebaceous cysts. These may be removed if they become greatly enlarged or secondarily infected.

Vulvitis

The most common cause of vulvar irritation is an infectious vulvovaginitis caused by *Candida albicans* or *Trichomonas vaginalis* or both. The vulva appears swollen and red and may be excoriated and secondarily infected. Mycotic vulvovaginitis is a common problem among diabetics, oral contraceptive users, and those receiving systemic antibiotics. Diagnosis is based on fresh-preparation identification of yeast or *Trichomonas*. Therapy is with antimycotic agents such as nystatin or butaconazole or, in the case of trichomoniasis, metronidazole for the patient and consort. Immediate relief is obtained by the additional use of topical creams containing hydrocortisone or miconazole. Condylomata acuminata, or venereal warts, occur as a presumed infectious vulvitis of viral origin (HPV). Such lesions are associated with an irritating vaginal discharge. These benign epithelial neoplasms may be few or many, in some cases even covering the entire perineum and extending onto the vagina or cervix. Therapy is topical application of podophyllin or trichloroacetic acid. On occasion, one may use 5-fluorouracil. Cautery or laser is used for the more extensive forms of the disease but requires an anesthetic.

Recently, there has been a near-epidemic of sexually transmitted vulvovaginitis caused by herpes progenitalis (herpes simplex Type II). This infection is characterized by vesicular eruptions that are extremely painful and are often secondarily infected when the patient is seen. Current therapy includes warm baths in water containing potassium permanganate, drying, and systemic analgesics. The duration of this infection is usually limited, but it may recur. The antiviral agent acyclovir reduces the severity of primary herpetic infections. Other data suggest that chronic acyclovir use may reduce the frequency and severity of recurrences. To date, however, there is no permanent cure, and approximately 20% of patients with a primary herpetic lesion have recurrent episodes.

Other sexually transmitted diseases may present as vulvar lesions. These include the primary chancre of syphilis or the moist, grayish patches (condylomata lata) of secondary syphilis. Lymphogranuloma venereum is a disease of viral origin, which may present with inguinal adenitis, multiple draining sinuses, and rectal stricture. Chancroid appears as a small papule 2 to 4 days after exposure and later becomes an indurated and punched-out lesion with soft edges and purulent surfaces.

Degenerative Diseases of the Vulva

There are three degenerative diseases of the vulva, all occurring most frequently after menopause. *Kraurosis vulvae* is a disease in which the vulva appears shrunken and dried. *Leukoplakia* presents initially as a hypertrophic lesion and later as an atrophic problem; the skin is whitened and leathery. *Lichen sclerosis et atrophicus* is the third form. It is a slowly changing, chronic, localized lesion but, unlike the other two problems, tends to involve the skin of the thighs. All cause itching, pain, dyspareunia, and frequent secondary infection. The incidence of vulvar carcinoma is increased with these lesions, and biopsy should be employed when necessary to exclude neoplasia. Treatment is symptomatic, with relief of pruritus a primary goal. Local excision may be necessary.

Carcinoma *in situ* of the Vulva

Carcinoma *in situ* of the vulva (VIN-III) may appear with leukoplakia, kraurosis vulvae, or lichen sclerosis et atrophicus, with or without pruritus. The diagnosis should be made only after adequate histologic study shows the criteria of intraepithelial changes characteristic of epidermoid carcinoma but without invasion. Treatment should be surgical excision in most instances. In patients with carcinoma *in situ* of the vulva, up to 35% may have a second malignant or premalignant genital lesion elsewhere.

Carcinoma of the Vulva

Vulvar cancers constitute approximately 3.5% of all genital malignancies, and the peak occurs in the seventh decade of life. In approximately half the patients, the cancer develops in areas of pre-existing leukoplakia, kraurosis vulvae, lichen sclerosis et atrophicus, or lichen sclerosis; others report a high incidence of syphilis and other vulvar venereal diseases among these patients. Most patients with vulvar carcinoma complain of a mass, ulceration, or irritation and pruritus. Bleeding and pain may be additional findings. Any firm tumor or ulceration must be biopsied and include the primary lesion as well as some adjacent normal tissue.

Carcinoma of the vulva is usually squamous (95%). Adenocarcinoma of the vulva usually arises from Bartholin's glands but may develop from paraurethral glands or embryonic cell rests. Melanocarcinoma, Paget's disease, and basal cell carcinoma all may be found on the vulva.

Vulvar cancer tends to spread by local extension and lymphatic metastasis. The primary lymphatic drainage of the vulva is via superficial inguinal lymph nodes ipsilateral and via Cloquet's node to the external iliac nodes and up the aortic chain. Contralateral vulvar drainage may occur, however, even from well-lateralized lesions. Vulvar lesions in the perineal, Bartholin's, or posterior fourchette areas may involve the rectovaginal septum, rectum, or vagina and may metastasize via the deep pelvic nodes. Blood-borne metastases are unusual.

The treatment of vulvar cancer is surgical. Radiotherapy generally has been of little use for primary or recurrent disease and is contraindicated. The prognosis is generally excellent for earlier lesions. The 5-year cure rate after surgical therapy of cancer of the vulva is approximately 60%. If the vulvar lesion involves the vagina, rectum, or urethra, pelvic exenteration may be the operation of choice.

THE VAGINA

The stratified squamous epithelium of the vagina is histologically similar to the epithelium of the cervix and the skin of the vulva and responds to estrogen by proliferation. Vaginal inflammation can occur from protozoan, fungal, bacterial, or viral infection and also from deficiencies of estrogen. Nonspecific bacterial infections, now termed *bacterial vaginosis* and thought to be sexually transmitted, also may exist. Gonorrhea is an occasional cause of vaginitis in the child. In all these categories, the cause of vaginal infection should be sought through wet preparation or culture, with appropriate treatment being instituted for the organism found. Often, there is vulvar inflammation that may require local therapy for immediate relief of symptoms.

Dysplasia and Intraepithelial Carcinoma of the Vagina

Dysplasia of the vaginal epithelium may be the source of abnormal genital smears even if the cervix is normal or absent. Intraepithelial carcinoma also may develop. These lesions may occur at the apex of the vagina in patients after hysterectomy or may be multifocal in areas remote from the vaginal apex. Diagnosis is suggested by genital cytologic and colposcopic examination and confirmed by biopsy. Therapy can be excision or partial or total colpectomy.

Carcinoma of the Vagina

Primary carcinoma of the vagina is a rare lesion, and most are epidermoid lesions. Postcontact bleeding is the usual presenting complaint. Many patients with invasive vaginal carcinoma have had other epidermoid lesions of the lower genital system previously. After appropriate staging, therapy is either irradiation or surgery (exenterative), with most favoring irradiation. Reasonable results are obtained with early-stage disease.

DEFECTS OF PELVIC SUPPORT

Overdistention (such as by childbirth) of the pelvic supporting structures may produce a number of defects in pelvic support. These problems include cystocele, urethrocele, rectocele, enterocele, and uterine prolapse. After hysterectomy, vaginal vault prolapse may occur. There may be attendant problems in urinary incontinence or exteriorization of pelvic structures. The common sensation of heavy pulling-down pressure in the pelvis is often present. The proper assessment includes urodynamic investigation of urinary dysfunction, careful search for occult enterocele, and surgical repair often combining abdominal and transvaginal approaches. Usually preservation of vaginal patency can be maintained with an excellent restoration of support.

BENIGN DISEASES OF THE CERVIX

The normal cervix is covered with squamous epithelium and is subject to a number of problems. Cervical infection is one of the most frequently encountered gynecologic lesions. Acute cervicitis is rarely seen other than in gonorrhea or *Chlamydia* infection. Pain and tenderness are rarely prominent symptoms, but a purulent discharge is seen frequently. Diagnosis is made by appropriate smears and cultures, and therapy with topical or systemic antibiotics is usually curative.

In chronic cervicitis, the mucus is mucopurulent and often profuse. Erosions and eversions of the cervix are often observed. An erosion is a true ulcer of the cervix, whereas an eversion is formed by proliferation downward of the columnar epithelium of the endocervical canal, forming a lowered squamocolumnar line. Diagnosis is based on cytologic examination and biopsy for exclusion of neoplasia, and these studies are more difficult when cervical infection is present. Colposcopy may be of aid in localizing areas for biopsy. After exclusion of malignancy, chronic cervicitis is usually treated by electrodesiccation, laser desiccation, or cryosurgery.

CANCER OF THE CERVIX

Invasive carcinoma of the cervix is now the second most common pelvic malignancy and represents 15% of cancers in women. In the past two decades, primarily through early detection, mortality from cervical cancer has declined significantly. Invasive carcinoma of the cervix theoretically should be a preventable disease, since regular examinations and frequent use of present technologies, particularly genital cytologic study, should enable detection of nearly all malignant lesions or preinvasive cervical carcinoma.

The average age of occurrence of carcinoma of the cervix is 49 years. However, many authors have reported cervical cancers in women as young as the teens and as old as the eighth decade. Epidemiologic relationships show peak occurrences among women of low socioeconomic status, those who begin coitus and childbearing at an early age, and those with multiple sexual partners. Cigarette smoking and heredity have a small role. The theory of a viral relationship has been advanced but not yet fully proven. Preinvasive carcinoma, or carcinoma *in situ* of the cervix, has been recognized for a number of years. It is suspected only on the basis of genital cytologic change, since *there are no gross lesions or symptoms of carcinoma in situ or dysplasia of the cervix*. The diagnoses of these lesions are made by histologic review of appropriate biopsy specimens.

Many patients with dysplasia or carcinoma *in situ* of the

cervix are now being treated with electrocautery, cryosurgery, or cone biopsy. Close follow-up after therapy is warranted. The primary caution is to exclude invasive carcinoma before such treatments are done. Another treatment for extensive or recurrent carcinoma *in situ* of the cervix may be abdominal or vaginal hysterectomy with excision of 2 to 3 cm. of the upper vagina. Radical hysterectomy and pelvic lymph node dissection are not indicated, and results are generally good.

Carcinoma of the Cervix

Approximately 95% of cervical cancers are squamous; the remaining 5% are usually adenocarcinomas. Microinvasive cancer of the cervix (Stage IA1 and above) denotes a minimal extent of invasion. A halo of carcinoma *in situ* is frequently found around an invasive cancer or on the vagina. There are few symptoms of early carcinoma of the cervix, the first symptom generally being bleeding. This may be postcontact or an irregular bloody discharge. More advanced cervical cancers cause symptoms referable to invasion of adjacent organs (bladder, rectum, or ureter) or to distant metastasis. Pain is a frequent symptom of advanced cervical cancer.

Although cytologic findings and clinical appearance may strongly suggest carcinoma of the cervix, the diagnosis can be made only on histopathologic study. Even in the presence of normal genital cytologic findings, cervical or vaginal ulcers or growths should be biopsied. False-negative genital cytologic study in the presence of ulcerative or exophytic cervical lesions is not uncommon.

The most common method of spread of cervical cancer and the most frequent cause of patient death is direct extension to involve the vagina, uterus, parametrium, pelvic sidewall, ureter, bladder, and rectum. Fistula formation is common, and bleeding may be a serious complication. Carcinoma of the cervix also has a propensity for lymphatic metastasis.

Treatment of cervical cancer can be accomplished effectively by surgical therapy or irradiation. Treatment, however, does not include simple hysterectomy or nonindividualized radiotherapy. No other major malignancy requires a more critical selection of technique or mode of therapy. The present operation for early cancer of the cervix (Stages I and IIA) is an extended or radical hysterectomy (Wertheim) that removes the parametrial tissues, the upper third of the vagina, and perhaps the adnexa. Pelvic node dissection is usually performed. Radical irradiation may be used in early-stage cancer of the cervix or in more extended disease. External irradiation followed by intracervical irradiation is the appropriate treatment. Results of treatment are generally good for earlier disease—86.4% for Stage I and only 8.8% for Stage IV. Patients who have been treated for cancer of the cervix must be followed for many years, since late recurrence is reasonably common.

BENIGN UTERINE DISEASE

Various benign uterine diseases occur, including leiomyoma uteri, adenomyosis, endometrial hyperplasia, and polyps. Abnormal bleeding, uterine enlargement, and pain are the primary symptoms associated with these diseases, but the major difficulty is achieving an accurate diagnosis.

Leiomyoma Uteri

Uterine leiomyomas are the most common cause of benign uterine enlargement and are seen in 20% of women, with a higher incidence among blacks. Leiomyomas originate from the smooth muscle cells of the myometrium and vary in size from microscopic to large enough to fill the entire abdomen. Such tumors may be single but are more often multiple. Compressed peripheral fibers form a pseudocapsule. Such tumors may be submucous, intramural, subserous, pedunculated, parasitic, cervical, or interligamentous.

The symptoms vary according to location; some may produce severe complaints, others none at all. The three most common symptoms are abnormal bleeding, pain, and uterine enlargement. Abnormal bleeding, usually cyclic but possibly profuse and prolonged, is most frequently due to submucous tumors that distort the overlying endometrium and interfere with normal hemostatic mechanisms. Occasionally, a submucous or cervical myoma may be extruded. Abnormal bleeding is the most common indication for hysterectomy for leiomyoma, but caution must be taken to exclude other causes, since a malignant lesion of the endometrium may coexist with a myoma. Often a curettage may be mandatory for making this differentiation. Rapid enlargement is another symptom of concern in patients with leiomyoma, because 0.05% to 0.08% may develop sarcomatous change. Estrogens, including the synthetic estrogens of oral contraceptives, may be associated in some patients with more rapid enlargement of leiomyomas. Myomas tend to regress after menopause, and any enlargement of these tumors after this age demands removal of the uterus. Slow enlargement of leiomyomas during the menstrual years frequently occurs with minimal symptoms, and surgical removal is not mandatory for slow growth or moderate size, unless other symptoms occur. Pelvic pressure, frequency of urination, and sciatic or hip pain may be symptoms of uterine leiomyoma. Tenderness is usually caused by degeneration, and cystic changes and calcification can occur. Significant pain or tenderness may warrant hysterectomy. Infertility is uncommon in patients with myomas, as is abortion, but either may occur.

Adenomyosis

Adenomyosis is invasion of the myometrium by the endometrium. It is a frequent cause of uterine enlargement and pain. Grossly, the uterus is enlarged, fibrotic, and thickened, and on cut section there are areas of endometrial growth and loculated menstruation within the myometrium. The classic signs and symptoms include acquired dysmenorrhea occurring in the 35- to 45-year-old patient; there often are menstrual irregularities with cyclic prolonged and profuse flow and an enlarged, tender uterus. Treatment is hysterectomy, although some types of hormonal suppression may provide temporary relief without removal of the uterus.

Endometrial Hyperplasia and Polyps

Hyperplasia of the endometrium, causing abnormal uterine bleeding, is a common problem of women in the perimenopausal years. It is seen occasionally in younger patients, particularly in adolescence. The basic problem is anovulation and failure of production of progesterone. Continued stimulation of the endometrium by estrogen produces proliferation, overgrowth, and hyperplasia. Areas of thickened endometrium may form polyps. Menstruation becomes irregular, with intervals of amenorrhea associated with other intervals of bleeding. Pelvic examination is usually not revealing, and biopsy or curettage is necessary to establish the diagnosis. Curettage also offers a therapeutic component. Because of the frequency of recurrence of hyperplasia, the administration of cyclic progesterone may limit recurrence. In various types of hyperplasias, notably the atypical adenomatous hyperplasias, there is a significant malignant potential, and the consideration of hysterectomy may be needed.

MALIGNANT DISEASES OF THE UTERUS

Adenocarcinoma of the endometrium, now the most prevalent gynecologic cancer, is seen most commonly among postmenopausal women. The peak incidence occurs in the 50- to 70-year-old age group, but it must be suspected as early as the third decade if there is an irregularity of menstrual bleeding. Irregular or postmenopausal bleeding is the cardinal symptom of endometrial cancer. Papanicolaou cytologic study may yield negative results, since the exfoliated cells may not reach the vaginal pool. Fractional curettage is the diagnostic method of choice, although screening by endometrial biopsy may be performed. On histologic examination, adenocarcinoma of the endometrium has wide variations in differentiation and in stromal invasion. The etiologic agent of endometrial cancer is unknown. There does appear to be a relationship to prolonged estrogen stimulation in some patients, as in patients with estrogen-producing ovarian tumors. Newer studies also suggest a higher incidence of endometrial adenocarcinoma in women given large-dose estrogen (only) replacement therapy for menopausal symptoms.

After appropriate staging, the treatment of adenocarcinoma of the endometrium is primarily surgical. Survival in patients with very early-stage disease and well-differentiated lesions is very good. External pelvic radiotherapy or transvaginal irradiation may be used for palliation or recurrent disease. Rarely, hormonal manipulations may be of benefit for metastases.

Sarcomas of the uterus may arise from the endometrium, myometrium, cervix, or uterine blood vessels or from a leiomyoma. These diseases are seen most frequently in the fifth decade. Treatment is primarily surgical, although radiotherapy may offer benefit.

PELVIC INFECTION

Acute pelvic infection may occur after pelvic surgery or from other causes, but the most frequent etiologic factors are gonorrhea and *Chlamydia* infection. The initial symptoms of acute pelvic infection usually occur within 3 to 6 days after inoculation, although they may be delayed until the onset of the next menses. Initial symptoms are referable to urethritis, skenitis, bartholinitis, and cervicitis and consist of vaginal discharge. Tubal involvement is a later symptom, and at that time organisms spread rapidly from the endocervix, across the endometrium, and involve the endosalpinx. It is in the fallopian tubes that the major infection and damage occur. The tubes become acutely inflamed and edematous, and the lumen fills with a purulent exudate. The tubular, peritubular, ovarian, and pelvic peritoneal surfaces are rapidly involved. Secondary infection with anaerobic bacteria is common. Pelvic abscess may develop.

The signs and symptoms of acute pelvic infection are those of pelvic peritonitis with bilateral lower abdominal pain and tenderness, temperature of 38 to 39° C., and signs of peritoneal irritation with direct and rebound tenderness and muscle spasm. On pelvic examination, purulent exudate may be seen in the cervix, and exquisite tenderness is often present with cervical manipulation and in the adnexal areas. Bilaterality of pain is an important point in differentiating acute pelvic infection from appendicitis. Therapy is based on the degree of peritonitis and fever. If significant peritonitis is present or the temperature is greater than 38.5° C., hospitalization is indicated, and intravenous antibiotic therapy is recommended. For women with serious episodes of pelvic infection, a number of therapeutic regimens have been proposed, including doxycycline plus cefoxitan, clindamycin plus gentamicin, or doxycycline plus metronidazole. Aggressive antibiotic treatment, analgesia, and parenteral fluid replacement are continued until the acute symptoms have subsided; then oral therapy is begun and continued for at least a week. If the presenting symptoms are not severe, the patient can be treated entirely as an outpatient, but close follow-up is warranted.

The patient with relatively asymptomatic gonorrhea can be treated with aqueous procaine penicillin G, 4.8 million units intramuscularly in divided doses at two sites, preceded by probenecid, 1 gm. by mouth. Approximately a week after the therapy is completed, a follow-up culture for "test of cure" should be done. The patient should be examined twice weekly to follow her progress and exclude pelvic abscess. Surgical therapy is not generally indicated for acute pelvic infection unless pelvic abscess drainage is required or differentiation from appendicitis is needed.

Chronic Pelvic Infection

Included among chronic pelvic infections are chronic salpingo-oophoritis, pyosalpinx, hydrosalpinx, and tubercular salpingitis. Chronic salpingo-oophoritis is one of the major complications of gonococcal and probably chlamydial infections. The patient may have few complaints or have recurrent and acute discomfort. The classic pattern of chronic pelvic infection is one of quiescent intervals interspaced with episodes of more acute inflammation. After the initial infection, anaerobic organisms invade and involve these tissues. These infections may be treated medically or surgically. The important elements of medical therapy are rest, heat, and antibiotic treatment. Analgesia may be required. Oral metronidazole, doxycycline, and tetracycline are the appropriate antibiotics utilized with modest increases in pain and symptoms from chronic pelvic infection. Symptoms in those patients who have recurrent pain or abnormal uterine bleeding from altered ovarian function caused by chronic pelvic infection are often difficult to relieve. In this instance, surgical extirpation may be needed, although it should be delayed until maximal medical control has been obtained.

BENIGN DISEASES OF THE OVARY

Benign ovarian tumors may be solid or cystic and may represent a "functional" process or neoplasia. They on occasion may become massively enlarged, although they usually are modest in size. A number of authors report that more than 90% of ovarian growths discovered in women under 30 years of age are benign. In the 30- to 50-year age group, 80% are benign. After 50 years of age, approximately half such ovarian growths are malignant. The various benign ovarian growths, excluding the frequently seen follicular and corpus luteum cysts, are endometrial cysts, simple cysts, serous and mucinous cystadenomas, and dermoids. Symptoms include slow abdominal enlargement, pain and tenderness from torsion of the pedicle, and rarely, aberrations of menstrual bleeding.

The benign, nonneoplastic ovarian cysts are usually of "functional" origin. These represent failure of the normal development and regression of ovulatory cysts. Most usually regress over a 4- to 8-week period. Of the nonfunctional benign cysts, the most frequently seen is the endometrial or "chocolate" cyst of pelvic endometriosis; this may achieve large size. Serous and mucinous cystadenomas arise from neoplastic nonmalignant changes in germinal epithelium and often reach large size. These tumors are usually multilocular, have smooth capsules, and usually replace the entire ovary. The benign teratoma, or dermoid cyst, is a common ovarian tumor, benign in more than 99% of patients. Approximately 20% of dermoids are bilateral, and thus if one ovary is involved, the other should be inspected carefully.

The solid benign ovarian tumors include the Brenner tumor, which is thought to arise from Walthard's inclusion rests in the cortex of the ovary; ovarian fibromas; and a number of rare and unusual tumors that may have hormonal activity. The most important decision confronting the surgeon who finds a solid ovarian tumor is differentiation of benign from malignant.

The treatment of benign ovarian growths is primarily surgical removal with conservation of all possible normal ovarian tissue in younger women. The functional cysts should regress within a relatively short interval and do not require removal unless rupture and hemorrhage have occurred. Endometrial or "chocolate" cysts usually require resection of all involved tissue. In any event, bilateral oophorectomy is rarely indicated in young women with ovarian masses unless one is *certain* that malignancy is present. In general, the author believes that if an undiagnosed mass larger than 6 cm. is found in a cycling patient or, if smaller, it persists for longer than 3 months, exploration should be done. Acute torsion or significant hemorrhage may require immediate resection.

OVARIAN CANCER

Most series report that ovarian cancer represents 4% to 6% of all cases of malignant disease in women. Most investigators include a number of types such as serous cystadenocarcinoma (60%), pseudomucinous carcinoma (15%), solid undifferentiated adenocarcinoma (10%), granulosa cell carcinoma (6%), and others at lesser percentages. The ratio of benign ovarian tumors to malignant ovarian tumors is 4:1 until the peak incidence of ovarian cancer at 40 to 60 years of age, when the ratio is 1:1.

The signs and symptoms of ovarian cancer may be only those of an enlarging tumor in the pelvis. Published reports indicate that half the patients complain of pain and abdominal swelling. A number of complaints include weight loss and abnormal bleeding. There may be ascites and even hydrothorax, and anemia is frequently found in advanced disease. Pelvic examination may reveal firm nodular implants. As noted, there are often no early symptoms of ovarian cancer. Annual bimanual examination is an important screening technique for this disease. Although not highly accurate for diagnosis, tumor "markers," if present, may be beneficial (CA 125, CEA).

The primary treatment of ovarian cancer is surgical. In general, this includes total abdominal hysterectomy, bilateral salpingo-oophorectomy, and omentectomy, although there may be residual tumor. The abdomen, including the diaphragm should be inspected carefully and appropriate lymph node sampling performed. Peritoneal washings should be obtained routinely. Chemotherapy has been a primary adjunctive technology, although radiotherapy has had limited success. With such treatment, approximately half the patients receive significant palliation, and the 5-year survival of Stage I ovarian cancer is only 66%. Unfortunately, only 20% of patients explored have disease limited to Stage I.

ECTOPIC PREGNANCY

An ectopic pregnancy is one in which the embryo implants and develops outside the uterine cavity. Ninety-five percent of ectopic pregnancies are tubal, with the greatest percentage of these occurring in the dilated ampulla. Less common sites of ectopic pregnancy are abdominal, ovarian, and interligamentary positions. Despite the fact that the ovum is implanted outside the uterine cavity, the uterine endometrium converts into a decidual structure similar to that of normal pregnancy. The size and consistency of the uterus also change in ectopic pregnancy, with the cervix and uterus softening and the corpus enlarging to 6 to 8 weeks' gestational size. All these changes are due to the production of placental hormones from the ectopic embryo. As ectopic placental function declines, as usually occurs in tubal pregnancy, the hormonal support declines, and irregular uterine bleeding begins.

The duration and eventual outcome of tubal ectopic pregnancy are determined primarily by the area of tube involved. If the ovum implants in the relatively large ampullary region of the tube, the pregnancy usually continues longer than one in the narrow isthmus. The ovular sac may extrude from the end of the tube, or the tube may rupture, particularly in the more narrow areas. Intra-abdominal hemorrhage may occur. The classic symptoms of ectopic pregnancy are a history of infertility or pelvic disease, light vaginal bleeding within 2 to 4 weeks after the first missed period, and sharp and fleeting lower abdominal pain. Eventually the patient experiences sudden severe abdominal pain and shock as the tube ruptures. On examination, the signs of early pregnancy such as cyanosis and softening of the cervix and uterine enlargement are noted. There may be a unilateral tender mass. Fever is a rare finding, but progressive anemia is observed frequently. Newer, more sensitive pregnancy tests are usually positive in most patients with unruptured tubal pregnancy.

The diagnosis of unruptured tubal pregnancy is not difficult to make when classic symptoms are present, but unfortunately, the symptoms are frequently atypical and the pelvic findings misleading. A high index of suspicion is the most valuable adjunct. Culdocentesis may reveal considerable dark old blood, and laparoscopy may allow visualization of the ectopic pregnancy. Other confounding diagnoses include complete spontaneous abortion, incomplete spontaneous abortion, or threatened abortion. Salpingitis and appendicitis usually present with signs of infection and without prior amenorrhea.

When this diagnosis is suspected, a sensitive pregnancy test should be done to determine whether human chorionic gonadotropin (hCG) is elevated. If the test is positive, a quantified assay should be obtained. If the hCG titer is in excess of 2000 mI.U. per ml., an intrauterine pregnancy, if present, should be seen by transvaginal ultrasonography. The finding of an intrauterine pregnancy in such a setting likely excludes ectopic pregnancy in all but the very rare patient who might have simultaneous intrauterine and ectopic pregnancies. Failure to note an ectopically placed pregnancy with ultrasonography is not diagnostic but warrants follow-up, probably with laparoscopy. In patients in whom the initial value of hCG is less than 2000 mI.U. per ml., alternate-day hCG assays for quantified values should be obtained. In normal pregnancy, hCG doubles every 48 hours during that interval of pregnancy.

Failure to show this rise supports the diagnosis of an abnormal pregnancy, either a missed abortion, an incomplete abortion, or possibly an ectopic gestation. All these studies should be utilized in the subtle case. Occasional patients may be treated successfully nonsurgically with methotrexate.

45

THE URINARY SYSTEM

David F. Paulson, M.D.

The urinary system consists of the paired kidneys, the paired ureters, the bladder, and the urethra. Diseases of the urinary system may be variously classified as congenital or acquired, benign or malignant, inflammatory or noninflammatory. It is important to have an understanding, therefore, of the signs and symptoms of urologic disease, of the diagnostic studies available to confirm or deny the presence of disease, and of the therapeutic modalities available to the clinician.

SIGNS AND SYMPTOMS OF UROLOGIC DISEASE

Usually, pain or bleeding is the initial indicator of disease involving the urinary tract. Renal pain is usually dull and aching and localized to the flank. This is most common when the pain is caused by inflammation; however, when produced by stone or acute bleeding, the pain may be sharp, localized to the flank, or radiate into the lower abdomen, the side, or the buttocks. The pain, when episodic, usually is associated with ureteral obstruction. Ureteral obstruction can produce symptoms of an acute abdomen with severe abdominal pain, nausea, and vomiting. As the pain or calculus that produces the pain moves distally in the ureter, the pain will radiate from the flank to the lower abdomen, occasionally radiating to the scrotum or labia majora and sometimes into the thigh. A calculus in the lower ureter or at the junction of ureter and bladder may cause urinary frequency with urgency and painful urination. Bladder pain usually is dull, aching, and localized to the suprapubic region.

PHYSICAL EXAMINATION AND DIAGNOSTIC STUDIES

While inspection of the abdomen may disclose a lower abdominal mass when the bladder is full and unable to empty, in adults, neither the distended bladder nor the hydrone-phrotic obstructed kidney is easy to define. In the child, the bladder is an intra-abdominal organ and is easily palpated. Further, because of the relative size differential in children and adults, the child's kidney is easily palpated and transillu-minated. When the kidney is tense from intrarenal bleeding or inflammation, sudden pressure in the area of the kidney in both adults and children may produce pain.

A urinalysis demonstrating either white blood cells, red

See the corresponding chapter or part in the *Textbook of Surgery,* 15th edition, pp. 1524–1551, for a more detailed discussion of this topic, including a comprehensive list of references.

blood cells, or bacteria will confirm the presence of infection or bleeding within the urinary tract. Renal function is determined by blood urea nitrogen and serum creatinine. The voided urine may be examined for the presence of malignant cells by Papanicolaou staining of the spun sediment.

IMAGING OF THE URINARY TRACT

Once a working diagnosis has been established by history, physical examination, and specific laboratory studies, it may be necessary to obtain disease-oriented imaging studies. Current techniques include excretory urography with nephrotomography, retrograde ureteral pyelography, arteriography, venacavography, computed tomography, ultrasonography, and magnetic resonance imaging. The most commonly used imaging study is the excretory urogram. This study depends on renal function and visualizes the urinary tract by concentration of intravenously injected organic iodine within the urinary tract. The contrast material is excreted primarily by the kidneys. The kidney and its collecting system become radiopaque as x-rays are absorbed by the iodinated agent. Retrograde ureteral pyelography and cystography involve the direct placement of iodinated contrast agents into the ureter or bladder. These studies should be avoided during acute infection, since instillation of the iodinated contrast material under pressure may precipitate a systemic infection by forcing bacteria into the lymphatics and venules of the bladder and kidney. Arteriography involves the injection of vascular contrast agents directly into the renal artery and allows an analysis of the vascular pattern of the kidneys. Renal angiography may be indicated whenever a vascular malformation is suspected or whether malignancy may be present. Digital venous angiography and venacavography are alternative methods of observing the vascular supply of the kidneys. Computed tomography, magnetic resonance imaging, and ultrasonography plus radioactive renography are noninvasive methodologies that permit visualization of the kidneys and identification of pathologic processes that may involve either the kidney or ureter.

NONSURGICAL/INFLAMMATORY DISEASES OF THE URINARY TRACT

The patient with acute urinary tract infections usually has symptoms related to site and severity of the infection. The most frequent urinary tract infection is *cystitis,* an infection within the bladder. Patients with cystitis have urinary frequency, painful urination, urgency, suprapubic pain, and hematuria. Pyelonephritis occurs when the infection itself involves the kidney. *Acute pyelonephritis* is accompanied by flank pain, fever, chills, and occasionally nausea and vomiting. Acute pyelonephritis differs from acute cystitis in that patients with bacterial cystitis usually do not have fever and chills. The diagnosis of urinary tract infection is supported by urinalysis demonstrating white blood cells and bacteria and confirmed by a positive culture.

Surgical diseases of the urinary tract are most commonly urinary tract calculi or malignancy. Congenital malformations are much less common, usually being diagnosed in infancy. The symptoms of urinary tract calculi are flank pain, cramping, and abdominal discomfort radiating to the groin, scrotum, or labia with microscopic hematuria. A plain film of the abdomen usually will identify the location of the stone and direct a form of intervention. The intravenous pyelogram determines whether the stone is totally or partially obstructing and identifies any associated anatomic abnormality. While calculus disease of the urinary tract was treated in the past primarily by open surgical removal of the offending calculus, new technology permits the treatment of almost all urinary tract calculi without the need for open surgery. Currently, urinary tract calculi involving the kidney and/or ureter may be managed alternatively by extracorporeal shock wave lithotripsy, based on the principle that shock waves, generated in a fluid media, can be focused through that fluid media and through the human body to impact and destroy calculi within the urinary tract. Percutaneous ultrasonic lithotripsy utilizes ultrasonic sound waves, transmitted down a hollow tube, to destroy calculi within the kidney or ureter. Laser energy, delivered through flexible catheters, also will pulverize stones within the ureter and/or kidney. Thus, using these noninvasive techniques, open stone surgery for the management of renal calculous disease is rarely performed.

Acquired diseases of the urinary tract consist primarily of malignant or traumatic disease. Malignant diseases of the urinary tract encompass carcinoma of the kidney, ureter, and bladder. Renal adenocarcinoma is the most common malignancy involving the kidney, occurring most often in the fifth decade of life, with an incidence three times higher in males than in females. Three histopathologic types of renal adenocarcinoma are identified: clear cells, granular cells, and spindle-shaped cells.

EVALUATION OF RENAL MASS LESIONS

Renal mass lesions should be evaluated carefully. Using a systematic approach to the identification of renal mass lesions, approximately 85% can be identified correctly by a combination of only two sequential examinations. The most frequent asymptomatic renal neoplasm is metastatic tumor, with carcinoma of the breast being the most common. Only 2.2% of asymptomatic space-occupying lesions of the kidney are primary renal cell malignancy. Renal cell carcinoma is treated by surgical removal of the kidney and the associated tumor, the adrenal gland, the surrounding perinephric fat, and Gerota's fascia, along with regional lymph nodes. Surgery is more effective when the disease is confined to the kidney itself or when it is extended minimally outside the renal capsule. Surgery is less effective once the disease is extended to adjacent structures or regional lymph nodes or when it has invaded the renal vein or vena cava. Surgical removal of the renal primary tumor in patients with metastatic disease has little value. While removal of the primary renal malignancy may provide temporary control of symptoms such as fever, pain, hematuria, anemia, and hypercalciuria, it does not reduce the likelihood of further dissemination of disease. Further, there is no evidence that removal of the primary tumor will either promote spontaneous regression of metastasis or improve the response of metastatic disease to other therapies.

Renal trauma may be classified as either blunt (nonpenetrating) or penetrating. Both blunt and penetrating trauma can be divided into two major classifications: those injuries which involve the parenchyma and those which involve the renal vasculature. In patients who have blunt trauma, fracture of the lower ribs, fracture of transverse processes, or scoliosis on an abdominal film, urologic evaluation is warranted, particularly in the presence of gross hematuria. Patients who have nonpenetrating injury with only microscopic hematuria are not candidates for intravenous pyelography. The incidence of being able to identify an abnormality that requires treatment is so low as to reject intravenous pyelography or contrast evaluation in this specific population. However, patients who have gross hematuria or penetrating injuries must be evaluated to determine the extent of the genitourinary injury. Much debate exists as to the optimal study. Intravenous pyelography has long been the standard screening study. However, computed tomography with contrast is a much more accurate imaging study to determine the extent of the lesion and any associated perirenal bleeding. Computed tomography also allows the clinician to determine the bilaterality of renal function and the amount of gross urinary extravasation.

In patients who have blunt renal trauma, the decision for exploration and repair is made only when the patient demonstrates hemodynamic instability. Even when major lacerations are identified, if the patient is hemodynamically stable, conservative observation is the best form of treatment. However, when the patient has penetrating injury or is felt to have vascular injury, exploration with repair is warranted. Penetrating injuries are associated with other intra-abdominal injuries in four of five patients. Thus, with the exception of those patients who have superficial stab wounds, it is recommended that patients who have penetrating injuries near the kidney should have an intravenous pyelogram and be considered for surgical exploration.

The ureters are protected by the fibrofatty tissue of the retroperitoneum. Their integrity can be threatened by a variety of congenital, inflammatory, traumatic, iatrogenic, and neoplastic diseases. With the exception of malignant disease or congenital obstruction involving the ureter, acquired obstruction by calculus disease usually is managed as described above. Malignant disease of the ureter may be intrinsic or extrinsic. When extrinsic, it is usually associated with malignant disease of other origin and is manifested by progressive renal failure. Intrinsic malignant disease of the ureter is usually manifested by gross or microscopic hematuria and can be identified by intravenous pyelography.

Obstruction of the ureter can be relieved without open surgical intervention. In the patient with either unilateral or bilateral obstruction, internal drainage can be established using a double-J Silastic catheter. These catheters may be inserted either transurethrally from below or percutaneously from above. The Silastic catheters may be left in place for 6 to 12 months with minimal encrustation. They may be removed percutaneously or transurethrally and replaced without difficulty.

Transitional cell carcinoma of the renal pelvis constitutes approximately 5% of all renal carcinomas. Between 80% and 90% of all patients with renal pelvic tumors have either gross or microscopic hematuria. Carcinoma of the ureter usually is a transitional cell tumor. Treatment of ureteral tumors traditionally has been nephroureterectomy with removal of the entire renal unit and ureter. Currently, there is argument to preserve the renal unit by means of local resection of the malignancy only, based on the belief that the salvage rate of patients with ureteral tumors depends more on the biologic aggressiveness of the tumor than on the aggressiveness of the chosen surgical therapy. Patients with high-grade lesions or lesions that have penetrated into the ureteral wall have little chance for cure, even with the most radical surgery. Preservation of the renal unit allows use of nephrotoxic chemotherapeutic agents if the patient later develops metastatic disease.

THE BLADDER

The urinary bladder is a storage organ. In simplest terms, disorders of bladder function can be segregated into disorders of storage and disorders of emptying. The disease processes that produce these disorders of storage or disorders of emptying can be identified by a combination of contrast and urodynamic studies. Urodynamic studies are neurophysiologic studies that assess the neuromuscular response of the bladder to filling and emptying. The normal bladder will fill to a volume of 400 ml. with no increase in pressure, no contractions of the bladder musculature, and without relaxation of the bladder sphincter. At approximately 400 ml., when the patient feels the necessity to void, the urodynamic study will record a spiking increase in bladder pressure and a coincidental relaxation of the bladder sphincteric musculature. When rising intravesical pressure overcomes falling urethral resistance, voiding begins and the bladder empties. Study of the coordinated filling of the bladder, relaxation and then contraction of the detrusor, increase in intravesical pressure during the relaxed and voiding phase, with simultaneous examination of the electrical activity of the urinary sphincters, is necessary to diagnose their neuromuscular disorders that affect either emptying or storage. While no blanket recommendations can be made as to the appropriate management of the various disorders of storage and emptying, when no specific anatomic defect or required surgical correction is identified, it is often possible either to enhance emptying or to facilitate storage by the use of various pharmaceutical agents. The common nonmalignant surgical diseases of the bladder are bladder fistulas, disorders of storage, and vesical trauma.

Bladder Fistulas

Bladder fistulas produce disorders of storage in that the urine is not retained within the bladder. The defect is between the bladder and either the small or large bowel (enteric fistula), the vagina, the uterus, or skin. They usually are of inflammatory, neoplastic, iatrogenic, or traumatic origin. Fifty percent of all vesicoenteric fistulas are secondary to sigmoid diverticulitis. Malignancy accounts for approximately 16% to 20% of all enteric fistulas, with 12% to 15% associated with Crohn's disease. Pneumaturia and fecaluria are the classic signs of vesicoenteric fistula. Pneumaturia is not pathognomonic of an enteric fistula, since gas per urethra may result from the fermentation of diabetic urine, from urinary tract infection by gas-producing organisms, or from urinary tract instrumentation. However, pneumaturia is the presenting sign in two-thirds of patients with vesicoenteric fistula. While fecaluria is diagnostic of vesicoenteric fistula, it occurs in only 20% to 50% of patients. When a fistula is suspected, contrast studies, such as intravenous pyelography, upper gastrointestinal studies, or a barium enema, may be necessary to identify the fistula. Surgical repair usually requires resection of the affected bowel segment and bladder *en bloc* with primary restitution of bowel and a primary bladder closure. Approximately 90% of all vesicovaginal fistulas are secondary to gynecologic procedures. The remaining 10% are a consequence of urologic surgery, extensive pelvic trauma, complications of internal/external radiotherapy, or a direct extension of malignant disease processes. Patients with small fistulas may have an intermittent watery vaginal discharge and appear to void normally, whereas patients with large fistulas may have total urinary leakage through their vagina with no urethral voiding. Most patients complain of a malodorous, watery vaginal discharge. Repair requires excision of the fistula with primary closure.

Disorders of Storage

One disorder of storage occurs when the bladder may not distend due to chronic inflammatory disease involving the bladder wall. In such instances, bladder augmentation using either ileum, cecum, or sigmoid may increase the bladder capacity and facilitate storage. Urinary incontinence is another disorder of storage, occurring most frequently in the aging female. Total incontinence is the continuous leakage of urine, with the bladder functioning only as a urinary conduit. However, the most frequently encountered form of urinary incontinence is that of stress urinary incontinence. This occurs in females through a loss of closing urethral pressure secondary to loss of pelvic floor support and shortening of urethral length. Stress incontinence is evidenced by leakage of urine during cough or straining. This must be segregated from urge incontinence, in which the patient gets spasm of the bladder musculature and leakage as a result of conscious stimuli. Techniques devised for the control of stress urinary incontinence in the female consist primarily of urethral lengthening procedures. These may be done either transvaginally or suprapubically. When there is damage to the sphincteric muscle in males, due to either previous surgery or trauma, artificial inflatable urinary sphincters under volitional control can be used to restore continence.

Vesical Trauma

Vesical trauma can be divided into trauma with and without pelvic fracture; penetrating injuries, either high- or low-velocity, and iatrogenic trauma. Each requires identification and repair. Retrograde urethrography and cystography should be used to determine the nature and extent of the bladder rupture. Once a bladder rupture has been identified, surgical exploration, identification of the defect, sharp excision of the devitalized tissue, and primary repair are appropriate.

CARCINOMA OF THE BLADDER

Approximately 90% of all bladder malignancies are transitional cell tumors, reflecting their origin from the transitional cells that line the bladder. Hematuria occurs in approximately 75% of patients with bladder malignancy. The disease may be confused with urinary tract infection, since hematuria also occurs in acute urinary tract infection. Bladder irritability is a presenting symptom in 30% of patients and is thought to be associated with muscle invasive disease. The treatment of transitional cell carcinoma is directed toward removal of all offending malignancy, with therapy based on the anatomic extent of disease. Tumor that has not invaded through the basement membrane of the epithelial surface (intraepithelial) may be controlled by either transurethral resection, fulguration, or use of intravesical agents that promote sloughing of the superficial mucosa. When the disease invades through the basement membrane, the disease must be treated by complete resection of the malignancy. This is best accomplished transurethrally. Radical cystectomy is advised for patients whose tumors demonstrate muscle invasion. Radical cystectomy in the male includes removal of the bladder, prostate, seminal vesicles, and all adjacent perivesical tissues, whereas in the female, radical cystectomy includes the bladder, uterus, tubes, ovaries, anterior vagina, and urethra. Survival rates depend on the grade and stage of the disease rather than on the use of adjunctive therapy, such as radiation, preoperative or postoperative, or chemotherapy, preoperative or postoperative.

When it is necessary to remove the bladder, the bladder may be replaced by either conduit or continent diversion. In conduit diversion, a segment of either large or small bowel is used merely as a conduit to establish rapid transit of the urine to the body surface, where the urine is collected. The continent reservoir utilizes either large or small bowel and provides an internal storage reservoir that is drained by intermittent catheterization of an external stoma created at the skin surface. An alternative to the continent diversion is orthotopic bladder replacement, in which an internal reservoir using either large or small bowel is created and anastomosed to the native urethra. Such a maneuver allows the patient to void volitionally through his or her own urinary passageway.

46

THE MALE GENITAL SYSTEM
John L. Weinerth, M.D., and Cary N. Robertson, M.D.

Unlike the female, parts of the male genital system are conjoined with regard to sexual and excretory functions—specifically, the prostate and the urethra. The components of the male genital tract are the prostate gland, seminal vesicles, Cowper's gland, the penis with its incorporated urethra, and the scrotum containing the testes, epididymides, vas deferens, and spermatic vessels. The male genital system functions for the purposes of sexual intercourse, reproduction, hormonal production, and urinary excretion.

The prostate gland, seminal vesicles, Cowper's gland, and gland of Littré produce secretions that serve to lubricate the system and provide a vehicle for storage and passage of spermatozoa. In addition, secretions of the seminal vesicles as a base and enzymes from the prostate gland and Cowper's gland conjoin to produce coagulation and subsequent liquefaction of the ejaculate. The penis is composed of two vascular erectile bodies. The corpora cavernosa also incorporate the corpus spongiosum, which contains the male urethra. The paired testes produce both testosterone and spermatozoa, the former in the Leydig's cells and the latter in the seminiferous tubules. The epididymides, lying in intimate contact with the testes, serve as an area of maturation and storage of sperm that are further transported along the efferent tract composed of the vas deferens and the ejaculatory ducts, emptying into the posterior urethra at the verumontanum of the prostate.

Since the *testis* arises from portions of the wolffian body on the genital ridge in close proximity to the kidney, the major blood supply of the testis arises from the aorta just below the renal arteries. Venous drainage of the testis is through multiple veins of the pampiniform plexus to the spermatic vein, usually single, emerging from the upper end of the cord and then following the internal spermatic artery through the retroperitoneum. On the right, the spermatic vein empties into the vena cava below the right renal vein, while on the left the spermatic vein empties into the main renal vein. Increased hydrostatic pressure, particularly on the left, may cause dilatation of the pampiniform venous plexus, producing a varicocele.

The *scrotal sac,* consisting of two lateral compartments fused in the midline, denoted by the median raphe, encloses the testes, epididymides, and terminal portions of the spermatic cords. The dartos, consisting of elastic fibers, connective tissue, and smooth muscle fibers, is intimately attached to the skin of the scrotum, rich in sebaceous glands, and provides for muscular contraction of the scrotal sac in response to tempera-

---

See the corresponding chapter or part in the *Textbook of Surgery,* 15th edition, pp. 1553–1572, for a more detailed discussion of this topic, including a comprehensive list of references.

ture changes or sexual excitation. The blood supply of the scrotum comes from the deep pudendal branches of the femoral artery and branches of the internal pudendal artery. The lymphatics of the scrotal halves anastomose freely, surround the penis, and drain to the inguinal and femoral nodes.

The *seminal vesicles* are paired, monotubular, convoluted structures lying beneath the base of the bladder and trigone. The seminal vesicles secrete a mucoid vehicle for the spermatozoa and also elaborate the body's only source of fructose, used as an essential nutrient for maintenance of spermatozoal viability.

The *prostate* is a fibromuscular glandular organ that surrounds the vesicle neck and the proximal portion of the male urethra. The prostate of a normal young adult male weighs approximately 20 gm., consisting of two portions, an anterior (inner) group of glands surrounding the urethra and a posterior (outer) portion. Normal prostatic function depends on androgens, principally testosterone, which is metabolized to dihydrotestosterone.

The anterior (inner) portion, consisting of the periurethral glandular structures, gives rise to the hyperplasia and hypertrophy of benign enlargement in bladder neck obstruction in older men. The posterior segment, a musculoglandular structure, is the most frequent origin of prostatic carcinoma. Operations that deal with benign hyperplasia and hypertrophy leave the posterior (outer) portion of the gland behind.

The male *urethra* consists of two major portions, the posterior urethra and the anterior urethra, each with two subdivisions. Beginning most proximally at the bladder neck, the posterior urethra consists of the prostatic portion and the membranous urethra. The prostatic and membranous portions of the urethra are relatively fixed by the puboprostatic ligaments and the inherent stability of the urogenital diaphragm.

The *penis* serves the dual function of sexual intercourse and excretion of urine. It consists of two parallel erectile compartments known as the *corpora cavernosa* that are situated dorsolaterally and the *corpus spongiosum* that invests the urethra ventrally, terminating distally in the erectile glans penis. The principal blood supply of the penis is through the dorsal arteries, deep to Buck's fascia, being derived from the internal pudendal arteries, branches of the internal iliac artery. The venous drainage is through the dorsal veins, the superficial dorsal vein emptying into the saphenous vein and the deep dorsal vein emptying into the prostatic plexus known as the *plexus of Santorini*.

Infertility can be the consequence of disturbance in either one or both of the primary testicular functions. It is estimated that 15% of marriages in this country are initially barren, with male factors accounting for about 50% of these barren marriages. The principal cause of male infertility is a spermatogenic defect estimated to account for 95% of cases of male infertility or sterility. Oligospermia by definition indicates a sperm count of less than 20 million per milliliter. Azospermia, complete absence of spermatozoa in the ejaculate, may be the cause of total occlusion of the sperm transport system, vas, seminal vesicles, ejaculatory ducts, or germinal arrest.

Infertility may be due to mechanical factors with no defects in spermatogenesis or delivery of spermatozoa. Surgery of the vesical neck, particularly transurethral resection, open wedge resection, or plastic reconstruction, or treatment of a congenital contracture may result in inability of the vesical neck to close with ejaculation, causing the ejaculate to pass in a retrograde fashion into the bladder rather than out through the urethra.

The most common congenital anomalies of the testes relate to anomalous location, although congenital absence of one or both testes may be observed. The term *cryptorchidism*, derived from the Greek *cryptos*, or "hidden," should be reserved for those testes which are truly obscure, usually within the abdominal cavity and not palpable on examination. Cryptorchid or intra-abdominal testes are observed unilaterally or bilaterally in 1% to 10% of male infants. Spermatogenic failure is progressive, and transposition of an intra-abdominal testis to the scrotum should be accomplished before the age of 2 years to ensure production of normal quantity and quality of spermatozoa. There is a very high incidence of carcinoma in abdominal testes, the incidence perhaps being as much as 20 times greater than that of carcinoma in a normally descended testis.

Pyogenic infections of the testis are almost always secondary to spread of infection through the male ductal system, the vas deferens, and the epididymis. Orchitis may be caused by viral infection in association with mumps, usually not until after the patient has reached pubescence. Tuberculous orchitis is almost always secondary to tuberculosis epididymitis, the primary focus within the urinary tract generally being within the kidneys or prostate. Orchitis must be differentiated from testicular tumor with hemorrhage and from torsion of the spermatic cord, both conditions demanding immediate surgical intervention.

Neoplasms of the testis itself are almost always malignant, with the only exception being rare fibromas of the tunica vaginalis and pure Leydig's cell tumors, which are usually benign. In contrast, extratesticular tumors within the scrotum are almost always benign, with the exception of rare rhabdomyosarcoma. The malignant germinal tumors of the testis arise from the totipotential cells of seminiferous tubules and are seen in all ages but predominate in persons between the ages of 20 and 35 years.

Torsion of the spermatic cord is due to an abnormally high attachment of the tunica vaginalis around the terminal cord, allowing the testicle to twist freely within the compartment. Incomplete torsion may cause partial strangulation, effects of which may be overcome if surgical intervention is accomplished within about 12 hours, whereas severe torsion with total compromise of the blood supply may cause loss of testes unless a surgical procedure is effected within about 4 hours. When torsion is treated on one side, the contralateral scrotum also should be explored to correct a similar abnormality often found. Torsion should be differentiated from acute epididymitis, but uncertainty should prompt exploration.

Treatment of epididymitis is medical with appropriate antibiotics. Occasionally, suppurative epididymitis may localize into an abscess and drain spontaneously; usually, surgical intervention should be avoided unless testicular abscess develops.

The *tunica vaginalis,* derived from the peritoneum as the processus vaginalis at the time of testicular descent, is a secretory membrane. Fluid is generated by the serous surface of the tunica vaginalis, fluid formation being enhanced by inflammation or trauma. Fluid within the tunica vaginalis is resorbed at a constant rate through the extensive venous and lymphatic systems of the spermatic cord. Hydrocele, the excessive accumulation of this serous fluid, results when there is increased production or decreased resorption due to inflammation or abnormal lymphatic drainage.

Prostatic infectious agents include the spectrum of gram-negative organisms, gram-positive cocci, gonococci, various mycotic organisms, mycobacteria, *Trichomonas, Chlamydia,* and *Candida* species. The ascending transurethral route of infection is usual, enhanced by urethral abnormalities. Hematogenous and lymphatic routes of access to the prostate, as well as descending infection from the upper urinary tract, have been described, especially with tuberculosis.

Benign prostatic overgrowth is a common cause of bladder outlet obstruction in men over 50 years of age. As the enlargement progresses, the prostatic urethra may become elongated, and the caliber of the prostatic portion of the urethra may actually increase. However, the adenomatous process causes compression of the prostatic urethra, restricting the free flow of urine, sometimes associated with actual mechanical intrusion of a median lobe at the vesical outlet.

The symptoms of benign prostatic hyperplasia are those of mechanical obstruction and the consequences of urinary stasis. With progressive residual urine, infection may occur with purulent cystitis. Similarly, vesical stasis of urine can predispose to the formation of bladder calculi with severe symptoms of dysuria and strangury. Treatment may be effective with new drugs affecting prostatic growth or internal sphincter activity. Surgical treatment still holds the dominant role.

There are standard surgical procedures for removal of the obstructing enlarged portion of the prostate gland. None of these procedures constitutes total prostatectomy; all of them are designed for removal of the adenomatous hyperplastic portion of the gland. These procedures most properly should be termed *prostatic adenectomy* rather than *prostatectomy,* since the true prostate, compressed laterally into a surgical capsule, is retained and may be the origin of later carcinoma.

Adenocarcinoma of the prostate is the most common malignant disease of men, and the incidence of cancer is increasing. One of the unique qualities of prostatic carcinoma is that many tumors produce enzymes, acid phosphatase, and prostatic-specific antigen (PSA) that can be detected in the serum of patients with both early and late disease.

Unfortunately, early symptoms of prostatic carcinoma are lacking. Since the majority of prostatic tumors occur in the periphery of the gland, encroachment of the urethra is a later manifestation of the disease. In essence, the diagnosis of prostatic carcinoma must be based on suspicion. Every man over the age of 50 should have an annual rectal examination and PSA. The finding of abnormal examination or elevated PSA suggests the diagnosis. The treatment of prostatic carcinoma at the present time is selected on the basis of accurate anatomic definition of the stage of the disease. It is the general feeling that local disease that has not escaped the confines of the prostate is best treated by surgical extirpation.

Radical prostatectomy involving removal of the entire prostate and the seminal vesicles can constitute cure. Prostatectomy can be accomplished in the classic perineal fashion or by the retropubic approach during which both pelvic lymphadenectomy and radical prostatectomy can be accomplished at the same time. Extended disease treatment is by hormonal manipulation or chemotherapy. Considering the rapid development of new chemotherapeutic agents, this is an area that may have the greatest impact over the next 10 years on the treatment of metastatic prostatic carcinoma and even as an adjunctive treatment for localized disease.

The most common distal urethral abnormality is urethral meatal stenosis, which usually can be recognized by inspection, suspected when the urinary stream is of poor caliber. In the area of the prostatic urethra, congenital valves usually occur, causing severe obstructive uropathy with decompensation of the urinary bladder, infection, and renal insufficiency unless prompt and adequate treatment is instituted.

Another anomaly of the urethra is called *hypospadias,* which involves varying degrees of failure of complete development of the distal urethra. The urethra may terminate just proximal to the glans (glanular hypospadias), at some point along the penile shaft (penile hypospadias), at the anterior margin of the scrotum (penoscrotal hypospadias), or in the perineum with a bifid scrotum (perineal hypospadias). Often associated with this defect is a severe ventral curvature of the penis, or *chordee,* which results from a fibrous band occurring in the projected course of the urethra.

Epispadias is the failure of development of the anterior wall of the urethra and concomitant failure of dorsal fusion of the penile corpora. *Complete vesical exstrophy,* a rare condition, is always associated by epispadias; epispadias alone with some degree of urinary continence is seen more commonly, although still infrequent.

Traumatic injury of the urethra commonly occurs in association with pelvic fractures but also can occur with injuries to the perineum, gunshot or stab wounds, or iatrogenic injury from instrumentation. Shearing injuries induced by external forces during blunt trauma cause rupture at the urogenital diaphragm in the region of the membranous urethra. Urinary extravasation is noted, often with extensive pelvic hemorrhage. The prostate and bladder may be displaced superiorly, well away from the distal urethra. The diagnosis of urethral rupture must be suspected in every instance of pelvic injury, and unless the patient is able to void clear urine in a normal fashion, a retrograde urethrogram should be undertaken in an aseptic fashion to determine the patency and competence of the urethra.

Carcinoma of the male urethra is rare, with fewer than 1000 cases being documented in the English literature. Malignant lesions occurring in the distal penile portion of the urethra are most often squamous cell carcinoma, while more proximal tumors are transitional cell lesions. Depending on the location of the lesion, partial urethrectomy with or without penectomy may be effective, as well as possible anterior exenteration and lymphadenectomy.

Cancer of the penis is a rare tumor in the United States. The most common form of cancer of the penis is squamous cell carcinoma, although basal cell carcinoma and melanoma have been described. Squamous cell carcinoma constitutes a more difficult challenge and is generally seen in association with chronic balanoposthitis from lack of circumcision, although occasional cases of penile carcinoma have been reported in circumcised persons. Diagnosis is established by biopsy. Treatment consists of partial or total penectomy; a proximal margin-free tumor of at least 1.5 cm. is desirable.

A localized induration of the fibrous investments of the penile shaft (Peyronie's plaque) was first described 100 years ago. A firm fibrotic thickening of the fascia of the corpora cavernosa is observed, usually involving the dorsolateral aspects of the penile shaft or the intracavernous septum between the corpora cavernosa, leading to deviation of the penis that interferes with intromission and coitus. If the patient is totally disabled and has long-term resistant disease, excision of the plaque with skin grafting with or without the insertion of a penile prosthesis is possible.

Prolonged pathologic and painful erection of the penis is termed priapism. Abnormal arterial/venous flow produces priapism and is observed with metastatic malignant diseases of various sorts, such as leukemia, pelvic trauma, sickle cell disease or trait, trauma to the corpora, or spinal cord injury. Prompt recognition and therapy are essential, since prolonged unrelieved priapism almost inevitably leads to subsequent permanent impotence from fibrosis of the corpora cavernosa.

While it is recognized that the aging process diminishes not only the libido but the capacity of erection as well, many men remain potent throughout their lifetime. Impotence may be due to psychological factors, drug effects, or systemic disease. Arteriosclerotic cardiovascular disease and diabetes may compromise circulation to the corpora, and in addition, many of the drugs used to treat hypertension and cardiovascular disease may have a secondary effect on the ability to maintain an erection. New therapies include intracorporal injection of vasoactive drugs and penile prostheses.

The intersex states include ambiguity of the external genitalia and inadequate and incomplete differentiation in gonadal and ductal structures. The most common mode of presentation of the intersex patient is by request for sexual differentiation in the neonatal nursery. Ambiguity of the external genitalia necessitates prompt and definitive assignment of sex, reassurance of parents, and early mobilization of medical and surgical measures required to establish the appropriate sex of the child. On occasion, the intersex patient may be seen rather late, often because of microphallus, undescended testes, labial fusion, or clitoral hypertrophy. The interested reader is referred to a number of definitive texts and monographs dealing with the various types of intersex.

47

DISORDERS OF THE LYMPHATIC SYSTEM

Richard L. McCann, M.D.

The lymphatic system is composed of lymphatic capillaries that collect interstitial fluid and are the site of interstitial fluid absorption throughout the body, transporting vessels, and lymph nodes. Lymphatic capillaries empty into the transporting vessels, which traverse the extremities and body cavities to empty into the venous system via the thoracic ducts. Lymph nodes periodically interrupt these transporting vessels, and the lymph is filtered within the lymph nodes, which serve a primary immunologic function. Lymphatic capillaries are similar to blood capillaries except that large gaps exist between adjacent endothelial cells, which allow particles as large as bacteria, red blood cells, and lymphocytes to pass through the walls. Some tissues such as epidermis, the central nervous system, the layers of the eye, and skeletal muscle have no lymphatic drainage. Other tissues are richly supplied with lymphatic vessels. One of these is dermis. The superficial lymphatic channels of the extremities consist of several valved channels that pass primarily on the medial aspect of the limb and course toward the groin or axilla, where they end in one or more lymph nodes. The vessels are of uniform caliber as they ascend, except for the ampullae, which are the site of the tricuspid valves. The channels form a plexiform network with frequent intercommunications. There is a separate deep lymphatic system with vessels that course deep to the muscular fascia running along with the neurovascular bundles. There is little, if any, communication between the superficial and deep lymphatic systems. Lymph vessels have a well-defined adventitia, a medium containing smooth muscle cells, and a thin intima. The lower extremity lymphatic channels join with the visceral channels to form the cisterna chyle adjacent to the upper abdominal aorta. The cisterna passes through the diaphragm to become the thoracic duct, which itself ascends on the right side of the mediastinum and crosses over to the left at the level of T5 and then joins the subclavian vein.

The circulation of lymph is a complex and incompletely understood process. Interstitial fluid is formed by the flux of plasma across the semipermeable capillary membrane. The exchange of fluid between the capillaries and the interstitial space depends on the hydrostatic pressure within the capillary as well as the osmotic pressure due to the presence of plasma proteins within the vascular space. Throughout the day there is a net efflux of fluid across the capillary membrane that is

---

See the corresponding chapter or part in the *Textbook of Surgery*, 15th edition, pp. 1573–1579, for a more detailed discussion of this topic, including a comprehensive list of references.

eventually returned to the circulatory space by way of the lymphatics. Normal lymph flow is 2 to 4 liters per day. This flow is greatly influenced by local and systemic factors, including protein concentration in the plasma and interstitial fluid, local arterial and venous pressures, and capillary pore size and integrity.

Edema formation occurs when there is an imbalance between the production of interstitial fluid and its transport by the lymphatic system. Excess production occurs when capillary pore size increases such as during local inflammation, if the venous pressure becomes too high because of acute venous obstruction, or if the colloid osmotic pressure becomes too low to reabsorb fluid across the capillary membrane, such as may exist in states of hypoproteinemia. Lymph propulsion is a complex process. Rhythmic contraction of the walls of the collecting ducts propels lymph toward the thoracic duct, as does compression due to active skeletal muscle contraction. Because of the presence of competent valves in these channels, lymph is propelled centrally. Increased abdominal pressure such as coughing or straining also compresses the lymphatic vessels, accelerating the flow of lymph upward.

Extremity swelling due to abnormalities in the lymphatic system are classified as primary and secondary. The primary lymphedemas are relatively common, occurring in 1 in 10,000 individuals, and are classified by age of onset of symptoms. Lymphedema congenita occurs shortly after birth; lymphedema praecox occurs about the time of puberty; and lymphedema tarda has its onset after the third or fourth decade.

The swollen extremity may be studied radiographically by lymphangiography, which requires a cutdown and cannulation of a lymphatic duct with injection of radiopaque contrast media. Alternatively, lymphoscintigraphy, in which a radiolabeled colloid is injected subcutaneously and its disappearance observed by gamma camera imaging, has been found to be more convenient, less expensive, and simpler, and it provides adequate sensitivity and specificity. Most commonly in primary lymphedema, hypoplastic or absent transporting vessels are seen.

Secondary lymphedema occurs due to inflammatory scarring, malignant tumor invasion, or radiation injury of previously functioning lymphatic beds. The most frequent tumors infiltrating lymph nodes causing lymphatic obstruction are carcinoma of the prostate in males and lymphoma in females. The most common cause of secondary lymphedema in Western countries is the combination of surgical excision of lymph nodes and radiation therapy for carcinoma of the breast.

Most patients with lymphedema can be managed nonoperatively with extremity elevation, the use of good-quality elastic support garments, and the use of massage therapy and sometimes mechanical devices for milking fluid toward more healthy regions of lymphatic drainage. Surgical therapy is reserved for disabling leg swelling and elephantiasis. The swollen, fibrotic subcutaneous tissues can be excised, with the resulting defect closed with a split-thickness skin graft. Attempts to bring lymphatic-bearing tissue into the area by pedicle transfer have been disappointing. Some success has been reported in microvascular bridging of lymphatic obstructions with microsurgical creation of lymphatic venous shunts or bridging vein grafts. These techniques remain experimental.

Lymphatic tumors and congenital malformations of lymphatic vessels usually present in infancy or childhood. The lesions usually grow slowly but may infiltrate the local tissues. Malignant degeneration is rare. Cystic hygroma is the most common tumor and is a lymphatic malformation consisting of endothelial-lined cysts. Radiation therapy is ineffective, and the most common treatment is local excision, avoiding injury to adjacent structures.

Lymphangiosarcoma is a rare lesion that may develop in a lymphedematous extremity regardless of the cause of the lymphedema. Malignant degeneration is more frequent in cases of secondary lymphedema. The lesions appear as purple-red nodules in the skin and are very aggressive and usually rapidly fatal.

48

VENOUS DISORDERS
M. Wayne Flye, M.D., Ph.D.

The pathophysiology of venous disease is, in many respects, more complex than that of arterial disease. With the exception of aneurysm formation, obstruction is responsible for virtually all the physiologic aberrations characteristic of arterial disease. Venous pathophysiology, on the other hand, involves both obstruction and valvular insufficiency. Moreover, the disability from venous disease includes not only regional problems but also those which result from the escape of thrombi into the pulmonary circulation.

Varicose veins with their associated symptoms and complications constitute the most common vascular disorder of the lower extremities. More than 20 million people in the United States alone are reportedly significantly affected. Most of these persons have either symptoms or complications from chronic venous insufficiency, and a substantial number suffer economic hardship from the resulting disability.

ANATOMIC AND PHYSIOLOGIC CONSIDERATIONS

Unlike arteries, veins are divided into a superficial and a deep system. Among the thick-walled *superficial veins* are the greater and lesser saphenous veins of the leg, the cephalic and basilic veins of the arm, and the external jugular veins of the neck. The *deep veins*, in contrast, are thin-walled and less muscular and are protected by the muscles and deep fascia. *Perforating veins* connect the deep and superficial systems by passing through the fascial layer that invests the deep system. Even modest motion, however, such as shifting weight, contracts the calf muscles, forcing blood toward the heart in the valved venous system. However, when venous valves are incompetent, the resulting hydrostatic column of blood is longer, and there is immediate retrograde venous filling with muscle contraction. The venous pressure of the lower leg, therefore, remains abnormally high, which predisposes to the development of dependent edema. According to the Starling concept, return of fluid escaping from the arteriolar end of a capillary to the circulation at the venular end is facilitated by lower venous pressures. In the normal situation, any dependent swelling that accumulates during the day usually disappears overnight when the body is horizontal. In the abnormal state, greater edema formation resolves more slowly, results in capillary underperfusion, and predisposes to chronic stasis changes.

See the corresponding chapter or part in the *Textbook of Surgery*, 15th edition, pp. 1581–1593, for a more detailed discussion of this topic, including a comprehensive list of references.

CLINICAL MANIFESTATIONS

Varicose veins, venous thrombosis, and venous valvular incompetence with venous stasis are present in half the adult population. *Varicose veins* are dilated, elongated, superficial veins. Dilatations of the smaller, cutaneous venules are somewhat different and are called *spider veins*. Factors contributing to their development are heredity, congenitally defective venous valves, trauma, hormonal factors in women, increased abdominal pressure in pregnancy, and arteriovenous fistulas. Symptoms may range from cosmetic dissatisfaction to intractable pain. Dull pain and aching usually begin in the afternoon after long standing and are promptly relieved by leg elevation. Itching is a manifestation of local cutaneous stasis and precedes the onset of dermatitis. A burning sensation over the varicose veins is probably caused by local pressure on cutaneous sensory nerves.

Thrombosis of the deep veins is the common pathway to both the immediate problem of pulmonary embolism and the chronic insidious disability produced by venous stasis disease. Factors predisposing to superficial and deep venous thrombosis include stasis of blood, local venous trauma, and systemic coagulation abnormalities (Virchow's triad). *Superficial thrombophlebitis* presents commonly as a linear, indurated, tender subcutaneous venous cord with local erythema. This type of thrombophlebitis occurs most commonly at the site of an intravenous infusion but also occurs frequently in the greater saphenous system below the knee in patients with varicose veins. The diagnosis of *deep venous thrombosis* (DVT), in contrast, is difficult. An accurate diagnosis on clinical grounds alone is possible only about one-half the time. Positive physical findings may include unilateral ankle edema, pretibial venous distention or an increased venous pattern of collateral veins over the upper thigh and groin, increased circumference of the calf or thigh, tenderness over the femoral vein or behind the knee, and discomfort with forceful dorsiflexion of the foot (Homan's sign).

Deep venous thrombosis causes significant swelling of the affected extremity by partially or completely occluding venous outflow. *Phlegmasia alba dolens* (milk leg) usually occurs in postpartum women and produces a cool, pale, swollen limb with impalpable pulses. Therapy for venous thrombosis generally will result in the return of arterial perfusion. In contrast, the near total venous occlusion of *phlegmasia cerulea dolens* (venous gangrene) produces rapidly rising pressure within the affected extremity and eventually obstruction of arterial inflow. This condition is diagnosed by sudden intense pain, massive edema, and cyanosis. If there is no immediate response to elevation of the extremity and heparinization, venous thrombectomy should be considered.

CHRONIC VENOUS INSUFFICIENCY. If recanalization of DVT traps the delicate venous valves, the valveless deep venous system develops venous hypertension, which is the central predisposing feature in the pathophysiology of the postphlebitic state. However, valvular incompetence alone is not enough to produce serious stasis sequelae but must occur in combination with incompetent perforator veins through which the high deep venous pressure in the upright position is transmitted to the superficial tissues. The location of these perforating veins from the malleoli up the lower half of the leg (gaiter area) determines the predilection of this area to the development of stasis changes and ulcers. When the deep venous hypertension is finally transmitted into the superficial veins and tissues, recurrent edema becomes "brawny" and associated with characteristic changes of skin pigmentation and susceptibility to trauma and ulceration. Within 10 years, 75% of patients with untreated thrombophlebitis will develop advanced stasis changes, and 50% will have had stasis ulcers.

DIAGNOSIS

While superficial varicosities are apparent on physical examination, additional studies are necessary to evaluate the patency of the deep venous system and valvular competency. In fact, the deep system is usually patent if there is no history of deep venous thrombosis. Historically, the *Perthes test* indicated deep venous obstruction when compression of superficial varicosities caused increasingly severe, crampy pain. The *Brodie-Trendelenburg test* was the first scientific attempt to evaluate valve function by observation of the speed of venous refilling. Currently, the first evaluation of a patient with suspected deep venous thrombosis or chronic venous insufficiency should be by noninvasive tests. The *duplex Doppler ultrasound* combines B-mode scanning to allow visualization of the vein to be examined with the directional Doppler to detect venous obstruction (forward flow) or valvular incompetence (reverse flow). However, the degree of venous insufficiency cannot be quantitated. Venography will be required to resolve confusing noninvasive results or to delineate the precise location of obstruction (ascending venography) or valvular incompetence (descending venography).

TREATMENT OF VARICOSE VEINS

Both surgical and nonsurgical methods are used in the management of superficial varicose veins. In general, the surgical excision of incompetent veins is the more definitive treatment, because the results are more satisfactory and lasting. Nonsurgical methods are generally reserved for patients who have medical contraindications to surgical treatment, deep venous insufficiency, or very minimal varicosities. Normal prominent superficial veins should not be disturbed or destroyed. These nonsurgical methods include sclerotherapy, elastic support, periodic elevation of the lower extremity, and exercise of the leg muscles. Advances in ablating symptomatic telangiectatic blemishes by sclerotherapy have now largely replaced minor surgical procedures. However, before any treatment is advised, the severity of the varicose problem must be assessed carefully, including determination of the functional status of the deep venous system.

SURGICAL TREATMENT. General indications for surgical

removal of all incompetent superficial veins and perforators are (1) symptoms of aching, heaviness, and cramps, (2) complications of venous stasis such as pigmentation, dermatitis, induration, superficial ulceration, and thrombosis of varicosities, (3) large varicosities subject to trauma, and (4) cosmetic concern. Patients with incompetence of all or most of the deep and perforator venous valves should not be considered for simple vein stripping because recurrence of varicosities is likely. Restoration of deep venous valvular competency by venous valve reconstruction or transposition may prove to be a logical choice for these patients. Finally, patients with deep vein obstruction, regardless of the condition of their venous valves, are the worst candidates for superficial venous ligation and stripping, because stripping of the superficial vein in such a patient may remove the major patent collateral vein and worsen the venous outflow problem. Surgery will not be required for those patients who obtain relief by elastic stocking support, and it should be recommended only for those patients in whom nonsurgical treatment (including compressive stockings or sclerotherapy) is not satisfactory.

TREATMENT OF VENOUS THROMBOSIS

Whereas superficial venous thrombosis is usually a benign, self-limited disease, involvement of the deep venous system is a major cause of morbidity and mortality. While any venous system may be involved, the lower extremities are affected most frequently. The incidence of venous thrombosis is particularly high in older patients undergoing surgery. In the United States alone, Hume and colleagues estimated that at least 140,000 fatal and 400,000 nonfatal cases of pulmonary embolism occur each year.

The treatment of *superficial venous thrombosis* depends on its etiology, extent, and symptoms. While localized thrombophlebitis usually requires only a mild analgesic, such as aspirin, and activity may be continued, more severe thrombophlebitis with increased pain and cellulitis should be treated with bed rest, elevation, and hot compresses. Purulence within the vein or suppurative thrombophlebitis requires immediate and complete excision of all the involved vein and appropriate systemic antibiotics. Upon resolution of symptoms, ambulation is begun with elastic stockings. Pulmonary emboli rarely originate from superficial thrombi. Also, DVT rarely develops in association with superficial venous thrombosis, but superficial involvement frequently occurs in patients with deep venous disease, especially in those with ankle ulceration.

DVT generally begins in the soleus venous plexus of the calf and ascends to the level of the groin. The patient must remain at absolute bed rest until symptoms have subsided and thrombus becomes fixed. Intravenous heparin in a dose to maintain a partial thromboplastin time (PTT) at 70 to 80 seconds for 7 to 14 days will prevent thrombus propagation and possibly pulmonary embolism while natural fibrinolysis occurs. Anticoagulation with sodium warfarin (Coumadin) should be continued for 3 to 6 months. Prevention of chronic venous insufficiency should begin as soon as the diagnosis of DVT has been made. Good, custom-fitted, toe-to-knee elastic stockings, worn whenever the patient is out of bed, must be combined with periods of elevation of the ankles above the heart level during the day to prevent edema. In patients who develop postphlebitic stasis ulcers, periodic application of Unna's paste boots from the toes to the knee is the mainstay of ambulatory treatment. Weekly reapplication of these compressive "boots," combined with elevation of the legs for at least 20 minutes several times each day, will allow healing of 90% of stasis ulcers. For nonhealing ulcers, removal of all superficial varicosities and complete subfascial ligation of all incompetent perforating veins is generally successful. Occasionally, abnormal venous hemodynamics may be improved by venous valvuloplasty or valve transplantation.

49

PULMONARY EMBOLISM

Mark W. Sebastian, M.D.,
and David C. Sabiston, Jr., M.D.

Pulmonary embolism is a common complication of a number of medical and surgical disorders. Its incidence continues to increase, and it is estimated that in the United States more than 600,000 patients develop this complication annually, with approximately 200,000 deaths. A greater number of the population now live longer and are subject to many medical problems that predispose to the development of thromboembolism. The pathogenesis of venous thrombosis is best conceptualized by *Virchow's triad*: (1) *stasis* due to reduced venous flow, (2) *intimal injury* predisposing to thrombosis, and (3) a state of *hypercoagulability*. Venous thrombosis occurs primarily in the iliofemoral and pelvic veins, as well as in the inferior vena cava. Surgical procedures that are especially apt to be complicated by pulmonary embolism include fractures of the hip, prostate operations, procedures on the lower extremities (including amputation), and soft tissue injuries of the legs and thighs. While pulmonary embolism clearly has a tendency to occur postoperatively, most series have shown that the majority of cases are *nonsurgical* in origin and develop as a complication of a serious underlying *medical* disorder. These include congestive heart failure, pulmonary disease, cerebrovascular accidents, carcinomatosis, hypercoagulable states, and many other conditions.

CLINICAL MANIFESTATIONS

The clinical manifestations of pulmonary embolism include three major features: dyspnea, pleural pain, and hemoptysis. The primary clinical signs are tachycardia, tachypnea, fever, rales, clinical evidence of thrombophlebitis, shock, and cyanosis. It should be emphasized that only a third of patients demonstrate clinical evidence of thrombophlebitis, and the remainder are *silent* with no abnormal physical findings in the legs. *Asymptomatic* pulmonary embolism is quite common, as has been documented repeatedly in postoperative patients undergoing routine pulmonary scans.

It is useful to assess each *patient's risk* of thromboembolism prior to major operations. *Low-risk* patients are those undergoing major surgical procedures who are under the age of 40 and all patients undergoing minor surgical procedures. *Moderate-risk* patients are those aged 40 or over undergoing surgical procedures of a duration of less than 30 minutes. *High-risk* patients are those over age 40 undergoing longer operative

See the corresponding chapter or part in the *Textbook of Surgery*, 15th edition, pp. 1594–1607, for a more detailed discussion of this topic, including a comprehensive list of references.

procedures and those with a history of deep venous thrombosis or pulmonary embolism, extensive malignant disease, prostatic operations, and orthopedic and other procedures on the extremities.

DIAGNOSIS

The plain chest film may show evidence of diminished vascular markings of the involved pulmonary vessels (Westermark's sign). However, this finding is seldom of sufficient prominence to be diagnostic. The electrocardiogram (ECG) is usually nonspecific, with only 20% of patients with proven emboli showing any significant ECG changes. When present, the electrocardiographic alterations include atrial fibrillation, ectopic beats or heart block, and enlargement of the T waves, ST-segment depression, and T-wave inversion. Right-axis deviation suggests the presence of massive embolism.

Of great importance is the measurement of arterial blood gases. In nearly all patients with significant pulmonary embolism, the arterial PO_2 is reduced, usually in the range of 50 to 70 mm. Hg, but it may be lower. In perhaps 10% of patients the PO_2 is greater than 80 mm. Hg. Retention of carbon dioxide is also common, causing an increase in PCO_2. *Pulmonary scanning* (ventilation-perfusion) is a very useful screening examination, particularly if the plain chest film is otherwise *completely normal*. Great caution must be exercised in interpreting any pulmonary scan on which there are changes in the plain chest film, since suspicious areas may be caused not only by embolism but by atelectasis, pneumonitis, neoplasm, fluid, emphysematous blebs, or pneumothorax. Ventilation-perfusion scan mismatch and intrapulmonary shunting are important features of pulmonary embolism and are caused primarily by regional atelectasis, bronchoconstriction, and pulmonary edema. A combination of $\dot{V}/\dot{Q}$ mismatch together with shunting produces hypoxemia, hyperventilation, increased pulmonary dead space, and an elevated alveolar-arterial gradient. If the perfusion scan is *normal*, clinically significant pulmonary embolism is excluded.

Pulmonary angiography is the most objective test for the diagnosis of pulmonary embolism and should be performed if the perfusion scan is not conclusive. In general, all patients with an abnormal pulmonary perfusion scan are candidates for pulmonary angiography. This is particularly important if the patient is to be given intravenous heparin, since a definite diagnosis of pulmonary embolism should be established in view of the complications that may follow heparinization. Contraindications include surgical procedures, gastrointestinal bleeding, blood dyscrasias, and many other conditions.

In cases of high clinical suspicion of pulmonary embolism with inconclusive $\dot{V}/\dot{Q}$ scan, diagnosis of deep venous thrombosis can be pursued via Doppler ultrasound of the lower extremities.

Venography is useful in establishing a firm diagnosis of thrombophlebitis in the legs with localization of the thrombi.

It is of particular significance in those patients in whom the diagnosis is in doubt or if interruption of the inferior vena cava is being considered. Radioactive fibrinogen scans of the legs also can be useful in the detection of developing thrombi, but the technique is less accurate in the iliofemoral region due to the background activity of the urinary bladder. Doppler flow studies are relatively simple and may be helpful. Recently, *magnetic resonance imaging* has been demonstrated to be quite sensitive in detecting venous thrombi and is quite reliable. It is especially helpful in demonstrating the pelvic veins, which are known to be difficult to visualize by venography.

PROPHYLAXIS

Prophylaxis of pulmonary embolism is important, especially in patients in high-risk groups. Many prophylactic measures have been recommended, but few have been supported convincingly by randomized studies. The simplest and safest method of prevention is simple *elevation* of the legs. Here gravity is quite effective in rapidly draining blood from the legs to prevent venous stasis. This can be shown easily by inspection of the legs elevated to 20 to 25 degrees and noting the complete collapse of the superficial veins. It has been used quite effectively, particularly when it is made certain that *constant elevation of the legs* is maintained throughout the postoperative course. This is best done in the conscious patient by explaining the necessity and reasons as well as the position directly to the patient. Leg exercises, elastic stockings, and compression devices have each been recommended. Considerable discussion continues to surround the role of prophylactic *low-dose heparin*. While some studies indicate successful prevention, others have been equivocal or negative. In postoperative patients it may cause increased bleeding. Moreover, the recent recognition that it may induce heparin sensitivity with the disastrous consequences of the *heparin-associated thrombotic thrombocytosis syndrome* has encouraged consideration of low-molecular-weight heparin (LMWH) in patients who are candidates for heparin prophylaxis. Another prophylactic measure involves sequential pneumatic compression of the lower extremities. These devices require proper placement preoperatively to offer benefit.

PROPHYLACTIC REGIMES

The *low-dose heparin* regimen consists of 5000 units of heparin administered subcutaneously every 12 hours and 2 hours prior to the surgical procedure. This dosage is continued until the risk of thromboembolism has significantly decreased. Care should be taken to observe postoperative bleeding. *Low-dose warfarin* can be administered preoperatively with maintenance of the prothrombin time 2 to 3 times the INR control value. Abnormal bleeding should be noted in the postoperative period. Antiplatelet agents including aspirin and dipyridamole (Persantine) have been used in prophylaxis with reports of success compared with placebos, but certainty the value of their use has not been established.

ANTICOAGULANT MANAGEMENT OF PROVEN PULMONARY EMBOLISM

Many patients with proven pulmonary embolism and a *stable* cardiovascular status are preferably managed by intravenous heparin by continuous pump-driven delivery. An initial intravenous bolus of 10,000 to 20,000 units should be given, with maintenance infusion of 800 to 1200 units per hour. The activated partial thromboplastin time (aPTT) should be evaluated at 4 to 6 hours and maintained between 1.5 and 2 times control. With an aPTT 2.5 times greater than normal, bleeding is apt to become a complication. Therapy is maintained with a gradual shift to warfarin therapy.

Warfarin anticoagulation can be achieved with the goal of maintaining the prothrombin time at 1.2 to 1.5 times INR control. This generally requires a loading dose of 10 to 15 mg. on the first day and 5 to 10 mg. on the second day. The maximal effect is usually reached in 1.5 to 2 days, and the average daily maintenance dose is between 5 and 10 mg. (range from 2 to 20 mg.). While the recommended duration of warfarin therapy is controversial, most advise a minimum of 6 weeks or continuance for 3 to 6 months. If thrombophlebitis persists, long-term anticoagulation is advisable. Should bleeding complications occur, FFP should be administered acutely. Vitamin K counteracts the effects of warfarin but requires 24 hours to show effect.

If the patient is in stable cardiovascular condition, the therapy is directed primarily toward continuous intravenous heparin, oxygen, and minimal amounts of inotropic agents and vasopressors as necessary. Surveillance is achieved on an intensive care unit. If the patient becomes unstable with hypotension, tachycardia, cardiac arrhythmias, cyanosis, low arterial oxygen saturation, and reduced urinary output, more intensive inotropic agents may be required, as well as tracheal intubation and placement on a respirator.

THROMBOLYTIC AGENTS

Although several thrombolytic agents have been available for many years, only recently has interest been renewed in their role in the management of pulmonary embolism. Three thrombolytic enzymes are being used, streptokinase, urokinase, and recombinant tissue plasminogen activator (rtPA), and may be especially indicated in patients with *massive* pulmonary embolism. Since this is a developing field, specific series and the results are cited. In a multitrial evaluation at eight centers, administration of rtPA was evaluated in 34 patients with acute massive pulmonary embolism. All patients received a bolus of intravenous heparin (5000 I.U.) followed by 1000 I.U. per hour. After 50 mg. of rtPA was given during a 2-hour period, the severity of the embolism as determined by pulmonary arteriograms declined. The mean pulmonary arterial pressures fell, and following an additional dose of 50 mg. of rtPA, the severity of the embolism had decreased by 38% with a further reduction in mean pulmonary arterial pressure.

Streptokinase therapy also may be appropriate in the management of both deep venous thrombosis and thromboembolism. Among 108 patients with phlebographically verified deep venous thrombosis treated with streptokinase, total or partial thrombolysis was demonstrated angiographically in 60 (55.6%). Twenty-two patients showed evidence of allergic reactions due to the foreign protein in streptokinase, and anaphylactic shock was observed in one patient. The dose of streptokinase is 250,000 units intravenously over a 30-minute period followed by 100,000 units hourly for 24 hours. Conventional heparin therapy is then administered intravenously. The incidence of bleeding is slightly higher with thrombolytic therapy compared with heparin or warfarin anticoagulation; nevertheless, its thrombolytic effect is often desirable or urgently needed. In one study using both agents, the results appeared more rapid and safer.

In a multicenter study of 2539 patients with pulmonary embolism it was determined that 1345 (53.5%) surveyed would have been acceptable for treatment with thrombolytic therapy. Risks of major blood loss were the most frequent contraindications to thrombolytic therapy and were found in 838 (33.3%) patients. Potential risk to the central nervous system was found to contraindicate thrombolytic therapy in 453 (17.9%). Similarly, risks of bleeding into special compartments were found to contraindicate thrombolytic therapy in 76 (3%).

SURGICAL THERAPY

Although anticoagulant therapy is usually successful in preventing further pulmonary emboli, occasionally absolute contraindications to anticoagulation or recurrent emboli may occur and raise the possibility of surgical management to prevent further embolization. While various forms of interruption of the inferior vena cava have been advocated, including complete ligation and application of clips and other devices for partial or complete occlusion, the most frequently utilized approach is the transvenous insertion of a conelike umbrella filter designed to prevent large emboli from passing into the upper inferior vena cava. This filter is relatively easily placed, and indications for its use include patients in whom anticoagulation therapy is not appropriate or those in whom fear of repeated embolism is sufficiently great. Although this technique has a low morbidity and mortality, the filters can migrate into the right atrium, right ventricle, and pulmonary artery. They also may perforate the vena cava and migrate to the iliac veins.

In patients with massive pulmonary embolism associated with cardiovascular instability and intractable shock, pulmonary embolectomy with extracorporeal circulation may be indicated. Under these circumstances, a proven diagnosis of pulmonary embolism by arteriography is highly desirable, if not mandatory. Occasionally, pulmonary embolectomy can be performed unilaterally without the use of the heart-lung machine. While the mortality of the procedure ranges as high as 50%, it can be lifesaving.

I

Chronic Pulmonary Embolism
Mark W. Sebastian, M.D.,
and David C. Sabiston, Jr., M.D.

While the vast majority of patients with pulmonary thromboembolism demonstrate resolution of the thrombi with the passage of time, about 0.1% of emboli do not undergo thrombolysis and chronic embolism ensues. Ultimately, these emboli may become so extensive that right ventricular and pulmonary artery hypertension occurs. The disorder may progress to chronic cor pulmonale with severe dyspnea, cyanosis, and right ventricular failure with a fatal outcome. Fortunately, those with emboli in the primary and secondary branches of the pulmonary arteries and with a *patent distal arterial circulation* can now be greatly improved by embolectomy. Distal pulmonary artery patency can be demonstrated by selective *retrograde* bronchial arteriography in which the contrast medium fills the bronchial vessels and passes through the pulmonary capillary circulation into the distal small pulmonary arteries. Postoperatively, patients demonstrate a decrease in pulmonary arterial pressure, increase in pulmonary arterial oxygen saturation, and relief of symptoms. In symptomatic patients, the natural history of this disorder is dismal, with only 20% of those with a mean pulmonary artery pressure greater than 50 mm. Hg alive at 2 years.

II

Fat Embolism Syndrome
Joseph A. Moylan, M.D.

Following fractures and other injuries, fat embolism continues as a major cause of pulmonary decompensation. The

See the corresponding chapter or part in the *Textbook of Surgery,* 15th edition, pp. 1607–1614, for Part I, and pp 1614–1617 (Part II), for a more detailed discussion of this topic, including a comprehensive list of references.

incidence of this syndrome remains 35% in patients involved in multisystem trauma, particularly that secondary to motor vehicle accidents, whereas there are two major theories describing the pathophysiologic mechanism of fat embolization, the mechanical theory and the physicochemical theory. Free fatty acids that arise from either the hydrolysis of neutral fats or the mobilization of fat stores by catecholamines produce alterations in the capillary alveolar membrane as well as in surfactant production. The result of this phenomenon is hemorrhage, edema, and alveolar collapse. Clinical investigation has shown the correlation between elevated free fatty acids and severity of the fat emboli syndrome.

This syndrome can be classified by using the respiratory distress index: $RDI = Pa_{O_2}/F_{I_{O_2}} (VF + PF)$, where VF equals 1 without mechanical ventilation or 1.5 with mechanical ventilation and PF equals 0 when positive end-expiratory pressure (PEEP) is less than 5 cm. H_2O or 0.5 when PEEP is greater than 5 cm. H_2O. The severity of pulmonary dysfunction estimated by this formula correlates with increasing levels of free fatty acids. Clinical studies have been supported by a number of animal experiments. The binding of free fatty acids by albumin also has been demonstrated experimentally as well as clinically to decrease the risk and incidence of fat embolism syndrome.

DIAGNOSIS. The primary clinical manifestations of this syndrome consist of changes in the cerebral, pulmonary, and cutaneous organ systems. Patients exhibit hypoxia, confusion, and petechiae as well as agitation, stupor, and tachypnea with progressive hypoxia. The peak incidence of this syndrome occurs from the second to fourth day following injury, and the diagnosis is usually made by a combination of laboratory and clinical parameters, including a history of multisystem injury, presence of posttraumatic shock, changes in respiratory and cerebral function, and the presence of petechiae. Radiologic changes may be present initially in only 30% of patients with the fat emboli syndrome, but over the subsequent 24 hours almost all develop radiologic abnormalities. Another important laboratory test is arterial P_{O_2}, which frequently falls to less than 60 mm. Hg on room air. Other studies include the presence of fat emboli, fat globules in the urine, and elevated free fatty acid levels.

PREVENTION AND TREATMENT. Prevention can be achieved by careful attention to risk factors following multisystem injuries, particularly the presence of a low circulating albumin level. Since albumin binds circulating free fatty acids, preventive treatment with albumin to maintain a circulating level of 3 gm. per 100 ml. is important. The role of steroids is controversial. Double-blind studies have failed to demonstrate any specific advantage on the outcome of the fat emboli syndrome. Therefore, steroids should not be used routinely, since they increase the risk of infection in a severely injured patient.

Endotracheal intubation and ventilatory support with a volume-cycled respirator with PEEP remain the primary therapy. PEEP increases functional residual capacity and directly decreases pulmonary shunting.

In summary, this syndrome is a frequent sequela of multisystem trauma producing confusion, tachypnea, and petechiae. This syndrome is caused by the vascular and membrane toxicity of unbound free fatty acids. Maintenance of an adequate serum albumin level in the early postinjury period is preventive. When the fat emboli syndrome develops, treatment includes careful attention to maintaining the Pao_2 by using early endotracheal intubation and volume-cycled ventilation with PEEP.

50

DISORDERS OF THE ARTERIAL SYSTEM

I

Introduction

David C. Sabiston, Jr., M.D.

Scientific and technical advances have combined to form the basis of the history of surgery, and prime examples of these are control of the arterial system and introduction of techniques to relieve arterial obstruction. During the past few decades, several quite significant developments have occurred, including the use of vascular autografts, arterial prostheses, extracorporeal circulation, and an improved understanding of the factors that affect endothelium and thrombosis. Considered together, these represent brilliant accomplishments.

Centuries ago hemostasis was achieved by the ancient Chinese with use of bandages and styptics; extremities could be amputated only at the site of gangrene where the blood vessels had thrombosed and would not be subject to hemorrhage when divided. Celsus advocated limited use of the suture to prevent bleeding, but this fell into disuse and was rediscovered by Paré in 1552 when he used ligature instead of the hot cautery in controlling hemorrhage. Carrel was the first to place the direct suture of blood vessels on a firm basis in a study published in 1906, for which he later won the Nobel Prize. The use of saphenous vein as an autograft was first performed by Goyanes in Madrid in 1906. Arteriography of the femoral arteries was introduced by Brooks in 1923; in 1927 Moniz performed carotid arteriography, and in 1929 an abdominal aortogram was first done by dos Santos. This was followed by the use of vascular grafts composed of plastic materials in the early 1950s and by development of extracorporeal circulation in 1953 by Gibbon.

See the corresponding chapter or part in the *Textbook of Surgery*, 15th edition, pp. 1618–1619, for a more detailed discussion of this topic, including a comprehensive list of references.

II

Anatomy

David C. Sabiston, Jr., M.D.

Blood is delivered from the heart by arteries to the tissues, and the arteries are classified as being large, medium-sized, and small vessels. Arteries less than 100 μm. in diameter are arterioles, and their histologic characteristics are largely dependent on the size of the vessels. For example, large arteries, which must withstand the greatest pressure, contain considerable elastic tissue to appropriately control differentials in pressure. Medium-sized arteries have less elastic tissue and more smooth muscle, and at the arteriolar level the elastic tissue is either scant or absent. Collagen is present in all three arterial systems and forms the strongest layer of the vascular wall for the larger vessels as well as the smaller arteries.

It is crucially important to be aware of the natural collateral circulation of tissues and organs, especially in the sequence of events that follows acute arterial occlusion. In addition, the duration of occlusion of an artery is of considerable significance. For example, with slowly progressive arterial occlusion there is sufficient time for collateral vessels to develop and become larger. Generally, as a smaller vessel is subjected to the need for increased flow (primarily due to the pressure gradient), the vessel is likely to become thin-walled and tortuous. This characteristic is easily demonstrated by arteriography, as in chronic occlusion of the abdominal aorta (Leriche's syndrome). Under these circumstances, adequate arterial collaterals develop that join the branches above the occlusion with distal vessels. It is surprising that slowly progressive occlusion of the entire abdominal aorta occurring over a period of time may produce minimal symptoms in some patients, whereas in others it produces the characteristic symptoms of intermittent claudication and impotence. Nevertheless, gangrene of the extremities is rare until late in Leriche's syndrome. However, acute occlusion of the abdominal aorta usually produces disastrous effects with the immediate appearance of severe ischemia, and if the occlusion is untreated, gangrene of the lower extremities ensues.

Of primary significance are the principles of collateral circulation in all aspects of medicine, especially in surgical procedures. All vascular circuits have some natural collateral circulation, although it may vary greatly in different tissues and organs. The subclavian artery usually can be ligated safely in the first portion, as in the performance of a subclavian-pulmonary anastomosis for congenital cyanotic heart disease (Blalock operation), because the collateral circulation around

See the corresponding chapter or part in the *Textbook of Surgery*, 15th edition, p. 1619, for a more detailed discussion of this topic, including a comprehensive list of references.

the shoulder is excellent. It is rare for ischemic symptoms to follow ligation of the subclavian at this site; indeed, with the passage of time, a pulse frequently reappears in the affected radial artery as additional collateral circulation develops. Moreover, three of the four major arteries of the stomach (the left and right gastric and left and right gastric epiploic) can be ligated without significant ischemia. In a number of other arteries the extensiveness of collaterals varies considerably, with ligation producing no ill effects in some patients and ischemic symptoms in others. Some arteries, such as the coronary, renal, and retinal arteries, have very inadequate natural collateral circulations. Acute occlusion of these vessels is usually followed by serious changes of ischemia and infarction.

III

Physiology of the Arterial System, Including Physiology of Nitric Oxide

Mark G. Davies, M.D., and Per-Otto Hagen, Ph.D.

The normal arterial wall consists of three layers: the intima, the media, and the adventitia. Endothelial cells are a confluent monolayer of thin, flattened, rhomboid-shaped cells lining the intimal surface of all blood vessels. Smooth muscle cells are found within the media in association with a matrix of connective tissue components (collagen, elastin, and occasional fibroblasts). In the adult human, the net mass of the endothelium is equivalent to approximately 1% of body mass and has a surface area of approximately 5000 sq. m. The endothelium, as constituted by the endothelial cells and the subendothelium, forms a relatively impermeable surface that limits passive transfer of cellular and fluid elements between the circulating blood and the body's tissue. The subendothelium provides structural integrity, mechanical strength, and elasticity to the vessel and contains primarily collagen fibers. Turnover is usually low within the subendothelium, even though endothelial cells secrete a variety of proteases such as metalloproteases, collagenases, elastases, and gelatinases. This is balanced by the secretion of a series of proteinase inhibitors to metalloproteases (TIMP), gelatinases, and collagenases. Modulation of the connective tissue matrix in the subendothelium by mediation of its synthesis and degradation allows the

---

See the corresponding chapter or part in the *Textbook of Surgery*, 15th edition, pp. 1620–1626, for a more detailed discussion of this topic, including a comprehensive list of references.

endothelium to control the activity of the underlying vascular smooth muscle cells and the structure of the vessel wall. In general, seven families of compounds have been associated with endothelium-mediated vasomotor responses: prostanoids, nitric oxide and nitric oxide–containing compounds, oxygen free radicals, endothelins, angiotensins, smooth muscle cell hyperpolarization factors, and other as yet, uncharacterized endothelium-derived constriction factors.

Smooth muscle cells are the principal cells found in the media of a vessel. They are embedded in a matrix of connective tissue elements and provide mechanical and structural support to the vessel. Physiologically active smooth muscle cells and the extracellular matrix provide intrinsic vascular dimensions and tone. In addition to their vasoreactive characteristics, smooth muscle cells are capable of synthesizing and secreting elements of the extracellular matrix, particularly proteoglycans. The biologic role of the proteoglycans is diverse, ranging from mechanical support functions, cell adhesion, and motility to proliferation. The exact mechanisms whereby smooth muscle cell proliferation is initiated, controlled, reduced, and eventually suppressed are not fully understood. Quiescent vascular smooth muscle cells are well-differentiated cells characterized by an abundance of contractile proteins, predominantly smooth muscle cell actin and myosin but little rough endoplasmic reticulum. Once activated, smooth muscle cells lose their differentiated state; they acquire abundant endoplasmic reticulum and commence the synthesis of extracellular matrix. *Endothelial-derived relaxing factor* (EDRF) is nitric oxide (NO). NO is synthesized from the conversion of L-arginine to citrulline by at least two categories of enzymes—constitutive nitric oxide synthases (cNOS, predominantly membrane-bound) and inducible nitric oxide synthases (iNOS, predominantly cytosolic), both of which are calcium- and calmodulin-dependent and utilize at least five cofactors (NADPH, tetrahydrobiopterin, FAD, FMN, and heme). It is now apparent that NOS activity is modulated by the Ca^{2+} flux into the cell, and recent studies suggest that NO can exert feedback inhibition on NOS to provide further control of its synthesis. This feedback inhibition may be through the interaction of NO with the heme cofactor or by NO-mediated protein phosphorylation of the synthetase. Protein phosphorylation by the cGMP-dependent kinases that are activated by NO-mediated increases in target cell cGMP is the basis of many of the effects attributed to NO. NO shares many of the vasoactive properties of prostacyclin in that it can relax smooth muscle and inhibit platelet aggregation. In the appropriate circumstances, NO can be converted in the endothelial cell to peroxynitrite, a potentially toxic molecule, and some have speculated that this molecule may play pivotal roles in the pathophysiology of several cardiovascular diseases. NO may only be one of several EDRFs present, and compounds such as nitrosothiols and dinitrosyl iron-cysteines, which are more stable than NO, may be responsible for a degree of the relaxation now attributed to NO. Additionally, such compounds would allow NO to be stored intracellularly. NO does not produce membrane hyperpolarization and thus is not the candidate factor for this effect.

The endothelium plays a primary role in the regulation of intravascular coagulation by four separate but related mechanisms: participation in and separation of procoagulant pathways, inhibition of procoagulant proteins, regulation of fibrinolysis, and production of thromboregulating compounds. The focal point for the coagulation cascades is the generation of the enzyme thrombin, which cleaves fibrinogen to form insoluble fibrin clot. The endothelium participates in this cascade by producing a number of cofactors, including high-molecular-weight kininogen (HMWK), factor V, factor VIII, and tissue factor. The basic barrier function of the endothelium separates intravascular coagulation factors (factor VII_a) from tissue factor in the subendothelium and also prevents exposure of platelets to the proaggregating constituents of the subendothelium such as collagen and von Willebrand's factor. Endothelial cells produce and express on their extracellular surfaces small amounts of the proteoglycan heparan sulfate, which serves to localize and increase the intrinsic activity of antithrombin III and LACI (lipoprotein-associated coagulation inhibitor). Endothelial cells inhibit procoagulant proteins with the protein C pathway, an autoregulatory pathway that involves protein C, protein S, and thrombomodulin; it inactivates factors V_a and VIII_a. For fibrinolysis to occur, plasminogen must be converted to plasmin. Endothelial cells bind plasminogen and synthesize the plasminogen activators as single-chain proteins and secrete and then bind them to allow their assembly into functional complexes. There are two forms of plasminogen activators (PA): the urokinase type (uPA) and tissue PA (tPA). *In vivo*, normal endothelial cells express tPA only. However, if stimulated by a variety of cytokines and circumstances, endothelial cells preferentially synthesize uPA and downregulate tPA synthesis. In addition to these two fibrinolytic enzymes, endothelial cells also secrete two PA inhibitors, PAI-1 and PAI-2. Finally, the endothelium is also a source of thromboregulators, which can be defined as physiologic substances that modulate the early phases of thrombus formation: eicosanoids (prostacyclin and thromboxane A_2), NO, and ectonucleotidases. Due to its strategic position, the endothelium is important in the mediation and modulation of both inflammatory and immunologic responses. The process of cell adherence, cell activation, and cell migration involves an interplay between the expression of adhesion molecules by the endothelial cells, leukocyte activation, and local cytokine activity. In general, when endothelial cells are stimulated by either cytokines or thrombin, they also express ELAM-1 (endothelial cell leukocyte adhesion molecule 1) and ICAM-1 (intracellular adhesion molecule 1). Once activated, endothelial cells also produce an enhancement factor, platelet-activating factor (PAF), that modulates the rapid expression of these adhesion molecules. In general, endothelial cells only express major histocompatibility complex (MHC) Class I antigens and when stimulated can express MHC Class II antigens, which modulate the interaction of endothelial cells with circulating lymphocytes. Once endothelial cells express the MHC-II anti-

gen, they can be considered to act as antigen-presenting cells
and can induce a T-cell response. Finally, stimulated endothelial cells can express GMP-140, a surface receptor that preferentially binds platelets. The binding of platelets increases the
local availability of PAF and further accelerates the endothelial
cell expression of adhesion molecules.

In addition to the variety of extracellular matrix proteins
produced by the endothelium, the endothelial cells also produce several regulatory substances that can either be growth
promoting or growth inhibiting. Endothelial cells synthesize
platelet-derived growth factor (PDGF), basic fibroblast growth
factor (BFGF), and insulin-like growth factor 1 (IGF-1). The
precise action of each peptide and the localization of each
receptor subtype are currently being defined; however, it does
appear that many are required to regulate cell proliferation.
In addition to these factors, other endothelium-derived factors, such as endothelin, angiotensin II, and oxygen free radicals, have been shown to be mitogenic for both endothelial
and smooth muscle cells. The endothelium inhibits cell growth
in the wall by the production of the various extracellular
matrix substances [collagen (Type V), glycoproteins, and the
glycosaminoglycans]. Both NO and prostacyclin inhibit cellular proliferation. Endothelial cells are capable of synthesizing
and releasing transforming growth factor β (TGF-β), which in
turn stimulates endothelial cell production of proteoglycans,
collagen, and fibronectin and regulates the receptors for these
proteins. TGF-β also can decrease the secretion of proteases
and increase the formation of protease inhibitors by the endothelial cells, which result in the stabilization of the connective
tissue matrix and the development of mature histologic features.

IV

Arterial Substitutes

Gregory L. Moneta, M.D., and John M. Porter, M.D.

Intensive research has led to development of reasonably
satisfactory arterial substitutes that have in large part been
responsible for the explosive growth of arterial surgery. Arterial substitutes include arterial and saphenous vein allografts,
umbilical vein allografts, arterial and venous autografts, xenografts, and various prosthetic grafts. Because of rejection, degeneration, aneurysm formation, rupture, and infection, xenografts and allografts currently have few clinical applications.

See the corresponding chapter or part in the *Textbook of Surgery*, 15th
edition, pp. 1626–1637, for a more detailed discussion of this topic,
including a comprehensive list of references.

Exceptions include limited use of bovine carotid xenografts for dialysis access and occasional use of umbilical vein allografts for infrainguinal arterial reconstructions.

ARTERIAL AUTOGRAFTS

Arterial autografts have limited but well-defined clinical applications. The obvious disadvantage of arterial autografts is lack of availability and length of usable arteries. Internal mammary autografts provide excellent patency in coronary artery bypass grafting. Internal iliac artery autografts are preferred for renal artery reconstruction in children.

VENOUS AUTOGRAFTS

Venous autografts are the most clinically important small-caliber arterial substitute. Greater saphenous vein is the most frequently used venous autograft for infrainguinal arterial reconstruction. Lower extremity bypasses using autogenous saphenous vein may be performed with two techniques. In reverse vein grafting the vein is removed, reversed to permit arterial flow in the direction of the venous valves, and then sutured in place. Alternatively, an intact ipsilateral vein may be left in its anatomic position and the valves mechanically disrupted by one of a variety of intraluminal devices, so-called *in situ* bypass.

Femoropopliteal saphenous vein autograft primary patency ranges from 80% to 90% at 1 year to up to 75% to 85% at 5 years for both *in situ* and reverse vein bypasses. Saphenous vein grafting to tibial arteries produces patencies 10% to 15% lower than femoropopliteal grafting. Patency is higher when bypass surgery is performed for claudication rather than limb salvage, when there is a widely patent outflow tract, and when the operation is performed with a good-quality vein. Cigarette smoking and the use of a small vein (<4 mm. after distention) adversely affect patency. Postoperative antiplatelet drugs appear to improve graft patency, although the evidence is presently inconclusive.

Pathology of Venous Allografts

Many pathologic alterations within the vein graft may lead to late graft occlusion. These include localized stenoses from clamps, fibrosis of venous valves, and late vein graft atherosclerosis. Fibrointimal hyperplasia, a myoproliferative process that appears to follow the conversion of normally quiescent myointimal and medial smooth muscle cells into actively proliferating secretory myofibroblasts, is the most significant process affecting autogenous vein grafts. The precise mechanism is unknown. It occurs in at least 10% of saphenous vein grafts and is the cause of failure in 15% to 30% of aortocoronary grafts occluding during the first year.

PROSTHETIC GRAFTS

The most widely used prosthetic grafts in clinical use are fabricated from Dacron or polytetrafluoroethylene (PTFE).

Dacron Grafts

Dacron grafts are manufactured by weaving or knitting multifilament texturized polyester yarns. Woven grafts are tightly interlaced with small interstices and low porosity. They leak minimally at implantation but are stiff and difficult to handle. Knitted grafts are softer with larger interstices and must be preclotted prior to implantation. Most modern Dacron grafts have velour surfaces, loops of yarn extending almost perpendicular to the fabric surface. Velour improves the graft handling characteristics and is a scaffold for graft adherence to tissue.

Polytetrafluoroethylene (PTFE) Grafts

PTFE is a semi-inert polymer composed of solid nodes of PTFE with interconnecting fibrils. The surface has an electronegative charge and is thus hydrophobic and more resistant to thrombosis.

Clinical Use of Prosthetic Grafts

Prosthetic grafts function well in arterial reconstructions proximal to the inguinal ligament. Patencies for aortofemoral bypass at 5 and 10 years are 80% to 90% and 60% to 70%, respectively. Axillobifemoral and femorofemoral bypass patency rates are up to 75% at 5 years.

PTFE grafts have received the most interest as an alternative to autogenous vein in infrainguinal reconstructions. When used in the femoral to above-knee popliteal position, the most favorable, PTFE grafts give patency results only about one half that of autogenous vein. They are even more inferior to autogenous vein for infrapopliteal bypass.

Prosthetic Graft Healing

Prosthetic grafts in humans never heal with a living neointima. With the exception of para-anastomotic areas, the luminal surfaces always remain covered with a compacted layer of fibrin.

Complications of Prosthetic Grafting

The most frequent complications of prosthetic grafting are anastomotic neointimal hyperplasia, anastomotic false aneurysms, and infection. Para-anastomotic neointimal hyperplasia is similar to that described for autogenous vein. Both Dacron and PTFE grafts are affected. Anastomotic false aneurysms are of uncertain etiology. Improper suture technique, arterial degeneration, infection, and compliance mismatch may all be important. Graft infection occurs in 1% to 2% of prosthetic grafts. Standard treatment is graft excision with revascularization through clean tissue planes. Morbidity and mortality can be reduced by performing extra-anatomic revascularization before graft excision.

FUTURE CONSIDERATIONS

Current research in graft design and fabrication is directed toward the development of a satisfactory prosthetic graft for small artery bypass and a graft and delivery system for transluminal minimally invasive treatment of aortic aneurysms. Continued improvement in the results of vascular grafting will require better prostheses and, perhaps more important, improved understanding of the processes of fibrointimal hyperplasia, atherosclerosis, thrombosis, and arterial healing.

V

Aneurysms
David C. Sabiston, Jr., M.D.

Aneurysms are localized or diffuse dilations of blood vessels. Most aneurysms involving arteries are *true* aneurysms containing all components of the arterial wall (intima, media, and adventitia). A *false* aneurysm ("pulsating hematoma") is the term applied when the aneurysmal sac is composed only of adventitia. Aneurysms may be either *saccular* or *fusiform*; the saccular aneurysm arises from a distinct portion of the arterial wall with a *stoma*, whereas the fusiform aneurysm is a generalized dilation of the entire circumference of the vessel. Aneurysms tend to form at specific sites and are either *congenital* or *acquired* in origin. Acquired aneurysms may be caused by arteriosclerosis, trauma, infection (mycotic), syphilis, or medial cystic necrosis. Most aneurysms can be managed surgically with excellent results.

See the corresponding chapter or part in the *Textbook of Surgery*, 15th edition, p. 1638, for a more detailed discussion of this topic, including a comprehensive list of references.

ANEURYSMS OF THE SINUS OF VALSALVA

David N. Campbell, M.D., John H. Calhoon, M.D., and Frederick L. Grover, M.D.

Sinus of Valsalva aneurysms are dilatations of the aortic sinuses of Valsalva that may rupture into a cardiac chamber, the pulmonary artery, or the pericardium. These aneurysms occur secondary to acquired or congenital disease.

ACQUIRED ANEURYSMS OF THE SINUS OF VALSALVA

Acquired sinus of Valsalva aneurysms occur secondary to subacute bacterial endocarditis, Marfan's syndrome, chronic dissection of the aorta and other degenerative lesions of the aortic root, atherosclerosis, and syphilis. Those associated with endocarditis are repaired usually at the time of aortic valve replacement by obliterating the orifice of the aneurysm. Atherosclerotic aneurysms usually are repaired with a Dacron patch. Those aneurysms caused by cystic medial necrosis or degenerative lesions of the aortic root usually require total replacement of the aortic root and valve with a composite graft and reimplantation of the coronary arteries. This can now be accomplished with a 5% operative mortality.

CONGENITAL ANEURYSMS OF THE SINUS OF VALSALVA

ETIOLOGY AND PATHOPHYSIOLOGY. The pathologic process of congenital aneurysms involves a separation between the aortic media and the heart at the anulus fibrosus of the aortic valve. There is a higher incidence in the Asian population, but the reason is unknown. The incidence varies from 0.23% to 0.69% of all cardiac procedures. These aneurysms frequently rupture into an intracardiac chamber, producing a sudden left-to-right shunt. The most common sinus involved is the right sinus, which commonly ruptures into the right ventricle and less frequently into the right atrium. The noncoronary sinus is the next most frequent site, and it usually ruptures into the right atrium. There have been unusual reports of rupture of the left sinus into all four chambers and the pulmonary artery. Associated intracardiac defects are frequently present, the most common of which are ventricular septal defect and aortic regurgitation.

CLINICAL PRESENTATION. The majority of patients are asymptomatic until the fistula ruptures. With rupture, the usual symptoms are dyspnea, palpitations, and chest pain.

See the corresponding chapter or part in the *Textbook of Surgery,* 15th edition, pp. 1638–1642, for a more detailed discussion of this topic, including a comprehensive list of references.

The symptoms are sometimes associated with dizziness, peripheral edema, and orthopnea and are usually accompanied by a precordial thrill, with a continuous murmur heard loudest over the second to fourth intercostal spaces to the left of the sternal border for those that communicate with the right ventricle and over the right third and fourth intercostal spaces for those that rupture into the right atrium. Pulse pressures are increased, and the murmur of aortic regurgitation may be present. Approximately one third of patients have a sudden onset of symptoms, sometimes associated with strenuous activity. Patients whose fistulas rupture into the pericardium present in cardiogenic shock with signs of cardiac tamponade.

Nonruptured aneurysms rarely cause symptoms due to compression of adjacent structures. Obstruction of the right ventricular outflow tract produces signs of right-sided heart failure. Aneurysms can cause acute myocardial infarction or unstable angina by compressing a coronary artery. Left ventricular obstruction has occurred when an aneurysm protrudes into the left ventricle. Ventricular tachycardia and heart block also have been reported, as well as thrombosis and cerebrovascular emboli.

Chest roentgenograms usually reveal increased pulmonary vascular markings with enlargement of the right side of the heart and prominence of the main pulmonary arteries. Common electrocardiographic changes are left ventricular hypertrophy, right ventricular strain, axis shift, and biventricular hypertrophy. By use of transesophageal color-flow Doppler echocardiography techniques, it is possible to visualize the aneurysm and to identify a fistula, if present, in more than 95% of patients. Cardiac catheterization has been helpful in delineating the anatomy of the aneurysm and identifying and quantitating the shunt but is no longer necessary in many cases.

TREATMENT. The presence of a fistula involving the sinus of Valsalva is considered an indication for operation because of progressive heart failure leading to death. Those patients who have an asymptomatic nonruptured aneurysm of the sinus of Valsalva should be managed conservatively but followed closely.

The fistula can be approached via the chamber into which it ruptures, through the aorta, or by a dual approach via the aorta and the chamber of entry of the fistula. Right ventricular fistulas also can be approached through the pulmonary artery. The dual approach is probably best. The advantage of the aorta-cameral approach is that the fistula can be probed from the aorta into the chamber involved and closed at both its origin and termination with an apparent decrease in recurrent fistula. The aortic valve can be inspected and protected from improperly placed sutures and repaired or replaced if significant insufficiency is present. The ventricular septum can be inspected carefully for the presence of a ventricular septal defect, which, if present, is closed.

RESULTS. In one review, the operative mortality was 12.7%, with failure to close the fistula in 1.6% and a favorable result in 85.7% of patients. Seventy per cent of the patients who died had an associated cardiac abnormality. More recent series report an operative mortality of 0% to 13% with an almost negligible reoperation rate. Death is most often related to uncontrolled sepsis in the acquired aneurysms. Actuarial survival at 25 years has been reported at 86%.

TRAUMATIC ANEURYSMS OF THE AORTA

Walter G. Wolfe, M.D.

The incidence of traumatic rupture of the aorta has increased markedly with the development of high-speed motor vehicle accidents. The method of injury is trauma of the chest, which may produce rib or sternal fractures, pulmonary contusion, and/or pulmonary lacerations. The high-speed automobile accident produces a deceleration injury that appears to be tearing of the aorta, which is also seen in patients who fall from appreciable heights. In sudden deceleration of the body at the time of impact with differential rates of deceleration of the thoracic organs, the thoracic aorta and the great vessels can cause a tear that involves the intima and the media. The tear may be partial or complete. Eighty per cent of patients with rupture of the aorta into the pleural space die at the scene of the accident. Associated injuries are an important component of high-speed motor vehicle accidents and include head injuries, closed and compound long bone fractures, and injury to the viscera including the liver and spleen.

The diagnosis should be suspected in an individual who has had a sudden decelerating accident, especially if there is a widened mediastinum and/or fracture of the first rib. In these patients, aortography should be done to establish the diagnosis of a traumatic rupture of the aorta. In acute transection, when the diagnosis is established, the patient is resuscitated and other critical injuries are assessed and treated.

Immediate repair of the aorta is recommended. Generally, the operation is done through the left chest with repair and/or grafting of the transected aorta. Bypass or shunting procedures may be used, with avoidance of systemic heparinization because of problems with associated injuries and bleeding.

MANAGEMENT OF CHRONIC TRANSECTION. Some patients survive transected aorta and present with an enlarging aneurysm, which is considered a chronic transected aortic aneurysm. Usually the finding of this lesion is an indication for surgical therapy, since over time it increases in size and ruptures later. The results and mortality for managing future transections are usually less than 10%, and death is usually related to associated injuries. Complications include bleeding and paraplegia, which may be associated with spinal injury at the time of the accident. On rare occasions, the ascending aorta may be injured, and the approach is through a median sternotomy with cardiopulmonary bypass and repair of the

See the corresponding chapter or part in the *Textbook of Surgery,* 15th edition, pp. 1642–1647, for a more detailed discussion of this topic, including a comprehensive list of references.

transected ascending aorta. Occasionally there may be associated valvular injuries also, which must be corrected.

DISSECTING ANEURYSMS OF THE AORTA

Walter G. Wolfe, M.D.

Dissecting aortic aneurysms are classified as DeBakey Type I, Type II, or Type III; Type I or Type II originates in the ascending aorta, and Type III originates in the distal subclavian. Other classifications divide these into ascending and descending dissecting aneurysms. They also may be acute or chronic. Aortic dissection is one of the most common catastrophic events involving the aorta and is a common cause of sudden death that may go undiagnosed without an autopsy. Acute dissection of the ascending aorta usually produces aortic insufficiency and may rupture into the mediastinum and/or pericardium, producing tamponade. Varying degrees of coronary as well as cerebral insufficiency may be seen. Dissection of the descending aorta may rupture into the left chest and commonly involve the entire length of the distal aorta, thereby involving the viscera to varying degrees.

CLINICAL PRESENTATION. Pain is the most frequent symptom in patients presenting with acute aortic dissection located in either the ascending or descending aorta. The patients are usually seriously ill and may have severe aortic insufficiency with pulmonary edema as well as diminished pulses. Differential diagnosis is myocardial infarction, rupture of sinus of Valsalva, aneurysm, cerebral vascular accident, acute surgical abdomen, pulmonary embolism, or arterial thrombosis at the bifurcation of the aorta. A high index of suspicion is necessary. The chest film usually reveals a widened mediastinum. The diagnosis is made by aortography, computed tomography, or, on occasion, transesophageal Doppler echocardiography. Survival of undiagnosed, untreated dissection is extremely low. By 48 hours, only 50% of the patients are alive. Management of this condition is control of hypertension if it is present.

If an aortic dissection originates in the ascending aorta, immediate operation with grafting of the ascending aorta with correction of the aortic insufficiency is the main operative intervention. In those patients with descending dissection, if the blood pressure is controlled and the patient is pain-free and there is no evidence of rupture or leak in the pleural space, continued observation with medical management and control of hypertension can be the primary therapy. If there is evidence of expansion or leak, left lateral thoracotomy with partial cardiopulmonary bypass and grafting of the descending thoracic aorta should be done.

See the corresponding chapter or part in the *Textbook of Surgery,* 15th edition, pp. 1647–1655, for a more detailed discussion of this topic, including a comprehensive list of references.

Treatment of chronic dissections is similar, with resection and grafting of the aneurysm with use of Dacron in both the ascending and descending thoracic aorta. Usually, in the chronic state in the ascending aorta, if there is aortic insufficiency, a valve replacement is necessary. Long-term follow-up has been excellent in those patients treated appropriately. Surgical mortality for acute ascending dissections is between 10% and 20%, and the long-term survival approaches 50%. In patients with descending aortic dissections, the mortality again is 10% or less with excellent long-term outlook.

ANEURYSMS OF THE THORACIC AORTA

Walter G. Wolfe, M.D.

The thoracic aorta consists of the ascending aorta, aortic arch, and descending thoracic aorta. The etiologic factor of thoracic aortic aneurysms today is most commonly atherosclerosis. However, cystic medial degeneration, myxomatous degeneration, and dissection trauma with a false aneurysm occurring most commonly at the ligamentum may be seen. Syphilitic aortitis is unusual today, but formerly it was a common cause. The incidence of thoracic aortic aneurysms increases with age, at which time cystic medial necrosis may accompany degenerative changes seen with atherosclerosis. Marfan's syndrome is best known through the finding of cystic medial necrosis as the etiologic basis for its degenerative nature and aneurysm formation in these patients.

Thoracic aneurysms present as an asymptomatic finding on chest film or perhaps with chest pain or pressure as a presenting symptom. Patients may experience hoarseness, superior vena caval syndrome, and tracheobronchial obstruction. Aneurysms of the ascending aorta may present with aortic insufficiency and cardiac failure. Diagnosis is made by use of the chest film, computed axial tomography, or arteriography. Surgical therapy for thoracic aneurysms began in 1953 with the method of local excision. Today the techniques are well established with use of cardiopulmonary bypass, deep hypothermia where necessary with resection and grafting of the aneurysm, and repair of the associated structures. The mortality is approximately 10%.

ASCENDING AORTIC ANEURYSMS. These aneurysms are usually degenerative and include the aortic root, anulus, and leaflets. Certain aneurysms may be seen at the sinus of Valsalva, which may rupture into one of the chambers of the heart. Anuloaortic ectasia, another commonly presenting condition, also involves the sinuses and the anulus; it is usually accompanied by aortic insufficiency and commonly seen in Marfan's disease. Usually, the operation of choice is the

See the corresponding chapter or part in the *Textbook of Surgery*, 15th edition, pp. 1655–1658, for a more detailed discussion of this topic, including a comprehensive list of references.

Bental operation with replacement of the aortic valve and ascending aorta with a composite graft with reimplantation of the coronary arteries.

TRANSVERSE AORTIC ARCH. The transverse aortic arch constitutes that portion of the aorta including the innominate, carotid, and subclavian vessels. Patients with this disorder are difficult to manage, and the operation performed is usually through a median sternotomy on cardiopulmonary bypass and deep hypothermic circulatory arrest. The aneurysm is replaced, and reconstruction of the arch vessels is done with use of a Dacron graft. This treatment has a mortality of 10% to 15% with occasional significant neurologic complications occurring because of prolonged circulatory arrest.

DESCENDING THORACIC AORTA. The descending thoracic aorta is that segment from the left subclavian to the diaphragm. The incidence of aneurysms is second only to those seen in the infrarenal abdominal aorta. The etiologic factor is most commonly atherosclerosis. The patient may present with chest pain, hoarseness, cough, and occasionally hemoptysis or dysphagia. The treatment is resection and grafting of the aneurysm, usually with use of a synthetic woven Dacron graft. The operation is done through the left chest with the use of femorofemoral bypass, heparin-bonded shunts, or left atrial aortic bypass. These techniques are used to reduce left ventricular strain as well as to maintain good flow to the viscera and spinal cord. The most serious complication of operation on the descending thoracic aorta is paraplegia. Today, aneurysms of the descending thoracic aorta can usually be treated with a mortality of less than 10%. The long-term survival has been excellent, with 5-year survival approaching 70%.

ANEURYSMS OF THE CAROTID ARTERY

Richard H. Dean, M.D.

The most frequent site of carotid artery aneurysms is the common carotid artery, particularly its bifurcation. The middle and distal portions of the internal carotid artery are the next most common sites. Aneurysms at the bifurcation are usually fusiform, whereas those located in the internal carotid artery are usually saccular. Atherosclerosis is responsible for 46% to 70% of all carotid artery aneurysms. Trauma and previous carotid artery surgery are less common causes.

The most common serious risk associated with carotid artery aneurysms is transient ischemic attacks and stroke. Most such central nervous system defects are caused by embolization of laminated thrombus lining the wall of the aneurysm. Less commonly, cerebral symptoms are caused by diminished

See the corresponding chapter or part in the *Textbook of Surgery*, 15th edition, pp. 1658–1660, for a more detailed discussion of this topic, including a comprehensive list of references.

flow through the carotid artery secondary to its compression by the mass of an adjacent saccular aneurysm. Rupture of carotid artery aneurysms is rare.

Elongation with kinking of the carotid artery is the most frequently found lesion masking as a carotid artery aneurysm. Usually, this lesion presents as a pulsatile mass at the base of the right neck, typically in hypertensive elderly women. This mass is easily distinguished from an aneurysm by the fact that the pulsation is along the long axis of the vessel.

Duplex sonography with B-mode imaging usually confirms or excludes the presence of an aneurysm of the extracranial carotid artery. However, high internal carotid artery aneurysms cannot be assessed accurately by this method owing to the limitations in visualizing that region. Computed tomography or magnetic resonance imaging is a useful substitute for B-mode imaging for the diagnosis of such lesions when they are located high in the neck. Angiography remains the definitive diagnostic test on which to base therapy. Visualization of the entire length of both extracranial and intracranial components of the carotid artery and the vertebrobasilar system is required for any treatment strategies to be adequate.

Because most carotid bifurcation aneurysms are associated with a redundant internal carotid artery, resection of the aneurysm and reanastomosis of the internal carotid artery are employed in about 50% of cases. Most of the other aneurysms are treated by resection and interpositional placement of either a saphenous vein graft or a polytetrafluoroethylene graft. Occasionally, a saccular aneurysm can be treated by resection and lateral arteriorrhaphy or patch angioplasty. When resection of the aneurysm is impossible, ligation of the internal carotid artery remains the only therapeutic option. If test clamping of the vessel is tolerated, ligation can be performed at a single stage. If it is not tolerated, extracranial-to-intracranial bypass can provide improved collateral perfusion to allow ligation. Gradual occlusion (over several days) with a Crutchfield clamp also continues to be useful. With either technique, anticoagulation for 10 days to 2 weeks is necessary to reduce the frequency of propagation of the distal clot into the collateral cerebral circulation.

CAROTID BODY TUMORS

Richard H. Dean, M.D.

Carotid body tumors are uncommon paragangliomas located at the carotid bifurcation. Most are benign, but approximately 5% metastasize. Cells of the carotid body producing such tumors are of mesodermal and third branchial arch and neural crest ectodermal origin. Although most are found as single tumors without association with tumors at other sites,

---

See the corresponding chapter or part in the *Textbook of Surgery*, 15th edition, pp. 1660–1662, for a more detailed discussion of this topic, including a comprehensive list of references.

occasionally they may have an autosomal dominant pattern of familial occurrence.

Most commonly, a carotid body tumor presents as a painless mass that is palpable at the carotid bifurcation. Large tumors may become painful and produce dysphagia, hoarseness, or even disturbance of tongue function by pressure or involvement of adjacent cranial nerves. Diagnostic studies may include computed tomography of the neck, but the definitive diagnostic study remains selective cerebral arteriography. The characteristic arteriographic appearance is that of an oval, hypervascular mass located between and widening the angle between the origins of the internal and external carotid arteries.

The preferred *treatment* of carotid body tumors is resection. Most small tumors can be removed without entering or resecting the carotid bifurcation. Since the cells producing the tumor are located in the outer region of the media, the tumor can usually be resected by entering and developing a subadventitial plane in the respective vessels of the carotid bifurcation. Large tumors may require resection of the bifurcation area and either patch closure of the defect or placement of an interposition graft. A few tumors are unresectable, and in these instances, radiation therapy may have some value. Resection can be achieved with minimal morbidity and mortality. Current results should include a combined incidence of major neurologic deficits and operative deaths that is less than 2%.

SUBCLAVIAN ARTERY ANEURYSMS

David C. Sabiston, Jr., M.D.

Atherosclerosis and trauma are the most common causes of subclavian aneurysms, and they may develop with the thoracic outlet syndrome as poststenotic dilatation of the subclavian artery. A common complication of these aneurysms is the presence of mural thrombi, and thromboembolism of the upper extremity may be a serious problem. Rupture of the aneurysm also may occur. Appropriate treatment is excision of the aneurysm with restoration of arterial continuity, which may require the use of a graft.

See the corresponding chapter or part in the *Textbook of Surgery*, 15th edition, p. 1662, for a more detailed discussion of this topic, including a comprehensive list of references.

VISCERAL ARTERIAL
ANEURYSMS

David C. Sabiston, Jr., M.D.

Visceral arterial aneurysms include those of the splenic, celiac, gastroduodenal, pancreaticoduodenal, and gastroepiploic arteries. Splenic artery aneurysms are the most common, particularly in females during pregnancy, and rupture is a recognized complication. Approximately half the women with these aneurysms have had six or more pregnancies. Whereas most are due to medial degeneration of the arterial wall. Fibromuscular dysplasia is also an etiologic factor. Mycotic aneurysms usually follow sepsis and are often the result of splenic emboli caused by subacute bacterial endocarditis. Pain in the left upper quadrant that may radiate to the left subscapular region is the most common symptom. Rupture is the most serious complication. A diagnosis can be made at times by the presence of a calcified lesion on the abdominal film and confirmed by arteriography. In one series of 40 ruptured splenic artery aneurysms, 10 were fatal. Operation is generally recommended when the aneurysm is discovered, especially those which are 2 cm. or greater in diameter. The procedure is excision of the aneurysm with ligation of the artery proximally and distally. Splenectomy is not necessary, since there is adequate collateral circulation for preservation of the spleen.

Aneurysms of the celiac artery are relatively uncommon, with clinical manifestations primarily being vague abdominal discomfort, with rupture as the most serious complication. These aneurysms generally should be excised when diagnosed.

Hepatic artery aneurysms rarely present with signs and symptoms similar to those of gallbladder disease. Occasionally, hematemesis or melena may follow erosion of the aneurysm into the gastrointestinal tract. Free rupture into the peritoneal cavity is the most serious complication and is frequently fatal because of massive blood loss. Surgical extirpation is recommended when the diagnosis is made. About 20% of these lesions are located within the liver and may be difficult to excise. Resection with use of a venous graft for preserving arterial continuity for prevention of hepatic ischemia is the operation of choice. Gastroduodenal, superior mesenteric, and pancreaticoduodenal artery aneurysms are uncommon, and most present with rupture as the first indication of a problem. Resection is the procedure of choice, and in some instances multiple exclusion ligation can be performed.

Renal artery aneurysms are generally located in the main renal artery or the bifurcation of the primary branches. A few are intrarenal and may be difficult to expose. Saccular

---

See the corresponding chapter or part in the *Textbook of Surgery*, 15th edition, pp. 1662–1665, for a more detailed discussion of this topic, including a comprehensive list of references.

aneurysms are more frequent than are fusiform, and the primary risk is free rupture into the peritoneal cavity. Clinical manifestations include symptoms of hypertension and upper abdominal pain. Multiple aneurysms also occur. The diagnosis is established by arteriography, and the management is excision of the aneurysm following diagnosis.

AORTIC ABDOMINAL ANEURYSMS

David C. Sabiston, Jr., M.D.

Because of their tendency to rupture, aortic abdominal aneurysms are dangerous if not treated appropriately. Dubost excised the first aortic abdominal aneurysm in 1951 and replaced it with an aortic hemograft from a cadaver. Since then, thousands of patients have had successful corrections, and today the aorta is generally replaced with a Dacron graft.

Untreated abdominal aortic aneurysms have a dismal natural history, and for this reason, nearly all aneurysms 5 to 6 cm. or more in diameter should be corrected soon after diagnosis. Prior to correction of aortic abdominal aneurysms, 102 patients seen at the Mayo Clinic before 1950 were followed, with 67% surviving 1 year, 49% surviving 3 years, and 19% surviving 4 years, with similar findings reported by others. If an aortic abdominal aneurysm is *symptomatic*, approximately 30% of these patients succumb within 1 month, and 75% are dead by 6 months. These statistics indicate the importance of early operative correction.

The symptoms of aortic abdominal aneurysm vary from those which are *asymptomatic* to those with sudden rupture with excruciating pain and profound shock due to blood loss retroperitoneally or into the peritoneal cavity. The *physical examination* of patients with asymptomatic aneurysms reveals the presence of a pulsating mass generally located between the xiphoid process and the umbilicus. About 95% of these aneurysms arise distal to the renal arteries. The inferior mesenteric artery arises from the abdominal aorta, usually at the site of the aneurysm, and is frequently severely stenotic or totally occluded owing to atherosclerosis in the aortic wall. This causes prominent development of collateral vessels, which anastomose with the inferior mesenteric artery distal to the obstruction. The iliac arteries also may be involved with aneurysms either unilaterally or bilaterally, and the femoral arterial system may show evidence of atherosclerotic disease with diminished or absent pulses in the groin and in the popliteal, posterior, tibial, and anterior tibial arteries. Increased attention has been given to the occurrence of inflammatory aortic abdominal aneurysms. These are characterized by aneurysms surrounded by dense periaortic inflammation

See the corresponding chapter or part in the *Textbook of Surgery*, 15th edition, pp. 1665–1673, for a more detailed discussion of this topic, including a comprehensive list of references.

and at times involvement of surrounding structures such as the duodenum, renal vein, and ureter. This problem occurs in about 7% to 10% of patients undergoing aneurysmectomy.

The size of the aneurysm together with its exact anatomic location are usually revealed by appropriate diagnostic studies. The wall of the aneurysm may be calcified, showing the "eggshell" appearance on the abdominal film, and the lateral film is quite helpful in confirming this point. Ultrasonography is a useful diagnostic procedure that provides objective information concerning the diameter of the aneurysm. Computed tomography is also helpful and permits delineation of the aortic lumen and aneurysmal thrombus with contrast enhancement. Aortography is the most definitive diagnostic technique and reveals the luminal size and extent of the aneurysm, the site of its anatomic location, and its relationship to the renal arteries and lesions within them, as well as to the distal circulation, including the presence of aneurysms, stenoses, and arterial occlusion. It is important to recognize the presence of *suprarenal* involvement of the aneurysm, because this is likely to change the surgical approach and increase the risk factors of operation. Although aortography is not essential, it is quite helpful, especially in localizing sites of renal and peripheral vascular disease.

Aortic abdominal aneurysms are associated with a number of complications, and these constitute the most significant problems. Since size is known to be related to rupture, it is important to recognize that with aneurysms greater than 8 cm. in diameter, the mortality ranges between 72% and 83% if such lesions are simply followed. Other complications include distal embolization of the iliofemoral arterial system with thrombi from the aneurysm, sudden thrombosis of the terminal aorta, infection, chronic consumptive coagulopathy, development of an aortic-intestinal fistula, and development of an aortic–vena caval arteriovenous fistula. In the preoperative assessment, careful attention should be given to cardiac function with a Holter monitor recording for 24 hours if there is concern regarding the presence of ischemic myocardial disease. In some patients, the extent and effects of coronary atherosclerosis may warrant myocardial revascularization before resection of the aortic aneurysms. The treatment of aortic abdominal aneurysms is surgical, with correction of the aneurysm and replacement with a prosthetic Dacron graft. The operation is usually performed through a midline incision extending from the xiphoid process to the symphysis pubis. An incision in the left flank with a retroperitoneal approach also has been recommended for patients who have had previous abdominal procedures when dense adhesions might represent a serious technical problem. In these circumstances, the retroperitoneal approach can be preferable in the management of smaller aneurysms and those located in the midportion of the abdominal aorta between the renal arteries and bifurcation. However, prolonged postoperative incisional pain may be a complication in some patients with this approach. The intestines are drawn toward the right and carefully protected while the retroperitoneum is incised over the aneurysm. After thorough identification of the site of the aneurysm and its relationship to the renal arteries, the aorta proximal to the aneurysm is occluded, as are the iliac vessels distally. The aneurysm is incised, and a Dacron graft is then inserted with an end-to-end anastomosis. A bifurcation graft is used when there is aneurysmal involvement of iliac arteries. The excess aneurysmal sac is excised, and the remainder is used to close over the graft to protect it from adherence to the duodenum and small intestine postoperatively. Prophylactic antibiotics are administered several hours preoperatively and for several days after operation.

For ruptured aortic abdominal aneurysms, emergency operation must be performed immediately. Blood loss should be replaced rapidly with restoration of a normal blood pressure and blood volume. A Swan-Ganz catheter should be inserted to monitor pulmonary arterial wedge pressure such that volume replacement fluids and blood can be administered appropriately. If the patient has been resuscitated, the ruptured aneurysm can be managed successfully. Renal failure and cardiac problems often complicate the postoperative course and are related to the severity and length of preoperative hypotension and shock. Aggressive postoperative management, including careful monitoring of cardiovascular dynamics, is helpful in achieving a favorable result. In most series, the mortality of ruptured aneurysms varies between 30% and 50%.

The most common serious associated problem is *myocardial insufficiency,* and careful monitoring is necessary, particularly in patients with a known history of coronary artery disease. Paralytic ileus is a common complication that should be managed by the use of a nasogastric tube. Occasionally, bleeding may occur from the graft and require blood replacement or reoperation for control. Infection of the graft, usually at the suture lines, is another postoperative problem that occurs in approximately 1% to 2% of patients. The treatment is quite extensive and usually requires reoperation with removal of the original graft and insertion of an axillobifemoral graft in a subcutaneous tunnel away from the previous graft site. If a new arterial prosthetic graft is placed at the site of the former graft, it usually becomes infected and necessitates another procedure. Other postoperative problems include changes in *sexual function* such as retrograde ejaculation and reduction or loss of sexual potency. These facts should be made known to patients preoperatively. Spinal cord paralysis is uncommon with aortic abdominal aneurysm, since the circulation to the spinal cord is rarely involved with lesions of the abdominal aorta, in contrast to those in the thorax.

Replacement of aortic aneurysms with a plastic prosthesis is associated with excellent results, and the mortality is less than 5% for elective procedures, with figures of 1% or less being reported. Fatalities are usually due to associated atherosclerotic lesions, including myocardial infarction, cerebrovascular disease, and renal disease. In a recent study, the 5-year survival was 72% for patients less than age 70 years at the time of operation. Thus nearly all patients with aneurysms 5 cm. or more in diameter should undergo elective operation to reduce the morbidity and mortality. For ruptured aneurysms, an emergency operation is the only hope for survival.

Recently, attention has been directed toward a less invasive procedure for insertion of aortic grafts by the transfemoral route, making an abdominal incision unnecessary.

FEMORAL ARTERY ANEURYSM

Raymond G. Makhoul, M.D.

Femoral artery aneurysms, the second most common type of peripheral aneurysms, can be grouped into two categories: true and false aneurysms. True aneurysms involve all three layers of the arterial wall and are largely secondary to atherosclerotic degeneration. They have a high association with abdominal aortic and popliteal aneurysms and occur bilaterally about 50% of the time. Those femoral artery aneurysms limited to the common femoral artery are called *Type I*, while those involving the orifice of the deep femoral artery are termed *Type II*. Femoral false aneurysms are most commonly iatrogenic, occurring after percutaneous cannulation of the femoral vessels, or anastomotic, secondary to the gradual disruption of an anastomosis of a graft to the native artery. Iatrogenic false aneurysms occur with a frequency of 0.6% to 1.0% of catheterizations and are associated with the use of large-bore catheters, anticoagulant therapy, or inadvertent cannulation of the superficial or deep femoral arteries. They consist of perivascular hematoma with a central area that remains fluid. Femoral anastomotic aneurysms are seen 1.5% to 3.0% of the time and are most frequently associated with previous aortobifemoral bypass grafting.

CLINICAL MANIFESTATIONS AND DIAGNOSIS

Approximately 25% of atherosclerotic femoral aneurysms are asymptomatic, while the remainder present with symptoms ranging from arterial ischemia, local compression of the femoral nerve or artery, or groin pain. The ischemic symptoms may be secondary to embolism or thrombosis of the aneurysm. Rupture is rare and occurs in less than 2% of patients. Diagnosis is usually made by physical examination of a pulsatile groin mass, and ultrasound is the most useful confirmatory test. Iatrogenic false aneurysms are usually symptomatic and present as a pulsatile groin mass. Color-flow duplex ultrasound is very useful in the diagnosis of these lesions. These aneurysms may thrombose spontaneously, rupture, expand rapidly, or produce femoral vein or nerve compression. Anastomotic false aneurysms present as pulsatile groin masses,

See the corresponding chapter or part in the *Textbook of Surgery*, 15th edition, pp. 1673–1675, for a more detailed discussion of this topic, including a comprehensive list of references.

with symptoms secondary to local compression or leg ische-mia due to embolism or thrombosis. Ultrasound is used to make the diagnosis, and arteriography is performed prior to repair.

TREATMENT

Surgical repair is indicated for all symptomatic atherosclerotic femoral aneurysms and for those which are asymptomatic and greater than 2.5 cm. in diameter. The surgical technique involves replacement of the aneurysm with a graft, usually synthetic. For aneurysms involving the deep femoral artery (Type II), reimplantation of that vessel may be necessary. The results of femoral artery aneurysm resection are excellent, with a very low morbidity and mortality.

Iatrogenic false aneurysms are best treated with ultrasound-guided compression. With this technique, thrombosis of the perivascular hematoma can be achieved about 90% of the time, with a very low incidence of recurrence. Surgery is indicated for very large or ruptured aneurysms and consists of direct suture repair of the unsealed puncture site.

Anastomotic false aneurysms tend to embolize or thombose and thus should be repaired surgically. Very small aneurysms (<2 cm.) may be followed with relative safety, however. Repair of these aneurysms involves obtaining proximal control of the aortobifemoral graft limb and then interposing a new segment of graft material between the old graft and the femoral artery.

POPLITEAL ANEURYSMS

Raymond G. Makhoul, M.D.

Popliteal aneurysms are the most common type of peripheral arterial aneurysms. The etiology of popliteal aneurysms is atherosclerosis in 95% of cases. Other rare causes include popliteal artery entrapment by the gastrocnemius muscle, bacterial infection, collagen disorders, and trauma. These aneurysms typically present in the seventh decade of life, with a male-to-female ratio of approximately 30:1.

Popliteal aneurysms occur bilaterally in about 50% of cases, and there is an increased incidence of associated abdominal aortic, iliac, and femoral aneurysms in these patients. Conversely, the incidence of popliteal aneurysm in patients presenting with abdominal aortic aneurysm is about 6%.

CLINICAL MANIFESTATIONS AND DIAGNOSIS

The majority of popliteal aneurysms present with symptoms. Leg ischemia, ranging from claudication to limb-threat-

See the corresponding chapter or part in the *Textbook of Surgery*, 15th edition, pp. 1675–1678, for a more detailed discussion of this topic, including a comprehensive list of references.

ening gangrene, is the most common manifestation and is due to thrombosis of the aneurysm, embolization to the tibial vessels, or a combination of these. Less commonly, large popliteal aneurysms may cause local compressive symptoms such as venous obstruction or nerve impingement with pain and tenderness. Unlike abdominal aortic aneurysms, rupture is rare, occurring less than 5% of the time. The diagnosis of popliteal aneurysm is principally clinical and requires a high degree of suspicion. Particular attention should be paid to those patients with a contralateral popliteal aneurysm or a strong family history of aneurysmal disease. Most popliteal aneurysms present as pulsatile popliteal masses or as firm, nonpulsatile masses if they are thrombosed. Some may be diagnosed by plain x-ray if there are vascular calcifications in the wall. The diagnosis is best confirmed with ultrasound, which documents the size of the aneurysm and the presence or absence of mural thrombus. Arteriography is indicated prior to operative repair of these aneurysms.

TREATMENT

The treatment for all *symptomatic* aneurysms is surgical. For *asymptomatic* aneurysms, there is some controversy. A reasonable approach is that operative therapy should be considered when they reach 2 cm. in size in a patient who is a good operative risk. The aim of operation for popliteal aneurysm is to eliminate the aneurysm from the circulation while restoring blood flow to the leg. The surgical procedure of choice is ligation above and below the aneurysm with bypass, preferably using autogenous saphenous vein. Occasionally, with large aneurysms causing local compressive symptoms, resection of the aneurysm with grafting may be necessary. This operation, however, is associated with a higher morbidity due to the associated dissection in the popliteal space. In patients with acute thrombosis of a popliteal aneurysm and limb-threatening ischemia, intra-arterial thrombolytic therapy in addition to operative repair may be an option. This therapy, usually consisting of urokinase infusion, is aimed at clearing the tibial and pedal vessels of thrombus and may be administered either preoperatively or intraoperatively. The long-term results of surgery for popliteal aneurysm depend on the nature of the aneurysm (symptomatic versus asymptomatic), the quality of the distal runoff vessels, and the type of graft employed.

VI

Thrombo-Obliterative Disease of the Aorta and Its Branches*

David C. Sabiston, Jr., M.D.

Atherosclerosis is the most frequent cause of occlusive disease of the major branches of the aorta. The most susceptible site for stenosis or occlusion is at the *origin* of vessels where the *turbulence* is maximal. When branches of the aortic arch such as the innominate, carotid, and subclavian vessels become stenotic or occluded, the symptoms produced are caused by ischemic disturbances due to reduction in blood flow.

The surgical management is by prosthetic bypass grafts. More specific indications such as those involving the carotid, subclavian, and axillary arteries are separately described.

TAKAYASU'S ARTERITIS†

David C. Sabiston, Jr., M.D.

Takayasu's disease was described originally by a Japanese ophthalmologist and is a nonspecific arteritis that affects the thoracic and abdominal aorta and its major branches. Although uncommon in the United States, it is often seen in Asia and occurs predominantly in young females but also in older women and men as well. The arteritis involves all layers of the arterial wall with proliferation of connective tissue and degeneration of elastic fibers. Granulomatous lesions may be present with associated fusiform or saccular aneurysms. This arteritis may be localized to the aortic arch and great vessels (group I) or to the local thoracic and abdominal aorta (group III) or involve the entire aorta (group II).

Symptoms and signs include those which are systemic with production of fever, malaise, and arthritis. Pericardial pain, tachycardia, and vomiting also may occur. Some believe this disorder to be an autoimmune disease, and steroids may be beneficial. The late manifestations are those of ischemia to the arterial circulation of the brain and upper extremities. Surgical treatment often has proved disappointing because the site of endarterectomy or bypass subsequently may be involved in recurrent disease. Operation is occasionally recommended for patients with disabling symptoms.

---

*See the corresponding chapter or part in the *Textbook of Surgery*, 15th edition, p. 1678, for a more detailed discussion of this topic, including a comprehensive list of references.

†See the corresponding chapter or part in the *Textbook of Surgery*, 15th edition, pp. 1679–1681, for a more detailed discussion of this topic, including a comprehensive list of references.

CAROTID ARTERY OCCLUSIVE DISEASE

Richard H. Dean, M.D.

Although the association of carotid artery disease and stroke had been suggested for over 130 years, intensity of interest developed with the introduction of reliable, safe arteriography and techniques of operative correction.

Three causes of transient ischemic attacks (TIAs) and stroke stem from occlusive disease of the extracranial carotid artery. These are thrombosis and propagation of distal clot, low flow-related ischemic events, and embolization from the atherosclerotic lesions at the carotid bifurcation. The most frequent cause is embolization from the atherosclerotic lesion with occlusion of an intracerebral branch. The clinical presentations of carotid artery occlusive disease can be categorized into three general groups: asymptomatic lesions, lesions producing TIAs, and those lesions that have produced cerebral infarction.

Asymptomatic patients are those who have a hemodynamically significant lesion or nonocclusive ulcerated lesion of the carotid artery but no history of cerebral symptoms.

The importance of an asymptomatic carotid artery stenosis should be emphasized, since serial studies using serial duplex scanning show an annual 4% rate of recurrent symptoms. Progression of a lesion to more than 80% stenosis, however, has a 35% risk of ischemic events or total occlusion within 6 months.

By definition, TIAs are temporary neurologic deficits lasting less than 24 hours and followed by complete recovery. When in the area supplied by the carotid artery, they are usually discrete motor and/or sensory dysfunctions. Contralateral facial, arm, and/or leg motor weakness or sensory loss is the classic presentation. Since the left hemisphere is dominant in 95% of the population, left hemispheric TIAs also may cause either receptive or expressive aphasia. Probably the most classic TIA of carotid artery origin is transient visual loss or blurred vision (amaurosis fugax) in the ipsilateral eye. It is classically described as a curtain being drawn down over the eye or as a quadrant field defect and is caused by embolization to the retinal branches of the ophthalmic artery, the first major intracranial branch of the internal carotid artery. In addition, the first clinical manifestation of carotid artery disease may be a permanent neurologic deficit or stroke. Depending on the area of cerebral cortex affected, the defect may range from minimal, with ultimate recovery of the lost function, to massive, causing death.

Initial evaluation of an asymptomatic cervical bruit is best achieved with duplex scanning. Cerebral arteriography is required if a severe lesion is found and in all patients evaluated

---

See the corresponding chapter or part in the *Textbook of Surgery*, 15th edition, pp. 1681–1685, for a more detailed discussion of this topic, including a comprehensive list of references.

following the onset of TIAs or stroke. In the last two groups, computed tomographic scanning of the head also is required to assess the cerebrum for the presence and size of infarcts and to exclude other pathologic intracranial processes.

Carotid *endarterectomy* is indicated for treatment of patients with asymptomatic lesions that reduce the luminal diameter 80% or more, patients with hemispheric TIAs, and patients with either retained or regained significant residual functioning cortex after a completed stroke associated with carotid bifurcation occlusive disease.

Current results of carotid endarterectomy should include less than a 5% combined cerebrovascular morbidity and operative mortality. Most current series have combined morbidity and mortality in the asymptomatic patient group of less than 3%. Obviously, the preoperative neurologic status of the patient affects the incidence of immediate perioperative events as well as the late results.

SUBCLAVIAN STEAL SYNDROME

Anthony D. Whittemore, M.D.,
and John A. Mannick, M.D.

The subclavian steal syndrome occurs when there is reversal of flow in the ipsilateral vertebral artery distal to a stenosis or occlusion of the proximal subclavian or, more rarely, the innominate artery. Because of the reduction of pressure in the subclavian artery distal to the obstruction, blood flows antegrade up the contralateral vertebral artery, into the basilar artery, and retrograde down the ipsilateral vertebral artery to supply collateral circulation to the upper extremity. Thus blood supply is presumably "stolen" from the basilar system and may compromise regional or total cerebral blood flow.

Classically, the subclavian steal syndrome should be suspected in a patient who manifests symptoms of vertebral basilar arterial insufficiency and is found to have a difference in the brachial systolic blood pressure of at least 30 mm. Hg between the two arms associated with a bruit in the supraclavicular area on the affected side. The neurologic symptoms reported in these patients most commonly include vertigo, limb paresis, and paresthesias, but the subclavian steal phenomenon frequently may be clinically asymptomatic. The diagnosis of subclavian steal is established with retrograde catheter angiography, during which the tip of the catheter is positioned in the aortic root and a delayed filming sequence demonstrates retrograde flow in the ipsilateral vertebral vessel.

Since the subclavian steal syndrome is rarely symptomatic in the absence of associated extracranial lesions and, contrary to internal carotid artery lesions, rarely causes stroke, the

---

See the corresponding chapter or part in the *Textbook of Surgery*, 15th edition, pp. 1685–1689, for a more detailed discussion of this topic, including a comprehensive list of references.

more threatening extracranial lesions should be repaired either initially or concomitantly with reconstruction for subclavian steal. In patients in whom the subclavian steal syndrome appears to be responsible for symptoms of vertebrobasilar insufficiency in the absence of other lesions in the extracranial cerebral arterial circulation, however, surgical correction of the lesion appears warranted.

A number of surgical procedures have been recommended for correction of subclavian steal, including simple ligation of the ipsilateral vertebral artery, aortosubclavian artery bypass graft, and subclavian endarterectomy utilizing a mediastinal or transthoracic approach. The carotid-subclavian bypass carried out through a transverse cervical incision is associated with less morbidity than the transthoracic approach. The clavicular head of the sternocleidomastoid muscle is divided, and the exposed scalene fat pad is swept inferiorly to expose the phrenic nerve coursing from lateral to medial over the anterior surface of the anterior scalene muscle. With gentle medial traction of the phrenic nerve, the scalene muscle is divided near its insertion on the first rib, allowing mobilization of the midsegment of the subclavian artery. The common carotid artery just deep to the sternal head of the sternocleidomastoid muscle and medial to the internal jugular vein is mobilized for a sufficient distance to accommodate a short arteriotomy. A 6- to 8-mm. graft is sutured end to side to the common carotid artery, delivered deep to the internal jugular vein, and anastomosed end to side to the subclavian artery. Thirty-day operative mortality is generally in the range of 2%, and 5-year graft patency rates approach 95%, with relief of symptoms in the vast majority.

The subclavian-carotid transposition has become the procedure of choice for many surgeons since the mid-1980s. The subclavian artery is divided just distal to its proximal stenosis or occlusion, and the proximal end is oversewn. The distal end is transposed and sutured end to side to the common carotid artery to perfuse both subclavian and vertebral systems. While the procedure requires more extensive mobilization of the proximal subclavian vessel, the necessity for a graft is obviated. Overall patency rates after 5 years approach 99%, with minimal operative morbidity and mortality.

THROMBOTIC OBLITERATION OF THE ABDOMINAL AORTA AND ILIAC ARTERIES (LERICHE'S SYNDROME)

David C. Sabiston, Jr., M.D.

Leriche's syndrome is the result of thrombotic obliteration of the terminal abdominal aorta, often involving the iliac vessels, due to underlying atherosclerosis on which thrombus is superimposed. The process is usually one of slow but progressive involvement. The duration of the pathologic process provides ample time for multiple collateral vessels to develop between the aorta proximally and the iliofemoral system distally, thus allowing reasonable circulation to the lower extremities. However, with the passage of time and continuously increasing obstruction, symptoms appear.

SIGNS AND SYMPTOMS. Symptoms characteristic of Leriche's syndrome include (1) fatigue in both lower limbs and thighs, which often has been described as weariness rather than typical intermittent claudication, (2) atrophy of both lower limbs without atrophic changes in the skin or nails, (3) pallor of the legs and feet, and (4) inability of males to maintain a stable erection owing to inadequate arterial flow to the penis.

Physical findings include absence of pulsations in the abdominal aorta and in the distal arteries. This disorder is often well tolerated for 5 or even 10 years, but ultimately, ischemia and gangrene ensue. Therefore, surgical therapy should be performed when symptoms are marked and before severe ischemic changes occur in the legs.

Clinical examination and arteriography usually confirm the diagnosis and reveal occlusion of the terminal aorta and often of one or both iliac arteries. Extensive collateral circulation is usually present. An arterial bypass graft from the proximal aorta to the distal aorta with an end-to-end anastomosis is the treatment of choice. If one or both iliac vessels are involved, a *bifurcation* graft is employed. The results are usually quite good. Patients should be advised preoperatively that retrograde ejaculation may occur after operation. Patients also should be strongly advised to cease smoking postoperatively because occlusion of the prosthetic graft is much more likely to occur if smoking continues.

See the corresponding chapter or part in the *Textbook of Surgery*, 15th edition, pp. 1689–1691, for a more detailed discussion of this topic, including a comprehensive list of references.

ILIAC ARTERIAL OCCLUSION*

David C. Sabiston, Jr., M.D.

Obstruction in the iliac arteries may be due to stenosis or occlusion causing symptoms or claudication of the hips and thighs. The distal pulses usually are diminished or absent in the involved extremity. Arteriography is diagnostic for both the site and magnitude of arterial obstruction. Even when the symptoms are unilateral, the arteriogram often demonstrates disease in the asymptomatic limb. Bypass grafting with a plastic prosthesis is the operation of choice and should be performed when symptoms are sufficiently severe to interfere with the patient's lifestyle.

FEMOROPOPLITEAL AND FEMORAL INFRAPOPLITEAL BYPASS†

Richard L. McCann, M.D.

Patients with arterial obstruction in the lower extremities usually present with *pain*. A careful analysis of the location, quality, and intensity of the pain and factors that aggravate and relieve the pain yields important clinical information. The term *claudication* (from Latin *claudicatio,* "a limp") is applied to the sharp, cramping-type pain felt in specific muscle groups when blood flow becomes inadequate to meet the metabolic requirements during exercise. The distance walked before onset of this pain is strikingly reproducible, and the pain is promptly relieved simply by cessation of ambulation. The location of the claudication is related to the site of principal arterial obstruction. Claudication in the buttock and thigh muscles indicates proximal aortoiliac obstruction, whereas calf claudication usually indicates disease in the superficial femoral artery. When blood flow is inadequate for meeting the metabolic demands of the tissues at rest, continuous pain may be described. This pain, in contrast to claudication, is usually felt in the toes and forefoot. Rest pain is an ominous symptom and demands prompt evaluation not only because of the considerable discomfort involved but also because it indicates such severe vascular compromise that the involved limb may soon evolve to frank gangrene in the absence of successful intervention.

It is important to recognize that atherosclerosis is a systemic metabolic disorder, and overt manifestations of concomitant

---

*See the corresponding chapter or part in the *Textbook of Surgery*, 15th edition, p. 1691, for a more detailed discussion of this topic, including a comprehensive list of references.

†See the corresponding chapter or part in the *Textbook of Surgery*, 15th edition, pp. 1692–1700, for a more detailed discussion of this topic, including a comprehensive list of references.

cerebrovascular or coronary vascular disease are often present in patients with lower extremity ischemia. The importance of associated coronary and cerebrovascular disease is emphasized by the fact that in many long-term studies, 75% of patients requiring lower extremity revascularization fail to survive more than 10 years and almost all the deaths were from myocardial infarction or cerebrovascular accident.

The vascular physical examination is used to confirm the suspicions elicited by the clinical history. Pallor of the skin may be present, particularly with elevation of the legs, and this is often associated with rubor of dependency, which is thought to be due to cutaneous reactive vasodilatation in response to chronic ischemia. Proximal obstruction not only decreases mean arterial pressure but also decreases the perceived pulse amplitude because the pulse pressure is diminished distal to a site of obstruction. The dorsalis pedis and posterior tibial pulses are usually not palpable in patients with lower extremity ischemia. Noninvasive vascular laboratory examinations are useful in providing a quantitative description of the vascular status of the lower extremities. The most useful examinations include determination of segmental blood pressures by use of a Doppler velocity detector, the use pulse volume recordings, and more recently, imaging by ultrasound techniques. Of particular importance is the response of these indices to a standardized exercise stress. It is important that the noninvasive vascular laboratory should not be used in isolation. It is used to complement the information obtained from the clinical history and vascular physical examinations. These help to establish a baseline for longitudinal comparisons, particularly before and after active interventions.

Studies of the natural history of intermittent claudication have shown that patients with this as the sole manifestation of lower limb ischemia have a low risk of limb loss. More than 75% of patients remain stable or even improve with conservative management alone. Medical treatment includes complete abstinence from the use of tobacco, control of body weight, and a program of graduated exercise. Patients who do stop smoking, even at this late stage, improve the prognosis for limb retention significantly. Regular walking exercise also produces a measurable improvement in walking distance in patients with intermittent claudication. The mechanism responsible for this improvement in exercise tolerance is not fully understood but may be due to adaptive changes in the muscle enzyme systems producing more efficient oxygen extraction and utilization. Of many pharmacologic agents that have been used in patients with claudication, only the hemorrheologic agents such as pentoxifylline have proved to be of any benefit, and benefit from this class of drugs is moderate. Strict compliance with these nonsurgical treatments often yields a doubling or more of claudication distance and may be the only treatment required. However, in patients in whom nonsurgical treatment fails to alleviate the disability imposed by intermittent claudication and in whom symptoms interfere with gaining a livelihood or impose an intolerable limitation of lifestyle, surgical treatment can be offered if it is understood that the goal is improvement in exercise capacity rather than limb salvage. In contrast, patients with rest pain, ischemic ulcerations, or limited gangrene are usually candidates for vascular reconstruction because the threat of immediate limb loss is much greater. Arteriography is necessary only if it has been decided that revascularization is indicated. The entire vascular tree from the aorta to the foot should be visualized to ensure that all significant stenoses and occlusions are corrected.

Percutaneous balloon angioplasty, in which a balloon-tipped catheter is passed percutaneously to a site of stenosis or obstruction in the arterial system of the lower extremities and inflated to enlarge the lumen, is very effective in treating short (<10 cm.) lesions. The addition of laser energy and miniature cutting devices to actually remove plaque has not proven to be more effective than simple balloon angioplasty alone. Metallic stents that are expanded within the arterial lumen and which remain in the vessel wall in the expanded state to enlarge the lumen have been introduced recently for treatment of lower extremity lesions and may improve the results of balloon angioplasty. Even though the restenosis rate is relatively high, this does not preclude either repeat angioplasty or subsequent bypass surgery, but angioplasty has not been successful in treating long occlusions or long stenoses with multiple sites of disease in the femoral artery. It is this type of lesion that usually produces severe ischemia and threat to the viability of the limb, and these lesions continue to be best treated by surgical bypass.

For patients treated surgically, most undergo vein bypass grafting. Endarterectomy is occasionally useful, as is enlargement of the orifice of the profunda femoris when it has been severely restricted by atherosclerotic disease. There has been considerable debate regarding the most appropriate graft material used in lower extremity bypass procedures. It has been demonstrated clearly that autogenous venous reconstructions are significantly more durable than are reconstructions performed with either a synthetic vascular conduit or modified biologic grafts. Results with synthetic grafts become progressively worse compared with autogenous venous grafts the closer that the distal anastomosis is to the foot.

With respect to the saphenous vein, two techniques have become established. In the *in situ* technique, the saphenous vein is not dissected from its bed except for the proximal and distal segments, which are mobilized and used to create the proximal and distal end-to-side anastomoses of the bypass. In the intervening segment the side branches must be ligated to prevent the occurrence of hemodynamically significant arteriovenous fistulas. The valves also must be destroyed or cut with specially designed valvulotomes in order to allow flow toward the foot. Advocates of this technique claim that it allows the use of smaller grafts because the small end of the vessel is attached to the smaller artery and the large end of the graft to the larger artery. With use of this technique, excellent patency and limb-salvage rates have been achieved. However, comparable concurrent series using the more traditional reversed saphenous vein graft also have shown improved results. Proponents of this technique also claim improved vein utilization rates and avoidance of reliance on synthetic grafts because in patients who do not possess an intact ipsilateral vein, a satisfactory graft can be constructed by use of the vein from the contralateral limb or by fragments of larger veins from either leg or even from the arm.

The increase in patency and limb-salvage rates in patients treated for lower extremity peripheral vascular obstructive disease has been one of the most dramatic improvements in vascular surgery. Current results now show 90% 1-year and 70% multiyear patency rates, with limb salvage a little bit higher. These improvements have been achieved by an increased appreciation of the fragility of the saphenous vein and the importance of gentle technique in its preparation for use by either the *in situ* or the reversed technique. In addition, the increased appreciation of the clear superiority of autogenous venous grafting over synthetic or modified biologic grafts also has had a role in this improvement.

PERCUTANEOUS TRANSLUMINAL ANGIOPLASTY

Jose A. Perez, M.D., Alyson J. Breisch, M.D., and R. Duane Davis, Jr., M.D.

Since the performance of the first successful percutaneous transluminal angioplasty (PTA) by Dotter and Judkins in 1964, this technique has gained rapid acceptance for the treatment of obstructive peripheral arterial disease. This enthusiasm is somewhat tempered by remaining uncertainties about the long-term durability of these procedures when compared with surgical bypass. In general, PTA confers a lower long-term patency; however, its use is justified by its reduced cost, lower risks, excellent acute success rate, and ease of reapplication. Currently, PTA is often used as an adjunctive procedure to surgical revascularization.

Using the available literature to directly compare the relative efficacy of PTA with the results of bypass surgery is largely invalidated by intrinsic differences between the two patient populations. To date, only one prospective, randomized trial has compared PTA to bypass surgery in 263 claudicating men with short focal peripheral arterial obstructions. Although the initial success rate for PTA was lower (85% versus 93% for operation), those patients with a successful angioplasty had as durable a hemodynamic result at a median follow-up period of 4 years (improvement in ankle-brachial index and functional status questionnaire).

PTA is associated with a total complication rate of 5% to 10%. The number and extent of complications depend on the vascular bed being treated, the severity and diffuseness of the

---

See the corresponding chapter or part in the *Textbook of Surgery*, 15th edition, pp. 1700–1711, for a more detailed discussion of this topic, including a comprehensive list of references.

atherosclerotic process, the experience of the operator, and the completeness with which complications are reported. Fortunately, mortality is extremely rare (0.2%) and usually caused by balloon-mediated rupture of a large vessel or a complicating myocardial infarction. Acute vessel closure or distal embolization results in limb loss in 0.2% of cases. PTA failures that caused acute limb ischemia or inadequate hemostasis required surgical repair in approximately 2% of all cases.

The indications for PTA have gradually broadened as technological improvements and operator experience have resulted in increasing success rates. As is true for surgery, the use of PTA to treat intermittent claudication should be offered only to patients who have significant functional limitation inadequately reduced by conservative measures. Ischemic rest pain, ulceration, gangrene, impaired wound healing, and impending limb loss are clear indications for intervention when lesion morphology is deemed amenable to percutaneous techniques. The use of adjunctive PTA to improve proximal inflow or distal runoff has proved to be valuable for simplifying and enhancing the durability of surgical bypass grafts.

RESULTS OF PTA IN PERIPHERAL VASCULAR DISEASE

AORTIC. Recent series report a high initial success rate of 93% to 100% using PTA to treat isolated stenoses of the infrarenal abdominal aorta. The long-term patency of 93% for up to 4 years compares favorably with surgical results.

ILIAC. PTA has become the procedure of choice for treating focal stenoses of the common and external iliac arteries. The initial success rate averages 90%, with good long-term durability after successful dilation noted in several series reporting an average 4-year patency of 65%. Standard PTA of total iliac occlusions, however, has resulted in lower initial success rates (65%) and clinically significant emboli complicating 3% to 20% of cases.

FEMOROPOPLITEAL. Femoropopliteal PTA can be expected to have an initial success rate of 89% with a long-term patency of 65% at 2 years and 58% at 5 years. The best results are obtained in patients with stenoses and at least two patent tibial runoff vessels (78% patency at 3 years) and the worst in patients with occlusions and one or no patent tibial vessels (25% patency at 3 years). Similarly, patients presenting with claudication fare much better than those presenting with critical limb ischemia.

TIBIOPERONEAL. Although recent series have reported a 90% acute success rate in tibioperoneal vessels, PTA is much less durable (60% patency at 1 year) than in more proximal vessels.

INFRAINGUINAL BYPASS GRAFT. Early graft failure results from initial hyperplasia that develops focally at anastomoses or at the sites of venous valves. Later graft failure is commonly the result of progressive atherosclerosis. Early detection of a failing graft by duplex ultrasound surveillance can identify the short focal stenosis (<5 cm. long) that responds well to PTA. Longer, more diffuse lesions and chronic occlusions are best treated with surgical revision.

RENAL. The indications for renal PTA (PTRA) are similar to those used for surgery and include renovascular hypertension, progressive renal failure, and volume overload in the setting of renal artery stenosis. The best results are obtained in patients with fibromuscular dysplasia. Nonostial atherosclerotic lesions also respond well to PTRA but have a higher restenosis rate. True ostial renal artery lesions are composed mostly of aortic plaque and are poorly suited to treatment with routine PTRA due to the inherent high elastic recoil. Complications are more frequent with PTRA than when performing PTA in other vascular beds.

NEW DEVICES FOR PERIPHERAL INTERVENTION

STENTS. Intravascular stents are used as an adjunct to routine PTA to prevent acute closure due to elastic recoil and plaque dissection. The greatest experience has been in the iliac vessels, where stenting has allowed safe percutaneous revascularization of more diffuse lesions. Early experience with stenting of ostial renal artery lesions appears encouraging.

ATHERECTOMY/LASERS. The present state of these technologies greatly limits their general applicability and usefulness for the treatment of peripheral arterial disease. Except for unusual lesion morphologies, percutaneous atherectomy or lasers have not proved superior to routine PTA.

ARTERIAL INJURIES

William H. Baker, M.D., and Steven S. Kang, M.D.

MECHANISMS OF INJURY. Arteries can be injured by penetrating or blunt trauma. Knife wounds transect arteries much as a surgical scalpel does, leaving little devitalized tissue on either side of the wound. Contrariwise, gunshot wounds involving high-velocity missiles may produce tissue damage for some distance on either side of the obvious wound and require extensive débridement.

Blunt trauma directly compresses and damages the vessel. For example, an artery that is crushed may be intact but have a damaged intima that will cause thrombosis. Rapid deceleration, as occurs when an automobile hits a stationary object, can stretch an artery or produce a shearing force to cause an intimal tear. If the artery is torn sufficiently to weaken the entire blood vessel, severe hemorrhage may occur.

See the corresponding chapter or part in the *Textbook of Surgery*, 15th edition, pp. 1711–1723, for a more detailed discussion of this topic, including a comprehensive list of references.

The adventitia of the artery usually contains the flow of blood, albeit temporarily.

PATHOPHYSIOLOGY. When an artery is completely severed, the ends characteristically constrict and retract into the adjacent tissue. The bleeding usually arrests spontaneously, since there is circumferential arterial constriction and the formation of a thrombus in each of the two ends. A partially severed artery cannot retract and constrict. Hemorrhage under these circumstances may be greater than with a completely severed artery. If contained by adjacent soft tissue, a pulsatile hematoma or pseudoaneurysm may develop. A partially severed artery may or may not develop a thrombus that obstructs flow, and thus distal pulses may be palpable. Blunt arterial injury produces intimal damage that can lead to acute or delayed thrombosis.

RECOGNITION OF ARTERIAL INJURY. The diagnosis of arterial injury is obvious in a patient with ischemia or loss of pulses distal to the site of injury. Critical ischemia of an extremity is noted by the five Ps: pulselessness, pallor, pain, paresthesia, and paralysis. In a patient with palpable pulses and no distal ischemia, arterial injury is confirmed by the presence of other "hard" signs: arterial bleeding, an expanding or pulsatile hematoma, or a bruit or thrill. A handheld Doppler and blood pressure cuff can be used to compare pressures in all extremities. A reduced systolic pressure in the injured extremity suggests the presence of arterial injury.

ANGIOGRAMS. Angiograms are rarely necessary for the diagnosis of a completely occluded artery but are extremely helpful in the diagnosis of partially severed or bluntly injured arteries. A patient with a single wound and no pulses distal to this wound does not require angiography for diagnosis. The patient with multiple gunshot wounds or a shotgun wound in an extremity requires angiography for localization of the exact site(s) of injury. Patients with multiple long bone fractures form the same category. Performance of an angiogram delays treatment, and this should be factored into the treatment plan of the multiply injured patient.

OPERATIVE TREATMENT. All major arterial and venous injuries are treated optimally with vascular reconstruction. Active bleeding is controlled temporarily with firm pressure, and the patient is rushed to the operating room. Patients with critical ischemia should have the damage repaired within hours of injury. Patients without either hemorrhage or critical ischemia may have the repair of injury triaged until later in their total care.

The incision should be planned to allow proximal and distal control of the arterial injury. For example, the thorax is prepared and draped in the case of injuries that may involve the abdominal aorta. This will allow clamping of the thoracic aorta should tamponade of the retroperitoneum be lost during exploration. When the arterial injury is identified and controlled, all devitalized artery is débrided. The artery is then preferably sutured end to end. If a graft replacement is required, autogenous vein from an uninjured extremity is used to bridge the gap. Prosthetic material is seldom used except in repair of the abdominal or thoracic aorta. If there has been extensive soiling of the wound, the risk of infection is obviously greater. In patients with critical ischemia of the extremity, a fasciotomy must be considered. If there is tense muscle in the operating room, this is done prophylactically. If a four-compartment fasciotomy is not performed immediately, the patient must be monitored constantly for evidence of a compartment syndrome. In questionable cases, compartmental pressures can be measured.

POSTOPERATIVE CARE. The pulses distal to the site of arterial repair should be evaluated frequently by trained personnel. Should any question arise, Doppler pressures can be followed. Decreasing pulses or pressures should prompt a return to the operating room.

SPECIFIC PROBLEMS

IATROGENIC. Cardiologists and radiologists alike use the arterial system for diagnostic and therapeutic access to patients. These arterial punctures are usually well tolerated, but in a rare instance, bleeding after angiographic study may require operative control. Thrombosis at the site of arterial puncture may produce an occluded artery. Hemorrhage from an axillary artery puncture may cause compression of the nerves in the axillary sheath. Operative decompression of this syndrome is urgently required.

ORTHOPEDIC. Orthopedic injuries such as knee dislocations can cause secondary trauma to an artery. Whereas fractures may directly puncture and damage the artery, dislocated bones usually stretch the arteries so that the intima alone is damaged. In instances of either partial severance or intimal injury, the pulses may be palpable immediately after injury. These arteries then occlude later, and critical ischemia may develop. These patients should be managed by either early routine arteriography or close observation.

VEINS. Venous injuries are repaired whenever possible. An end-to-end interrupted anastomosis is preferred. Although flow is slower and the incidence of thrombosis is increased, most authors agree that the long-term results of repair are superior to those of ligation. Pulmonary embolism occurs infrequently in these patients.

RENAL ARTERY. The kidney tolerates but an hour or two of warm ischemia time. Injuries of the renal artery that are repaired after several hours may or may not produce a functioning kidney. Nonetheless, in a young patient, repair is usually undertaken.

CAROTID. The patient with a carotid artery injury who presents with a severe stroke is usually not reconstructed because restoration of a normal pressure to the damaged brain may cause worsening of the neurologic deficit. Patients with either no or moderate deficits are reconstructed, since most authors believe the results merit such actions.

LATE SEQUELAE. If an arterial injury is not recognized or is improperly treated, the patient may develop chronic ischemia. In the extremity, this may require amputation or may lead to intermittent claudication. Late reconstruction is indeed possible if the extremity is viable and potentially may be returned to useful function. Partially severed arteries may develop pseudoaneurysms. These may continue to grow until they compress the adjacent organs or rupture. Partial injuries that involve both the artery and vein may cause formation of an arteriovenous fistula. Not only will they have all the complications of a false aneurysm, but these patients also will have an increase in venous return and potentially may develop congestive heart failure. This increase in venous return may give signs and symptoms of venous hypertension in the affected extremity.

ACUTE ARTERIAL OCCLUSION

Thomas J. Fogarty, M.D., and Amitava Biswas, M.D.

ETIOLOGY

Acute arterial occlusion occurs as a result of embolization or *in situ* thrombosis. Most arterial emboli originate in the heart as a result of underlying cardiac disease. Embolization from rheumatic mitral stenosis has decreased significantly. The primary cardiac disorder is atherosclerotic disease manifested by myocardial infarction, atrial fibrillation, congestive heart failure, and ventricular aneurysm. There has been a significant increase in the incidence of *in situ* arterial thrombosis, and this pathology now represents 85% of acute arterial occlusions.

PATHOPHYSIOLOGY

The majority of surgically treatable emboli lodge in the lower extremities. The highest incidence is in the femoral artery, followed by the iliac, aortic, and popliteal vessels; embolism of the renal, brachial, mesenteric, and cerebral arteries is less common. Regardless of the source or histologic structure of an embolus, it is the location and sequelae following an embolism that determine the viability of an extremity.

It is important to remove all distal thrombosis and to recognize that discontinuous thrombus is present in approximately one third of patients. Under these circumstances, backbleeding from collaterals may be quite forceful despite the presence of additional distal thrombus. If this is not recognized, suboptimal restoration of the circulation follows. Routine distal exploration with balloon catheters should be done independently of the status of backbleeding.

See the corresponding chapter or part in the *Textbook of Surgery*, 15th edition, pp. 1723–1730, for a more detailed discussion of this topic, including a comprehensive list of references.

PREOPERATIVE EVALUATION AND CARE

Patients with acute embolic occlusion should be assumed to have significant associated heart disease. Evaluation of cardiac function should proceed simultaneously with evaluation of peripheral vessels.

Appropriate therapy is initiated while emergency preparation for operation is made. Digitalis, antiarrhythmic agents, morphine, diuretics, and heparin can be administered as needed without delaying surgical intervention.

INSTRUMENTATION

The balloon embolectomy catheter is flexible and available in graduated sizes for use in major vessels of any caliber. At its proximal portion the syringe fitting provides the means for fluid exchange into a soft, distensible balloon located at the distal tip of the instrument. Embolectomy is performed by inserting the catheter into the acutely occluded vessel as far as possible. The balloon is inflated and withdrawn in the inflated position while the same surgeon manipulates both the syringe and the catheter. Alternatives to the conventional balloon catheter, such as the spiral balloon embolectomy catheter and the wire loop graft thrombectomy catheter, are used to remove particularly adherent thrombus in grafts or native vessels. Experience is the most significant factor in reducing the incidence of complications.

OPERATIVE PROCEDURE

The procedure is initiated with local anesthesia, and the field should be surgically prepared from the toes to the nipple line; aortoiliac emboli require preparation of both extremities. A distal exploration is conducted with routine passage in the superficial femoral artery (3- to 4-French catheter) and in the profunda (2- to 3-French). Any uncertainty about adequate removal of thrombi should be resolved by arteriography or angioscopy. Angioscopy allows directional access to the tibial vessels and minimizes the need for distal incisions. After removal of the thrombotic material, the distal arterial system should be irrigated copiously with heparinized saline solution.

In patients with *advanced* ischemia, concomitant major venous occlusion also may be present and may require venous thrombectomy. After removal of the arterial emboli, the distal arteries and veins are irrigated with heparinized saline. Heparin is administered at operation and in the immediate postoperative period. Massive swelling that may embarrass arterial inflow is most common in patients who present with advanced ischemia before surgical intervention. Capillary damage and compromised venous outflow are factors in this swelling, and fasciotomy is required in these situations. If immediate improvement by limited fasciotomy is not obtained, the skin incisions should be extended and deeper fascial compartments opened widely. Immediately following restoration of arterial continuity in extremities with advanced ischemia, significant alterations in electrolytes and acid-base balance may occur, which can cause electrocardiographic changes and hypotension. Buffering agents and antiarrhythmic agents can be employed at the time of clamp release.

EMBOLIC OCCLUSION IN THE PRESENCE OF SIGNIFICANT CHRONIC OCCLUSIVE DISEASE

A careful history and examination of the uninvolved extremity often can provide a reliable assessment of the peripheral circulation before the acute episode. Initially, it is advisable only to attempt to return the circulation to the acute preocclusive state. However, definitive procedures may be performed adjunctively, particularly if there is a concern about the viability of the extremity and the patient was active and in reasonable health before the occlusion. Reconstructive procedures such as localized endarterectomy or femorofemoral grafts can be done under local anesthesia. Catheter therapy, such as adjunctive dilation or atherectomy, can be employed at the time of thrombectomy or embolectomy and is being utilized with increasing frequency.

UPPER EXTREMITY, RENAL, MESENTERIC, AND CAROTID ARTERY EMBOLI

The management of emboli to these areas is similar to that described for the lower extremity. The vessels supplying the viscera and brain are friable and thin-walled, and catheter manipulation should be undertaken with considerable care. Unless emboli are observed within the first 6 hours of onset, surgical intervention in the internal carotid system should not be considered because of the risk of potentially fatal hemorrhagic infarction.

MORBIDITY AND MORTALITY

The aim of surgical intervention for arterial emboli is restoration of the peripheral circulation to its preocclusive state. Evaluation of results is based on the restoration of pulses, relief of symptoms, and return of normal color and temperature. The possibility of maintaining a viable, functional extremity after acute arterial occlusion should exceed 90%. The condition of the extremity rather than the duration of occlusion represents the primary determinant of operability. Failure of the initial exploration after an apparent success is an indication for re-exploration. The most common cause for failure relates to technical factors, which often can be corrected if they are recognized.

The presence of a stronger than normal "water hammer" pulse after an apparently successful embolectomy has been associated with a high incidence of reocclusion; this indicates obstruction at the small artery and arteriolar level. Adjunctive intraoperative use of lytic agents is indicated in these circumstances.

THROMBOLYTIC AGENTS

Thrombolytic agents can be useful in the treatment of acute arterial occlusion. The systemic use of lytics has largely been abandoned because of the high incidence of hemorrhagic complications. Delivering the lytics at the site of thrombosis has proven more effective than systemic use and is associated with fewer complications. However, catheter-mediated thrombolysis is rarely a definitive therapy. Additional procedures such as direct surgery, dilation, and/or stent placement are always required. In my experience, time delay to reperfusion, cost, multiple angiograms, and the potential for hemorrhage have limited their use. Heparinization with surgical balloon embolectomy remains the most effective form of treatment for acute arterial occlusion.

ARTERIOVENOUS FISTULAS

H. Kim Lyerly, M.D., and David C. Sabiston, Jr., M.D.

One of the most fascinating lesions in medicine is an arteriovenous fistula. Fistulas may be either congenital or acquired and are of variable etiology, anatomic distribution, and clinical presentation. They are associated with numerous pathophysiologic changes at the local site and systemically. An arteriovenous fistula can be defined as a connection, other than the capillary bed, between the arterial and venous systems. This definition encompasses a vast array of conditions, including some occurring in the normal development of the circulation, congenital malformations, acquired lesions, and iatrogenic shunts.

Congenital lesions may have single or multiple communications and are respectively denoted as *arteriovenous fistulas* or *arteriovenous malformations*. Lesions with a single communication usually represent either a normal fetal communication that fails to resolve or a developmental abnormality. Lesions with multiple communications usually represent persistent communications that normally exist during the early phase of the development of the arterial and venous systems. Hemangiomas are multiple abnormal venous communications.

Single communications usually are found in acquired lesions and are termed *arteriovenous fistulas*; frequently, they consist of a distinct communication between an artery and a vein bypassing the capillary bed.

See the corresponding chapter or part in the *Textbook of Surgery*, 15th edition, pp. 1731–1737, for a more detailed discussion of this topic, including a comprehensive list of references.

PATHOPHYSIOLOGY

Fistulas involving a large artery that conducts massive amounts of blood flow usually are associated with extensive cardiovascular changes. Under these circumstances, much blood is shunted through the fistula because the venous side offers very little resistance. With large volumes of blood shunted directly into the venous circulation, a sequence of events follows that is directly related to the volume of blood flowing through the fistula. Cardiac output may be increased in patients with arteriovenous fistulas, and compression of the fistula, which diminishes the flow through the fistula, is followed by a diminished heart rate (Branham's or Nicoladoni's sign) and a lower cardiac output. If the fistula is acute with a large volume of blood flowing through it, the heart may not be able to compensate adequately.

The hemodynamic disturbances associated with arteriovenous fistulas often produce structural changes in the arterial wall. The venous wall of large fistulas becomes thin, closely simulating the sac of a false aneurysm. The walls of small fistulas may become thickened and assume the appearance of an artery. Thrombi are also apt to form in the dilated parts of these fistulas and may harbor bacterial organisms.

CLINICAL FEATURES

At the site of the fistula, aneurysmal dilatation is usually present with involvement of both the artery and vein caused by turbulence due to the high- to low-pressure interface within the fistula. In response to the low arterial pressure distal to the site of the fistula, an extensive collateral circulation develops that connects the arteries proximal to the fistula with those distal. This collateral circulation can become massive and often causes an increase in temperature in both skin and muscle. When the fistulas occur in an extremity, the limb may increase in length. Other local features are demonstrated by the presence of a thrill at the site of the lesion, especially if it is located near the surface. On auscultation, a bruit that continues through most, if not all, of the cardiac cycle is audible.

The diagnosis can be established by arteriography and ultrasonography. In acquired fistulas, a single communication often occurs at the site of the fistula and can be localized either by direct visualization of the communication or by the initial venous opacification at the site of the fistula. Congenital lesions with multiple communications often have a radiographic appearance that is much more complicated. Indirect signs of an abnormal arteriovenous communication, including increased flow in the afferent arteries, decreased flow in the peripheral arteries, and rapid venous filling, are usually present. However, the multiple communications may not be visible because they are often of microscopic size, and overlying opacified arteries and veins add to the complexity of the radiographic pattern. Selective angiography of the afferent artery or arteries may be helpful in delineating the extent of the fistula. Sometimes localized dilated contrast-filled spaces indicate the site of the fistula with some precision. On other occasions, small fistulas are revealed as faint, diffuse opacifications between major arterial and venous channels. Other indications may include abnormal vessels arising from the parent artery, horizontal branches connecting parallel veins, and venous retia.

Although ultrasonography may not be expected to reveal the actual fistula, the detection of aneurysms may call attention to a previously unsuspected fistula as well as determine the diameter and morphologic features of the proximal vessels. Color-flow imaging also may reveal patterns suggestive of increased turbulence at sites of increased flow. Computed tomography (CT) and magnetic resonance imaging (MRI) may be used to demonstrate the location and extent of arteriovenous communications, including the involvement of specific muscle groups and bone.

TYPES OF FISTULAS

In the extremities, congenital arteriovenous communications are quite common, especially in the legs, and varicose veins often result. Congenital arteriovenous communications have been reported in all organs of the body and frequently are difficult to manage because multiple communications exist between arteries and veins. Congenital pulmonary arteriovenous fistulas are common and often are multiple. These are usually seen as well-circumscribed lesions on the chest film; if large, they may be accompanied by cyanosis due to the right-to-left shunting. The symptoms include exertional dyspnea, easy fatigability, cyanosis, and clubbing of the fingers. Approximately 10% to 15% occur in children. Complications of these lesions include cerebrovascular accidents, brain abscesses, hemoptysis, and intrapleural rupture. A continuous bruit with systolic accentuation during deep inspiration is heard in approximately two thirds of patients. Pulmonary arteriography confirms the diagnosis. Hereditary telangiectasis (Rendu-Osler-Weber disease) is quite common and may be familial in origin.

Some hemangiomas represent a specific type of lesion composed of large venous spaces under low pressure with no clinical angiographic evidence of significant arteriovenous shunting. They may occur anywhere in the body. Venous lesions are often asymptomatic but may be disfiguring in a large, exposed area. Localized symptomatic lesions may be treated by excision, although, as previously mentioned, they may be more extensive than is evident clinically.

Acquired fistulas are found most frequently in the extremities and often are secondary to penetrating trauma with accompanying varices, edema, and pigmentation. Unlike congenital communications, a single or limited number of abnormal communications occur that can be demonstrated by angiography or color-flow Doppler. Vascular insufficiency of digits and ulceration also may be present in the more severe forms. A palpable thrill and an audible coarse machinery–like bruit are usually present at the site of the fistula.

Certain surgical procedures are associated with iatrogenic fistulas, including operations on the kidney and intervertebral discs. Disc procedures may be associated with fistulas in the iliac vessels or with aortocaval fistulas. Iatrogenic fistulas following thyroid procedures, coronary artery bypass grafting, distal splenorenal shunts, small bowel resection, Fontan's operation, and pelvic surgery have each been described.

The wall of the aneurysm may be involved with atherosclerosis, and an erosion can occur into accompanying veins, the prominent example being that of an aortocaval fistula from an abdominal aortic aneurysm. Such a lesion may place a patient precipitously in congestive heart failure and require an emergent surgical procedure. Proximal and distal control of the aorta allows the artery to be opened and the fistula controlled by a finger placed on the communication. Compression with sponge sticks proximal and distal to the fistula allows repair of the vein. After the vein is repaired, the preferred method for restoring arterial continuity is with a graft. Aortocaval fistulas of neoplastic origin also have been reported.

It is interesting that the most common acquired arteriovenous fistula is that associated with vascular access for permitting renal dialysis in the management of renal insufficiency. Arteriovenous fistulas also have been constructed surgically to increase blood flow and patency to a vascular anastomosis, such as venous reconstruction procedures.

Closure of the communication is generally recommended, since most arteriovenous fistulas are potentially symptomatic. Early surgical attempts to correct these lesions consisted primarily of ligation of the involved artery proximal to the fistula. Gangrene can result because blood reaching the distal extremity by arterial collaterals is apt to drain retrograde through the fistula directly into the venous system, thus depriving the limb of adequate distal arterial blood flow. The first successful treatment of an arteriovenous fistula was proximal and distal ligation of both the artery and the vein.

An accurate diagnosis and determination of the extent of the lesion are necessary prior to correction. Acute fistulas with high flow causing cardiovascular collapse or distal ischemia require immediate repair, whereas long-standing lesions with extensive involvement of surrounding tissue require thoughtful preoperative planning. The site of the communication always should be localized carefully by arteriography; however, CT scanning, MRI, and color-flow Doppler imaging are being used increasingly to diagnose arteriovenous communications. The ideal surgical management usually includes direct closure of the fistula with restoration of arterial and venous continuity. However, when this is not possible, quadripolar ligation is acceptable when sufficient arterial collateral circulation for adequately supplying the tissues distally exists. Complete excision is reserved for fistulas involving small nonessential arteries, such as the radial or ulnar arteries when adequate collaterals are present. Rarely, small fistulas have closed spontaneously.

Some arteriovenous fistulas are too extensive for appropriate and complete surgical excision. For these, palliative surgical procedures are used to control disabling ulceration and infection or life-threatening hemorrhage. Ligation of major feeding arteries is not recommended because distal ischemia may result and the intravascular access required to allow embolization becomes limited. Staged treatment with intervals between embolizations allows portions of major malformations to be obliterated and repeated treatments in persistent areas. Often this combination of embolization followed by surgical excision is effective in managing these difficult malformations. Other types of therapy include injection of sclerosing solutions or irradiation. The complex communications seen with congenital arteriovenous malformation often require a multidisciplinary approach including selective intraarterial embolization in conjunction with surgical therapy. Asymptomatic lesions may not require treatment; nevertheless, a fistula represents a hazard. Absolute indications for treatment include hemorrhage, secondary ischemic complications, and congestive heart failure from arteriovenous shunting; relative indications include pain, nonhealing ulcers, functional impairment, and cosmetic deformity. If treatment is required, careful planning is mandatory.

THROMBOANGIITIS OBLITERANS (BUERGER'S DISEASE)

H. Brownell Wheeler, M.D.

Thromboangiitis obliterans (Buerger's disease) is an uncommon form of peripheral arterial insufficiency that typically occurs in heavy smokers between 20 and 35 years of age. It occurs predominantly in men. This diagnosis should be considered in any young smoker with severe peripheral ischemia, particularly if the upper extremities are involved or there is a history of migratory superficial phlebitis. Arteriography early in the disease usually reveals segmental obliteration of the medium-sized arteries of the forearm and calf, with a normal appearance of proximal vessels. Digital arteries frequently are involved. Careful clinical evaluation is necessary to rule out other causes of peripheral ischemia, especially atherosclerosis.

NATURAL HISTORY. The clinical course of thromboangiitis obliterans is prolonged and painful but relatively benign. If a patient ceases smoking, prolonged remission usually occurs. However, many patients are addicted to tobacco and continue to smoke despite all advice. They have repeated attacks and may require multiple distal amputations. Cases of mesenteric and cerebral involvement have been reported, but life-endangering complications are infrequent. Long-term life

---

See the corresponding chapter or part in the *Textbook of Surgery,* 15th edition, pp. 1738–1740, for a more detailed discussion of this topic, including a comprehensive list of references.

expectancy is only slightly less than that of the general population.

ETIOLOGY. The striking association with cigarette smoking suggests a strong etiologic relationship, but a specific cause for thromboangiitis obliterans has never been demonstrated. Any factor that causes vasospasm, thrombosis, or local inflammation may contribute to the development of the syndrome in a susceptible patient. It is likely that some immunologic process activated by cigarette smoking plays a major etiologic role in Buerger's disease.

INCIDENCE. Thromboangiitis obliterans is observed more frequently in Asia, Eastern Europe, and the Middle East than in the United States. Currently, thromboangiitis obliterans occurs in less than 1% of all patients with severe peripheral ischemia in the United States. In Israel and Eastern Europe, the corresponding incidence is approximately 5%, whereas in Japan it is 16%.

MANAGEMENT. The main clinical problem in thromboangiitis obliterans is pain management. Narcotics are usually necessary but must be used cautiously because of the frequency of drug addiction. Peripheral or sympathetic nerve blocks may provide temporary pain relief, especially when the disease is accompanied by severe vasospasm. When nerve blocks prove helpful, cervical or lumbar sympathectomy also may benefit such patients. Every effort should be made to have the patient stop smoking, since indefinite remissions often follow abstinence from cigarettes. Meticulous conservative treatment of ischemic lesions is usually followed by healing, especially in the upper extremity. No specific medication has found wide acceptance, but prostaglandins, anticoagulants, vasodilators, antiplatelet agents, and pentoxifylline have all been advocated. Arterial reconstruction is usually impossible because of the distal nature of the disease but should be considered in segmental proximal occlusions. Amputation at the lowest possible level is indicated for intractable pain or gangrene.

RAYNAUD'S SYNDROME

James M. Edwards, M.D., Gregory J. Landry, M.D., and John M. Porter, M.D.

Raynaud's syndrome defines a condition characterized by episodes of vasospasm that cause closure of the small arteries and arterioles of the distal parts of the extremities in response to cold exposure or emotional stimuli. Classically, the episodes consist of intense pallor of the distal extremities followed by cyanosis and rubor upon rewarming, with full recovery requiring 15 to 45 minutes.

Pallor is caused by severe spasm of the arteries and arteri-

See the corresponding chapter or part in the *Textbook of Surgery*, 15th edition, pp. 1740–1747, for a more detailed discussion of this topic, including a comprehensive list of references.

oles, which causes cessation of capillary perfusion. After some minutes, the capillaries and probably the venules dilate. This is followed by relaxation of the arteriolar spasm with entry of a trickle of blood into the dilated capillaries, where it rapidly becomes desaturated and produces cyanosis. Rubor follows the entry of increasing amounts of blood into dilated capillaries. The episode terminates with the entry of a normal volume of blood through the relaxed arterioles.

Patients with Raynaud's syndrome may be divided into two distinct pathophysiologic groups: obstructive and spastic. Patients with *obstructive* Raynaud's syndrome have sufficiently severe arterial obstruction to cause significant reduction in resting digital artery pressure. In such patients, a normal vasoconstrictive response to cold is sufficient to overcome the diminished intraluminal distending pressure and cause arterial closure. Patients with *spastic* Raynaud's syndrome do not have significant palmar-digital artery obstruction and have normal digital artery pressure at room temperature. Arterial closure in these patients is caused by the markedly increased force of cold-induced arterial spasm. A number of studies have suggested altered adrenoceptor activity in patients with spastic Raynaud's syndrome. Although conclusive data are lacking, abnormalities in both alpha$_2$ adrenoceptors and presynaptic beta receptors have been implicated in the cause of Raynaud's syndrome.

CLINICAL DESCRIPTION. In spastic Raynaud's syndrome, both hands are affected equally, and frequently the thumbs are spared. About 10% of patients have a primary lower extremity involvement. Obstructive Raynaud's syndrome appears to be about equally distributed between males and females; the symptomatic onset occurs after the age of 40 years, and the area of involvement is frequently limited to one or several fingers. Typically, younger women present with spastic Raynaud's syndrome, and idiopathic Raynaud's without associated disease is most common in this age and sex group. Older males who develop Raynaud's usually have the obstructive type associated with digital artery occlusion, usually from atherosclerosis. Most episodes of digital vasospasm are induced by cold exposure, although emotional stimuli also may produce episodes. Fingertip ulceration occurs only in the presence of widespread palmar or digital artery obstruction. Ischemic ulceration is never caused by vasospasm alone.

EVALUATION. Historical information should be sought regarding symptoms of connective tissue disease, including arthralgia, dysphagia, skin tightening, xerophthalmia, or xerostomia. Symptoms of large-vessel occlusive disease, exposure to trauma or frostbite, drug history, and history of malignancy also should be sought. The skin of the hands and fingers should be inspected for ulcerations or fingertip hyperkeratotic areas suggesting healed ulcers. The hand and fingers should be examined for evidence of an associated autoimmune disease. The physical examination is frequently completely normal in patients with Raynaud's syndrome. The diagnosis is made primarily from the history.

Increasingly sophisticated vascular laboratory techniques

have been used to evaluate Raynaud's syndrome. Digital blood pressure response to 5 minutes of digital occlusive hypothermia has proved to be 87% specific and 90% sensitive in diagnosing Raynaud's syndrome but does not differentiate between obstructive and spastic causes. Digital photoplethysmography with digital blood pressure determination detects digital artery obstruction. The extent of laboratory evaluation varies somewhat depending on the findings of the history and physical examination. Minimal evaluation should include a hand radiograph for calcinosis or tuft resorption, complete blood count, sedimentation rate, rheumatoid factor, and antinuclear antibody for aiding in the detection of any associated autoimmune disease. Arteriography is recommended only in patients presenting with ischemic digital ulceration, because a small percentage of these patients develop these ulcers as a result of embolization from a surgically correctable proximal lesion.

TREATMENT. Most patients with Raynaud's syndrome have only mild symptoms that respond well to cold and tobacco avoidance. Patients who work in cold areas may not respond to any treatment until their occupational exposure is reduced. At the present time, nifedipine is the first-line drug for Raynaud's syndrome. Patients with spastic Raynaud's syndrome are more likely to respond to medication than are those with obstructive Raynaud's syndrome.

In the small number of patients with a proximal cause of upper extremity arterial insufficiency, surgical correction may be indicated. In patients with digital ulceration caused by palmar and digital arterial occlusions, the healing rate with conservative therapy is 85%. Thoracic sympathectomy has fallen into disfavor due to mediocre long-term results. Lumbar sympathectomy, however, remains an option in patients with lower extremity symptoms.

ACKNOWLEDGMENTS

Supported by Grant RR00334 from the General Clinical Research Centers branch of the Division of Research Resources, National Institutes of Health, and Grant 8839 from the Medical Research Foundation of Oregon.

CIRCULATORY PROBLEMS OF THE UPPER EXTREMITY

Milton M. Slocum, M.D., and Donald Silver, M.D.

ARTERIAL INSUFFICIENCY

Arterial flow to the upper extremity may be reduced by atherosclerotic stenoses or occlusions, thromboembolism,

See the corresponding chapter or part in the *Textbook of Surgery*, 15th edition, pp. 1748–1750, for a more detailed discussion of this topic, including a comprehensive list of references.

trauma, tumor, inflammatory processes, or compression of the subclavian-axillary arteries in the region of the thoracic outlet. Penetrating arterial injuries are more common in the upper extremities (53%), whereas blunt traumatic vascular injuries occur most often in the lower extremities (89%). Between 3% and 5% of all arterial emboli lodge in the arteries of the upper extremities. Brachial and axillary catheterizations cause thrombotic occlusions of the respective arteries in approximately 0.5% to 10% of the cases. Arteritis is an increasingly frequent cause of upper extremity and hand ischemia. The larger proximal arteries may be obstructed by giant cell arteritis or idiopathic arteritis, whereas the palmar and digital arteries are affected more frequently by collagen-related vasculitis— especially scleroderma.

Management of the upper extremity ischemia includes treatment of an arteritis with steroids and, at times, other forms of immunosuppression. If bypass grafting is required, the inflammatory process should be controlled before grafting. Arterial occlusions are treated according to the etiologic basis: damaged arteries can be repaired or replaced with vein grafts; thromboembolic occlusions can be extracted with an embolectomy catheter, usually with local anesthesia, or lysed with fibrinolytic agents followed, when necessary, with thromboendarterectomy or bypass grafting.

VENOUS INSUFFICIENCY

The manifestations of venous insufficiency include edema, distention of superficial veins, tightness, aching, a reddish-blue discoloration, and pain. Most of these symptoms are caused by occlusions of the axillary, subclavian, or innominate veins. More distal venous occlusions rarely produce significant edema or chronic symptoms. Tumors, mediastinal fibrosis, trauma, and indwelling central venous catheters are the common causes of thrombosis in the large central veins.

The extent of the venous thrombosis should be documented by duplex ultrasonography or by phlebography. Management of the patient with symptomatic upper extremity venous obstruction varies according to the cause of the obstruction. If there is obstruction of venous outflow but no thrombosis, the sites of obstruction should be eliminated; for example, the thoracic space is decompressed, tumors are resected or irradiated, abscesses are drained. If there is acute thrombotic occlusion, the thrombus can be lysed with fibrinolytic agents or can be contained with heparin. The cause of the thrombosis should be eliminated. If restoration of patency of the venous system cannot be achieved with fibrinolytic agents and/or operative decompression, symptoms caused by the thrombotic compression can be relieved with saphenous vein bypasses of the obstruction, e.g., axillary-jugular bypass, brachial-subclavian bypass, and the like.

LYMPHEDEMA

Primary lymphedema of an upper extremity is rare. Secondary lymphedema occurs in up to 10% of women who have had radical mastectomies, usually in conjunction with radiation therapy, for breast cancer. Secondary lymphedema is a potential complication of any axillary dissection. Most often the lymphedema can be controlled with elevation of the arm, elastic sleeves, salt restriction, good skin care, and prompt management of infection. Resistant lymphedema may require the use of a lymphedema pump. Uncontrollable edema usually requires operative procedures for improvement of lymph flow and/or reduction in the size of the extremity.

ASSOCIATED CIRCULATORY PROBLEMS

Causalgia describes the burning, agonizing pain and vasomotor disturbances that occur in 2% to 5% of patients after peripheral nerve injuries. Sympathetic blockade is an excellent diagnostic and therapeutic procedure. If sympathetic blocks provide relief for only short periods, operative sympathetic denervation may be required. Active physical therapy is an important part of the postsympathectomy management.

Causalgia-like pain also may occur after an injury to an extremity in which there is no demonstrable nerve damage. These patients have pain, edema, vasomotor disturbances, soft tissue dystrophy, and atrophy of bone. This disorder has been termed *posttraumatic reflex sympathetic dystrophy*. Management consists of treating the local injury with supportive measures and controlling, if necessary, the pain with analgesics and/or sympathetic blockade.

Acrocyanosis is characterized by painless coolness and cyanosis of the distal portions of the extremities caused by spasm of the small arteries. This symptom complex does not cause any serious disability, and management consists only of protection from cold and trauma.

VISCERAL ISCHEMIC SYNDROMES

William R. Flinn, M.D., and John J. Bergan, M.D.

Mesenteric ischemia is rare, but accurate diagnosis and successful treatment remain challenging in these cases. Mesenteric ischemia may be acute or chronic and may be produced by arterial or venous disorders. Regardless of its cause, when mesenteric ischemia proceeds to intestinal infarction, patient mortality rates range from 50% to 80%, which makes visceral ischemia one of the most lethal vascular problems. Table 1 provides a brief outline of the causes and management of the syndromes of acute mesenteric ischemia.

See the corresponding chapter or part in the *Textbook of Surgery*, 15th edition, pp. 1750–1759, for a more detailed discussion of this topic, including a comprehensive list of references.

TABLE 1. Syndromes of Acute Mesenteric Ischemia

Diagnosis	Presentation	Arteriogram	Treatment	Surgical Findings
Embolism	Abdominal apoplexy Cardiac source Hx of previous emboli	Sharp cut-off, "meniscus" in SMA beyond first jejunal branches	Embolectomy Thrombolytic therapy*	Jejunal "sparing," viable transverse, descending colon Normal pulse in proximal SMA
Arterial thrombosis	Pain out of proportion to PE Hx of postprandial pain, weight loss Severe PAD	Occlusion of celiac, SMA, IMA at their origins	SMA bypass with sufficient viable gastrointestinal length	Ischemia of entire midgut Absent pulse in SMA
Nonocclusive ischemia	Severe cardiopulmonary dysfunction Digitalis, vasopressors	Normal SMA trunk, severe spasm, "pruning" of branch vessels	Intra-arterial vasodilator (papaverine) Surgical exploration for peritonitis	Variable distribution of ischemia, skip areas Normal SMA pulse
Mesenteric vein thrombosis	Younger patients with severe unexplained abdominal sx. Hx of DVT	Normal celiac, SMA Thrombus or nonvisualization on venous phase	Heparin → warfarin Thrombolytic therapy* Surgical exploration PRN	No predictable pattern of ischemia SMA pulse normal Venous thrombi in cut edges of mesentery

*Selected cases.

627

ACUTE MESENTERIC ISCHEMIA

Patients with acute mesenteric ischemia classically present with pain suggestive of a severe underlying abdominal disorder but no findings on physical examination to suggest local or generalized peritonitis. This "abdominal pain out of proportion to physical findings" often results in a delay in the diagnosis. Patients with cardiac disorders, severe peripheral arterial disease, and cardiodynamic instability are at higher risk for acute mesenteric ischemia. While many patients may have a marked leukocytosis or evidence of metabolic acidosis, there is no reliable serologic marker for mesenteric ischemia. When the diagnosis of acute mesenteric ischemia is considered in any patient, arteriography should be performed promptly, since further delay often results in gut infarction and death. Prompt arteriographic diagnosis also may provide an opportunity for catheter-directed thrombolytic or vasodilator therapy in selected patients. Diagnosis of acute mesenteric ischemia due to mesenteric venous thrombosis may require computed tomographic (CT) scan or other imaging techniques. When surgical treatment is required, an attempt should first be made to revascularize the gut when macrovascular occlusion has occurred. Selection of the appropriate revascularization procedure—embolectomy or bypass—may be dictated by the arteriographic findings or the clinical distribution of ischemia noted at the time of surgery. After revascularization, resection of nonviable bowel is performed with anastomosis or exteriorization of remaining segments. In cases of acute mesenteric ischemia treated with surgery, a "second-look" exploration should be performed 24 to 36 hours after initial treatment, since the ischemia-reperfusion injury to the bowel may progress even after successful revascularization.

CHRONIC MESENTERIC ISCHEMIA

Chronic mesenteric ischemia is produced most often by atherosclerotic occlusive lesions of the main mesenteric arteries, the celiac, superior mesenteric artery (SMA) and inferior mesenteric artery (IMA). This problem occurs most often in women with a mean age of 60 years. These patients usually have a long history of postprandial abdominal pain that leads to "food fear" and meal avoidance. As a consequence, these patients have almost all experienced marked weight loss. In most cases this leads to an extensive, often repeated gastrointestinal evaluation for a presumed malignancy. Patients with coexistent aortoiliac occlusive disease are at higher risk for visceral arterial involvement. When the diagnosis of chronic mesenteric ischemia is considered, mesenteric duplex ultrasound scanning, when available, may be a useful noninvasive technique to detect the presence or absence of severe occlusive lesions (Table 2).

Arteriography provides a definitive diagnosis and, in symptomatic patients, usually reveals severe stenosis or occlusion of two or more main mesenteric vessels. Arteriography is also important for identifying associated aortic disease and

TABLE 2. Syndromes of Chronic Mesenteric Ischemia

Diagnosis	Presentation	Arteriogram	Treatment
Chronic atherosclerotic mesenteric occlusion	Postprandial abdominal pain, "food fear" Weight loss	Severe stenosis or occlusion of celiac, SMA, IMA	Mesenteric bypass grafting Mesenteric endarterectomy PTA*
Celiac compression syndrome	Abdominal pain Infrequent weight loss Hx of drug abuse or psychiatric disorder	Focal stenosis of celiac artery Normal arteriogram/duplex scan in deep inspiration	Division of median arcuate ligament of the diaphragm Careful patient selection
Mesenteric venous thrombosis	Younger patients Nonspecific abdominal pain	Venous phase of selective SMA Duplex ultrasound scan CT scan	Heparin Warfarin Thrombolytic therapy*

*Selected cases.

clarifying reconstructive alternatives. In selected patients, balloon angioplasty of severe mesenteric stenoses may be performed, but most will require surgical revascularization. Mesenteric artery bypass and transaortic endarterectomy have been the most successful surgical procedures. Retrograde bypass from the infrarenal aorta (or from an aortic prosthesis when concomitant aortic replacement is indicated) and antegrade bypass from the supraceliac aorta are preferred techniques. In elective cases, comprehensive revascularization, e.g., reconstruction of all three main mesenteric vessels, is recommended, but in all cases lesions of the SMA must be treated.

Isolated stenosis of the celiac artery secondary to extrinsic compression from the crura of the diaphragm has been termed the *celiac artery compression* or the *median arcuate ligament syndrome*. This anatomic variant has been reported to cause symptoms of chronic mesenteric ischemia in small numbers of patients. This diagnosis can be confirmed noninvasively by duplex scanning, which reveals flow abnormalities that return to normal with deep inspiration. Surgical division of the crural fibers produces successful relief of the extrinsic compression. However, selection of appropriate patients for surgical treatment has been difficult because isolated foregut ischemia is difficult to reconcile physiologically and many of these patients have associated societal dysfunction.

Mesenteric venous thrombosis is also listed as a cause of chronic mesenteric ischemia, since nearly a third of cases have had symptoms for more than a month. Unlike the arterial causes of mesenteric ischemia, mesenteric venous thrombosis may affect much younger patients, often as a manifestation of an underlying congenital coagulation disorder such as a deficiency of antithrombin III, protein C, or protein S. This diagnosis should be considered in patients with confusing abdominal symptoms, since, untreated, the outcome can be equally catastrophic.

Syndromes of mesenteric ischemia that go on to mesenteric infarction are associated with a mortality rate that is comparable to or greater than ruptured abdominal aortic aneurysms. Fortunately, the incidence of ruptured aortic aneurysms is decreasing due to early detection and elective treatment. However, no similar trend has been demonstrated for mesenteric ischemia. Only early diagnosis and effective treatment before gut infarction occurs offer any hope for improved survival in these patients.

RENOVASCULAR DISEASE

J. Caulie Gunnells, Jr., M.D., and
Richard L. McCann, M.D.

Hypertension produced by obstruction of the renal arteries is termed *renovascular hypertension* and is the most common form of potentially curable high blood pressure. This form of hypertension is usually difficult to control medically, and patients with this disorder are at a continuing potential risk for irreversible damage to the kidneys as well as other critical organ systems such as the eye, heart, and brain if inappropriate or ineffective pharmacologic modalities are utilized in a futile attempt to control blood pressure.

Furthermore, if the mechanical obstruction producing the hypertension is progressive, there may be inexorable loss of renal function. It is now well accepted that mechanical intervention utilizing modern revascularization techniques of surgical bypass or balloon angioplasty provides a very appropriate and effective relief of this form of hypertension, and as well this type of intervention may lead to preserved or improved renal function in many patients.

Estimates of the prevalence of renovascular hypertension vary from less than 5% to more than 20% of the adult hypertensive population in the United States. The true incidence is difficult to determine accurately owing to wide variability in criteria among investigative groups for patient selection for clinical investigation.

Systemic arterial blood pressure is controlled by a number of factors, including cardiac output, peripheral vascular resistance, and blood volume along with the activity of the renin-angiotensin-aldosterone system (RAS) together with the integrating function of the sympathetic nervous system. Renal ischemia stimulates secretion of the enzyme renin, which acts on renin substrate, a plasma protein that is synthesized in the liver.

This reaction cleaves the decapeptide angiotensin I, a substance with little physiologic activity. Angiotensin I is acted on by another enzyme, angiotensin-converting enzyme, causing the production of the octapeptide angiotensin II. The latter's two major physiologic activities—direct vasoconstriction and stimulation of production of aldosterone by the adrenal gland—cause sodium retention, increased intravascular volume, and potassium excretion. Thus hypertension is produced by the two complementary mechanisms of vasoconstriction and augmentation of intravascular volume.

The availability of laboratory techniques to measure levels of plasma renin activity in both peripheral and renal venous blood, along with the appropriate utilization of angiotensin-converting enzyme inhibitors to enhance or augment renin secretion, has contributed greatly to the evaluation of patients

---

See the corresponding chapter or part in the *Textbook of Surgery*, 15th edition, pp. 1759–1767, for a more detailed discussion of this topic, including a comprehensive list of references.

suspected of having renovascular hypertension. Furthermore, specific pharmacologic blockade of angiotensin II receptors is now possible, and these agents are useful for both diagnosis and treatment.

The most common cause of renovascular hypertension is atherosclerosis, which is the etiologic basis of the lesions in two thirds of patients with this disorder. Atherosclerotic lesions are most apt to occur near the origin of the renal vessels from the aorta and are often segmental and short. The second most frequent cause of renovascular hypertension is fibromuscular dysplasia of the renal arteries. This group of lesions may involve disease in any of the three vascular coats, but the most common is fibrous dysplasia of the medial layer. This lesion usually occurs in young women and causes serial constrictions alternating with areas of increased diameter, which on angiography produce a corrugated effect termed the *string of beads*. A new group of vascular lesions, collectively termed *atheroembolic renal artery disease*, has recently been identified as an important cause of renovascular hypertension. The concomitant development of emboli involving the renal circulation may contribute to hypertension as well as compromised renal function.

Considerable difference of opinion persists regarding which patients within the larger population with arterial hypertension should be evaluated for renovascular disease. Patients with renovascular disease tend to have sudden or abrupt onset of hypertension, often before age 35 or subsequent to age 55. Patients with renovascular hypertension often have sustained severe diastolic blood pressure (greater than 115 mm. Hg) or a pattern of accelerated or malignant hypertensive disease. Patients who exhibit failure of antihypertensive drug therapy or who lose previous control and those with deteriorating renal function despite adequate blood pressure control should be considered for investigation of renovascular disease. In patients with renovascular disease, physical examination may reveal an abdominal or epigastric bruit. Patients with all these findings are relatively rare, but when several of these are present, they demand strong consideration for further investigation to establish a diagnosis of functionally significant renal artery stenosis.

The definitive study for renovascular disease is renal angiography. Since this is an invasive and expensive examination, it is necessary to select patients from the larger hypertensive population who have a higher probability of harboring renovascular disease as a contributing etiologic factor to their hypertension. A number of screening evaluations with variable sensitivity have been proposed. The value of measuring plasma renin activity has been enhanced recently by the finding that plasma renin activity can be increased in patients with renovascular hypertension by acute inhibition of angiotensin-converting enzyme by pharmacologic agents such as captopril. The predictive value of both peripheral plasma renin activity and renal vein renin ratio determinations can be enhanced significantly by administration of this drug. Similarly, the utility of radioisotope renography is increased by concomitant administration of angiotensin-converting enzyme inhibitors.

The goal of treatment of patients with renovascular disease is amelioration of the high blood pressure together with preservation and occasionally improvement in renal function. Whereas medical therapy of hypertension of renovascular origin may obviate the risk of operation, it requires a high degree of patient compliance, constant medical supervision, and lifelong administration of antihypertensive medication. Medical therapy also has been demonstrated to be less effective than is restoration of renal blood flow in terms of long-term preservation of renal function.

Balloon catheter dilation of renal artery stenoses can be used in some patients. In patients with fibromuscular disease, particularly of the medial fibroplasia type, balloon angioplasty has a high rate of success, and recurrence is unusual. The experience with atherosclerotic disease has not been as favorable, and some studies suggest that less than half of patients with atherosclerotic obstruction of the renal artery are improved after a follow-up of less than 2 years. Ostial lesions of the renal artery in particular respond poorly to attempted balloon dilation.

If the affected kidney has been severely damaged by ischemia and contributes little to total renal function, the most appropriate procedure may be nephrectomy. A renal length of 7 cm. and severe arteriolar nephrosclerosis with hyalinization of all or most glomeruli on biopsy suggest an unsalvageable kidney, the removal of which may ameliorate hypertension and improve prognosis for maintenance of renal function in the remaining kidney. Aortorenal bypass by use of an autogenous saphenous vein graft is the most frequently selected surgical procedure for renal artery stenosis. When there is severe disease of the aortic wall, however, it may be difficult to attach a graft at this location, and a more peripheral origin such as the splenic or hepatic artery may be used to revascularize the left and right kidneys, respectively. Severe branch vessel disease may be corrected surgically through "benchwork surgery" after the kidney has been temporarily removed from the body and cooled.

Good long-term results with 70% to 90% improvement in hypertension is expected. The effect of revascularization on preservation of renal function is less certain but clearly of major importance. Mortality is rare and occurs almost exclusively in patients with widespread systemic atherosclerotic disease, in whom renal revascularization is only a part of a larger vascular reconstruction.

VII

Venous Injuries
Norman M. Rich, M.D.

In contrast to repair rather than ligation of injured arteries widely practiced since the Korean conflict, similar management of venous injuries has been more controversial. It is ironic that Murphy stated in 1897 that ". . . closure of wounds in the veins by suture is now an acceptable surgical practice."

Two major concerns prevented development of repair of injured veins: perceived increased incidence of thrombophlebitis and fear of pulmonary embolism. Many injured veins can be ligated with few or no immediate problems and no recognized long-term disability. Until the last 35 years, the effectiveness of venous repair remained uncertain. Thrombosis was recognized to be much more common in the lower-pressure venous system compared with the good results achieved following repair of arterial injuries. Also, in contrast to arterial repair, in which simple palpation of a peripheral pulse is usually adequate for determining success or failure, effectiveness of venous repair is more difficult to evaluate because there is no simple method for determining patency of venous reconstruction.

Acute venous hypertension, particularly in lower extremities, following ligation of major veins contributes to an increased amputation rate. In addition, the degree of disability from chronic venous insufficiency is not recognized by many. This disability may not become evident for months or even many years following injury. It has been recognized throughout history that important surgical progress has occurred during periods of armed conflict when surgeons are required to treat large numbers of patients with similar injuries within a relatively short period of time. This connection between military surgery and vascular surgery has been particularly noteworthy in the twentieth century. An analysis including importance and effectiveness of repair of venous injuries during the American experience in Southeast Asia was started at Walter Reed Army Medical Center in 1966 as the Vietnam Vascular Registry. A preliminary report demonstrated a significant 27% incidence of venous injuries. An early report emphasized the need for the repair of injured veins. A more aggressive approach for the repair of injured veins, particularly in lower extremity venous trauma, was advocated in 1974.

Venous repair may be particularly important in large-caliber lower extremity veins, specifically the popliteal vein. Venous repair may be necessary in the presence of massive soft tissue injury and is mandatory in replantation of extremities. Repair

---

See the corresponding chapter or part in the *Textbook of Surgery,* 15th edition, pp. 1767–1774, for a more detailed discussion of this topic, including a comprehensive list of references.

of injured veins should be considered routinely with large-caliber veins in an attempt to prevent acute or chronic venous insufficiency. Important central veins such as the portal vein, the superior mesenteric vein, and the vena cava should be repaired. Lateral suture repair of a lacerated vein is frequently the most rapid and safest method of halting hemorrhage from an injured vein. Although the general status of the patient with multiple injuries must be considered, it is possible to also repair veins by end-to-end anastomoses and by interpositional grafts, including compilation venous grafts, spiral venous grafts, and ringed prostheses. The challenge of obtaining successful venous reconstruction remains. Identification of the ideal substitute that will have a high degree of success with long-term patency in the low-pressure venous system is a major obstacle.

Recent studies provide data that refute the fear of producing a higher incidence of venous thrombosis and pulmonary embolization by attempting repair of injured veins. The dangerous sequence has been surprisingly unusual. It is conceivable that small emboli may not be recognized clinically; however, the absence of clinically detectable pulmonary emboli has been uniformly documented both in the Vietnam Vascular Registry and other reports. Civilian and military experiences have had similar and contrasting aspects emphasized in part by the difference in the types of wounds sustained.

INCIDENCE. Many surgeons have considered venous injuries to be unimportant and the true incidences undetermined. The notable early exception is the report by Gaspar and Treiman of a group of 228 patients with vascular injuries in Los Angeles. About 22% or 51 patients had venous injuries. Meyer (1987) identified 36 patients with major extremity venous injuries. Aitken (1989) reviewed the cases of 26 patients with lower limb venous trauma.

ETIOLOGY. Many wounding agents have been associated with venous trauma. Iatrogenic injuries to the venous system have increased over the past 30 years as a result of rapid development of angiographic and therapeutic techniques. Fractures have been associated with venous injuries.

DIAGNOSTIC CONSIDERATIONS. Doppler ultrasound may be useful. Color duplex expands the options. Impedance plethysmography, phlebography, and radionuclide studies have helped diagnosis of venous occlusions.

SURGICAL MANAGEMENT. General management of injured patients should be of primary concern. Venous injury can be managed by ligation, lateral suture repair, end-to-end anastomosis, venous patch graft, and venous replacement graft.

POSTOPERATIVE CARE. Specific attempts should be made after the operation to minimize or eliminate edema of the involved extremity.

RESULTS. There are an increasing number of reports emphasizing the success of repair and reconstruction of injured major-caliber veins. Successful venous repair recorded in the Vietnam Vascular Registry stimulated civilian surgeons to duplicate the success. Sharma (1990) emphasized the high degree of success associated with meticulous technique in venous reconstruction. Controversy continues. While Sharma (1992) emphasizes repair, Yelon and Scalea (1992) note that ligation is acceptable. Additional documentation of clinical experience and additional research support are indicated.

51

DISORDERS OF THE LUNGS, PLEURA, AND CHEST WALL

I

Anatomy
Walter G. Wolfe, M.D., and R. Eric Lilly, M.D.

The anatomy of the lung is fundamental in understanding and management of difficult clinical problems involving the pulmonary system. The lung is of additional importance because of its position as a target organ for many complications that occur following a host of surgical procedures. Complications occur with passage of tubes through the nasal pharynx. Vocal cord injury and injury to the larynx and trachea occur with intubation and may be involved in traumatic injuries of the neck and thorax. Consequently, a knowledge of anatomy is essential because of the seriousness of overlooked injury and the surrounding structures including the great vessels and esophagus. The interruption or loss of function of the laryngeal mechanism that protects patients from the dangers of aspiration may be the most serious pulmonary complication occurring in surgical patients. Contamination of the airway by either aspiration or bacteria produces pneumonia and sepsis.

Knowledge of the airways and their hyperreactivity, such as seen in patients with asthma, as well as of fluid overload and sudden mucosal edema producing small airway obstruction is extremely important. The mucociliary blanket protects the alveoli by moving mucus and particles from the conducting airways so that they can be expelled by cough. Interference with this mechanism subjects the patient to pulmonary complications. Consequently, loss of ciliated cells and the increased production by mucous cells have a significant role in the ability of these surgical patients, especially smokers, to clear secretions in the postoperative period.

Alveolar epithelium and the endothelium of the capillaries are susceptible to toxic substances, the most common used in the intensive care unit being oxygen. Therefore, protecting patients on long-term ventilation from oxygen toxicity is mandatory.

The blood supply to the lung, including the pulmonary circulation and the bronchial circulation, is of utmost importance. Obliteration of pulmonary arteries through either pulmonary emboli or inflammatory processes may have serious consequence to the alveoli and gas exchange. In inflammatory or cyanotic conditions in which there is a prominent bronchial circulation, significant hemoptysis may occur. Also, the blood

See the corresponding chapter or part in the *Textbook of Surgery*, 15th edition, pp. 1775–1786, for a more detailed discussion of this topic, including a comprehensive list of references.

supply of primary bronchogenic tumors of the lung is usually via the bronchial circulation. Knowledge of the bronchial circulation as well as of the pulmonary arterial circulation is important because of resurgence of lung transplantation and problems that occur with healing of the bronchial anastomosis.

In summary, the anatomy of the lung and its metabolic functions continue to be essential in surgical therapy not only for the management of the conditions that occur primarily in the lung, such as inflammation, abscess, and carcinoma, but also because the pulmonary system remains a significant target organ for morbidity and mortality in patients undergoing operations in all surgical specialties.

II

Clinical and Physiologic Evaluation of Pulmonary Function

Richard A. Hopkins, M.D., Walter G. Wolfe, M.D., and Farid Gharagozloo, M.D.

PULMONARY FUNCTION

Understanding the factors that contribute to and alter pulmonary ventilation and gas exchange requires a detailed knowledge of lung function at the alveolar level. Ventilation serves to replenish the gas in the lungs for maintenance of the high-oxygen–low-carbon-dioxide pressure, with production of maximal gradients. *Distribution* of gas is the delivery of air to the alveolar units by way of the bifurcating tracheobronchial tree. *Diffusion* is the transfer of gas molecules across the alveolar membranes in the region of high concentration. The blood-air surface of over 90 sq. m. in adult humans is condensed in a lung volume of only 5 L. This is made possible by the small radius and the large number (300 million) of alveoli. *Perfusion* is the means by which desaturated blood is brought into intimate contact with the alveolar-capillary bed.

LUNG VOLUMES. *Respiratory excursion* is the amount of air inspired and expired; this is termed *tidal volume* (VT). The amount of gas contained in the lung at the end of quiet expiration is termed the *functional residual capacity* (FRC). When the patient makes a maximal inspiration and increases the lung volume compared with that contained at the peak tidal volume, the inspiratory *reserve capacity* or *volume* (RV) is

---

See the corresponding chapter or part in the *Textbook of Surgery*, 15th edition, pp. 1787–1801, for a more detailed discussion of this topic, including a comprehensive list of references.

reached. With forcible expiration, with exhalation of as much air as possible from the lung, the volume expired from the maximal inspiration to maximal expiration is the *vital capacity* (VC). The amount of air remaining in the lungs after maximal expiration is the *residual volume* (RV). These lung volumes may be measured in the spirometer, except for the RV and FRC. The FRC must be measured by other techniques. One of three different methods—inert gas dilution and washout, whole-body plethysmography, or radioisotope techniques—may be employed.

MAXIMAL BREATHING CAPACITY. *Maximal breathing capacity* (MBC) is defined as the largest volume of air that can be moved in and out of the chest per minute. The term *MBC* is reserved for the maximal breathing capacity of an individual, whereas the term *maximal voluntary ventilation* (MVV) indicates the maximal volume of gas breathed per minute under specific testing conditions. The analysis of VC and of MBC permits differentiation of ventilatory abnormality into obstructive versus restrictive disease, since MBC is markedly decreased in obstructive disease.

FLOW RATES. Measurement of dynamic properties of the lungs, i.e., flow rates, is extremely important. The patient inhales maximally and then exhales forcibly into the spirometer while the device records the volume versus the time. A common test of maximal expiratory airflow is the volume of air expired in 1 second (FEV_1). This number is decreased in the presence of bronchial obstruction, but the value also may be decreased in restrictive disease. For this reason, the FEV_1 is usually related to the total exhaled VC. This ratio of FEV_1 to VC may be decreased in the presence of airway obstruction but normal in restrictive lung disease.

GAS DIFFUSION. A single-breath carbon monoxide (DL_{CO}) diffusion capacity should be considered a screening test. In this test, the patient is required to inhale low, nontoxic concentrations of carbon monoxide, hold the breath for 10 seconds, and then exhale. This test is rapid, simple, safe, and painless. DL_{CO} is an estimate of the pulmonary capillary surface area. There are several factors that affect diffusion in a single alveolus. The thickness of the alveolar lining membrane is important as well as the thickness of the layer of plasma between the capillary wall and the red blood cell. In addition, the permeability of the erythrocyte to carbon monoxide or oxygen must be considered along with the reaction rate of hemoglobin with carbon monoxide or oxygen. In a single-breath diffusion capacity with use of carbon monoxide, the presence of carbon monoxide hemoglobin in the pulmonary arterial blood diminishes the rate of carbon monoxide transfer.

The measurement of arterial blood gases is probably the most frequently used pulmonary function test. The interpretation of PaO_2 depends on the oxygen tension in the inspired air. After calculating the alveolar oxygen tension, the alveolar-arterial oxygen tension gradient can be determined; if the PaO_2 and the $(A-a) DO_2$ are normal, there is no disturbance in oxygen transport.

The measurements of $PaCO_2$ provide an immediate indication of the patient's alveolar ventilation. A $PaCO_2$ of less than

37 mm. Hg indicates hypocapnia, whereas hypercapnia is
defined as greater than 43 mm. Hg (i.e., normal range, 38 to
42 mm. Hg). Any level of hypercapnia indicates severe disease
representing functional loss of perhaps more than 50% of the
lung. *Acidosis* is defined as a pH of less than 7.37, and *alkalosis*
indicates a pH of greater than 7.43. Evaluation of acid-base
requires interpretation of both respiratory and metabolic determinants of pH; potential aberrations include respiratory
acidosis, respiratory alkalosis, metabolic acidosis, and metabolic alkalosis.

CLOSING VOLUMES. The *closing volume* is the remaining
lung volume at the end of expiration below which alveolar
collapse begins to occur, with production of "physiologic"
shunting. In the normal young individual, this closing volume
is well below the FRC. Age alone is associated with a decrease
in the elastic properties of the lung such that although FRC
gradually increases with age, so does the effective closing
volume. Placing a patient supine, even at a young age, or
other mechanical factors such as obesity may produce an
elevation in closing volume and relative hypoxemia. Hypoxemia is common postoperatively because of this *closing
volume effect*. The presence of interstitial pulmonary edema
accentuates this effect. When end-expiratory pressure is applied, FRC returns to normal and corrects the closing volume
abnormality.

PREOPERATIVE EVALUATION

Pulmonary complications are not infrequent following
major operative procedures. Age, obesity, type of surgical
procedure, cigarette smoking, and anesthesia impair pulmonary function and are preoperative risk factors.

Pulmonary function should be evaluated in relation to the
operative procedure planned. Patients can be divided into
the following groups: (1) those undergoing thoracotomy for
removal of lung tissue, (2) those undergoing thoracotomy
without excision of pulmonary tissue, (3) those undergoing
abdominal surgery, and (4) those undergoing procedures on
extremities or elsewhere. It is apparent that each group responds somewhat differently to the effects of the operation,
anesthesia, and pulmonary function. Every effort should be
made postoperatively to obtain maximal pulmonary function
as soon as possible for ensuring rapid return of the FRC to
the preoperative level. Supplemental oxygen should be used
as necessary for prevention of hypoxemia. In general, if the
VC and FRC are returned to the preoperative level and hypoxemia is prevented, the ventilation-perfusion ratio will be corrected.

**RISK IN PATIENTS WITH PRE-EXISTING PULMO-
NARY DISEASE.** Obstructive pulmonary disease is the most
important risk factor in the patient undergoing operation. The
more severe the disease, the greater is the risk of postoperative
complications. Restrictive lung disease is usually better tolerated; however, these patients cannot afford to lose much functioning lung. Because of better expiratory flow rates, cough is

better preserved than with obstructive disease. In general, an FEV_1 of 1 to 2 L. is not associated with an increased operative risk; with an FEV_1 less than 800 ml., there is clearly increased risk for severe pulmonary complications; those with less than 500 ml. have the greatest risk. The presence of carbon dioxide retention is a marker for the patient at dramatically increased risk.

Thoracotomy and pulmonary resection are not well tolerated in patients with obstructive airway disease. Not only is there a loss of functional tissue in a patient with pulmonary disease, but the thoracotomy alters the mechanical and gas exchange properties of the lung. This may be accentuated if lung tissue is removed during operation. Thoracotomy produces pain in the postoperative period, which reduces the patient's ability to cough for clearance of secretions. If the airway disease is severe, the patient may not be able to tolerate the loss of even a single pulmonary segment. Thus, in these patients, preoperative evaluation is extremely important, and preparation of the patient by cessation of smoking and the use of a number of drugs for improvement of airway function and ventilation is extremely helpful in decreasing operative risk.

In individuals with pulmonary hypertension and carbon dioxide retention, resective procedures may be contraindicated. For example, if FEV_1 is less than 2 L. and the MVV or MBC is less than 50%, patients usually do not tolerate pneumonectomy. Therefore, predicting postresection lung function can be helpful in preventing a surgically cured but pulmonary-crippled patient. A good estimate of postoperative pulmonary function can be obtained by comparing the quantitative perfusion lung scan with the patient's preoperative FEV_1. Ferguson and colleagues have demonstrated that measurement of $D_{L_{CO}}$ is an important discriminator for postoperative morbidity and mortality following pulmonary resection.

It has been reported that routine pulmonary function tests cannot predict which patients develop complications following pulmonary resection. These observations have underlined the inaccuracy of predicting complications or mortality of thoracotomy and pulmonary resection based on pulmonary function testing alone. The postoperative complications and mortality seen with a thoracotomy stem from a functional defect in the cardiopulmonary unit. The heart and the lungs, together with hemoglobin, comprise the integrated cardiopulmonary unit responsible for sustaining O_2 availability for tissue metabolism. The successful functioning of the cardiopulmonary unit is determined by the oxygen uptake (V_{O_2}) and CO_2 production (V_{CO_2}). These parameters can be measured during cardiopulmonary exercise testing. Cardiopulmonary exercise testing simulates the postresection conditions of increased pulmonary blood flow, CO_2 excretion, and O_2 uptake required of the remaining lung. Patients with a $V_{O_{2max}}$ exceeding 20 ml. per kg. per minute have low morbidity following thoracotomy, patients with a $V_{O_{2max}}$ of 15 to 20 ml. per kg. per minute appear to be at moderate risk (25% complication rate), those with a $V_{O_{2max}}$ of 10 to 15 ml. per kg. per minute are at high risk (32% complication rate), and patients with a

VO_{2max} of less than 10 ml. per kg. per minute have an unacceptably high complication rate of 80% following pulmonary resection.

OPERATIVE AND POSTOPERATIVE CHANGES. The effects of anesthesia may increase venous admixture, increase ventilation and perfusion mismatching, change the cardiac output, and alter the mechanical properties of the chest wall or the lung itself, whether or not paralysis is used during anesthesia. Mucociliary transport may be decreased, and the hemoglobin concentration and function may change. Diaphragmatic function may be impaired, and the position of the patient during operation may compound some of these difficulties. The dependent basilar segments, for example, are usually underventilated and therefore have a greater tendency to develop atelectasis. In general, the patient is ventilated with positive pressure, and the dependent areas of the lung, which have the smallest airway diameters and are the least compliant, are poorly ventilated. The more compliant and less perfused areas receive the greatest ventilation. This produces ventilation-perfusion mismatching and hypoxemia and atelectasis. The FRC decreases in almost all anesthetized surgical patients as well as in injured patients regardless of whether the injury is a result of the operation or of trauma. It follows, therefore, that the FEV_1 and VC are also reduced. These changes are maximal in the first and second postoperative days but remain abnormal for a week following operation. Decrease in the FRC causes airway closure and ventilation-perfusion mismatching with resulting hypoxemia, which may be accentuated in the older patient. The patient should be encouraged to sit upright as soon as possible. Lung function is clearly improved with early ambulation. This is especially important in the obese and elderly. Early ambulation increases FRC and also helps to reduce the risk of pulmonary embolism. Pulmonary embolism in the postoperative period is a dangerous postoperative complication in these higher-risk patients with impaired pulmonary functions. Care must be taken to prevent aspiration.

III

Bronchoscopy
Mark Tedder, M.D., and Ross M. Ungerleider, M.D.

Fiberoptic technology has revolutionized the field of bronchoscopy by markedly expanding its diagnostic capabilities.

See the corresponding chapter or part in the *Textbook of Surgery*, 15th edition, pp. 1801–1805, for a more detailed discussion of this topic, including a comprehensive list of references.

A firm understanding of the indications for bronchoscopy, all anesthetic techniques, the technical aspects of the intervention (with both flexible and rigid instruments), and the management of potential complications is imperative to the clinician. Common indications include a mass on chest film, foreign-body aspiration, persistent atelectasis, and the preoperative assessment of resectability.

BRONCHOSCOPIC EXAMINATION. Continuous pulse oximetry, telemetry, and blood pressure are monitored prior to sedation and throughout the procedure. The need for pre-bronchoscopic intubation must be individualized and should depend on the likelihood of a major airway complication (e.g., presence of massive hemoptysis, copious secretions), the patient's pulmonary status, and the extent of the planned intervention.

A compulsive examination is essential to maximize the amount of information gained from a bronchoscopy, such as cord mobility, airway position and patency, branching pattern, and mucosal and extramucosal abnormalities. Endobronchial washings (selective or nonselective) should be sent for appropriate studies as indicated. Standard biopsy forceps, brushes, curettes, or needles are commonly used to evaluate endobronchial lesions and peribronchial tissues. Several newer bronchoscopic techniques have been applied, such as laser therapy, phototherapy, cryotherapy, immunotherapy, and brachytherapy. The ultimate roles that these modalities will achieve in treating various pulmonary diseases has yet to be determined.

RIGID BRONCHOSCOPY. Only 2% of bronchoscopies are performed using the rigid bronchoscope, and 90% of these are performed by surgeons. Certain clinical scenarios are best approached with rigid bronchoscopy. This remains the procedure of choice for pediatric bronchoscopy (especially foreign-body removal) and for the evaluation of massive hemoptysis (600 ml. in 24 hours). Stricture dilation, stent placement, laser therapy, phototherapy, and cryotherapy also may be performed through the rigid bronchoscope. Its durability, the large instrument channel, and the secure airway it provides are advantages the rigid has over the flexible bronchoscope.

FLEXIBLE BRONCHOSCOPY. Since its introduction less than 30 years ago, flexible bronchoscopy has become commonplace in the evaluation of numerous pulmonary disorders. Because these instruments are highly maneuverable and smaller in size than most rigid bronchoscopes, they can be used to reach areas in the endobronchial tree not accessible by their rigid counterparts. Furthermore, patient tolerance, the ability to be performed in the outpatient setting, and topical anesthesia are additional advantages of flexible bronchoscopy.

COMPLICATIONS. Bronchoscopy is generally considered a safe procedure. Most complications are preventable when appropriate attention is given to preoperative preparation, identification of high-risk patients, and the performance of a careful bronchoscopic examination. A comprehensive survey of bronchoscopic complications ($n = 24,521$) revealed the morbidity and mortality to be 0.08% and 0.01%, respectively. Most complications are minor and relate to anesthesia, cardiopulmonary embarrassment, technical difficulties, or biopsy.

Bleeding following bronchoscopy with biopsy is usually minor and self-limiting. Interventions may include epinephrine injection, tamponade by lodging the tip of the bronchoscope into the appropriate segment, packing with prothrombotic agents, selective balloon tamponade, angiography with embolization, and pulmonary resection, depending on the severity of the hemorrhage. Almost 50% of pneumothoraces require decompression with either a dart or a chest tube.

IV

Diagnostic Thoracoscopy
Joseph B. Shrager, M.D., and Larry R. Kaiser, M.D.

Although the concept of thoracoscopy dates to the early twentieth century, only in the past decade has the technique been applied to a wide variety of thoracic diseases. Most disorders encountered by general thoracic surgeons have been managed successfully with the thoracoscope. The advantage of thoracoscopy over thoracotomy is the ability to perform the same procedure as done by the "open" approach but with decreased morbidity. This advantage has been clearly established for some of the procedures, while data are forthcoming concerning others. Thus the appropriate role of thoracoscopy in thoracic surgery remains to be fully defined.

Due to the rigidity of the chest wall, thoracoscopy does not require insufflation of gas to create a space in which to manipulate instruments. Single lung ventilation on the side opposite the procedure, allowing ipsilateral lung collapse, is sufficient. The technique provides excellent exposure to the entire hemithorax, rivaling "open" exposure for recessed structures such as the sympathetic chain and thoracic duct.

For most thoracoscopic procedures, the patient is placed in a lateral decubitus position as for thoracotomy, and three 2- to 3-cm. incisions are made and deepened over an adjacent rib. The videotelescope is placed through a port, which is usually through the most inferior incision, while instruments or fingers are placed directly through the two superior incisions, allowing operative manipulations. The two superior incisions generally are placed in the line of a standard thoracotomy incision, such that if conversion to thoracotomy is required, the incisions simply can be joined. The inferior incision is usually the site of postoperative chest tube placement. Video monitors are placed on either side of the table as for laparoscopic cholecystectomy.

See the corresponding chapter or part in the *Textbook of Surgery,* 15th edition, pp. 1806–1814, for a more detailed discussion of this topic, including a comprehensive list of references.

The most common application of video-assisted thoracic surgery (VATS) is in the diagnosis and treatment of pleural disease. Recurrent pleural effusion, if the etiology is thought to be malignant but fluid cytology has been negative for malignant cells, frequently can be both diagnosed and treated by thoracoscopy. Examination of the pleural space may allow identification of lesions to be biopsied for diagnosis, while pleurodesis may be performed by insufflation of talc. This creates an inflammatory reaction that causes adhesions between the visceral and parietal pleurae, thus obliterating the space in which further fluid might accumulate. In patients with effusions of known malignant origin but in whom pleurodesis through a chest tube has failed, thoracoscopic pleurodesis may be more successful. If a malignant effusion is loculated and cannot be drained completely with a chest tube, thoracoscopy allows complete drainage and pleurodesis simultaneously.

Infected pleural fluid frequently becomes loculated, rendering complete drainage with chest tubes difficult, but infected pleural fluid, or empyema, may be drained successfully under direct vision thoracoscopically. The thick, fibrinous exudate that frequently develops can be evacuated completely by VATS. If performed early in the course of the infection, the lung usually expands postoperatively to fill the entire hemithorax. However, if there is delay in achieving complete drainage, a constricting "peel" may form around the lung and require decortication, often with a minithoracotomy. Similarly, hemothorax is usually posttraumatic, and drainage through a chest, if clotted, may be done easily thoracoscopically, thus preventing later trapping of underlying lung by organized thrombus.

The treatment of parenchymal lung disease also has been affected by the availability of VATS. Prior to VATS, many patients with interstitial pulmonary processes were treated empirically because of the perceived morbidity of a thoracotomy. The availability of the less morbid VATS approach to lung biopsy has prompted earlier and more frequent referral of these patients. Some hold that biopsy through a small inframammary incision without rib spreading also causes minimal morbidity and is the preferred approach for lung biopsy in interstitial lung disease. This is the optimal approach in the critically ill, ventilator-dependent patients for whom changing the endotracheal tube to a double-lumen tube may represent a substantial risk. For the usual ambulatory patient in stable condition, the VATS approach is preferred, allowing visualization of the entire lung and directed biopsy of abnormal areas. Further, it decreases postoperative pain.

In the patient with spontaneous pneumothorax, which generally follows rupture of congenital apical blebs, many have employed a VATS approach instead of thoracotomy. The classic indications for operation have been a second episode of pneumothorax or bilateral pneumothoraces. The operation employed generally has been resection of the blebs and creation of a pleural symphysis by one of several means. This has been described for standard thoracotomy or transaxillary thoracotomy. The same procedure can be performed by VATS by stapling the apical blebs and abrading the parietal pleural surface with a surgical sponge. A randomized study demonstrated that VATS management of spontaneous pneumothorax is equally effective and causes less postoperative morbidity compared with treatment by thoracotomy. Patients generally leave the hospital on the first or second postoperative day.

Secondary pneumothorax, or pneumothorax from a process other than congenital blebs, also may be treated by VATS. Since these patients often have significantly compromised pulmonary function (from, for example, emphysema), they are apt to benefit even more from the VATS approach than the younger, healthier primary pneumothorax patients. The underlying lesion in these patients is somewhat more complex, and one must identify the site of leakage prior to repair. The leaking site is repaired by stapling, fibrin glue, laser, or argon beam coagulator.

The primary indication for operation in patients with bullous disease, aside from the presence of pneumothorax, is the presence of a giant bulla causing compression of adjacent, relatively normal lung. If there is a significant amount of parenchyma that appears compressed on preoperative chest film and computed tomography (CT) and is likely to expand after elimination of the compressing bulla, these patients are likely to improve symptomatically after operation to ablate the bulla. Previously, it was feared that thoracotomy in these severely compromised patients might prove fatal. With the advent of VATS, the procedure can be performed safely and usually with immediate postoperative extubation by application of the argon beam coagulator, which causes the wall of the bulla to contract but remain intact. The base of the bulla is then stapled with a bovine pericardium as a buttress. This latter innovation provides a low incidence of prolonged air leaks.

The solitary pulmonary nodule is another lesion often treated by thoracoscopic resection. The primary question posed by a solitary pulmonary nodule ("coin lesion") is whether or not it is malignant. Despite historical and radiologic features that may suggest whether a nodule is more likely to be benign or malignant, a benign diagnosis unfortunately can never be firmly established without a histologic diagnosis. Furthermore, the small tissue fragments obtained by bronchoscopy or transthoracic needle biopsy only provide a specific benign diagnosis in about 10% of patients. Therefore, transthoracic needle biopsy is only performed in two situations: in a patient with multiple unresectable nodules that are thought to be malignant and when a tissue diagnosis is needed in a patient who has an absolute contraindication to operation. In the other instances, complete excision of the nodule by VATS is recommended.

VATS excision of a pulmonary nodule is performed using the standard three incisions. A preoperative chest computed tomographic (CT) scan is obtained to carefully localize the lesion. On entry into the chest, the visceral pleurae are inspected for changes that may denote an underlying lesion. Palpation with a finger placed through one of the incisions may then confirm the position of the lesion. The mass is then grasped, and the involved portion of the lung containing it is separated from surrounding lung with a stapler. The specimen is placed in an endoscopic bag prior to removal from the chest to prevent deposition of tumor cells in the wound.

There is controversy concerning the management of a lesion believed to be a carcinoma. The Lung Cancer Study Group examined the question of limited resection versus lobectomy for early lung cancers in a prospective, randomized trial, and at 5 years there was a decreased survival in those with less than a lobectomy. It is preferable to perform VATS wedge excision for biopsy and then perform a lobectomy by VATS or convert to open thoracotomy for performance of a lobectomy. Only in a patient whom it is felt cannot tolerate a thoracotomy is wedge excision alone appropriate. Prospective, randomized trials are required to assess whether VATS or open thoracotomy is better in these cases.

Finally, VATS has been used in the staging of bronchogenic carcinoma. Cervical mediastinoscopy, the accepted standard of pathologic staging, does not allow access to lymph nodes in the subaortic window or in the posterior subcarinal space. Since VATS permits access to these areas, some patients with enlarged lymph nodes in this location on CT may benefit by preoperative biopsy by VATS. The occasional patient may be spared an avoidable thoracotomy by introducing the thoracoscope to document the absence of diffuse pleural disease.

Primary lesions of the anterior mediastinum also have proven amenable to VATS techniques, including thymoma, lymphoma, and teratoma. For thymoma in myasthenia gravis, where complete thymectomy is critical, a combined transcervical and VATS exposure may be used. For the nondiscrete mediastinal mass, biopsy for tissue diagnosis may be obtained by VATS. Posterior mediastinal masses also have been resected successfully by VATS, including schwannomas and bronchogenic cysts.

Pericardial effusions can be managed by VATS, since excellent exposure of the pericardium is obtained from either the right or the left side. The accepted operation for recurrent pericardial effusion is creation of a pericardial window, and this can be performed by either a subxiphoid or a VATS approach. Both are considered minimally invasive, and a prospective study is necessary to determine if there is a clear advantage of one over the other.

Although some groups have described total esophagectomy by a VATS approach and others have reported staging of esophageal cancer by VATS lymph node biopsy, the primary application of VATS to esophageal disease has been for management of achalasia. VATS esophageal myotomy for achalasia has been performed in multiple patients with excellent results. The ability to perform the procedure without thoracotomy may prompt earlier referral of these patients for definitive therapy, replacing repeated pneumatic dilation. A final application of VATS to the esophagus is in excision of leiomyoma, the most common benign lesion of the esophagus. Its submucosal location renders it eminently resectable by VATS.

Other procedures performed successfully by VATS techniques include dorsal sympathectomy for hyperhidrosis and reflex sympathetic dystrophy and thoracic duct ligation for chylous pleural effusion. The sympathetic chain is well visualized, and resection can be performed proximally to the superior cervical ganglion. Thoracoscopic clipping of the thoracic duct where it enters the chest at the aortic hiatus has provided immediate relief for chylothorax unresponsive to nonoperative therapy. Finally, VATS has been shown to provide excellent exposure of the thoracic spine for procedures including drainage of abscesses, biopsy of lesions, discectomy, and anterior release of kyphoscoliosis.

These applications of the new technology of VATS are not performed without complications. A recent review of 266 thoracic VATS procedures, however, reported no deaths, only 10 prolonged air leaks, and bleeding requiring transfusion in only 5 patients. No consistent pattern of major complications from VATS has been reported.

In summary, video-assisted thoracic surgery has proven to be quite useful in the diagnosis and treatment of multiple thoracic diseases. Many of these procedures can be performed as safely, with equal efficacy, and with less morbidity than by thoracotomy. With the strides in the development of VATS, it has been used for many conditions. Some procedures for which there was early enthusiasm are now being performed less frequently, while others have withstood the test of time. Critical comparisons between VATS procedures and corresponding open techniques are being performed, and such studies are required to provide answers to questions raised by these procedures. Nevertheless, VATS has clearly found a place in the modern practice of thoracic surgery and is likely to have an ever-increasing role in the management of diseases of the chest.

V

Tracheostomy and Its Complications

Hermes C. Grillo, M.D., and Douglas J. Mathisen, M.D.

The indications for tracheostomy are relief of upper airway obstruction, control of secretions, and, in patients requiring mechanical ventilation, support for respiratory failure. The use of rigid bronchoscopes or the laser to dilate or core-out benign and malignant strictures of the airway and flexible bronchoscopy and minitracheostomy for pulmonary toilet

See the corresponding chapter or part in the *Textbook of Surgery*, 15th edition, pp. 1815–1820, for a more detailed discussion of this topic, including a comprehensive list of references.

may diminish the frequency of tracheostomy for the first two indications.

The timing of tracheostomy for long-term mechanical ventilation is controversial. The authors' policy has been to perform tracheostomy *early* if long-term ventilation can be predicted or if, after 7 to 10 days, it appears extubation is not likely in the next 3 to 4 days. Critical to this policy is the reversibility of most complications of tracheostomy versus irreparable injury to the glottis from prolonged endotracheal intubation. This is especially true of glottic injuries from an endotracheal tube too large for the glottis or pressure necrosis posteriorly by the tube. This concern is substantiated in a study that showed an increasing incidence of complex laryngeal injuries the longer oral endotracheal intubation was utilized (especially with large tubes).

There are many techniques of tracheostomy. The technique the authors prefer involves a horizontal skin incision, separation of the strap muscles in the midline, and division of the thyroid isthmus to allow accurate identification of the second and third tracheal rings. A longitudinal incision is then made through these cartilages. The trachea is spread, and a tracheostomy tube is inserted, secured to the skin, and tied around the neck. The tracheostomy tube should be the smallest size compatible with the patient's trachea and utilize a low-pressure, high-volume cuff.

Many authors refer to a high incidence of complications from tracheostomy. Usually, these statements are made in reference to the emergent procedure, performed under less than ideal conditions, and possibly with tubes of inferior design and quality. A precise, carefully performed tracheostomy should be associated with few complications. Careful identification of anatomic landmarks should avoid injury to recurrent nerves, esophagus, and nearby vascular structures. By use of the second and third rings, the risk of subglottic stenosis from injury of the cricoid cartilage or innominate artery hemorrhage from the tube's pressing against this structure, which can occur if the tracheostomy is placed too low, can be minimized. High-volume, low-pressure cuffs have markedly reduced cuff stenosis, but constant vigilance must be exercised to not overinflate low-pressure cuffs, thereby converting them into high-pressure cuffs. Avoidance of excessively large tubes, large openings in the trachea, and excessive leverage on the tubes by heavy rigid connecting tubing should minimize stomal stenosis. Conscientious nursing care prevents many potential problems by ensuring that tubes are tightly secured for avoidance of dislodgment; that proper levels of humidification are provided for avoidance of drying and crusting of secretions; and that cuffs are not overinflated, thus risking herniation and obstruction by the cuff. Tracheoesophageal fistula is avoided by eliminating the use of large, hard nasogastric tubes and cuffed airway tubes. The combination acts in a pincer manner, eroding the tracheoesophageal walls. Gastrostomy tubes or soft, small Silastic feeding tubes are preferable.

Despite improvements in tube and cuff design and attention to surgical technique, postintubation tracheal stenosis still occurs. *Every patient with signs of upper airway obstruction— wheezing or stridor, dyspnea on effort, or episodes of obstruction from secretions—who has been intubated previously with either an endotracheal tube or tracheostomy tube must be considered to have obstruction until it is proved otherwise.* These patients are often treated for asthma with steroids because of wheezing despite a clear chest film.

Patients too ill or inappropriate for resection and reconstruction are best managed by tracheostomy or a T-tube placed *through the old stoma or stenotic segment—never through viable trachea, which may preclude future repair.* Tracheal dilation by rigid bronchoscopes or use of the laser is only a temporary measure, since restenosis usually occurs.

Resection and reconstruction is preferred for the management of postintubation stenosis. At the Massachusetts General Hospital, 503 patients were treated for postintubation stenosis (etiologic basis of stenosis: stomal, 35%; cuff, 50%; both, 7.6%; uncertain, 7.4%). Good to excellent results were attained in 440 patients (87.5%); 3 (6.2%) had satisfactory results; there were 20 failures and 12 deaths.

Subglottic stenosis and acquired tracheoesophageal fistulas are best managed by single staged operation but represent challenging problems.

VI

Pulmonary Infections
Stewart M. Scott, M.D., and Timothy Takaro, M.D.

PYOGENIC LUNG ABSCESS

Pyogenic lung abscess results when septic debris is aspirated. It is more likely to occur in patients unconscious from alcoholism, general anesthesia, epilepsy, cerebrovascular accidents, or drowning. Thus the debris goes to the most dependent bronchi, that is, the superior segment of the right lower lobe and the posterior segment of the right upper lobe.

Microorganisms commonly responsible for pyogenic lung abscess are anaerobic bacteria, alpha- and beta-hemolytic streptococci, staphylococci, nonhemolytic streptococci, and *Escherichia coli*. Clinically, cough, foul-smelling sputum, fever, pleuritic chest pain, weight loss, and night sweats occur. The chest x-ray typically shows a cavity with an air-fluid level. In contrast, staphylococcal pneumoceles in infants appear as thin-walled cysts, often with pleural effusion, empyema, or

---

See the corresponding chapter or part in the *Textbook of Surgery,* 15th edition, pp. 1820–1830, for a more detailed discussion of this topic, including a comprehensive list of references.

pyopneumothorax. Lung abscesses in immunosuppressed patients are often multiple and usually hospital-acquired. Treatment is prolonged administration of penicillin G or clindamycin. Bronchoscopy is indicated to exclude cancer and identify causative organisms, to remove any foreign body present, and to drain the abscess through the bronchus. Surgical therapy is indicated if a large, thick-walled abscess fails to respond to antibiotics or if a malignant lesion is suspected. The mortality rate for pyogenic lung abscess in immunocompetent patients is 5% to 6% but is much higher in immunosuppressed patients.

FUNGAL AND ACTINOMYCETIC INFECTIONS OF THE LUNG

Actinomycosis is caused by the anaerobic bacterium *Actinomyces israelii*, clusters of which form "sulfur granules" in sinuses and abscesses. Actinomycosis may be cervicofacial, thoracic, or abdominal. Thoracic actinomycosis originates from normally resident oropharyngeal organisms. Empyema and chronic chest wall sinuses are typical. Pulmonary lesions appear as infiltrates or hilar masses like bronchogenic carcinoma. Treatment requires high doses of penicillin G for a prolonged period and surgical excision when possible.

Nocardiosis is caused by *Nocardia asteroides*, an aerobic, gram-positive, acid-fast organism that mimics tuberculosis, actinomycosis, pneumonia, and lung abscess. It is often an opportunistic infection. Long-term trimethoprim-sulfamethoxazole or minocycline is required.

Histoplasmosis, caused by *Histoplasma capsulatum*, is endemic in the Mississippi Valley. Acute infection produces diffuse infiltration or scattered nodules. While most persons are asymptomatic with AIDS, the infection can be severe and should be treated aggressively. Clinically, an asymptomatic solitary nodule with concentric rings of calcium on chest x-ray is common. Chronic cavitary histoplasmosis resembles tuberculosis. The organism is found in sputum or tissue. Acute histoplasmosis is treated with amphotericin B or itraconazole. Chronic cavitary histoplasmosis is treated with amphotericin B, itraconazole, or ketoconazole. Surgical treatment is reserved for chronic thick-walled cavities that do not respond to treatment.

Coccidioidomycosis, caused by *Coccidioides immitis*, is found in the desert areas of southern California, Nevada, Arizona, and New Mexico. The organism appears in tissue as a large spherule packed with endospores. Lung lesions can be "thin-walled cavities" or suppurative, infiltrative, or chronic granulomas, making coccidioidomycosis difficult to distinguish from tuberculosis and histoplasmosis. Hemoptysis may occur, as well as cough, weight loss, fever, and chest pain. Skin tests and complement fixation are usually positive, and organisms can be found in the sputum. Acutely ill patients require therapy with amphotericin B or fluconazole. Surgery is sometimes necessary for severe hemoptysis or thick-walled cavities (>2 cm.).

North American blastomycosis is caused by the single-budding yeast *Blastomyces dermatitidis*, endemic to the central United States and Canada. Cutaneous lesions are common. Pulmonary symptoms are nonspecific. On chest x-ray lesions may be cavitary, nodular, fibrotic, or disseminated. The diagnosis is made from sputum or serologic testing. Treatment consists of itraconazole, amphotericin B, or ketoconazole. An operation is performed only if bronchogenic carcinoma is suspected.

Cryptococcosis, usually an opportunistic infection, is caused by *Cryptococcus neoformans*, a yeast cell with a thick capsule. Subclinical infections occur. X-rays are nonspecific. It is the most common fungal infection in renal transplant patients and also common in AIDS. Treatment with fluconazole or 5-fluorocytosine and amphotericin B is indicated for active progressive meningitis.

Aspergillus fumigatus, causing aspergillosis, is a ubiquitous fungus colonizing pre-existing lung cavities and forming aspergillomas, which are masses of necrotic hyphae with a typical x-ray appearance: a crescent-shaped radiolucency outlining a fungus ball that moves freely within a cavity. Hemorrhage is a common complication for which surgical excision is often necessary. Antimycotic drug therapy is unsatisfactory. Aspergillosis is an opportunistic infection in transplant patients and in patients with leukemia and lymphoma but not with AIDS.

Candidiasis is an opportunistic infection caused by *Candida albicans*, a normal inhabitant of the gastrointestinal and female genital tracts. It occurs when host defenses are altered. Colonization occurs from indwelling catheters used for hyperalimentation or dialysis. Amphotericin B alone or with 5-fluorocytosine is the best treatment available. Surgical intervention is necessary to eradicate large vegetations occurring on natural or prosthetic heart valves.

Less common fungal infections include pulmonary sporotrichosis, which usually responds to itraconazole but may require surgery. Zygomycosis (mucormycosis), also rare but serious, occurs in debilitated patients. Its treatment also consists of amphotericin B and sometimes surgery. *Pseudallescheria boydii*, a secondary invader of damaged lung tissue, is treated with miconazole and sometimes surgery. South American blastomycosis (paracoccidioidomycosis), as a pulmonary granuloma or cavity, responds to itraconazole.

AIDS-ASSOCIATED PULMONARY INFECTIONS

Opportunistic infections in AIDS patients are due to *Pneumocystis carinii*, cytomegalovirus, atypical mycobacteria, *Toxoplasma gondii*, *Candida*, herpes simplex virus, cryptococcus, and cryptosporidium. *Pneumocystis* pneumonia occurs in 80% of AIDS patients. The protozoan stains with silver methenamine in sputum or biopsied lung tissue. Trimethoprim-sulfamethoxazole and pentamidine isethionate are equally effective. Kaposi's sarcoma, a hallmark of AIDS, is viral-induced and occurs as a painless purple nodule in the lungs and airway.

VIIA

The Pleura and Empyema
Stewart M. Scott, M.D., and Timothy Takaro, M.D.

The pleura is a serous membrane that lines two independent pleural spaces. These spaces extend into the neck, the retrosternal areas, the costophrenic sinuses, and the interlobar fissures.

PLEURAL EFFUSIONS

The classic signs of pleural effusion are dullness, diminished breath sounds, and mediastinal displacement. An effusion of 500 ml. or less may not be apparent on x-ray. Infections, tumor, and congestive failure account for 75% of effusions (Table 1). If the pleural fluid is a transudate, that is, fluid low in protein, it is probably due to systemic disease such as congestive heart failure or cirrhosis. An exudative effusion is more likely to be associated with a diseased pleura, as seen with malignancies and infections. Characteristics of commonly encountered effusions are outlined in Table 1.

SPONTANEOUS PNEUMOTHORAX

Spontaneous pneumothorax is almost always due to rupture of a subpleural cyst or bulla. It occurs in the healthy young adult, in older patients with emphysema, and even in the newborn requiring vigorous resuscitation. The patient may be asymptomatic or dyspneic with chest pain. Breath sounds are diminished or absent. The diagnosis is confirmed by chest roentgenogram. A small (20% or less), asymptomatic pneumothorax will absorb. This is facilitated by supplemental oxygen. Closed thoracostomy is adequate for most large pneumothoraces. If the air leak persists, excision of the ruptured bulla and pleurectomy by video-assisted thoracoscopic surgery (VATS) or open thoracotomy are indicated.

Tension pneumothorax is the result of a valvelike mechanism that allows air to enter the pleural space from the lung parenchyma when airway pressure is elevated. This occurs during episodes of coughing and in patients on ventilators.

See the corresponding chapter or part in the *Textbook of Surgery,* 15th edition, pp. 1830–1838, for a more detailed discussion of this topic, including a comprehensive list of references.

TABLE 1. Differential Characteristics of Pleural Effusions

	Congestive Failure	Malignancy	Pneumonia and Other Nontuberculous Infections	Tuberculosis	Fungal Infection, Actinomycosis, Nocardiosis	Rheumatoid Arthritis and Collagen Disease	Pulmonary Embolism	Trauma	Chylothorax	Esophageal Rupture
Clinical	Signs and symptoms of congestive failure	Older patient, poor health prior to effusion	Signs and symptoms of respiratory tract infection	Younger patient, exposure to tuberculosis good health prior	Exposure in endemic area	History of joint involvement may or may not be present, subcutaneous nodules	Postoperative patient, immobilized patient, venous disease	History of trauma	History of trauma, known malignancy	History of instrumentation of or of vomiting
Gross appearance	Serous	Often sanguineous	Serous	Usually serous, may be sanguineous	Serous or purulent	Turbid or yellow-green	Often sanguineous	Sanguineous	Chylous or milky	Serous; may contain food particles Squamous epithelial cells
Microscopic examination	0	Cytology positive in 50%	May or may not be positive for bacilli	Positive for acid-fast bacilli in 30% to 70% of cases, cholesterol crystals	May or may not be positive for fungi	0	0	0	Fat droplets	
Cell count	10% 10,000 erythrocytes; 10% over 1000 leukocytes	65% bloody, over 40% over 1000 leukocytes, mainly leukolymphocytes	Polymorphonuclear clear cells predominate	Leukocytes mainly lymphocytes; eosinophils more than 10%; excludes Tbc	Polymorphonuclear leukocytes or lymphocytes	Lymphocytes predominate	Erythrocytes predominate	Erythrocytes	0	Red blood cells and white blood cells
Culture	0	0	May or may not be positive	Less than 25% are positive	May or may not be positive	0	0	0	0	0

Specific gravity	90% under 1.016 (unless pulmonary embolism)	75% over 1.016	Over 1.016	75% over 1.016	Over 1.016	Over 1.016	Over 1.016	Over 1.016	Over 1.016	Over 1.016
Protein	75% less than 3 gm.	90% 3 gm. or more	3.0 gm. or more	Usually 5.0 gm. or more	3.0 gm. or more	3.0 gm. or more	3.0 gm. or more	3.0 gm. or more	Less than half plasma	3.0 gm. or more
Glucose	0	15% have 60 mg. per 100 ml. or less	Occasionally less than 60 mg. per 100 ml. or less	Less than 50% have 60 mg. per 100 ml. or less	0	78% below 30 mg. per 100 ml. (rheumatoid)	0	0	0	0
pH	Greater than 7.20	May be 7.20 or less	May be less than 7.20	May be less than 7.20	Greater than 7.20	May be 7.20 or less	Greater than 7.20	Greater than 7.20	Greater than 7.20	Usually less than 7.20; may be less than 6.00
Amylase	0	10% are elevated	0	0	0	0	0	0	0	Elevated
Lactic acid dehydrogenase	Not elevated	May be elevated	May be elevated	May be elevated	May be elevated	May be elevated	May be elevated	0	0	0
Other	Right-sided in 55% to 70%	If hemorrhagic fluid, 65% will be due to tumor, tends to continue to form after removed; hyaluronic acid >1 mg./ml. in mesothelioma	Associated with infiltrate on roentgenogram	Less than 5% mesothelial cells; will be the cause in 75% of men under 25 years; 50% of men over 25 years; adenosine deaminase 70 I.U./L.	Skin and serologic tests may be helpful	Rapid clotting time; lupus erythematosus cell or rheumatoid factor titer >640	Source of emboli may or may not be helpful	0	Fat content higher than plasma	0

Modified from Bessone, L.N., Ferguson, T.B. and Burford, T.H.: Chylothorax. Ann Thorac Surg., 12:527, 1971; Light R.W.: Pleural Diseases. Philadelphia, Lea & Febiger, 1983; and Kinosewitz, G.T.: Pleuritis and pleural effusions. In Bone, R.C. (Ed): Pulmonary and Critical Care Medicine. St. Louis, Mosby–Year Book, 1993.

Severe respiratory distress results when the lung collapses, and increased intrapleural pressure causes the mediastinum to shift. Emergency needle aspiration is necessary followed by closed thoracotomy.

HEMOTHORAX

Trauma is the most frequent cause of blood within the pleural cavities, but hemothorax also occurs with pulmonary infarction, pleural and pulmonary neoplasm, torn pleural adhesions accompanying pneumothorax, and anticoagulant therapy. Blood within the pleural and pericardial cavities is partly defibrinated. It will be absorbed unless it becomes infected, in which instance a fibrothorax may develop that can compromise pulmonary function. A small, self-limited hemothorax requires only observation. For moderate blood loss (500 ml. or greater), the pleura should be drained completely by closed thoracostomy. If active bleeding persists (200 ml. per hour or more), a thoracotomy for control of bleeding is necessary. Massive bleeding may require vigorous blood volume replacement, which can be augmented by reinfusion of the partially defibrinated blood collected from the chest tubes.

CHYLOTHORAX

Chylothorax, the accumulation of lymph in the pleural space, is the result of trauma to the thoracic duct or tumor. Gunshot wounds, stab wounds, and automobile injuries account for most occurrences, but it sometimes occurs following cardiac and thoracic surgery. Spontaneous chylothorax in an adult is ominous and suggests a malignancy. Considerable fluid can escape from the thoracic duct, and symptoms may be due to impaired nutrition or compression of the lung. Conservative treatment includes decompression of the thoracic lymphatics by hyperalimentation or oral medium-chain triglycerides and drainage of the pleural space. If chylothorax persists after 3 to 4 weeks, an attempt to ligate the thoracic duct can be made, talc pleurodesis can be tried, or a pleuroperitoneal shunt used.

EMPYEMA

Pleural empyema is a collection of pus in the pleural cavity. It is almost always secondary to some underlying disease, usually pneumonia, but it occurs with lung abscess, ruptured bullae, bronchopleural fistulas, esophageal rupture, and abscessed lymph nodes. It also occurs when infection is introduced by trauma, surgery, or needle aspiration. The most common bacteria are *Staphylococcus aureus*, *Streptococcus*, and a variety of gram-negative organisms including anaerobic flora. Treatment consists of (1) control of the underlying disease, (2) evacuation of the empyema and eradication of the empyema sac, and (3) re-expansion of the lung. Regardless of the underlying condition, adequate drainage is necessary, and usually an intercostal tube of generous caliber is necessary. The tube should be placed in the most dependent portion of the empyema space. This may require resection of a short segment of rib to identify the extent of the cavity and to break up adhesions. Empyemas sometimes follow thoracic surgical procedures, usually pneumonectomies. If a bronchopleural fistula is present and develops early following a surgical procedure, an attempt can be made to close the fistula. Fistulas late in onset are likely to be associated with residual tumor or disease and should be treated with open drainage.

PLEURAL TUMORS

Primary pleural tumors are essentially mesotheliomas, of which there are the localized benign and the diffuse malignant types. Both may contain fibrous and epithelioid elements, making it difficult at times to distinguish benign from malignant and mesothelioma from carcinoma. Patients with benign localized fibrous mesotheliomas may be asymptomatic or they may have arthralgia, clubbing of the fingers, or fever. The tumor that ordinarily arises from the visceral pleura is easily excised, after which symptoms usually disappear. Diffuse malignant mesotheliomas cause chest pain and bloody pleural effusion. Both visceral and parietal pleura are involved, and the extent of the tumor is variable. Metastases are uncommon, but prognosis is poor and death usually occurs within 2 years regardless of treatment used. The causal relationship between exposure to asbestos dust and malignant mesothelioma is strong.

Metastatic tumors are far more common than primary pleural tumors. The most frequent are tumors of the lung, breast, pancreas, and stomach. As with malignant mesothelioma, bloody pleural fluid containing malignant cells is usually present. Treatment is palliative.

VIIB

Surgical Management of Pulmonary Emphysema
James R. Mault, M.D.

Pulmonary emphysema is a major health problem for more than 4.5 million Americans and is the most common cause of respiratory disability. Supportive medical therapy is the

See the corresponding chapter or part in the *Textbook of Surgery*, 15th edition, pp. 1838–1844, for a more detailed discussion of this topic, including a comprehensive list of references.

mainstay of treatment for the majority of patients with dyspnea due to emphysema. However, in properly selected patients, surgery may improve pulmonary function, chest wall mechanics, and lifestyle.

Emphysema is defined as an anatomic alteration of the lung characterized by an abnormal and permanent enlargement of the air spaces distal to the terminal bronchiole, accompanied by destructive changes of the alveolar walls. Pulmonary *bullae* are defined as emphysematous spaces of greater than 1 cm in diameter in the inflated lung, and a bulla that occupies one-half the hemithorax or greater is called a *giant bulla.*

Indications for surgical management of patients with these various classifications of emphysema can be distinguished by the presence or absence of chronic dyspnea. In patients without dyspnea, surgery is required for acute complications such as spontaneous pneumothorax. In patients with chronic dyspnea, a selected subset may benefit from operation by resection of bullae that compress surrounding tissue and allow re-expansion of preserved lung.

Primary spontaneous pneumothorax (PSP) is due to rupture of a periacinar bleb in young patients with otherwise normal lung tissue and accounts for 85% of all spontaneous pneumothoraces. The typical patient is a 20- to 40-year-old, tall, thin male with a history of tobacco use. A positive family history of PSP is obtained in 10% of patients. Secondary spontaneous pneumothorax (SSP) occurs in patients with underlying lung disease. Compared with PSP, this population of patients is much older (range 45 to 75 years). The majority of cases are due to bullous emphysema but also include tuberculosis, *Pneumocystis carinii* pneumonia, and lung cancer.

Patients with primary or secondary spontaneous pneumothoraces present with an acute history of chest pain and/or shortness of breath. Primary evaluation includes a careful history and physical examination. Tension pneumothorax should be treated immediately with needle decompression without further studies. Inspiratory and expiratory plain chest radiographs are diagnostic of pneumothorax.

Initial treatment for spontaneous pneumothorax is dictated by the patient's symptoms and extent of pneumothorax. The stable, nondyspneic patient with a unilateral pneumothorax estimated to be less than 15% of the hemithorax may be observed in the hospital and monitored by daily chest radiograph. Tube thoracostomy should be performed in patients with persistent symptoms and unilateral pneumothorax greater than 15% of a hemithorax, all patients who present with simultaneous bilateral pneumothoraces or previous pneumonectomy, and those who fail observation. The chest tube should be connected to a water-sealed drainage system with 20 cm. H_2O suction. With re-expansion of the lung and resolution of air leak, the chest tube may be removed and the patient discharged after follow-up chest radiograph confirms full lung inflation. The recurrence rate of spontaneous pneumothorax after nonoperative management of the first episode is 45% with PSP and 35% with SSP. In patients with SSP who represent a significant operative risk, chemical pleurodesis (using 2 gm. sterile talc or other sclerosing agent) performed prior to chest tube removal has been shown to reduce recurrence in SSP by one half.

Indications for operation after spontaneous pneumothorax are massive air leak preventing lung re-expansion, simultaneous bilateral pneumothoraces, previous contralateral pneumothorax or pneumonectomy, and unresolved, persistent air leaks for 48 to 96 hours. Patients with a first recurrence of spontaneous pneumothorax have an excessively high risk of second recurrence and should receive an operation. Patients with occupational hazards for pneumothorax, such as pilots and scuba divers, should be treated operatively during hospitalization for the first episode. Spontaneous pneumothorax can be corrected via open thoracotomy or thoracoscopically by resection of bleb(s) and pleurodesis.

The clinical evaluation for bullectomy begins with a careful history and physical examination to clearly define the cause of dyspnea in the patient being considered for surgery. A distinction must be made between patients who have primarily emphysema (pink puffers) from those with chronic bronchitis (blue bloaters). Patients with chronic bronchitis are characterized by a productive cough, frequent respiratory infections, carbon dioxide retention, and bronchospasm and are correspondingly poor candidates for pulmonary surgery.

All patients should undergo standard pulmonary function testing with room air blood gas measurement. Blood gas measurements are necessary to exclude patients with carbon dioxide retention and hypercapnia at rest. Radiographically, apical bullae occupying more than 50% of a hemithorax with lower crowding of lung marking and pulmonary vasculature predict a good operative result. Computed tomography (CT) is an essential component in the evaluation of these patients and can quantitatively define the size and number of bullous lesions.

The operative strategy for bullous disease is directed at removal of the space-occupying disease while preserving all vascularized and potentially functional lung tissue. This is best accomplished by limited resections. With recent advances in stapling devices, resection and closure of bullae have been accomplished successfully with minimal air leaks when staple lines are reinforced by bovine pericardium or parietal pleura. In patients with bilateral bullous disease, simultaneous bilateral bullectomy can be performed safely via median sternotomy. Resection of bullous emphysema also has been performed thoracoscopically using endoscopic stapling techniques as well as laser coagulation. Patients with giant bullae who are unsuitable for open or VATS resection may receive intracavitary drainage in a single-stage procedure. Lastly, patients with end-stage emphysema also may undergo single or bilateral lung transplantation.

In most series, perioperative mortality averages 1% to 3% and is usually attributed to respiratory failure, pneumonia, or cardiovascular disorders. Morbidity is common after surgery for emphysema and consists of prolonged air leaks, delayed lung expansion, and infection. In short-term follow-up, most patients show significant improvements in spirometric parameters, while approximately two thirds of patients experience significant improvements in exercise tolerance.

The goal of surgical therapy for diffuse emphysema is to reduce the total lung volume occupying the chest cavity and re-establish diaphragmatic excursion and chest wall motion. The lung reduction technique is performed through a median sternotomy and involves excision of 20% to 30% of the volume of each lung.

VIII

Bronchiectasis
Donald D. Glower, M.D.

Bronchiectasis was first described by Laënnec in 1819, and the first successful operation for bronchiectasis was performed by Krause in 1898. While bronchiectasis has become relatively uncommon since the introduction of antibiotics, surgical treatment still has a role today.

Bronchiectasis is defined as persistent abnormal dilatation of the bronchi, generally below the subsegmental level. Bronchiectasis has been classified into three types, cylindrical, varicose, and saccular, based on radiographic appearance of the bronchi. Commonly involved segments include the left lower lobe, the right middle lobe, the lingula, and the right lower lobe.

In 74% of patients, bronchiectasis is an acquired disease caused by impaired clearance of bronchial secretions and subsequent bronchial injury. Congenital disorders that may produce bronchiectasis include congenital bronchomalacia due to Williams-Campbell syndrome, tracheobronchomegaly due to Ehlers-Danlos or Mouier-Kuhn syndrome, congenital ciliary dysmotility, alpha$_1$-antitrypsin deficiency, intralobar bronchopulmonary sequestration, and congenital immunodeficiency.

Symptoms generally occur in the second or third decades of life, and there is a female-to-male predominance. Patients generally have a persistent cough productive of purulent sputum, and patients also may suffer from hemoptysis and repeated pulmonary infection. Physical findings are variable but may include rales over the involved lung fields.

The chest radiograph is generally abnormal but nondiagnostic. High-resolution computed tomography usually demonstrates abnormally dilated bronchi extending into the lung parenchyma. Bronchography may have a role to define the bronchial anatomy for potential pulmonary resection. Bron-

---

See the corresponding chapter or part in the *Textbook of Surgery*, 15th edition, pp. 1844–1847, for a more detailed discussion of this topic, including a comprehensive list of references.

choscopy may be indicated for tracheobronchial toilet or in
assessing the airway at the level of potential pulmonary resection; however, bronchoscopic findings are usually not diagnostic of bronchiectasis.

The mainstay of treatment for bronchiectasis is conservative
medical therapy with oral antibiotics such as amoxicillin, either on a short-term basis for acute exacerbations or as long-
term therapy. Chest physiotherapy and postural drainage are
also generally beneficial. Operation, either lobectomy or segmentectomy of involved segments, is reserved for those patients who continue to have significant symptoms despite a
prolonged medical trial. For patients with bilateral disease,
the side with greater involvement is resected first, and a
second thoracotomy is performed only if symptoms persist
for 6 to 12 months.

Prior to modern therapy, patients with bronchiectasis generally died from sepsis, pulmonary infection, or cor pulmonale.
Today, only 18% to 36% of patients ultimately require operation. Most patients treated with either medical or surgical
therapy ultimately obtain improvement in symptoms.

IX

Surgical Treatment of Pulmonary Tuberculosis
Jon F. Moran, M.D.

Pulmonary tuberculosis remains the leading infectious killer
in the world, causing 3 million deaths annually. *Mycobacterium
tuberculosis,* an aerobic, nonmotile, slow-growing bacillus, is
responsible for the majority of pulmonary mycobacterial disease. Other species of mycobacteria can rarely cause pulmonary infection, and these are referred to as *atypical mycobacteria.* Atypical mycobacteria are more frequently resistant to
chemotherapy. *Mycobacterium avium-intracellulare* and *Mycobacterium kansasii* are the two atypical organisms that most
often cause clinical pulmonary infection. Surgical treatment of
pulmonary mycobacterial infection is rarely required because
antituberculous chemotherapy is so effective.

PATHOLOGY. The pathologic response within the lung to
the various mycobacteria is identical. *M. tuberculosis* is a virulent organism requiring a minimal airborne inoculum for infection to occur in normal tissue. The pneumonic process
caused by mycobacteria is characterized by caseous necrosis

See the corresponding chapter or part in the *Textbook of Surgery,* 15th
edition, pp. 1847–1853, for a more detailed discussion of this topic,
including a comprehensive list of references.

with formation of a granuloma. Most mycobacterial infections are contained at the early pneumonic stage by the body's own immune response. Miliary tuberculosis arises from massive hematogenous spread with thousands of 1- to 2-mm. (millet seed–sized) tubercles throughout the body.

Adult pulmonary tuberculosis is the most common pattern of mycobacterial infection and is called *reinfection* or *postprimary tuberculosis*. Adult tuberculosis begins as a segmental pneumonia in the apical or posterior segment of an upper lobe or the superior segment of a lower lobe. Bilateral disease is common. The pneumonic infiltrates progress to caseous necrosis with cavity formation when the necrotic area erodes into an adjacent bronchus. The visceral and parietal pleurae adjacent to the disease are involved by an intense inflammatory reaction with obliteration of the pleural space.

DIAGNOSIS. There is an important distinction between mycobacterial infection and mycobacterial disease. Infection implies the entrance of an organism into the body without symptoms. The diagnosis of mycobacterial disease depends on the confirmation of active disease by radiographic and bacteriologic studies. Symptoms of pulmonary tuberculosis include a chronic cough, easy fatigability, weight loss, hemoptysis, and fever with night sweats. The most frequent radiographic findings in pulmonary tuberculosis are apical infiltrates with frequent cavitation. Standard tuberculosis skin testing involves the intracutaneous injection of 5 tuberculin units of purified protein derivative (PPD) on the volar aspect of the forearm. This is termed an *intermediate PPD,* and greater than 10 mm. of induration after 48 to 72 hours defines a positive test. The isolation of mycobacterial organisms from the sputum is required to confirm the diagnosis of mycobacterial disease. The presence of acid-fast organisms on smear allows for a rapid presumptive diagnosis, although cultures are necessary to document the species of mycobacteria. Mycobacterial cultures require 3 to 6 weeks to grow. Antimycobacterial chemotherapy is often begun while awaiting final cultures. Sensitivity testing for a variety of antituberculous drugs is particularly important in patients being considered for surgical therapy.

CHEMOTHERAPY. Chemotherapy for pulmonary mycobacterial infection requires the administration of two or three drugs simultaneously to avoid the emergence of drug-resistant organisms. The two currently recommended regimens for treatment of pulmonary tuberculosis are (1) a 6-month course of isoniazid and rifampin with pyrazinamide during the first 2 months and (2) a 9-month course of isoniazid and rifampin. Atypical mycobacterial infections may require the use of other antibiotics. Complications of resectional surgery for mycobacterial disease are reduced in patients who have been converted to sputum-negative status.

SURGICAL TREATMENT. When an operation is required for pulmonary mycobacterial disease, resection of the diseased portion of the lung is the procedure of choice. Thoracoplasty and other procedures intended to collapse the infected portion of lung are rarely indicated and are of historic interest only.

Guidelines for pulmonary resection in mycobacterial disease are listed below:

1. Persistently positive sputum cultures with cavitation following an adequate period of chemotherapy with two or more drugs to which the organism has been proved sensitive require surgical intervention.

2. Localized pulmonary disease caused by *M. avium-intracellulare* (or another mycobacterium broadly sensitive to chemotherapy) is an indication for resection.

3. A mass lesion of the lung in an area of mycobacterial infection is an indication for resection for simultaneous diagnosis of the mass lesion and treatment of the mycobacterial disease.

4. Massive hemoptysis is an indication for resection of the infected portion of the lung that is the source of hemorrhage. Pulmonary hemorrhage is a rare but often fatal complication of pulmonary mycobacterial disease. Massive hemoptysis is defined as greater than 600 ml. per 24 hours. Asphyxiation rather than hypovolemia is the usual cause of death from hemoptysis. The site of bleeding is almost invariably a cavitary lesion. Tuberculosis remains the most common cause of massive hemoptysis.

5. A bronchopleural fistula secondary to mycobacterial infection that does not respond to tube thoracostomy often requires surgical treatment.

OPERATIVE MANAGEMENT. Use of a double-lumen endotracheal tube can make resection for tuberculosis easier and safer. A double-lumen tube protects the dependent lung from contamination by secretions from the infected upper lung while the patient is in the lateral position. In the setting of severe hemoptysis, a double-lumen tube protects the dependent lung during resection of the bleeding portion of the upper lung. The extent of pulmonary resection is guided by the principle that all gross evidence of disease should be resected. For active mycobacterial disease, a lobectomy is usually required. A wedge resection can be used for a mass lesion that is being excised to exclude carcinoma. Pneumonectomy is required only to remove a totally destroyed lung.

Patients requiring operation generally have associated problems that predispose them to complications. Administration of effective antimycobacterial drugs, judicious timing of operation, careful operative technique, and meticulous postoperative care are the important factors in avoiding complications from pulmonary resection for mycobacterial disease. The incidence of bronchopleural fistula after resection for mycobacterial disease is about 3%. An apical space problem complicates approximately 20% of resections for mycobacterial disease, but only 10% to 15% of these patients develop a bronchopleural fistula or empyema. Resectional surgery for mycobacterial disease is now employed in a selected group of patients who have failed chemotherapy or have a serious complication. Mortality for pulmonary resection of mycobacterial disease varies from zero with low morbidity when surgical intervention is elective to 15% or greater when resection is performed as an emergency. Long-term prognosis after resection is excellent, with 90% of patients surviving and remaining free of mycobacterial disease.

X

Benign Tumors of the Trachea and Bronchi
David Harpole, Jr., M.D.

Benign tumors of the trachea and bronchi consist of various histologic masses that can be derived from any of the cells in the respiratory tract. Although these comprise less than 1% of respiratory cancers and only 15% of tracheal tumors, a detailed description is warranted to aid in early recognition of these potentially obstructive masses.

Benign tumors have a predominance in males and a peak incidence in the fifth and sixth decades of life. These masses develop over years, are usually less than 2 cm. in size, and tend to have a smooth contour. Early symptoms of airway irritation include cough and hemoptysis, while later symptoms of dyspnea and wheezing occur once the mass has grown to a size that threatens the airway. The most proximal tracheal masses can cause stridor, and masses with a large extrinsic component may intermittently obstruct as the individual's position is changed from prone to supine. Occasionally, patients present with recurrent pneumonia and atelectasis due to chronic luminal obstruction. Radiologic examinations can demonstrate tracheal or bronchial luminal narrowing, postobstructive atelectasis, or tumor calcification; however, it is difficult to differentiate benign from malignant etiology.

Differentiating benign lesions with cytology is difficult, so a histologic diagnosis requires bronchoscopy. This procedure should be performed in the operating room using a rigid bronchoscope for control of the airway in patients with threatening obstruction, because bronchoscopic manipulation can cause edema, hemorrhage, or bronchoconstriction. Most benign tracheal masses require a segmental resection of the airway for adequate treatment (chondroma, fibroma, pleomorphic adenoma, and ectopic thyroid). Pedunculated tumors resected with a bronchoscope often leave a foci of tumor behind, and recurrence is a significant problem. During the resection, a sterile, armored endotracheal tube is placed through the incision and into the distal airway. Either a standard volume ventilator or a high-frequency jet ventilator can

See the corresponding chapter or part in the *Textbook of Surgery*, 15th edition, pp. 1854–1860, for a more detailed discussion of this topic, including a comprehensive list of references.

be used. Once the anastomosis has begun, the original endotracheal tube can be replaced past the lesion. Tracheal lesions above the clavicle call for a cervical incision, those of the midtrachea need a cervical and a proximal sternal division, while lower tracheal lesions are approached through a right posterolateral thoracotomy. Care must be taken to adequately localize the length of the lesion and plan the operative approach; intraoperative bronchoscopy is often necessary. Primary anastomosis is possible after resection of 2 to 3 cm. of trachea; however, if a larger resection is necessary for an adequate margin, a tracheal mobilization procedure is needed. A tracheal anastomosis after an extensive resection should be covered with an appropriate myoplastic flap.

Squamous papillomatosis is the most common benign lesion in adults and children. There is no obvious gender predominance, and these are most commonly observed in the larynx with voice change. Endoscopic anatomy reveals multiple cauliflower-like tumors, which on histologic examination are irregular papillary or villous fibrous masses covered with squamous epithelium. There is an association with human papillomaviruses, and malignant transformation can occur. Local bronchoscopic excision is complicated, with a 90% recurrence rate, but newer modalities, such as bronchoscopic fulguration, cryotherapy, and laser ablation, allow for multiple treatments with minimal morbidity and mortality.

Hamartomas contain cartilage along with lymph tissue, fat, and epithelial elements. Eighty per cent of hamartomas are located in the periphery of the lung, often immediately subpleural. A thoracoscopic wedge resection is curative.

Hemangiomas are the most common lesion of the trachea and bronchi observed in children. These may occur anywhere in the conducting airways but are most common in the subglottic region, where they may threaten the airway. The size and symptoms may vary with engorgement. These lesions are more common in females and are easily recognized, so a biopsy is unnecessary and may create severe hemorrhage. The treatment of choice is observation, because many will regress spontaneously.

XI

Bronchial Adenomas
David Harpole, Jr., M.D.

Bronchial adenomas are not true adenomas but are malignant tumors that grow more slowly than the typical non-

---

See the corresponding chapter or part in the *Textbook of Surgery*, 15th edition, pp. 1860–1865, for a more detailed discussion of this topic, including a comprehensive list of references.

small cell lung cancers. These lesions comprise 1% to 2% of lung cancers. There are three types: carcinoid tumors, adenoid cystic carcinomas, and mucoepidermoid carcinomas.

Carcinoid tumors comprise 85% of bronchial adenomas. They are seen in all ages and are equally distributed in both sexes. These tumors are APUD (amine precursor uptake and decarboxylation) tumors. The cytoplasm contains neurosecretory granules that contain active peptide hormones, including serotonin, bradykinin, corticotropin, and others. Typical carcinoids consist of clusters of monotonous polyhedral cells, while 10% to 15% of carcinoids are more aggressive or "atypical," with frequent mitoses and nuclear pleomorphism. Carcinoids share ultrastructure and immunoreactivity with small cell neuroendocrine cancer of the lung and are grouped as Kulchitsky Type I (typical carcinoid), Kulchitsky Type II (atypical carcinoid), and Kulchitsky Type III (small cell lung cancer). Most carcinoid tumors are located in the main airways and cause a variety of symptoms (cough, hemoptysis, or stridor). Peripherally located carcinoids are often asymptomatic, unless they secrete an active peptide hormone (carcinoid syndrome: flushing, wheezing, and diarrhea). There is no characteristic x-ray picture; however, histologic diagnosis is often possible utilizing bronchoscopy.

Complete resection is the treatment for all typical and most atypical carcinoids without mediastinal lymph node metastases. Peripheral lesions most often require a lobectomy to include the regional lymph nodes. Central lesions may require a larger resection such as a sleeve resection of the mainstem bronchus. The 5-year survival after resection is 90% for typical and 50% for atypical carcinoids.

Adenoid cystic carcinoma (cylindroma) is a common malignant tumor of the salivary glands that grows slowly and has been observed in all ages, comprising 10% of bronchial adenomas. Adenoid cystic carcinomas are located in the central airways with three distinct patterns of growth: cribriform, tubular, and solid. Perineural lymphatic and submucosal invasion is often observed. Definitive histologic diagnosis is obtained with bronchoscopy. Complete resection is curative; however, only 60% of cases have histologically negative margins. Preoperative radiation therapy has been used successfully for large invasive tumors, and patients can live many years with metastatic disease.

Mucoepidermoid carcinoma represents 1% to 5% of bronchial adenomas of the trachea and proximal bronchi. The tumor consists of squamous, intermediate, and glandular elements and is classified as low-grade or high-grade. Most tumors are low-grade. Symptoms of cough, hemoptysis, and airway obstruction predominate, and bronchoscopy is needed for a histologic diagnosis. Complete surgical resection is curative for most low-grade lesions. Adjuvant radiotherapy after resection appears to improve survival in high-grade cancers.

XII

Carcinoma of the Lung

Thomas A. D'Amico, M.D.,
and David C. Sabiston, Jr., M.D.

PATHOLOGY

Lung cancer, the most common cause of death by malignancy, is divided into two categories for the purposes of staging, estimating prognosis, and selecting therapy: small cell lung cancer (SCLC) and non-small cell lung cancer (NSCLC). The three major histologic types of NSCLC are adenocarcinoma (50%), squamous cell carcinoma (30%), and large cell carcinoma (10%). Adenocarcinomas are often peripheral lesions and tend to invade the pleura. Squamous cell carcinomas originate centrally, grow toward the mainstem bronchus, and invade bronchial cartilage, pulmonary parenchyma, and lymph nodes. Large cell carcinomas are peripheral lesions that are unrelated to bronchi. SCLC is characterized by more rapid growth, stronger likelihood of metastases at the time of diagnosis, and greater responsiveness to chemotherapy and radiation therapy.

Several studies have established a clear relationship between the magnitude of tobacco use and the incidence of lung cancer. Most carcinogens act synergistically with cigarette smoke (including passive smoking) as etiologic agents in the pathogenesis of lung cancer.

DIAGNOSIS AND STAGING OF LUNG CANCER

The primary objective in the diagnosis and staging of lung cancer is to identify patients who are candidates for curative pulmonary resection. A complete history and physical examination are performed, with particular attention to possible manifestations of the primary tumor. Symptoms relating to carcinoma of the lung depend on the anatomic location of the tumor, extension into surrounding structures, metastatic spread, and the systemic effects of paraneoplastic syndromes. By the time the diagnosis of carcinoma of the lung is made, most patients have regional lymph node involvement or distant metastases.

Symptoms referable to the thorax may result from endobronchial growth, extrinsic growth, or regional spread of the primary tumor. The most common symptom is cough, which results from endobronchial erosion and irritation. Intratho-

See the corresponding chapter or part in the *Textbook of Surgery*, 15th edition, pp. 1865–1876, for a more detailed discussion of this topic, including a comprehensive list of references.

racic extension of lung tumors may involve surrounding structures, such as the recurrent laryngeal nerve and the esophagus. Local extension of a tumor at the apex of the lung may produce the superior sulcus (Pancoast) tumor syndrome.

A solitary pulmonary nodule is the classic radiographic presentation of lung cancer. The chest radiograph usually demonstrates a mass arising in the hilum or the lung field. Computed tomography (CT) of the chest is useful in the evaluation of the primary tumor and regional lymph node involvement. CT scans include the apices of the thorax superiorly and extend inferiorly to include the liver and the adrenal glands. It is generally accepted that a maximum diameter of 10 mm. is acceptable for considering hilar and mediastinal nodes to be uninvolved, suggesting operability. Flexible fiberoptic bronchoscopy, an important adjunct in the staging of lung cancer, may establish histologic diagnosis and exclude endobronchial involvement.

The TNM staging system for carcinoma of the lung provides a consistent, reproducible description of the anatomic extent of disease at the time of diagnosis. The TNM subsets are subsequently grouped in a series of stages of disease to identify groups of patients with similar prognosis and therapy.

SURGICAL MANAGEMENT OF NSCLC

Pulmonary function tests are used to determine the feasibility of pulmonary resection. Estimation of postoperative pulmonary function is based on calculation of the preoperative function and the projected resection of pulmonary parenchyma. When the forced expiratory volume at 1 second (FEV_1) and forced vital capacity are less than 30% of predicted values, thoracotomy is generally contraindicated. If the value of the predicted postoperative FEV_1 is at least 60% of the predicted value, the patient is considered able to tolerate resection. Contraindications to pulmonary resection at the time of thoracotomy include pleural metastases, extensive mediastinal lymph node involvement (N_3 disease), or direct extension of the tumor (T_4 disease). In addition, pulmonary resection is aborted when complete resection would result in inadequate pulmonary reserve, as determined by preoperative pulmonary function studies.

Complete resection of the tumor and all grossly involved regional bronchial and mediastinal lymph nodes, including *en bloc* resection of adjacent structures involved by direct extension of the primary tumor, is undertaken when feasible. Incomplete resection or resection that would leave a patient with an inadequate functional pulmonary reserve should not be performed. The procedure selected must provide removal of the entire tumor, with adequate margins, while preserving the maximum amount of functional lung tissue. At the time of thoracotomy, a systematic lymph node evaluation is undertaken and recorded to ascertain complete pathologic staging.

The most commonly performed pulmonary resection for lung cancer is lobectomy. Pneumonectomy is performed when lobectomy does not provide complete resection and when the loss of pulmonary parenchyma will be tolerated. Patients with small peripheral lesions may be candidates for segmentectomy, which has been advocated to provide complete resection while preserving more functional parenchyma. Wedge resection may be performed in high-risk patients or in patients with small lesions without lymph node involvement. Limited pulmonary resection is associated with a higher recurrence rate when compared with lobectomy.

The treatment of choice for Stage I disease is lobectomy, although wedge resection or segmentectomy may be performed for small peripheral tumors. Patients with Stage I carcinoma of the lung can expect 3- and 5-year survival rates of approximately 85% and 70%, respectively. Neither chemotherapy nor radiation therapy is recommended following complete resection of Stage I lung cancer.

Surgical therapy for Stage II carcinoma includes resection of the primary tumor; *en bloc* resection of the hilar, interlobar, lobar, and segmental lymph nodes; and systematic mediastinal lymph node dissection to exclude the presence of mediastinal metastases. Patients with Stage II disease experience 5-year survival rates of 40% to 50%. The rate of recurrence after resection of Stage II disease is greater than 50%, and most recurrences are distant metastases.

Stage IIIa NSCLC is associated with a relatively poor prognosis. In patients with tumor invading the chest wall (T_3), complete resection of the tumor with involved adjacent tissue provides the most effective treatment; 5-year survival after complete resection is 40%. Preoperative identification and histologic confirmation of N_2 disease usually contraindicate surgical resection; however, when unsuspected N_2 disease is encountered, pulmonary resection is performed if complete excision can be achieved, with 5-year survival up to 40%. Patients with Stage IIIb NSCLC (T_4 or N_3 disease) are generally considered unresectable. Optimization of pulmonary status preoperatively in patients with borderline cardiopulmonary function and meticulous postoperative care contribute to minimizing morbidity and mortality in patients who undergo pulmonary resection for carcinoma of the lung. Complications after pulmonary resection include atelectasis, persistent air leaks, bronchopleural fistula, infection (pneumonia, empyema, sepsis), myocardial infarction, atrial arrhythmias, pulmonary embolism, prolonged pulmonary insufficiency, chylothorax, and chronic thoracic pain. The mortality varies with the extent of resection: 1.4% for wedge resection or segmentectomy, 2.9% for lobectomy, and 6.2% for pneumonectomy.

ADJUVANT THERAPY FOR NSCLC

Approximately 60% of patients with NSCLC have distant metastases at the time of initial diagnosis. Postoperative chemotherapy may be responsible for significantly longer disease-free survival in patients with Stage III (and perhaps Stage II) NSCLC. The efficacy of postoperative chemotherapy and radiotherapy in patients with extensive lymph node involvement or positive surgical margins in reducing systemic recurrences and prolonging disease-free survival also has been demonstrated. Adjuvant therapy is not associated with improved overall survival and has not been shown to be beneficial in patients with Stage I NSCLC.

The capability of induction therapy (consisting of chemotherapy alone or chemotherapy in combination with radiation therapy) to improve survival in marginally resectable patients and to allow resection to be performed in categorically unresectable patients is being evaluated in numerous studies. In summary, current survival is significantly better in patients with Stage III NSCLC who receive preoperative chemotherapy and undergo complete resection as compared with historical controls.

Thoracic irradiation for cure is reserved for patients with Stage IIIb disease, selected patients with Stage IIIa disease, and patients with medical contraindications to thoracotomy. Adjuvant radiotherapy, applied to patients with completely resected Stage II or Stage III NSCLC, has been shown to decrease local recurrence but has no significant effect on survival. However, postoperative irradiation may provide a survival advantage in patients who have resection and are found to have metastases to hilar or mediastinal lymph nodes. Thus the purpose of adjuvant radiotherapy is the prevention of local tumor recurrence, especially when lymph node sampling of the mediastinum at thoracotomy is incomplete.

MANAGEMENT OF SCLC

Locoregional therapy directed toward the primary tumor is ineffective in prolonging survival because the majority of patients present with distant metastases or rapidly relapse with metastatic disease. Multimodal therapy is required for both locoregional control and systemic treatment of SCLC. The goals of therapy are to prolong survival and to alleviate symptoms while minimizing treatment-associated toxicity. Despite encouraging response rates to aggressive combination chemotherapy, the 2-year survival rate is only 10%.

After ascertaining the histologic diagnosis of SCLC, staging is performed, including thorough neurologic examination and CT evaluation of the chest, abdomen, and brain. For most patients with limited-stage disease, treatment is initiated with six cycles of combination chemotherapy. Radiotherapy to the chest is usually employed after three initial cycles of chemotherapy and is continued for 4 weeks. Among patients with limited-stage disease, thoracotomy for pulmonary resection is recommended in the subset of patients with Stage I SCLC. Postoperatively, patients receive six cycles of adjuvant chemotherapy and radiation therapy. For patients with extensive stage disease, six cycles of chemotherapy are administered. Therapy for local control is not employed; quality-of-life issues are paramount.

XIII

Mesothelioma

David J. Sugarbaker, M.D., Michael F. Reed, M.D., and Scott J. Swanson, M.D.

Mesothelioma is a rare malignancy affecting the pleura (81.8%), peritoneum (14.4%), or pericardium (0.9%) and extremely rarely the tunica vaginalis, testis, or ovarian epithelium. In the United States, approximately 3000 new cases are diagnosed annually, and the incidence is rising. The primary etiologic agent for mesothelioma is asbestos, specifically the amphibole group (crocidolite, amosite, anthophyllite, tremolite, and actinolite). Chrysotile exposure is not associated with risk of mesothelioma. Risk groups are those with industrial exposures such as insulators, pipe fitters, shipyard workers, brake mechanics, railroad workers, and individuals in construction trades. The latency period is 30 to 40 years.

The tumor begins as discrete nodules that coalesce and form a rind encompassing the pleura and often invading the diaphragm, pericardium, fissures, and chest wall but frequently sparing lung parenchyma. Relentless local spread is typical and is usually the cause of death. The three histologic types are epithelial (50%), sarcomatous (16%), and mixed (34%). Accurate diagnosis requires open biopsy or thoracoscopy to obtain tissue. Immunoperoxidase staining is essential, especially to differentiate epithelial mesothelioma from adenocarcinoma.

Most frequently affected are men between 50 and 70 years old. Presenting symptoms are nonpleuritic chest pain (60%), dyspnea (50%), or both. Pleural effusion occurs at some point in 90%. Also common are weight loss, fever, and cough. Physical examination demonstrates dullness to percussion and diminished breath sounds.

Thrombocytosis (>400,000 per cu. mm.) occurs in 60% of patients. Plain radiographs show pleural plaques early in the disease course and later can demonstrate pleural thickening, effusion, ipsilateral volume loss, and mediastinal shift. Computed tomography is used to evaluate spread into the extrapleural soft tissue, the mediastinum, or the diaphragm. Magnetic resonance imaging provides additional anatomic information if resection is contemplated.

Positive prognostic factors are age less than 55 years, good performance status (0–1), female sex, longer duration of symptoms, Stage I disease, the epithelial variant, absence of malignant cells in the pleural fluid, parietal without visceral pleural involvement, and no lymph node metastases. Negative factors are weight loss (>10%) and chest pain.

See the corresponding chapter or part in the *Textbook of Surgery*, 15th edition, pp. 1876–1883, for a more detailed discussion of this topic, including a comprehensive list of references.

Without treatment, patients survive less than 12 months. Single-modality therapy (surgery, chemotherapy, or radiation therapy) does not improve survival. A combination of these three (trimodality therapy) may increase survival. The roles for surgery are biopsy for diagnosis, thoracentesis and pleurodesis for palliation of recurrent effusions in debilitated patients, pleurectomy with decortication in unresectable patients who can tolerate surgery, and cytoreduction by extrapleural pneumonectomy for Stage I patients who can tolerate radical pulmonary surgery. Extrapleural pneumonectomy involves *en bloc* resection of the parietal and visceral pleura, lung, pericardium, and diaphragm. The diaphragm and the pericardium (for right-sided resection) are reconstructed with prosthetic patches.

XIV

Thoracic Outlet Syndrome
John G. Adams, Jr., M.D., and Donald Silver, M.D.

The *thoracic outlet syndrome* is the preferred term for those disorders produced by compression of neurovascular structures in the thoracic outlet. The symptoms of the thoracic outlet syndrome vary depending on the nerves or vessels involved. Neurologic symptoms predominate in 90% to 95% of cases. The syndrome occurs most often in the young to middle-aged female, although all groups may be afflicted. Neurologic symptoms consist of pain, weakness, paresthesias, and numbness usually in the fingers and hands in an ulnar distribution. However, symptoms may occur anywhere in the upper extremity, neck, or shoulder girdle. Late neurologic deficits include sensory loss, motor weakness, and atrophy.

Symptoms of arterial compression include ischemic pain, numbness, fatigue, paresthesias, coldness, and weakness in the arm or hand. These symptoms are accentuated by exercise and exposure to cold. Thrombosis may occur in the compressed or poststenotic dilated areas of the subclavian artery. Distal embolization may be associated with vasomotor symptoms in the fingers consisting of episodic pain with pallor and/or cyanosis. Ulceration or gangrene of the fingertips may occur. Venous compression may produce arm swelling, pain, and cyanosis. The patient frequently complains of a sensation of heaviness or tightness in the arm. Distended superficial veins may be present.

The diagnosis is generally made by history and physical examination, although a number of ancillary tests are usually

---

See the corresponding chapter or part in the *Textbook of Surgery,* 15th edition, pp. 1883–1888, for a more detailed discussion of this topic, including a comprehensive list of references.

indicated. A careful neurologic examination may reveal motor or sensory deficits in the distribution of the brachial plexus, especially of the ulnar nerve. Occasionally, symptoms may be reproduced by pressure or light percussion in the supraclavicular fossa. Signs of arterial involvement may include weakened distal pulses or supraclavicular bruits. A chest film may reveal cervical ribs. Nerve conduction velocities should be obtained to exclude a carpal tunnel syndrome. The 3-minute elevated arm stress test is a useful diagnostic maneuver. The patient is asked to slowly open and close the hands while keeping both arms abducted, externally rotated and flexed to 90 degrees at the elbow. Normal patients may experience fatigue but rarely have pain or paresthesias. The test may reproduce symptoms in patients with the thoracic outlet syndrome. The Adson, hyperabduction, and costoclavicular maneuvers are often positive in normal patients and are usually not helpful in establishing the diagnosis of a thoracic outlet syndrome.

For all patients, except those with symptomatic complete vascular occlusions, distal embolization, or a postcompression aneurysm, initial management should consist of a trial of weight reduction and an exercise program directed toward improving posture, strengthening the elevators of the shoulder girdle, and avoiding hyperabduction. These measures relieve symptoms in 50% to 70% of patients. Nonoperative management appears to be most successful in the obese, young to middle-aged female with poor posture. When patients do not respond to a 4-month or longer trial of conservative treatment, surgical intervention should be considered. Currently, supraclavicular decompression of the thoracic outlet is favored. This operation consists of anterior scalenectomy, middle scalenectomy, removal of a cervical rib if present, and on occasion, first rib resection. Resection of the first rib via a transaxillary approach is also popular and produces similar results. However, the transaxillary operation is associated with a higher incidence of complications. Vascular reconstruction may be required in those few cases with vascular thrombosis or arterial aneurysm.

XV

Congenital Deformities of the Chest Wall

Jeffrey S. Heinle, M.D., and David C. Sabiston, Jr., M.D.

Congenital deformities of the chest wall represent a spectrum of deformities ranging from minor cosmetic defects to

See the corresponding chapter or part in the *Textbook of Surgery*, 15th edition, pp. 1888–1895, for a more detailed discussion of this topic, including a comprehensive list of references.

gross deformities incompatible with life. The defects have both physiologic and psychological consequences and are often associated with other abnormalities. Currently, surgical intervention offers excellent cosmetic results and symptomatic improvement with minimal morbidity and mortality, and patients presenting with these defects should be considered for surgical repair.

PECTUS EXCAVATUM

Pectus excavatum, or funnel chest, is the most common of the congenital deformities of the chest wall, accounting for 90% of the defects and having an incidence of approximately 1 in 125 to 300 live births. It is characterized by a concave, posteriorly displaced sternum due to overgrowth of the costal cartilages. Most commonly the defect begins at the junction of the manubrium and the body of the sternum and becomes progressively deeper toward the xiphoid. The manubrium and the first and second costal cartilages are typically normal. The defect usually presents at birth but can become manifest or exaggerated during growth surges. In the most severe cases, posterior concavity of the sternum leads to displacement and compression of the heart and reduction in volume of the left pleural space. Pectus excavatum is more common in males than in females, with a male-to-female ratio of approximately 2 to 3:1. It is most commonly sporadic in nature, although familial occurrence has been reported. It may be associated with congenital heart disease, Marfan's syndrome, and other skeletal defects, including scoliosis. The classic physical features include the characteristic central depressed sternum, rounded sloped shoulders, dorsal kyphosis, protuberant abdomen, and paradoxical sternal retraction on inspiration. Patients most often present because of the cosmetic defect but are frequently found to have other symptoms, including impaired cardiopulmonary function and scoliosis. Pulmonary complaints include dyspnea and respiratory infections. Restrictive alterations in chest wall mechanics and abnormalities in pulmonary function tests, including decreased vital capacity, decreased total lung capacity, decreased maximal ventilatory volume, and decreased maximal breathing capacity, have been documented.

After surgical correction, patients frequently note an improvement in self-image and a subjective increase in exercise capacity. Objective improvement in cardiac function postoperatively due to relief of the sternal compression has been documented. Postoperatively, worsening of the forced expiratory volume at 1 second (FEV_1), vital capacity, and total lung capacity have been noted, while a significant improvement in maximal ventilatory volume, total progressive exercise time, and maximal oxygen consumption also has been documented. Following surgical correction there is a consistent increase in maximal exercise capacity at every level of workload, a lower heart rate at every workload, and an increase in exercise duration. Because of the significant cosmetic and psychological improvement, subjective increase in exercise tolerance, documented improvement in the cardiac and respiratory status, and prevention of the development of scoliosis following surgical intervention in these patients, surgical correction should be considered for all patients with a moderate to severe deformity. Because there may be spontaneous improvement in the pectus deformity in infants, the optimal age for repair is early childhood (3 to 5 years old). Preoperative evaluation should include a posteroanterior and lateral chest roentgenogram and pulmonary function tests. Prophylactic antibiotics are administered in the perioperative period.

The basic principles of surgical repair include exposure of the sternum and costal cartilages, subperichondrial resection of all involved costal cartilages, correction of the posterior displacement of the sternum using transverse osteotomies, and fixation of the sternum in a slightly overcorrected position. The use of a closed-suction substernal drain significantly reduces the incidence of seroma and fluid collections. Operative mortality is rare (0% to 0.5%), and overall morbidity is low (approximately 5% to 6%). Subcutaneous or substernal seromas and fluid collections occur in about 6% of patients, pneumothorax in 1% to 5%, wound infection in 1% to 2%, and pneumonitis in 4%. Pulmonary toilet needs to be encouraged postoperatively because of the common finding of atelectasis. Postoperative cosmetic results are excellent or good in over 90% of patients, and 98% report improvement in exercise tolerance. Recurrence of the deformity occurs less than 10% of the time and is related to the age at repair.

PECTUS CARINATUM

As opposed to pectus excavatum, pectus carinatum is a protrusion deformity of the breast. It is less common than pectus excavatum and is due to an overgrowth of the costal cartilages, which forces the sternum anteriorly. The anterior protrusion usually involves the lower portion of the sternum, and a lateral depression of costal cartilages accentuates the sternal prominence. This lateral depression can cause compression of the heart and reduce thoracic volume. It usually manifests in midchildhood and may worsen during the growth spurt of adolescence. Males are more commonly affected than females in a ratio of approximately 4:1. It can be found as an isolated anomaly or in association with congenital heart disease or other skeletal anomalies.

As with pectus excavatum, there is a significant psychological component to the deformity. Because of the cosmetic appearance and psychological implications, surgical correction should be considered for all but the minimal deformities. Surgical repair is performed when the patient presents with the deformity, preferably prior to adolescence. The operative technique is similar to that of pectus excavatum, with exposure and subperichondrial resection of all involved costal cartilages. Reefing sutures are placed in the perichondrium to move the sternum posteriorly. A substernal drain is placed to prevent seroma formation. Excellent cosmetic results are obtained with essentially no mortality and low morbidity.

Four per cent of patients will develop postoperative complications, including pneumothorax (2.6%), wound infection (0.7%), atelectasis (0.7%), and local tissue necrosis (0.7%). Recurrence of the defect requiring operative revision occurs in less than 2% of the cases.

STERNAL CLEFTS

Sternal clefts are an uncommon spectrum of defects ranging from simple clefts to complete defects of the sternum and pericardium with herniation of the heart through the defect. The severe forms of the defect, thoracic and cervical ectopia cordis, involve a sternal cleft in which there are no overlying somatic structures and the heart is exposed. The apex of the heart is characteristically positioned anteriorly and cephalad. Intrinsic cardiac anomalies are frequent, and this deformity is frequently fatal. Surgical management is aimed at construction of an anterior chest cavity with tissue coverage of the heart while avoiding posterior displacement of the heart back into the limited thoracic cavity and subsequent hemodynamic compromise.

Thoracoabdominal ectopia cordis involves an inferiorly cleft sternum in which the heart is covered by a thin layer of skin. The heart lacks the severe anterior and superior rotation of thoracic and cervical ectopia cordis, and successful surgical repair and long-term survival are possible. A form of this lesion, Cantrell's pentalogy, involves the association of a lower sternal defect with defects in the supraumbilical abdominal wall, diaphragm, and pericardium along with a congenital intracardiac defect. Initial repair addresses the repair of the intracardiac defect as well as the skin defects overlying the heart and abdominal cavity. The simplest and least severe of these defects is the cleft sternum, which involves primarily the upper sternum and manubrium. Only the sternum is involved in this variant; there is an intact pericardium and normal skin coverage over the defect. This lesion is usually asymptomatic and uniformly correctable. Repair is performed to cover and protect the heart by reapproximating the sternal bands.

POLAND'S SYNDROME

Poland's syndrome is a peculiar spectrum of deformities including unilateral hypoplasia of the thorax and upper extremity with absence of the ipsilateral pectoralis major muscle. These patients usually have little functional disability but present because of the cosmetic deformity. The goal of reconstruction is to restore the natural contour of the chest wall while stabilizing the chest wall deficiency. This reconstruction can be performed with excellent cosmetic results and little or no morbidity or mortality.

Lesions of the Chest Wall

Cemil M. Purut, M.D.

Chest wall tumors are rare neoplasms primarily of bone and soft tissue. Malignant tumors outnumber benign lesions. Slightly more than half the lesions are primary rather than metastatic. Complete surgical excision of the tumor is usually required to effect a cure. The prognosis after surgical therapy is generally good, provided that the margins are found to be free of tumor, but the prognosis is poor if the resection has been incomplete.

INCIDENCE

Tumors of the chest wall comprise approximately 2% of all tumors of the body. Approximately 60% of primary tumors of the chest wall are malignant, and most are of bony origin. Chondrosarcomas are most prevalent, followed by fibrosarcomas, multiple myelomas, Ewing's sarcomas, and osteosarcomas. Malignant fibrous histiocytomas, synovial sarcomas, liposarcomas, rhabdomyosarcomas, undifferentiated sarcomas, and malignant hemangioendotheliomas are less common.

The most common benign lesions of the chest wall are fibrous dysplasia of bone (30%) followed by chondromas/ osteochondromas (20%), while desmoid tumors, neurofibromas, and rhabdomyomas comprise the remainder.

SIGNS AND SYMPTOMS

Most tumors are slowly growing and initially asymptomatic; 75% of patients present only with an asymptomatic, palpable chest wall mass, and pain is a late finding. Metastatic tumors tend to produce symptoms earlier, presumably because of their more rapid doubling time. A history of chest wall trauma may be elicited in some cases but usually is unrelated to the diagnosis. Primary and metastatic tumors of the ribs and cartilage are usually hard and fixed, whereas tumors of soft tissue origin may be less firm and more mobile. Note should be made in the physical examination of constitutional symptoms such as cachexia that would suggest the existence of malignancy.

DIAGNOSIS

The chest film is first test of choice, but computed tomography (CT) is better for determining depth of muscular invasion

---

See the corresponding chapter or part in the *Textbook of Surgery*, 15th edition, pp. 1896–1898, for a more detailed discussion of this topic, including a comprehensive list of references.

because this will help determine the feasibility of chest wall reconstruction. Bone scans should be performed in all patients presenting with bony lesions to exclude synchronous, asymptomatic lesions elsewhere in the body. Bronchoscopy is useful only when there is direct extension of a primary pulmonary lesion into the thoracic wall. Pulmonary function testing should be performed in all patients in whom suspicion of pulmonary dysfunction exists and in whom lung is to be resected.

Small (less than 4 cm.) tumors should undergo excisional biopsy with wide (2 to 4 cm.) margins. Large tumors should undergo incisional biopsy using a surgical approach that does not compromise later reconstruction of the chest wall. The specimen obtained should be nonnecrotic and sufficient to allow for sharing of tissue, special stains, and electron microscopy. Frozen sections are not necessary unless the adequacy of the specimen is in question. Hemostasis should be obtained carefully, since a large and expanding hematoma may spread tumor cells.

TREATMENT
Benign Tumors

Osteochondromas of childhood that are painful or disfiguring need to be resected, and those arising in adulthood always should be resected. *Chondromas* that are less than 4 cm. in diameter may be considered benign, although exclusion of malignancy may sometimes be difficult. Therefore, all chondrosarcomas should be resected with wide margins. *Fibrous dysplasia* usually presents as a solitary, slowly growing, painless mass localized on the posterolateral aspect of a rib. Tumors that are disfiguring or painful should be excised.

Malignant Tumors

Chondrosarcomas are slowly growing, painful tumors that typically arise from the costochondral junction or sternum. Men in the third or fourth decade of life are the most common victims. Mottled calcification may be apparent on chest x-ray. Wide excision with 4- to 5-cm. margins is curative in 97% of patients at 10 years.

Ewing's sarcoma is a highly vascular tumor occurring primarily in young males. These tumors tend to produce symptoms early—primarily pain and generalized malaise. The tumor spreads early, primarily by the hematogenous route, although lymph node metastases occur. Approximately 50% of patients have metastatic disease at the time of presentation. Physical signs such as fever, leukocytosis, and elevated sedimentation rate may be present, and pleural effusions are common. Radiographically, the tumor may have an onion skin appearance due to elevation of the periosteum and multiple layers of new bone formation.

Osteogenic sarcoma primarily affects male children and young adults. Presentation is usually characterized by a rapidly enlarging, painful, firm mass attached to the underlying bone. The radiographic appearance is one of a sunburst due to periosteal elevation by the nonossified tumor. The lungs are the usual first site of metastasis. The tumor is responsive to both chemotherapy and radiotherapy. Surgical resection with wide margins is appropriate for local control of disease.

PRINCIPLES OF CHEST WALL RESECTION

Double-lumen endotracheal intubation often facilitates operation. The skin incision should be planned carefully in order to include the old biopsy scar yet allow primary closure when appropriate. Skin that has been invaded by tumor must be resected with at least a 3-cm. margin, and uninvolved skin must be dissected free to the limits of resection. The tumor capsule must not be violated. The muscle is divided 4 cm. from the edge of the tumor. The rib margins should be 6 cm. Adhesions to the lung should not be separated but remain attached as the underlying lung is divided. At least one grossly normal rib should be excised above and below the primary tumor. In all patients, negative margins are of utmost importance, and resection should not be discontinued prematurely because of concern over the subsequent difficulty of reconstruction of the chest wall.

PRINCIPLES OF CHEST WALL RECONSTRUCTION

Chest wall reconstruction is undertaken to prevent paradoxical movement of the chest wall and to protect underlying organs. Defects of 5 cm. or less, or of three or fewer ribs, do not require special reconstructive closure techniques. Rib resections that are covered by the scapula likewise usually require no reconstruction. Large bony defects of the chest wall may be repaired with either autologous tissue such as fasciae latae or harvested rib or with synthetic material such as Marlex mesh, Prolene mesh, or Gore-Tex. Myocutaneous flaps of the latissimus dorsi, pectoralis major, transverse rectus abdominis, serratus anterior, or external oblique muscles may be used to repair soft tissue defects. The choice of flap depends on the extent and location of the defect.

XVI

Extracorporeal Membrane Oxygenation

James R. Mault, M.D., and Robert H. Bartlett, M.D.

Extracorporeal circulation can be used for days or weeks to support the life of patients with severe cardiac or pulmonary failure. That procedure, referred to as *extracorporeal membrane oxygenation* (ECMO), involves cannulation of major vessels without thoracotomy, carefully titrated partial anticoagulation with heparin, and continuous high-flow extracorporeal circulation through a membrane lung. ECMO is not a therapy but a mechanical support system that allows time for the damaged heart or lungs to heal in a milieu of normal perfusion and gas exchange while "resting" the damaged organs from the effects of mechanical ventilation. ECMO has been the most successful in neonatal respiratory failure and is considered standard therapy for that condition. It is also used for respiratory failure in children and adults.

INDICATIONS

ECMO is indicated when conventional management of respiratory failure fails and mortality risk is high. In the neonate, the underlying pathophysiology is pulmonary arterial vasospasm, causing pulmonary hypertension and right-to-left shunting through the ductus arteriosus or foramen ovale. The lung is intrinsically normal, and recovery rate is excellent. Shunting results in arterial hypoxemia measured by alveolar arterial oxygen gradient ($AaDo_2$). ECMO should be considered when the $AaDo_2$ is greater than 600 mm. Hg despite optimal therapy. ECMO is also indicated for barotrauma manifested by uncontrolled air leaks or poor compliance, with mean airway pressure greater than 20 cm. H_2O.

The underlying pathophysiology in children and adults includes interstitial edema and inflammation leading to necrosis and fibrosis, so patient recovery is related to the extent of irreversible pulmonary injury. For children and adults, ECMO is indicated when the $AaDo_2$ is consistently greater than 600 mm. Hg (representing more than 30% transpulmonary shunt) despite optimal therapy. Barotrauma with air leaks or compliance less than 0.5 cc. per cm. H_2O pressure is also an indication.

ECMO is contraindicated in patients with severe brain injury, poor prognosis for a normal quality of life, active

---

See the corresponding chapter or part in the *Textbook of Surgery*, 15th edition, pp. 1898–1905, for a more detailed discussion of this topic, including a comprehensive list of references.

bleeding, and irreversible pulmonary injury (usually associated with mechanical ventilation longer than 10 days).

THE ECMO CIRCUIT AND MANAGEMENT

Although most of the clinical application of ECMO is currently in newborn infants, the basic principles of extracorporeal circulation, gas exchange, and systemic oxygen delivery apply to patients of all sizes and ages. The circuit includes a servo-regulated roller pump, membrane lung, heat exchanger, tubing, and connectors. Right atrial blood is drained via a right internal jugular catheter to the extracorporeal circuit. Blood is pumped by the servo-regulated pump through the membrane lung and back into the patient. The sizes of catheters, tubing, and membrane lung are designed to be capable of total cardiopulmonary support, even though partial support will be adequate for most patients. Typical flow rates are 80 to 120 ml. per kg. per minute. In *venoarterial* ECMO the blood is perfused through the carotid, femoral, or axillary artery into the aortic arch, providing both heart and lung support. In *venovenous* ECMO, oxygenated blood is returned to the venous circulation, relying on native cardiac function for perfusion, and therefore supports gas exchange only. Cannulation is performed at the bedside in the intensive care unit. Once on ECMO, supporting drugs are reduced or discontinued and the ventilator is turned down to allow "lung rest." Extracorporeal circulation is continued at low ventilator settings until the lung recovers, typically 4 days for newborn infants. Perfusion is monitored by the mixed venous saturation, which measures the adequacy of oxygen delivery in relation to metabolic needs. The patient is heparinized to maintain the whole-blood activated clotting time between 180 and 200 seconds. The extracorporeal flow is gradually decreased as native lung function increases. When flow is approximately 20 ml. per kg. per minute, a trial off bypass at low ventilator settings is attempted. If pulmonary function is adequate, the cannulas are removed.

RESULTS

ECMO is performed in patients with a predicted mortality of approximately 80%. Yet, as of July 1995, the survival rate for 10,000 patients in the Neonatal ECMO Registry was 81% and represents significant salvage from acute respiratory failure. Survival of children and adults receiving ECMO is approximately 50%. When death occurs in newborn infants, it is caused by anoxic brain injury from the perinatal period or intracranial bleeding. When death occurs in children and adults, it is caused by multiple organ failure and sepsis or diffuse pulmonary fibrosis.

Physiologic complications occur in approximately two thirds of patients, including intracranial bleeding (14%), surgical site bleeding (13%), seizures (13%), hemolysis (11%), and positive cultures (6%). Mechanical complications occur in approximately one quarter of patients, including oxygenator change (5%), tubing rupture (1%), and cannula problems (10%).

In follow-up examination, 75% of the survivors are normal. Abnormalities are related to neurolgic and pulmonary systems and are generally caused by the primary disease rather than the ECMO procedure. Twenty per cent of newborn infants have a detectable neurologic abnormality, and 10% have bronchopulmonary dysplasia. Both these problems improve with time. Follow-up in children and adults demonstrates the findings of pulmonary fibrosis and restrictive disease, which usually return to normal within 1 year.

THE FUTURE OF EXTRACORPOREAL LIFE SUPPORT

ECMO is the treatment of choice for infants with severe respiratory failure who fail to respond to conventional management. In the next decade, the use of heparin-coated circuits will decrease the risk of bleeding, and venovenous catheterization will simplify vascular access. Both these improvements will permit the earlier use of ECMO in respiratory failure, which will probably improve outcome results in children and adults. With these technical improvements, the use of ECMO for respiratory failure will become a standard adjunct to conventional mechanical ventilation rather than a salvage procedure when mechanical ventilation fails or causes lung injury. The lesson learned from neonatal experience is that avoiding high-pressure, high-oxygen mechanical ventilation by means of extracorporeal life support results in recovery of the lung and patient survival.

52

THE MEDIASTINUM

R. Duane Davis, Jr., M.D.,
and David C. Sabiston, Jr., M.D.

The mediastinum is an important and complex anatomic division of the thorax defined by the following borders: the thoracic inlet superiorly, the diaphragm inferiorly, the sternum anteriorly, the vertebral column posteriorly, and the parietal pleura laterally. The characteristic location of many tumors and cysts of the mediastinum has led to the artificial division into three subdivisions: the anterosuperior, middle, and posterior. The anterosuperior mediastinum is anterior to the pericardium and the pericardial reflection extending over the great vessels. The posterior mediastinum is posterior to the pericardium and the pericardial reflection. The middle mediastinum is contained within the pericardial sac.

The contents of the anterosuperior mediastinum include the thymus gland, the aortic arch and its branches, the great veins, lymphatics, and fatty areolar tissue. The middle mediastinal contents include the heart, pericardium, phrenic nerves, tracheal bifurcation and main bronchi, the hila of each lung, and lymph nodes. The posterior mediastinum contains the esophagus, vagus nerves, sympathetic nervous chain, thoracic duct, descending aorta, the azygous and hemiazygous systems, lymphatics, and fatty areolar tissue.

MEDIASTINAL EMPHYSEMA

Air within the mediastinum produces mediastinal emphysema or pneumomediastinum. The source of the air may be from the esophagus, trachea, bronchi, neck, or abdomen. Common causes of pneumomediastinum include penetrating wounds and perforations of these structures, blunt trauma that leads to fractured ribs or vertebrae, and barotrauma caused by either blunt trauma or positive-pressure ventilation. Spontaneous pneumomediastinum does occur and usually is seen in patients with exacerbation of bronchospastic disease. The clinical manifestations include substernal chest pain, which may radiate into the back, and crepitation in the region of the suprasternal notch, chest wall, and neck. With increasing pressure, the air can dissect into the neck, face, chest, arms, abdomen, and retroperitoneum. Rarely does sufficient pressure develop to impair venous return and cause hemodynamic instability. Frequently, pneumomediastinum and pneumothorax occur simultaneously. The diagnosis of pneumomediastinum is confirmed by the presence of air in the mediastinum on chest film. Because the morbidity of an un-

---

See the corresponding chapter or part in the *Textbook of Surgery*, 15th edition, pp. 1906–1929, for a more detailed discussion of this topic, including a comprehensive list of references.

corrected esophageal leak increases dramatically with time, a Gastrografin swallow should be obtained early to evaluate for an esophageal perforation. Treatment is directed toward correcting the inciting cause. Although careful observation for the development of circulatory compromise is necessary, surgical decompression is rarely needed.

MEDIASTINITIS

Infection of the mediastinal space is a serious and potentially fatal process caused by perforation of the esophagus due to instrumentation, foreign bodies, penetrating or, more rarely, blunt trauma, spontaneous esophageal disruption (Boerhaave's syndrome), leakage from an esophageal anastomosis, tracheobronchial perforation, mediastinal extension from an infectious process originating in the pulmonary parenchyma, pleura, chest wall, vertebrae, great vessels, or neck, and following operations using median sternotomy. Wound infections after median sternotomy for cardiac operations occur in 2% of patients; half of these involve the mediastinum. Mediastinitis is manifested clinically by fever, tachycardia, leukocytosis, and pain that may be localized to the chest, back, or neck. The lateral chest film and computed tomographic (CT) scan may assist in the diagnosis by identifying air-fluid levels, abnormal soft tissue densities, and sternal dehiscence. Use of endoscopy, bronchoscopy, and contrast studies of the esophagus is helpful in identifying esophageal and tracheal-bronchial etiologies. Treatment of mediastinitis requires correction of the inciting cause and aggressive supportive therapy with appropriate antimicrobial coverage. Correction of inciting causes, when identifiable, with débridement of necrotic tissue and surgical drainage is necessary. A number of techniques for treating postoperative mediastinitis have been used, but the best results with the shortest hospital stays have occurred using tissue flaps (rectus or pectoralis muscle and omentum) to cover the mediastinum after obtaining surgical control of the wound infection.

SUPERIOR VENA CAVA OBSTRUCTION

A number of benign and malignant processes may cause obstruction of the superior vena cava, leading to increased pressure in the venous system draining into the superior vena cava and producing the characteristic features of the superior vena caval syndrome: edema of the head, neck, and upper extremities; distended neck veins with dilated collateral veins over the upper extremities and torso; cyanosis; headache; and confusion. These findings are more pronounced when the patient is in a recumbent position. Sudden occlusion may lead to rapid development of cerebral edema and intracranial thrombosis, which may lead to coma and death. Bronchogenic carcinoma of the right upper lobe is the most common etiology, but a large number of malignant mediastinal tumors also commonly cause this syndrome. Less than 25% of patients with superior vena caval obstruction have a benign etiology.

The syndrome occurs infrequently in children. Atrial-level repairs for transposition of the great arteries and malignant mediastinal neoplasms are the most common causes.

CT or magnetic resonance imaging (MRI) is usually sufficient to establish the diagnosis of superior vena cava obstruction. A histologic diagnosis is attempted before initiating therapy owing to the alteration in morphologic appearance of the tumor following treatment. Needle biopsy or biopsy performed under local anesthesia is used preferentially due to the hazards of cardiovascular compromise during general anesthesia. Radiation, corticosteroids, and chemotherapy are the usual modalities of treatment. When neurologic symptoms are present, urgent therapy is mandated. Surgical bypass using a variety of graft materials has been used with improving success. Percutaneous angioplasty using stents can be successful if the obstruction is not complete.

PRIMARY NEOPLASMS AND CYSTS

A large number of neoplasms and cysts arise from multiple anatomic sites in the mediastinum and present with myriad clinical signs and symptoms. The most common mediastinal masses are neurogenic tumors (20%), thymomas (19%), primary cysts (21%), lymphomas (13%), and germ cell tumors (10%). Many mediastinal masses occur in characteristic sites within the mediastinum. In the anterosuperior mediastinum, the most frequent neoplasms are thymoma (31%), lymphoma (23%), and germ cell tumors (17%). Posterior mediastinal lesions are usually neurogenic tumors (52%), bronchogenic cysts (22%), and enteric cysts (7%). Middle mediastinal masses are usually pericardial cysts (35%), lymphomas (21%), and bronchogenic cysts (15%). Malignant neoplasms represent 25% to 42% of mediastinal masses. Lymphomas, thymomas, germ cell tumors, primary carcinomas, and neurogenic tumors are the most common. The relative frequency of malignancy varies with the anatomic site in the mediastinum. Anterosuperior masses are most likely malignant (59%), as compared with middle mediastinal masses (29%) and posterior mediastinal masses (16%). Patients in the second through fourth decades have a greater proportion of malignant neoplasms; those in the first decade have a lower proportion. The incidence of various mediastinal masses varies in infants, children, and adults. In a series of 706 children with mediastinal masses, neurogenic tumors (35%), most commonly gangliomas, ganglioneuroblastomas, and neuroblastomas; lymphomas (25%), usually non-Hodgkin's; germ cell tumors (11%), predominantly benign teratomas; and primary cysts (16%) occurred most frequently. Pericardial cysts and thymomas are uncommon in children.

SYMPTOMS

Of patients with a mediastinal mass, 56% to 65% are symptomatic at presentation. Patients with a benign lesion are more often asymptomatic (54%) than are patients with a malignant

neoplasm (15%). While 75% of asymptomatic patients have a
benign histology, almost two-thirds of symptomatic patients
have a malignant lesion. The most common symptoms include
chest pain, cough, and fever. Although myasthenia gravis was
present in only 7% of patients from the overall series, in
patients with thymoma, 43% had myasthenia gravis. Infants
most likely present with symptoms or findings (78%) because
of the relatively small space within the mediastinum.

Symptoms may be related to compression or invasion of
mediastinal structures or production of hormones or antibodies causing systemic symptoms that characterize a specific
syndrome. The pathophysiology of some of the systemic syndromes is not well defined, although autoimmune mechanisms have been implicated.

DIAGNOSIS

The optimal goal of the diagnostic evaluation is the precise
histologic classification and staging of the lesion to determine
optimal therapy. Although the history and physical examination provide useful information, the diagnosis is rarely possible without further investigation. The routine chest film demonstrates the location, size, relative density, and degree of
calcification of the mediastinal mass, which greatly narrows
the differential diagnosis. CT scans increase the sensitivity
and specificity of the diagnostic evaluation because of the
improved spatial resolution, ability to examine areas poorly
interrogated by chest films (aortopulmonary window and subcarinal region), and through the use of contrast materials to
differentiate primary mediastinal lesions from a variety of
cardiovascular abnormalities that mimic a mediastinal mass
on chest film. CT scans reasonably indicate when a lesion is
resectable; however, the prediction of unresectability is not as
accurate. MRI also differentiates primary masses from vascular lesions. CT scans and MRI are useful in determining the
presence of spinal column involvement by posterior mediastinal tumors and airway compression by anterior and middle
mediastinal masses.

Examples of useful nuclear scans include [131I] *meta*-iodo-
benzylguanidine (MIBG), which identifies pheochromocytomas (particularly helpful when the tumor is located in the
middle mediastinum), and radioisotopic iodine scans, which
identify functioning ectopic thyroid tissue.

Monoclonal antibodies have been used to develop serologic
markers for a variety of mediastinal tumors, the most important of which are those used to measure alpha-fetoprotein
and beta-human chorionic gonadotropin. These tumor markers identify nonseminomatous germ cell tumors, and they
should be obtained in all males with a mediastinal mass in
the second through fifth decades.

Nonoperative methods of establishing a histologic diagnosis
are available, including fine-needle biopsy (22-gauge needle)
technique, which produces a cytologic specimen, and cutting-
needle techniques, which produces a histologic specimen. Although a cytologic determination of malignancy can be made

in 80% to 90% of patients, a precise histologic diagnosis is determined less commonly. Because the precise diagnosis, and in particular the subclassification of lymphomas, requires more tissue than can be obtained using needle techniques, more invasive procedures are often necessary. Mediastinoscopy provides access to paratrachial masses, while mediastinotomy and extended mediastinoscopy provide access to the anterosuperior mediastinum for biopsy of lesions. Thoracoscopic techniques are useful for biopsies and for resection of carefully selected benign tumors. Thoracotomy and median sternotomy provide greater exposure for biopsy or when resection is indicated. The majority of patients can undergo these diagnostic procedures safely. However, patients with large anterior and middle mediastinal masses that compress the trachea, bronchus, or superior vena cava may be susceptible to cardiopulmonary collapse. CT, MRI, and pulmonary flow mechanics are sensitive indicators of airway compromise and select patients at high risk for general anesthesia. In these patients, diagnosis should be established using needle biopsy techniques or biopsy under local or regional anesthesia. Occasionally, a diagnosis cannot be established prior to initiation of empirical therapy.

Because of the similar morphologic appearance by light microscopy of the undifferentiated malignant tumors of the anterosuperior mediastinum, the use of electron microscopy to examine cellular ultrastructure and immunohistochemistry to identify characteristic surface antigens and tumor secretory products may be necessary to establish a diagnosis and to subclassify the various non-Hodgkin's lymphomas.

NEUROGENIC TUMORS

Neurogenic tumors are the most common neoplasm found in the mediastinum, comprising approximately 21% of all primary tumors and cysts. These tumors are usually located in the posterior mediastinum and originate from the sympathetic ganglia (ganglioma, ganglioneuroblastoma, and neuroblastoma), the intercostal nerves (neurofibroma, neurilemoma, and neurosarcoma), and the paraganglia cells (paraganglioma). Although the peak incidence occurs in adults, neurogenic tumors comprise a proportionally greater percentage of mediastinal masses in children (35%). Whereas the majority of neurogenic tumors in adults are benign, a greater percentage of neurogenic tumors are malignant in children.

The most common neurogenic tumor is the neurilemoma, which originates from the perineural Schwann's cells. These tumors are well circumscribed and have a well-defined capsule. In contrast, neurofibromas are poorly encapsulated and originate as a proliferation of all the peripheral nerve elements. Both entities occur as manifestation of neurofibromatosis. Surgical excision results in cure.

Ganglioneuromas, ganglioneuroblastomas, and neuroblastomas originate from the sympathetic chain, are comprised of ganglion cells and nerve fibers, and are the most common neurogenic tumors of childhood. The degree of differentiation of the ganglion cells differentiates these tumors: well-differentiated—ganglioneuroma; poorly differentiated—neuroblastoma; and mixture—ganglioneuroblastoma. Surgical excision is usually curative for ganglioneuromas, Stage I and II ganglioneuroblastomas, and Stage I neuroblastomas. Radiation and multiagent chemotherapy are used in the treatment of higher-staged malignant tumors. Children less than 1 year of age and those with less extensive disease have the best prognosis.

Mediastinal paragangliomas are rare tumors, comprising less than 1% of mediastinal masses and less than 2% of all pheochromocytomas. The majority of these tumors occur in the paravertebral sulcus; however, a number occur in the middle mediastinum. Catecholamine production is less common than with adrenal paragangliomas, and when present, the product is usually norepinepherine. Catecholamine production causes the classic constellation of symptoms associated with pheochromocytomas, including periodic or sustained hypertension, often accompanied by orthostatic hypotension, hypermetabolism manifested by weight loss, hyperhydrosis, palpitations, and headaches. Measurement of elevated levels of urinary catecholamines or their metabolites, the metanephrines and vanillylmandelic acid (VMA), usually establishes the diagnosis. Tumor localization has improved remarkably through the use of CT and *meta*-iodobenzylguanidine (^{131}I-MIBG) scintigraphy, particularly when the tumors are hormonally active. When possible, resection is the appropriate therapy. Although many tumors appear morphologically malignant, only 3% of patients develop metastatic disease. Multiple paragangliomas occur in 10% of patients and more commonly in association with the multiple endocrine neoplasia or Carney's syndrome and when a family history is present.

THYMOMA

Thymoma is the most common neoplasm of the anterosuperior mediastinum and the second most common mediastinal mass (20%). The peak incidence is in the third through fifth decades, and thymoma is rare during childhood. Although symptoms due to local mass effects such as chest pain, dyspnea, and cough are most common, systemic syndromes are associated particularly with thymomas, most commonly myasthenia gravis and red cell aplasia. Myasthenia gravis occurs in 10% to 50% of patients with a thymoma. In patients with myasthenia gravis, 10% to 42% have a thymoma, with elderly and male patients having a higher incidence. The disease process is characterized by weakness and fatigue of the skeletal muscles associated with destruction of the postsynaptic nicotinic receptors. This process appears to be immune-related.

Whenever possible, the therapy for thymoma is surgical excision without removing or injuring vital structures. Even with well-encapsulated thymomas, extended thymectomy with eradication of all accessible mediastinal fatty areolar tissue should be performed to ensure removal of all ectopic thymic tissue. This approach has been shown to lower the number of tumor recurrences. The best operative exposure is obtained using a median sternotomy. The differentiation between benign and malignant disease is determined by the presence of gross invasion of adjacent structures, metastasis, or microscopic evidence of capsular invasion. In patients with tumor invasion through the capsule or into surrounding structures, postoperative radiotherapy is recommended. Multi-agent chemotherapy has been useful in patients with metastatic or recurrent disease.

Patients with thymoma and myasthenia gravis require careful perioperative management, using plasmapheresis in the 72 hours prior to surgery, discontinuation of anticholinesterase inhibitors, as well as good pulmonary therapy. Postoperatively, decisions regarding extubation are based on adequate respiratory mechanics.

GERM CELL TUMORS

Germ cell tumors are benign and malignant neoplasms thought to originate from primordial germ cells that fail to complete the migration from the urogenital ridge and come to rest in the mediastinum. These tumors are classified as teratomas, teratocarcinomas, seminomas, embryonal cell carcinomas, choriocarcinoma, and endodermal cell (yolk sac) tumors and are identical histologically to those originating in the gonads. They occur most commonly in the anterosuperior mediastinum. Teratomas are neoplasms comprised of multiple tissue elements foreign to the area in which they occur and derived from the three primitive embryonal layers. The peak incidence is in the second and third decades of life. There is no sex predisposition. The teratodermoid is the simplest form, comprised predominantly of derivatives of the epidermal layer (hair, sebaceous material, and dermal and epidermal glands). Teratomas are histologically more complex. The solid component of the tumor contains well-differentiated elements of bone, cartilage, teeth, muscle, connective tissue, fibrous and lymphoid tissue, nerve, thymus, mucous, and salivary glands, lung, liver, or pancreas. Malignant teratomas are differentiated by the presence of embryonal or primitive tissue. Surgical resection of benign teratomas, even partial, is the recommended therapy to prevent complications.

MALIGNANT GERM CELL TUMOR

Malignant germ cell tumors occur predominantly in males, with a peak incidence in the third and fourth decades. These tumors frequently cause symptoms due to local mass effects, including the superior vena caval syndrome. Serologic measurements of alpha-fetoprotein (α-FP) and beta-human chorionic gonadotropin (β-hCG) are useful for the following tasks: differentiating seminomas from nonseminomas, quantitatively assessing response to therapy in hormonally active tumors (plasma half-life of α-FP and β-hCG is 5 days and 12 to 24 hours, respectively), and diagnosing relapse or failure of therapy prior to changes that can be observed in gross disease. Seminomas rarely produce β-hCG (7%) and never produce α-FP; in contrast, over 90% of nonseminomas secrete one or both of these hormones. The differentiation between seminomas and nonseminomatous germ cell tumors is important due to the radiosensitivity of seminomas and the contrasting insensitivity of the other germ cell tumors. Seminomas are also more likely to remain intrathoracic than the other germ cell tumors. With seminomas, surgical therapy usually is limited to establishment of the histologic diagnosis. Radiotherapy is the basis of therapy, with the use of multiagent chemotherapy for patients with extrathoracic disease or tumor relapse. In contrast, the optimal treatment of nonseminomatous germ cell tumors is cis-platinum–based chemotherapy with subsequent resection of residual disease. Chemotherapy may be initiated based on the presence of an anterosuperior mediastinal mass in a male patient in the second through fifth decades with elevated β-hCG or α-FP, emphasizing the importance of measuring these hormones. The presence of residual disease after surgical resection portends a grave prognosis.

LYMPHOMAS

Although the mediastinum is frequently involved in patients with lymphoma sometime during the course of the disease (40% to 70%), it is infrequently the sole site of disease at the time of presentation. These tumors frequently produce symptoms due to local mass effects, in addition to characteristic symptoms such as cyclic fevers (Pel-Ebstein) and chest pain associated with alcohol consumption. These tumors occur most commonly in the anterosuperior mediastinum or in the hilar region of the middle mediastinum. Mediastinal involvement with Hodgkin's disease is most common, with nodular sclerosing and lymphocyte predominant subtypes. Patients with Stage IA and IIA disease are treated with radiation therapy, while those with Stage IIB, III, and IV disease are treated with chemotherapy. Controversy exists regarding therapy for patients with bulky mediastinal involvement due to the higher relapse rate following radiation treatment. Although some centers use chemotherapy as primary treatment, equivalent survival is achieved using chemotherapy as salvage treatment in patients who relapse following radiation. Non-Hodgkin's lymphomas are usually either of lymphoblastic morphology (60%) or large cell morphology with a diffuse pattern of growth (40%). Multiagent chemotherapy is the optimal treatment. Operative intervention is limited to providing adequate tissue for a precise histologic diagnosis. Because of the importance of precise immunotyping in the selection of chemotherapeutic regimen, needle biopsy techniques are usually inadequate due to the insufficient tissue sample obtained.

PRIMARY CARCINOMA

Primary carcinomas comprise between 3% and 11% of mediastinal masses. Their origin is unknown, but it is important to differentiate these tumors from the neoplasms that may have a similar morphologic appearance such as thymoma, lymphoma, metastasis, and bronchogenic cancers by using electron microscopy and immunohistochemistry. Primary carcinomas usually cause symptoms and are rarely resectable. Prognosis is poor, with mean survival less than 1 year after diagnosis with minimal benefit from chemotherapy and radiation therapy.

ENDOCRINE TUMORS

Although substernal extension of a cervical goiter is common, totally intrathoracic thyroid tumors are rare and account for less than 1% of mediastinal masses. Arising from ectopic thyroid tissue, these tumors occur most commonly in the anterosuperior mediastinum but also occur in the middle and posterior mediastinum. Symptoms are usually due to mass effect; however, hormone production can result in thyrotoxicosis. When functioning thyroid tissue is present, the radioactive iodine (^{131}I) scan is diagnostic. Importantly, the ^{131}I scan can determine if functioning cervical thyroid tissue is absent, which would contraindicate excision of an asymptomatic intrathoracic thyroid tumor. Because of thoracic derivation of the blood supply, intrathoracic thyroid tumors should be approached through a thoracic incision. Most tumors are adenomas, but carcinomas have been reported.

Mediastinal parathyroids occur in 10% of patients, but the majority are accessible through a cervical incision. Only 2% of patients with hyperfunctioning parathyroid glands require a sternotomy for resection. These glands are usually adjacent to or within the thymus. Using CT, MRI, thallium, and technetium scanning, venous angiography with selective sampling, and selective arteriography, preoperative localization of these tumors can be made in approximately 80% of patients. Preoperative localization should be attempted in those patients who have had a cervical exploration and continue to have hyperparathyroidism prior to performing a mediastinal exploration. Parathyroid carcinomas occur and tend to be more active hormonally.

Mediastinal carcinoid tumors arise from cells of Kulchitsky located in the thymus. Occurring more often in male patients, these tumors usually are located in the anterosuperior mediastinum. When active hormonally, these tumors usually produce ACTH, causing Cushing's syndrome. Hormonally inactive carcinoids tend to be larger and frequently are invasive locally. In addition, metastatic spread to mediastinal and cervical lymph nodes, liver, bone, skin, and lungs occurs in the majority of patients. Surgical removal, when possible, is the preferred treatment. Radiation therapy and chemotherapy have not been demonstrated to be effective in the treatment of malignant disease.

MESENCHYMAL TUMORS

Mediastinal mesenchymal tumors originate from the connective tissue, striatal and smooth muscle, fat, lymphatic tissue, and blood vessels present within the mediastinum, giving rise to a diverse group of neoplasms. Relative to other sites in the body, these tumors occur less commonly within the mediastinum. Mesenchymal tumors comprised 7% of the primary masses in the collected series. There is no apparent difference in incidence between sexes. The soft tissue mesenchymal tumors have a similar histologic appearance and generally follow the same clinical course as the soft tissue tumors found elsewhere in the body. Fifty-five per cent of these tumors are malignant. The vascular tumors are poorly encapsulated, and even benign tumors may be locally invasive. Between 10% and 30% are morphologically malignant, but only 3% develop metastases. Surgical resection remains the primary therapy in the treatment of patients with mesenchymal tumors, since poor results have been obtained using radiation and chemotherapy.

Other uncommon mediastinal masses include giant lymph node hyperplasia, extramedullary hematopoiesis, and chondromas.

PRIMARY CYSTS

Primary cysts of the mediastinum comprise 20% of the mediastinal masses in the collected series. These cysts can be bronchogenic, pericardial, enteric, or thymic or may be of an unspecified nature. More than 75% of patients are asymptomatic, and these tumors rarely cause morbidity. However, due to the proximity of vital structures within the mediastinum, with increasing size even benign cysts may cause significant morbidity. In addition, these masses need to be differentiated from malignant tumors.

Bronchogenic cysts are the most common primary cyst. They originate as sequestrations from the ventral foregut, the antecedent of the tracheobronchial tree. The bronchogenic cyst may lie within the lung parenchyma or the mediastinum. The cyst wall is composed of cartilage, mucous glands, smooth muscle, and fibrous tissue with a pathognomonic inner layer of ciliated respiratory epithelium. When bronchogenic cysts occur in the mediastinum, they are usually located proximal to the trachea or bronchi and may be just posterior to the carina. Often these cysts are poorly demonstrated by routine chest films but readily visualized using CT.

Pericardial cysts are the second most frequently encountered cysts within the mediastinum and comprise 6% of all lesions and 33% of primary cysts. These cysts classically occur in the pericardiophrenic angles, with 70% in the right pericardiophrenic angle and 22% in the left and the remainder in other sites in the pericardium.

Enteric cysts (duplication cysts) arise from the posterior division of the primitive foregut, which develops into the upper division of the gastrointestinal tract. These cysts are found less frequently than bronchogenic or pericardial cysts and comprise 3% of the mediastinal masses in the collected series. Occurring most commonly in the posterior mediastinum and in children, these lesions are composed of smooth muscle with an inner epithelial lining of esophageal, gastric, or intestinal mucosa. When gastric mucosa is present, peptic ulceration with perforation into the esophageal or bronchial lumen may occur producing hemoptysis or hematemesis. When enteric cysts are associated with anomalies of the vertebral column, they are referred to as *neuroenteric cysts*. Such cysts may be connected to the meninges, or less frequently, a direct communication with the dural space may exist. In patients with neuroenteric cysts, preoperative evaluation for potential spinal cord involvement is mandatory, usually using CT or MRI.

Thymic cysts may be inflammatory, neoplastic, or congenital lesions. Congenital cysts are thought to originate from the third bronchial arch and are not usually related to thymomas. These cysts are defined by the presence of thymic tissue within the cyst wall. An apparent increase in the incidence of thymic cysts following treatment of malignant anterior mediastinal neoplasms has been reported. Nonspecific cysts include those lesions in which a specific epithelial or mesothelial lining cannot be identified.

The optimal treatment of a mediastinal cyst is surgical excision primarily for diagnosis and to differentiate these cysts from malignant lesions, although the bronchogenic and enteric cysts frequently can cause significant symptoms, particularly in children. Patients with characteristic lesions and classic CT findings for pericardial cysts have been managed with needle aspiration and serial follow-up with CT rather than surgical excision.

I

Acute Suppurative Mediastinitis
Thomas J. Krizek, M.D., and Lawrence J. Gottlieb, M.D.

Acute suppurative mediastinitis is an infrequent but serious complication of cardiac surgery. An incidence of less than 1% is encountered in pediatric cardiac surgery and increases to a maximum of 2.5% in complicated, re-do surgery in adults, particularly when valve replacement or use of the internal mammary arteries is required.

The chest wall serves a dual purpose of being a rigid compartment for protecting the heart and lungs from injury while allowing flexibility to accomplish ventilation. Stress on the postoperative sternum, often accompanied by long and complicated surgery on patients whose systemic defense

---

See the corresponding chapter or part in the *Textbook of Surgery*, 15th edition, pp. 1929–1933, for a more detailed discussion of this topic, including a comprehensive list of references.

mechanisms are compromised, predisposes to postoperative infection.

The diagnosis is suspected in the patient whose pain increases in the postoperative period and is confirmed when purulent drainage from the wound occurs. Prophylactic antibacterials are used routinely, so infections are often caused by more resistant organisms. Staphylococci account for about 40%, and another 40% are from gram-negative and mixed-flora infection. Bacterial lodgment in the operative wound requires a level of 10^5 organisms per gram of tissue before infection becomes manifest; this level of bacteria in tissue may be isolated from systemically administered antibacterials, requiring that these infections be treated surgically.

The wound from which drainage is identified must be opened, and débridement requires that sutures, wires, blood clots, and bits of bone be removed. Irrigation under pressure is necessary to wash out the bacteria lodged in tissue, and antibacterial therapy must include topical agents such as silver sulfadiazine to complement systemic treatment. Minor infections may be managed on occasion by closure over irrigation catheters through which antibacterials can be instilled and effluent carried away. More complicated infections require that the wound be managed by an open technique until bacterial balance can be achieved, as measured by quantitative cultures of biopsy specimens of both soft tissue and bone.

Secondary closure requires a dual approach. The sternum, like most bones, heals best when rigid internal fixation techniques have been employed. The sternum should be débrided to healthy tissue and bacterial control confirmed by biopsy cultures. Miniplates are then applied to fix the sternum. The second part of the closure demands the use of adequate well-vascularized soft tissue to obliterate dead space and provide supple and protective coverage. The pectoralis major muscle singly or from both sides serves to close at least 80% of such wounds. The origin of the muscle, when freed, takes tension off the sternal repair and allows the muscle to be mobilized to or across the midline. Alternative coverage may employ the rectus abdominis muscle or omentum. When available, the skin of the chest provides surface closure; when not, skin grafts can be applied to muscle or omentum.

Suppurative mediastinitis has been reported to be fatal in more than 70% of cases managed without surgery. With adequate débridement, antibacterial control confirmed with quantitative cultures, and rigid internal fixation and adequate soft tissue closure, the mortality has been reduced to less than 3%.

II

Surgical Management of Myasthenia Gravis

Jeffrey A. Hagen, M.D., and Joel D. Cooper, M.D.

Myasthenia gravis is a neurologic disorder defined clinically on the basis of weakness or fatigability occurring with repetitive exercise that resolves with rest. It is believed to be an autoimmune disorder in which the number of functional acetylcholine receptors are reduced. The clinical course is characterized by frequent spontaneous remissions and relapses, with an unpredictable response to therapy, specifically with respect to the response to thymectomy.

Myasthenia gravis is uncommon, occurring in 0.5 to 5 per 100,000 population. The peak age of onset is 20 to 30 years of age in women and over 50 years of age in men. Women are affected more commonly than men, with a ratio of 3:2. Most cases are nonfamilial, but associations with various HLA types suggest a genetic predisposition. There is also an association between myasthenia gravis and other disorders of autoimmune etiology, such as Graves' disease, Hashimoto's thyroiditis, systemic lupus erythematosus, and pernicious anemia.

PATHOPHYSIOLOGY

The basic pathophysiologic alteration in myasthenia gravis involves a reduction in the number of functional acetylcholine receptors. Proposed mechanisms of this reduction in receptors include antibody-mediated receptor destruction, complement activation and receptor destruction, and specific antibody binding resulting in receptor blockade. The source of these autoantibodies is unknown. The thymus is believed to play a major role based on observations that histologic abnormalities of the thymus are detectable in 80% of the patients and that thymic B cells contain antibodies to acetylcholine receptors and on the beneficial effect observed following thymectomy.

CLINICAL FINDINGS

The hallmark of the diagnosis of myasthenia gravis is a weakness or fatigability that occurs with repetitive exercise and improves with rest. The muscle groups involved vary significantly from one patient to another and in a given patient over time. Ocular symptoms of ptosis and diplopia are the most common initial symptoms, occurring in one half of pa-

---

See the corresponding chapter or part in the *Textbook of Surgery,* 15th edition, pp. 1933–1942, for a more detailed discussion of this topic, including a comprehensive list of references.

tients. As the disease progresses, over 90% will develop ocular symptoms. Involvement of other cranial nerves is less common but may result in dysphagia, nasal regurgitation, and aspiration.

Generalized muscle weakness develops over time in 85% of patients. This weakness tends to involve the proximal muscles of the shoulder and hip region more than the muscles of the extremities. Sensory examination and deep tendon reflexes are normal.

NATURAL HISTORY

Early studies of the natural history of untreated myasthenia gravis suggests a mortality rate of 30% to 60%. However, these studies predated intensive care units and widespread use of mechanical ventilators. More recent data on untreated cases do not exist, but survival with current medical and/or surgical therapy is approximately 60% to 90% at 20 years. Spontaneous remissions occur in 10% to 20% of medically treated patients. The majority of these occur in the first year following diagnosis, but they have been observed to occur at up to 13 years.

DIFFERENTIAL DIAGNOSIS

The differential diagnosis of myasthenia gravis includes disorders of neuromuscular transmission such as botulism and the Lambert-Eaton syndrome. Botulism, a descending type of paralysis, is caused by the toxin from *Clostridium botulinum*. The result is a decrease in acetylcholine release from the motor neuron, in contrast to the impaired binding to receptors seen in myasthenia gravis. The Lambert-Eaton syndrome, a disorder also believed to be of autoimmune origin, typically presents with a proximal muscle weakness that in general spares the facial muscles. The majority of cases are associated with an underlying malignancy, with small cell cancer of the lung present in 70%. Both botulism and Lambert-Eaton syndrome can be differentiated from myasthenia gravis on the basis of electromyographic (EMG) testing.

DIAGNOSIS

The diagnosis of myasthenia gravis can be established in most cases on the basis of single-fiber EMG studies. These will be abnormal in 90% to 100% of patients with severe generalized symptoms but in only 60% to 75% with isolated ocular involvement. In those patients in whom EMG studies are normal, the diagnosis of myasthenia gravis can be made on the basis of a positive Tensilon (edrophonium) test, demonstrating improvement in strength following intravenous administration. The Tensilon test is positive in 85% of patients with ocular symptoms and in 95% with generalized disease. Acetylcholine receptor antibodies also can be utilized to establish the diagnosis, being detectable in the serum of 65% of patients with ocular symptoms and 90% of patients with generalized disease.

TREATMENT

Therapeutic options for patients with myasthenia gravis include anticholinesterase therapy, immunosuppression, plasmapheresis, and surgical thymectomy. The roles of these therapies and their sequence of utilization remain controversial.

Pyridostigmine (Mestinon) is the most commonly used cholinesterase inhibitor medication. By reducing the hydrolysis of acetylcholine, these compounds enhance neuromuscular transmission. Side effects of nausea, abdominal cramping, diarrhea, excessive salivation, and bradycardia often limit the use of these medications.

Immunosuppressive treatment with corticosteroids and azathioprine (Imuran) has been utilized with response rates of up to 80%. Because of the serious side effects of these compounds, their use is generally limited to refractory cases.

Plasmapheresis therapy, by removal of immunoglobulins and other plasma constituents, results in improvement in symptoms in up to 90% of patients. However, the duration of benefit is short-lived. Cost and side effects of repeated plasmapheresis limit the use of this therapy to short-term applications such as preparation of patients for thymectomy or treatment of myasthenic crisis.

Surgical thymectomy has long been shown to produce favorable responses in patients with myasthenia gravis. Options include transcervical thymectomy, transsternal simple thymectomy, and radical combined transcervical and transsternal thymectomy, as advocated by Jeretzki. To date, no clear benefit has been shown for one technique over another. The single most important principle of surgical thymectomy involves complete removal of the thymus.

RESULTS

Surgical thymectomy has been associated with complete remission rates of up to 50%, with clinical improvement noted in approximately 80% to 95%. In addition, a survival advantage has been demonstrated in at least two large retrospective series. Factors associated with improvement following thymectomy include young age at diagnosis, female gender, the presence of mild generalized symptoms, and duration of symptoms less than 1 year prior to thymectomy. The presence of a thymoma, while mandating thymectomy, is associated with lesser degrees of improvement.

53

SURGICAL DISORDERS OF THE PERICARDIUM

Michael E. Jessen, M.D.

ANATOMY AND PHYSIOLOGY. The *visceral pericardium* consists of a loose layer of fibrous tissue covered by mesothelial cells situated on the epicardium of the heart. Clear serous pericardial fluid secreted by this layer is contained within the *parietal pericardium,* a dense fibrous structure lined with an inner serous membrane. The pericardium anchors to surrounding structures (sternum, vertebral column, and diaphragm) and fuses to the great vessels, venae cava, and pulmonary veins. Up to 50 ml. of fluid may normally be present within the pericardium, returning via lymphatics in the parietal surface to the thoracic duct. The pericardium serves to (1) provide anatomic fixation of the heart during body motion, (2) reduce friction between the heart and surrounding structures, and (3) provide a barrier against local infections. Except in disease states, the pericardium exerts minor hemodynamic effects, and congenital absence or surgical removal does not cause symptoms. However, the pericardium does limit acute cardiac distention and contributes to *diastolic coupling*: the process whereby distention of one ventricle alters the distensibility of the other.

ACUTE PERICARDITIS. Acute inflammation of the pericardium presents with retrosternal chest pain, often worsening with deep inspiration and lying supine and improving with sitting upright. Dyspnea, cough, fever, chills, and weakness may be accompanying symptoms. Abnormal physical findings occur if a significant effusion accompanies this process and consist of muffled heart sounds and a pericardial friction rub. The chest x-ray may show an enlarged cardiac silhouette. The electrocardiogram (ECG) may reveal diminished QRS voltage and diffuse ST-segment elevation. Echocardiography may demonstrate an accumulation of pericardial fluid. Most cases are idiopathic, but pericarditis may be a sequela of (1) an infectious process (viral, bacterial, fungal, or tuberculous), (2) mediastinal irradiation, (3) acute myocardial infarction, (4) aortic dissection, (5) blunt or penetrating chest trauma, (6) direct tumor invasion, (7) uremia, (8) collagen-vascular disease, (9) drug therapy (e.g., hydralazine or procainamide), or (10) cardiac surgical procedure. Fever, pericarditis, and pleuritis appearing 2 to 4 weeks after cardiac operation constitute the *postpericardiotomy syndrome,* which is usually accompanied by leukocytosis and an elevated sedimentation rate. This process has been associated with the appearance of antiheart antibodies suggesting an autoimmune basis. Most cases of

---

See the corresponding chapter or part in the *Textbook of Surgery,* 15th edition, pp. 1943–1951, for a more detailed discussion of this topic, including a comprehensive list of references.

acute pericarditis will resolve spontaneously in 2 to 6 weeks, although recurrences can occur. Nonsteroidal anti-inflammatory agents are the first line of therapy, although short courses of steroids are used in severe or nonresponding cases. Anticoagulants should be avoided. Surgical therapy is unusual but may consist of pericardiocentesis or pericardial window for (1) relief of large effusion causing tamponade symptoms or (2) diagnosis and treatment of purulent pericarditis. Constrictive pericarditis is a rare complication of acute pericarditis, and drainage of asymptomatic effusions does not appear indicated. An exception is tuberculous pericarditis, where early pericardial resection can prevent future problems.

CONSTRICTIVE PERICARDITIS. Constrictive pericarditis represents the development of a thickened fibrotic pericardium that restricts the diastolic filling of the heart. It may arise secondary to an infectious process (particularly tuberculosis), mediastinal irradiation, or following cardiac surgical procedures, although most cases are idiopathic. Patients with this disorder present with fatigue, dyspnea, and physical findings of peripheral edema, ascites, and distended jugular veins. The jugular venous pressure may increase with inspiration (Kussmaul's sign). A chest x-ray may be normal or reveal pericardial calcification (most common with tuberculosis). Echocardiography may reveal wall motion abnormalities, and computed tomography (CT) or magnetic resonance imaging (MRI) may demonstrate pericardial thickening. Differentiating constrictive pericarditis from restrictive cardiomyopathy can be difficult, although features such as (1) loss of respiratory variation in right atrial pressure, (2) presence of pulmonary artery systolic pressure less than 50 mm. Hg and pulmonary capillary wedge pressure less than 18 mm. Hg, or (3) appearance of a right ventricular diastolic "square root sign" are more common in patients with constrictive pericarditis at catheterization. Mild cases may be treated with diuretics or corticosteroids, but more severe cases mandate total pericardiectomy. About 75% of patients with constrictive pericarditis achieve long-term benefit from pericardiectomy, although the operative mortality is 5% to 15%. Surgical results are worse if constriction is secondary to radiation.

PERICARDIAL EFFUSION AND CARDIAC TAMPONADE. Pericardial effusions can result from multiple causes, including neoplastic invasion, chronic infection (including tuberculosis), uremia, trauma, hypothyroidism, radiation, or following cardiac surgery. Slowly developing effusions can reach large sizes without symptoms, but rapid accumulation produces signs of tamponade, including hypotension, muffled heart sounds, and elevated jugular venous pressure (a combination known as *Beck's triad*). Chest x-ray usually reveals an enlarged cardiac silhouette, and echocardiography identifies the effusion and may suggest pending tamponade. The diagnosis can be confirmed by pericardiocentesis, although creation of a subxiphoid pericardial window allows more complete drainage and can provide a pericardial biopsy specimen. When evidence of tamponade is present, urgent decompression is required. Once stable, the underlying cause of the effusion must be identified and treated.

PERICARDIAL NEOPLASMS AND CYSTS. Congenital pericardial cysts or diverticula are rare abnormalities that are usually asymptomatic and require no treatment. Primary pericardial neoplasms are extremely rare. Most malignant neoplasms are mesotheliomas that may encase the heart and cause fatal myocardial restriction. Benign primary tumors include teratoma (the most common), hemangiomas, lipofibromas, lipomas, and fibromas. The pericardium is the site of secondary involvement in up to 10% of patients with malignancies. Almost any tumor can metastasize to the heart, although the most frequent cardiac metastases are from lung cancer, breast cancer, leukemia, and lymphoma. Up to 70% of patients with melanoma may develop cardiac metastases. Treatment may involve drainage of the associated pericardial effusion if symptomatic. Some patients have been managed by intrapericardial instillation of sclerosing agents.

SURGICAL TECHNIQUES. *Pericardiocentesis,* or aspiration of pericardial fluid, is done to establish a diagnosis or relieve symptoms of tamponade. It is done using a fine needle inserted at the xiphoid level or through the left fourth or fifth interspace. The needle can be inserted blindly or with an electrode connected to an ECG to detect contact with the heart. The preferred technique is to perform the procedure under fluoroscopic or ECG guidance to avoid laceration of the heart or coronary arteries. A small drainage catheter may be left in place after the procedure. When open pericardial drainage is required, a formal pericardiotomy with insertion of drainage tubes (either via the subxiphoid or left anterior thoracotomy approach) may be performed. Usually a pericardial biopsy is included. Thoracoscopic approaches and percutaneous balloon pericardiotomy have been described. Resection of a localized portion of pericardium is referred to as a *pericardial window. Pericardiectomy* is performed for constrictive pericarditis (and rarely for chronic effusions). Best exposure is provided by median sternotomy, although left anterior or bilateral thoracotomies can be used. Removal of as much pericardium as possible is advised while avoiding the phrenic nerves. The heart may be densely adherent, and occasionally, cardiopulmonary bypass may be needed to facilitate the operation and control bleeding.

54

THE HEART

I

Cardiopulmonary Resuscitation
Donald D. Glower, M.D.

Modern cardiopulmonary resuscitation (CPR), combining external cardiac massage with mechanical ventilation and electrical defibrillation, originated with the studies of Kouwenhoven, Jude, and Knickerbocker in 1960. Sudden death requiring cardiopulmonary resuscitation most commonly results from ventricular fibrillation due to coronary artery disease; other causes include anoxia, electrolyte abnormalities such as hypokalemia or hyperkalemia, bradycardia, asystole, heart block, ventricular tachycardia, or toxicity of such drugs as digitalis, procainamide, or quinidine.

Cardiac arrest is characterized by cessation of the normal circulation with progressive tissue hypoxia, anaerobic metabolism, acidosis, and ultimately cell death. Permanent neurologic injury typically occurs after more than 5 minutes of cardiac arrest at normal body temperature. Open-chest cardiac massage has been the most effective means of cardiopulmonary resuscitation, capable of nearly meeting normal oxygen requirements for the body. Closed-chest massage generally provides 5% to 15% of normal coronary and cerebral blood flow. Closed-chest compression restores the circulation by the mechanisms of direct cardiac compression and by the thoracic pump mechanism.

Cardiopulmonary resuscitation is divided into two phases: basic life support that may be conducted by nonmedical personnel and advanced cardiac life support generally requiring trained medical personnel. A 15-second period of observation is recommended to document the absence of consciousness, spontaneous breathing, and central arterial pulse. Once the diagnosis of cardiac arrest is established, the airway should be freed of obstructing foreign material and ventilation begun either using a valved mask system, mouth-to-mouth resuscitation, or endotracheal intubation with a ventilatory rate of 12 to 15 beats per minute with the nostrils occluded if the trachea is not intubated. If circulation is not present, manual compressions over the lower sternum are begun at a rate of 80 to 100 beats per minute.

In the hospital setting with advanced cardiac life support, the electrocardiograph is used to document cardiac rhythm. Ventricular fibrillation or tachycardia should be treated by electrocardioversion with 200 to 360 J with up to three shocks

See the corresponding chapter or part in the *Textbook of Surgery,* 15th edition, pp. 1952–1956, for a more detailed discussion of this topic, including a comprehensive list of references.

in rapid succession. Venous access is achieved, and epinephrine 1 mg. is given if initial defibrillation is unsuccessful.
Acidosis may be treated with intravenous sodium bicarbonate
1 mEq. per kg., and recurrent ventricular fibrillation is treated
with intravenous lidocaine 75 to 100 mg. with the possible
addition of bretylium 5 to 30 mg. per kg. Asystole or bradycardia should be treated with intravenous atropine 0.5 mg. repeated in 5 minutes or with intravenous epinephrine. Temporary pacing for bradycardia, asystole, or heart block may
be necessary. Hyperkalemia should be treated with calcium
gluconate, glucose, and insulin; correction of acidosis; and
potassium-binding resin. Treatable causes of electromechani-
cal dissociation, such as cardiac tamponade, hypovolemia,
tension pneumothorax, pulmonary embolism, and metabolic
disturbances, should be considered and corrected. If effective
circulation cannot be restored after 10 to 15 minutes of CPR,
consideration should be given to open-chest cardiac massage.

For both in-hospital and out-hospital cardiac arrests, 30%
to 60% of patients are resuscitated successfully. Recurrent
cardiac arrest occurs in 30% to 40% of survivors, and mean
survival after successful resuscitation is 3 to 6 years. Myocardial ischemia should be sought and treated in survivors, and
Holter monitoring and electrophysiologic stimulation studies
should be performed in patients with sudden death in the
absence of myocardial ischemia.

II

Penetrating Cardiac Injuries
Fred A. Crawford, Jr., M.D.

The incidence of penetrating cardiac injuries has increased
significantly, particularly those due to gunshot wounds. Penetrating cardiac injuries occur most often in the home (70%),
by a known assailant (83%), and are due to domestic or social
disputes (73%). Victims are commonly male (83%). Approximately 60% to 80% of individuals with such injuries die at the
scene or prior to arrival at a trauma facility. Factors influencing mortality include, in order of decreasing significance, (1)
coronary artery injury, (2) multiple-chamber injury or isolated
left atrial or left ventricular injury, (3) comminuted tear of a
single chamber, (4) single right-sided chamber injury, and (5)
tangential injuries that do not penetrate the endocardium.

DIAGNOSIS

Any patient with a penetrating injury to the chest, neck,
upper abdomen, or back should be suspected of having a

See the corresponding chapter or part in the *Textbook of Surgery*, 15th
edition, pp. 1956–1961, for a more detailed discussion of this topic,
including a comprehensive list of references.

cardiac injury. The right ventricle is the most common chamber injured, followed by the left ventricle, right atrium, left atrium, and great vessels. Patients with penetrating cardiac injuries present with either cardiac tamponade or hemorrhagic shock. Stab wounds to the heart may bleed a small amount and seal spontaneously but, if bleeding is significant, may cause cardiac tamponade. A relatively small amount of blood in the pericardium can produce acute cardiac tamponade because of the nondistensibility of the intact pericardium. These patients may present with classic findings of tamponade (hypotension, elevated venous pressure, and decreased heart sounds). If a significant amount of blood has been lost, the neck veins may not be distended, and the findings of tamponade are not so apparent. When hypotension and distended neck veins are present in a cooperative patient with a penetrating chest wound, one must assume some degree of cardiac injury, but the absence of classic findings of tamponade does not allow one to rule out a cardiac injury. Chest x-ray and electrocardiogram (ECG) are rarely useful unless ischemic ECG changes suggest a coronary artery injury. Echocardiography may be helpful, but quality studies may be difficult to obtain under conditions imposed by these patients. Pericardiocentesis is technically difficult, especially in uncooperative patients, and may produce both false-negative and false-positive results. However, the removal of a small amount of blood from the pericardial space in a patient with acute pericardial tamponade can result in significant but transient hemodynamic improvement. A subxyphoid pericardial window provides accurate diagnosis, but the surgeon must be capable of proceeding immediately to a thoracotomy should a cardiac injury exist.

If the cardiac injury is significant, either from a stab wound or more commonly from a gunshot wound, cardiac tamponade is uncommon, and the mode of presentation is most frequently that of hemorrhagic shock. Accordingly, the diagnosis of significant cardiac injury should be suspected in anyone with evidence of penetrating injury to the chest, obvious bleeding, or profound hypotension.

TREATMENT

Patients with penetrating chest trauma should undergo standard initial resuscitative measures, including airway control, insertion of large intravenous lines, and fluid replacement. Once the patient is stable and the diagnosis of cardiac injury is strongly suspected, he or she should be transported promptly to the operating room for thoracotomy and repair of the injury. Emergency room thoracotomy has been advocated for those patients who present *in extremis* or who deteriorate rapidly following arrival in the emergency room. A significant number of these individuals may be salvaged by prompt emergency room thoracotomy, and complications are relatively uncommon.

Penetrating cardiac injuries may be approached through either a left anterior thoracotomy or a median sternotomy incision. The left anterior thoracotomy requires no special equipment and is performed more easily in the emergency room than a sternotomy. On the other hand, most elective operative procedures on the heart utilize a median sternotomy incision, and this is the preferred approach when time permits. Cardiopulmonary bypass is rarely necessary in such patients but should be available. Once the pericardium is opened and blood evacuated, the injury usually can be controlled with digital pressure until the laceration is closed with interrupted sutures. Injuries to the atria or great vessels may be repaired similarly or may be repaired after applying a tangential side-binding clamp. Injuries adjacent to coronary arteries usually can be repaired by placing the sutures such that flow through the arteries is not compromised. Injuries to distal small coronary artery branches are best managed by ligation, but proximal coronary artery injuries should be repaired or the vessel bypassed with a saphenous vein or internal mammary artery.

Penetrating cardiac wounds also may result in injury to valves and in the development of intracardiac or extracardiac shunts. Most commonly the shunt occurs between the left and right ventricles, but it also may occur between the atria or between other great vessels or cardiac chambers. Intracardiac injuries are rarely appreciated on initial evaluation, but when suspected, preoperative or intraoperative echocardiography is useful in making the definitive diagnosis. Careful postoperative follow-up (physical examination and echocardiography) is mandatory to detect any residual defects. Small residual defects or insignificant shunts may be left alone and may close spontaneously, but larger shunts (greater than 1.5:1 left-to-right) may require reoperation to close the shunt. Gunshot wounds to the heart may result in the retention of foreign bodies in the pericardium, the wall of the heart, or a cardiac chamber. Indications for operative removal of such retained fragments include (1) large vessels, (2) symptomatic patients, and (3) intracardiac location, especially the left side. It is clear that not all retained missiles in or around the heart need to be removed.

Although the majority of the patients who sustain penetrating cardiac injuries die at the scene or prior to arrival at a treatment facility, survival can be obtained in some who arrive *in extremis* and without vital signs, and for those in whom vital signs are present on arrival in the emergency room, survival of 60% to 70% can be expected.

III

Patent Ductus Arteriosus, Coarctation of the Aorta, Aortopulmonary Window, and Anomalies of the Aortic Arch

J. William Gaynor, M.D., and David C. Sabiston Jr., M.D.

PATENT DUCTUS ARTERIOSUS (PDA)

The ductus arteriosus is a fetal structure derived from the left sixth aortic arch. The ductus extends from the main or left pulmonary artery to the descending aorta, inserting just distal to the origin of the left subclavian artery. *In utero,* most of the blood ejected by the right ventricle bypasses the high-resistance pulmonary circuit and flows almost exclusively through the ductus to the lower extremities and the placenta. During the transition from the fetal to adult circulation, the lungs expand with the first breath, which decreases the pulmonary vascular resistance, resulting in increased pulmonary blood flow and increasing arterial oxygen concentration. In normal, full-term neonates, functional closure of the ductus occurs in the first 10 to 15 hours of life as rising arterial oxygen tension causes constriction of muscle fibers in the wall. Prolonged patency of the ductus produces a left-to-right shunt with pulmonary congestion and left ventricular volume overload. With a large, nonrestrictive ductus, the level of the pulmonary vascular resistance is important in determining the severity of shunting. Shunting occurs throughout systole and diastole, resulting in diastolic hypotension and possibly impaired systemic perfusion.

PDA is not a benign entity, although prolonged survival has been reported. In the preantibiotic era, 40% of patients with PDA died of bacterial endocarditis, and most of the remainder died of congestive heart failure. Premature infants with PDA often have associated problems of prematurity that are aggravated by the left-to-right shunting and abnormal hemodynamics. In patients surviving to adulthood, severe pulmonary hypertension with reverse shunting through the ductus may develop.

The signs and symptoms of PDA depend on the size of the ductus, the pulmonary vascular resistance, the age at presentation, and associated anomalies. Full-term infants usually do not become symptomatic until the pulmonary vascular resistance decreases at 6 to 8 weeks of life, allowing a significant left-to-right shunt. Because premature infants have less

---

See the corresponding chapter or part in the *Textbook of Surgery,* 15th edition, pp. 1961–1975, for a more detailed discussion of this topic, including a comprehensive list of references.

smooth muscle in the pulmonary arterioles, vascular resistance decreases earlier, and symptoms may develop in the first week of life. A large, hemodynamically significant PDA usually presents in infancy with congestive heart failure. Afflicted infants are irritable, tachycardic, and tachypneic and take feedings poorly. The physical examination reveals evidence of a hyperdynamic circulation with a hyperactive precordium and bounding peripheral pulses. The systolic blood pressure is usually normal, but diastolic hypotension may be present. Auscultation reveals a continuous murmur, termed a *machinery murmur*, which is best heard in the pulmonic area and radiates toward the middle third of the clavicle. Absence of the characteristic murmur does not exclude the presence of a PDA, especially in premature infants. The chest roentgenogram may show cardiomegaly and pulmonary congestion. The diagnosis is best confirmed by echocardiography, and cardiac catheterization is reserved for patients with atypical findings, suspicion of associated anomalies, or pulmonary hypertension.

The presence of a persistent PDA in a child or adult is sufficient indication for surgical closure because of the increased mortality and risk of endocarditis. In symptomatic patients, closure should be performed when diagnosis is made. In asymptomatic children, intervention can be postponed if desired but should be done in the preschool years. If severe pulmonary hypertension has occurred with reversal of the ductal shunting, closure is associated with a higher mortality and may not improve symptoms.

When surgical therapy is indicated, either division or multiple-suture ligation of the ductus via a left anterior or a posterior thoracotomy may be performed. In neonates, single or double ligation of the ductus is usually the procedure of choice. Recently, there has been increasing interest in the nonoperative closure of PDA, and successful transcatheter techniques have been developed. Ligation of a PDA using thoracoscopic technique has been introduced and utilized with increasing frequency. However, these techniques are still investigational, and their role in the management of PDA has not been determined.

Surgical closure of PDA has become a very safe procedure. Operative mortality approaches zero, even in critically ill neonates. In premature infants, hospital mortality and long-term results depend primarily on associated pulmonary disease, coexisting anomalies, and the degree of prematurity. Most patients with PDA become functionally normal and have a normal life expectancy after closure.

COARCTATION OF THE AORTA

Coarctation of the aorta is a narrowing that diminishes the lumen and produces an obstruction to the flow of blood. The lesion may be a localized obstruction or a diffusely narrowed segment, which is termed *tubular hypoplasia*. Coarctation may occur at any site in the aorta, but the most common site is at the insertion of the ligamentum arteriosum. Externally there appears to be an obstructing indentation on the posterior wall of the aorta, whereas internally there is an infolding of the aortic media with a ridge of intimal hyperplasia.

Coarctation of the aorta represents 5% to 10% of congenital heart disease, and the autopsy incidence is 1 per 3000 to 4000 autopsies. With isolated coarctation, males predominate, but there is no sex difference in patients with more complex lesions. Several anomalies occur commonly in patients with coarctation of the aorta: bicuspid aortic valve, ventricular septal defect, PDA, and various mitral valve disorders.

Infants with severe narrowing may appear normal at birth and have palpable femoral pulses if a PDA allows blood flow around the obstructing shelf. Significant aortic obstruction develops as the PDA closes. The infants are irritable, tachypneic, and uninterested in feeding. A systolic murmur may be present over the left precordium and posteriorly between the scapulae. Moderate upper extremity hypertension and an arm-leg pressure gradient are usually present, even in neonates. These findings may be absent in critically ill infants with a low cardiac output. Hypotension, oliguria, and severe metabolic acidosis may be present in severely ill infants.

Older children and adults often present with unexplained headache, epistaxis, visual disturbances, hypertension, and exertional dyspnea. Many cases are discovered during evaluation of hypertension or unexplained murmur heard on routine examination. Findings on physical examination include hypertension, a systolic pressure gradient between the arms and legs, a systolic murmur heard over the left precordium and posteriorly between the scapulae, and diminished or absent femoral pulses. There may be evidence of collateral circulation in older children and adults involving branches of the subclavian arteries that are proximal to the obstruction.

The electrocardiogram in infancy may show right, left, or biventricular hypertrophy. In older children and adults, it may be normal or show evidence of left ventricular hypertrophy. A chest film may reveal rib notching secondary to the enlarged, tortuous intercostal vessels that are part of the collateral circulation. Two-dimensional echocardiography with spectral and color-flow Doppler echocardiography is the most useful method of diagnosis and allows evaluation of associated anomalies.

The natural history of untreated coarctation of the aorta depends on the age at presentation and associated anomalies. Symptomatic infants have a high mortality, depending on the severity of the coarctation and the presence of associated defects. Patients surviving until adulthood have a diminished life expectancy. The most common causes of death in untreated coarctation are spontaneous rupture of the aorta, bacterial endocarditis, cerebral hemorrhage, and congestive heart failure.

The presence of coarctation is generally sufficient indication for surgical correction. The major decisions are the timing and method of repair. Symptomatic infants usually require surgical intervention. A major advance in the treatment of the critically ill neonates with coarctation has been the introduction of prostaglandin E_1 therapy. Infusion of prostaglandin E_1 can reopen and maintain patency of the ductus arteriosus in many neonates and allows perfusion of the lower body with correction of the metabolic acidosis and oliguria. Stabilization of these severely ill infants allows surgical correction to be accomplished under more optimal conditions.

The timing of elective repair of coarctation of the aorta is an important determinant of surgical outcome. Repair in late childhood or adulthood, although providing relief of some symptoms, has an increased incidence of persistent hypertension. The current trend is for elective repair at an early age, and many authors believe that repair should be undertaken at the time of diagnosis in symptomatic and asymptomatic infants to prevent the development of complications.

Three surgical techniques have been developed for repair of coarctation of the aorta. The classic method of repair is resection of the area of obstruction with primary end-to-end anastomosis. Advantages of the classic repair include complete resection of the abnormal tissue, preservation of normal vascular anatomy, and no requirement for prosthetic material.

In the prosthetic patch aortoplasty, the area of constriction is incised, and a prosthetic patch is used to enlarge the lumen. Advantages of this technique include decreased operative time, decreased dissection, maximal augmentation of the area of stenosis, preservation of the collateral vessels, and no need for sacrifice of normal vascular structures. However, the use of prosthetic material may predispose to infection, and there are increasingly frequent reports of the formation of aneurysms and pseudoaneurysms. The subclavian flap aortoplasty is also utilized for repair of coarctation. The subclavian artery is ligated, incised, and turned down as a flap for enlarging the area of constriction. Advantages include avoidance of prosthetic material, decreased dissection, decreased aortic cross-clamp time, and increased anastomotic growth, since there is no circumferential suture line.

Outcome after surgical correction depends on the age at the time of operation, the method of operation chosen, and especially the presence of associated anomalies. The optimal management of associated anomalies remains controversial. PDA is frequently present and should be divided or ligated. Appropriate management of an associated ventricular septal defect is unclear, since there is a high incidence of spontaneous closure. Many infants improve sufficiently after repair of the coarctation to allow elective repair at a later date if the ventricular septal defect fails to close. Other options include pulmonary artery banding or primary repair of the ventricular septal defect at the time of coarctation repair.

Percutaneous transluminal angioplasty has been introduced as an alternative therapy for native and recurrent coarctation. The initial results were encouraging; however, aneurysmal dilatation following balloon angioplasty of native coarctation has been reported. Balloon dilation of recurrent coarctation has been successful, and there have been fewer reports of aneurysm formation. The long-term results of balloon angioplasty of coarctation in terms of restenosis and aneurysm formation are unknown, and the technique must be considered investigational.

Follow-up of surgical patients indicates that they are not rendered entirely normal. There is an increase in premature death rates, which is related to cardiovascular disease. Aortic stenosis or regurgitation secondary to a bicuspid aortic valve may develop and necessitate valve replacement. As has been emphasized, the long-term prognosis of many patients is determined primarily by the presence or absence of associated anomalies.

AORTOPULMONARY WINDOW

Aortopulmonary window is a rare congenital heart defect after abnormal septation of the truncus arteriosus into the aorta and pulmonary artery. Other terms for this anomaly include aortopulmonary fistula, aortic septal defect, aorticopulmonary septal defect, and aortopulmonary fenestration.

An aortopulmonary window is usually a single large defect beginning a few millimeters above the aortic valve on the left lateral wall of the aorta. Multiple defects have been rarely reported. The defect may occasionally be found more distally overlying the origin of the right pulmonary artery; and, rarely, absence of the entire aortopulmonary septum may be encountered. Origin of the right coronary artery and rarely the left from the pulmonary artery may occur and can complicate surgical correction. Associated anomalies include Type A IAA, ventricular septal defect, tetralogy of Fallot, and PDA. An aortopulmonary window allows a large left-to-right shunt, causing pulmonary hypertension and congestive heart failure. Irreversible pulmonary vascular disease may occur at an early age; patients with a large aortopulmonary window usually do not survive infancy. Children or young adults with an aortopulmonary window usually have developed significant pulmonary vascular disease. The clinical course is thought to be similar to that of untreated patients with a large ventricular septal defect.

Infants with aortopulmonary window usually present with congestive heart failure, growth retardation, and recurrent pulmonary infections. Physical examination reveals a systolic murmur and occasionally a continuous murmur suggestive of PDA. Chest film reveals cardiomegaly, with pulmonary vascular engorgement or congestive heart failure. Aortopulmonary window must be differentiated from PDA, persistent truncus arteriosus, ventricular septal defect with aortic regurgitation, and ruptured aneurysm of the sinus of Valsalva.

Cardiac catheterization reveals an oxygen saturation step-up at the level of the pulmonary artery, and the course of the catheter may suggest the diagnosis. Retrograde aortography provides accurate visualization of the defect. It is necessary to document the presence of normal aortic and pulmonic valves to confirm the diagnosis, and the location of coronary ostia must be carefully demonstrated before surgical intervention. Echocardiography may also be used to diagnose aortopulmonary window.

The presence of an aortopulmonary window is sufficient indication for repair unless severe pulmonary vascular disease has occurred. The preferred technique for repair is transaortic closure, either by direct suture or patch closure. Operative mortality is low for repair of isolated aortopulmonary window or aortic origin of a pulmonary artery in infancy. Long-term results are good if there are no associated anomalies. In older infants and children, the results depend on the severity and reversibility of the pulmonary vascular disease.

ANOMALIES OF THE AORTIC ARCH

Vascular rings are developmental anomalies of the aorta and great vessels that encircle and may constrict the esophagus and trachea. The natural history of vascular rings is obscured by the wide spectrum of anomalies and range of symptoms. Vascular rings should be suspected in any infant with stridor, dysphagia, recurrent respiratory tract infections, difficulty in feeding, or failure to thrive. Vascular rings are not necessarily inconsistent with prolonged survival. Infants with symptomatic rings most commonly present with respiratory difficulties, tachypnea, stridor exacerbated by feeding, and recurrent respiratory infection. The physical examination is usually nondiagnostic. The chest roentgenogram may be normal or show pneumonia or, occasionally, compression of the air-filled trachea. The barium esophagogram is the most valuable study for evaluation of patients with a suspected vascular ring. The combination of posterior compression of the esophagus with anterior tracheal compression is diagnostic of a vascular ring.

Although a few patients with symptomatic constricting vascular rings improve as they grow, the long-term prognosis of the medical therapy is poor. Despite the wide spectrum of anomalies, the principles of surgical therapy are simple. Surgical intervention should be undertaken at the time of diagnosis and is designed to divide the vascular ring, relieve the constriction, and preserve circulation to the aortic branches.

The most common anomaly producing a true vascular ring is persistence of the right and left fourth aortic arches with formation of a *double aortic arch*. The right or posterior arch is usually larger, and there is usually a left descending aorta and a left ductus arteriosus. The right carotid and subclavian arteries arise from the right arch, and the left carotid and subclavian arteries arise from the left arch. The diagnosis of double aortic arch can be made easily from the barium esophagogram. Surgical intervention is indicated at the time of diagnosis. The smaller anterior arch is divided at its junction with the descending aorta so that the left carotid and subclavian arteries arise from the ascending aorta.

Aberrant origin of the right subclavian artery is a very common anomaly but rarely causes symptoms. Anomalous origin of the right subclavian artery is not a true vascular ring. However, the aberrant artery may compress the esophagus, causing dysphagia. The diagnosis of aberrant origin of the right subclavian artery can be made by a barium esophagogram. In children, the artery simply may be ligated and divided without sequelae. In adults, division with anastomosis to the ascending aorta is usually necessary.

Pulmonary artery sling is a rare cardiac anomaly occurring when the left pulmonary artery arises from the right pulmonary artery and courses between the trachea and esophagus, but it is not a true vascular ring. Compression of the distal trachea and mainstem bronchi may occur. A barium esophagogram may show anterior pulsatile compression of the esophagus. Bronchoscopy is particularly useful in these patients for evaluation of associated tracheobronchial anomalies. Division of the anomalous artery with anastomosis to the main pulmonary artery anterior to the trachea may be performed. If tracheal stenosis is present, a tracheal resection may be required. Mortality is usually related to the severity of the tracheobronchial stenosis and associated defects. Survivors generally have a benign course, although occlusion of the left pulmonary artery may occur.

The results of surgical therapy in infants with vascular rings are good in terms of both survival and relief of symptoms. Operative mortality is low but not zero. Postoperative morbidity is often related to tracheomalacia secondary to vascular compression and to associated anomalies.

IV

Atrial Septal Defects, Ostium Primum Defects, and Atrioventricular Canals

Ross M. Ungerleider, M.D.

An atrial septal defect (ASD) is a hole in the atrial septum that enables mixing of blood from the systemic and pulmonary venous circulations. These holes may develop in a variety of locations that relate to the formation of the intra-atrial septation, and the embryology of this region should be reviewed carefully by the student. The most common atrial septal defects are (1) *secundum,* (2) *sinus venosus,* and (3) *ostium primum.* Atrial septal defects can occur in other locations, such as around the coronary sinus, but these are quite unusual and are not discussed in this chapter.

Secundum atrial septal defects occur in the fossa ovalis and relate to a deficiency of septum primum tissue or to lack of fusion between the septum primum and the limbus of the septum secundum. These defects are clearly in the wall between the two atria and can range in size from a small patent

---

See the corresponding chapter or part in the *Textbook of Surgery,* 15th edition, pp. 1975–1996, for a more detailed discussion of this topic, including a comprehensive list of references.

foramen to a large defect that gives the appearance of a common atrium. The lower boundary can extend inferiorly toward the eustachian valve of the inferior vena cava and superiorly to the superior limbus of the septum secundum. These are the most common atrial septal defects and can be seen in association with almost any other type of cardiac anomaly. Approximately 30% of secundum ASDs occur with other cardiac defects. Furthermore, intra-atrial communication at the level of the foramen ovale is essential for survival in certain forms of congenital heart disease, such as tricuspid atresia or total anomalous pulmonary venous return. In addition, enlargement of a defect at this location is a common palliative maneuver for patients with transposition of the great arteries (Rashkind balloon septostomy) to allow mixing of blood at the atrial level. Secundum atrial septal defects occur more frequently in females than in males with a ratio of 3:1. Familial inheritance on the basis of a dominant autosomal gene with incomplete penetrance has been reported and may help to explain the appearance of ASDs of the secundum variety within a family lineage. Nevertheless, most secundum ASDs are caused by unknown and random disturbances in development.

Sinus venosus defects are less common than secundum ASDs and account for about 10% of atrial septal defects. Sinus venosus ASDs are commonly associated with partial anomalous pulmonary venous return, especially of the right superior pulmonary veins draining into the lateral aspect of the superior vena cava. These defects occur high in the atrial septum and actually represent a deficiency between the "shared" posterior wall of the superior vena cava and the anterior wall of the left atrium. In part due to the commonly associated anomalous pulmonary venous return, the left-to-right shunt across these defects can be quite large.

Ostium primum atrial septal defects are located at the annulus of the tricuspid and mitral valves and represent a defect in endocardial cushion formation. This region of the atrium, referred to as the *triangle of Koch,* marks the location of the AV node and corresponds to the septation between the left ventricle and the right atrium. In this respect, this small region is referred to as the *atrioventricular septum,* and defects in this location are referred to as *atrioventricular septal defects.* An ostium primum ASD is a defect of the atrioventricular septum of the *partial* variety, since an intracardiac communication exists only at the atrial level. Because the endocardial cushions are involved in the formation of the mitral and tricuspid valves, these defects are often associated with a cleft in these valves, especially of the anterior leaflet of the mitral valve. When deficiency also occurs in the ventricular septum, the resulting defect is a *complete* atrioventricular septal defect or complete AV canal, which produces both an intra-atrial and intraventricular communication with a common AV valve that bridges the defect. Both partial and complete AV canal defects are sometimes seen in association with more complex and severe forms of congenital heart disease. It is not uncommon for these patients to also have a small secundum-type ASD as well as a patent ductus arteriosus. Some form of this defect may be present in as many as 30% of children with Down syndrome.

NATURAL HISTORY

The natural history of an atrial septal defect is related to the type of defect and any other associated anomalies. Most secundum atrial septal defects can exist for years without recognition, and they constitute one of the more common congenital heart defects that can have their initial presentation in adulthood. Likewise, sinus venosus defects with partial anomalous pulmonary venous return (PAPVR) are also frequently first recognized in late childhood or early adulthood. AV canal defects, because of the degree of physiologic shunting involved, are more commonly detected at an earlier age. Despite the relatively benign nature of most of these defects, long-term survival with an atrial septal defect is diminished compared with age-matched controls and becomes significant by the time these patients reach the third and fourth decades of life. Long-term complications attributable to atrial septal defects include the development of progressive congestive heart failure and atrial arrhythmias. Furthermore, the potential for paradoxical embolization is present at any time in patients with these defects. Pulmonary hypertension is reported but unusual as a late development in these patients. The functional status of patients with atrial septal defects deteriorates with age so that concomitant with the decline of life expectancy patients begin having increasing symptoms of easy fatigability, exercise intolerance, and palpitations. Patients with complete AV canal defects have a much more malignant natural history, with 80% of unoperated patients dying by 2 years of age. Those patients who survive often do so because of the development of pulmonary hypertension, which leads to inoperability at an early age.

PHYSIOLOGY

The direction of an intracardiac shunt is toward the most compliant downstream chamber. When the defect occurs at the level of the atrial septum, the compliance of the right and left ventricles dictates the amount and direction of shunt flow. The size of the atrial septal defect itself is not a factor as long as the defect is large enough to be unrestrictive to flow. Most atrial level shunts are in the left-to-right direction, since the right ventricle is more compliant (distensible) and offers less resistance to being filled with increasing volume during diastole. Shunt flow across an atrial septal defect can be in a right-to-left direction, especially as right ventricular compliance diminishes, such as is common if the ventricle hypertrophies in response to pulmonary stenosis. The impact of left-to-right shunting is increased flow through the lungs and a tendency for these patients to have frequent pulmonary infections. Patients who have right-to-left shunting present with cyanosis. If the cyanosis is a reflection of right-to-left shunting due to pulmonary hypertension, then it may be a sign that the patient's defect is no longer surgically correctable. Patients with partial (ostium primum) and complete AV canal defects also may have mitral regurgitation, which impacts on the physiology of their lesion.

PHYSICAL FINDINGS AND DIAGNOSIS

Patients with atrial septal defects may have very little in the way of physical findings. If the left-to-right shunt is greater than 1.8:1, there may be a visible left parasternal heave with a palpable right ventricular lift. Auscultation reveals prominence of the first heart sound, with fixed splitting of the second heart sound. A soft systolic ejection murmur will be present in the second or third left intercostal space, and a mid-diastolic tricuspid flow rumble also may be audible in the fourth or fifth left intercostal space. A chest x-ray shows mild to moderate cardiomegaly and prominence of a pulmonary artery shadow. In addition, there are increased pulmonary vascular markings. Patients with partial and complete AV canal defects may have cardiomegaly of a more pronounced degree due to the mitral insufficiency. An electrocardiogram (ECG) commonly shows an incomplete right bundle branch block in lead V_1 for patients with secundum level defects, whereas patients with ostium primum defects will show left-axis deviation. Diagnosis is usually confirmed by two-dimensional echocardiography with color-flow mapping. This technology also can provide excellent information about the atrioventricular valves. Cardiac catheterization is rarely necessary for patients with secundum or sinus venosus defects and is usually necessary in complete AV canal defects only when there is a concern about pulmonary artery hypertension. Patients with pulmonary vascular resistance greater than 12 units per sq. m. are considered to be inoperable. If the pulmonary vascular resistance is less than 6 units, the defect usually can be corrected safely.

TREATMENT

Spontaneous closure of atrial septal defects may occur early in life but is uncommon after the first year of life. It is also unlikely to occur in patients with hemodynamically significant shunts that produce right ventricular enlargement and symptoms. The safety of modern cardiopulmonary bypass techniques has enabled most atrial septal defects to be approached and repaired with a low morbidity and mortality. Secundum defects can be closed primarily or with a patch of pericardium or prosthetic material. More recently, some groups have reported closing secundum ASDs with devices that can be delivered in the cardiac catheterization laboratory from transvenously inserted catheters. Sinus venosus defects are always closed using a patch to redirect the anomalous pulmonary venous return toward the left atrium. Ostium primum defects also require a patch as well as repair of the involved atrioventricular valves. This usually entails repair of a cleft in the mitral valve. Figures depicting these repairs can be found in the textbook, as well as in several atlases. The adequacy of the surgical repair can be evaluated using intraoperative color-flow Doppler. Operative mortality for closure of uncomplicated secundum and sinus venosus atrial septal defects approaches 0% and should be no greater than 1% to 2%, even in older patients. Long-term results are very good, with survival statistics comparing with those of normal age-matched controls, especially if the repair is undertaken prior to 5 years of age. Outcome is less predictable if the repair is delayed past age 60. Repair of AV canal defects carries a somewhat higher risk, but uncomplicated partial AV canal defects should have a mortality risk that also approaches 0%. Mortality for repair of complete AV canal defects is highly inconsistent because of the wide variation and anatomic patterns with this anomaly but should range between 5% and 13%. This risk is influenced by the nature of the common AV valve and the adequacy of the right and left ventricles. The long-term outcome for patients after repair of AV canal defects is also related to the degree and nature of associated defects but in appropriately selected patients can be very good.

V

Disorders of Pulmonary Venous Return

Erle H. Austin III, M.D.

The most common disorder of pulmonary venous return, total anomalous pulmonary venous connection (TAPVC), results when all four pulmonary veins fail to connect directly to the left atrium. In this condition, which represents between 1% and 2% of congenital heart defects, saturated blood returning from the lungs must take a circuitous route to get to the heart. This route is via primordial venous connections that normally disappear during development. TAPVC is classified according to the abnormal connections that persist. In the supracardiac form (Type I, 50%), a common pulmonary vein that receives all four pulmonary veins drains by an anomalous left vertical vein (pre-existing cardinal vein) into the left innominate vein. Less often the common pulmonary vein connects directly into the superior vena cava. In the intracardiac form of TAPVC (Type II, 25%), the common pulmonary vein connects with the coronary sinus or, occasionally, directly into the right atrium. The infracardiac form (Type III, 20%) involves drainage of the common pulmonary vein by a vertical vein (pre-existing umbilicovitelline vein) that passes through

See the corresponding chapter or part in the *Textbook of Surgery*, 15th edition, pp. 1997–2004, for a more detailed discussion of this topic, including a comprehensive list of references.

the diaphragm and connects with the portal vein at the level of the sinus venosus. TAPVC also can occur with mixed independent connections to the systemic venous system or right atrium (Type IV, 5%).

The pathophysiology and natural history of this anomaly are importantly affected by the size of the interatrial communication and any anatomic obstruction to pulmonary venous return. In most patients (75%) a relatively restrictive patent foramen ovale exists. An unrestrictive secundum atrial septal defect is present in the remainder. Pulmonary venous obstruction can occur with all types of TAPVC but occurs uniformly with infracardiac TAPVC, in as many as 50% with supracardiac TAPVC, and in up to 22% with TAPVC to the coronary sinus.

In TAPVC, all the oxygenated pulmonary venous blood mixes with the desaturated systemic venous blood in the right atrium. A portion of this admixture passes into the right ventricle for circulation back to the lungs. The remaining portion crosses the interatrial septum to support the systemic circulation. If significant pulmonary venous obstruction exists, oxygen exchange and pulmonary blood flow are limited, resulting in cyanosis and congestive heart failure. If a patent foramen ovale also restricts flow across the interatrial septum, the circulatory derangement results in severe cyanosis, intractable heart failure, and death within the first hours or days of life. If there is no pulmonary venous obstruction, pulmonary blood flow is increased, and a large volume of oxygenated blood returns to the right atrium. In these patients, cyanosis is usually mild or unnoticed, and if the interatrial communication is large, the clinical effects and natural history are much less severe, resembling that of a significant atrial level left-to-right shunt.

TAPVC should be suspected in any infant with cyanosis and congestive heart failure and usually can be diagnosed definitively with two-dimensional echocardiography. Cardiac catheterization should be avoided if possible to avoid additional stress to critically ill neonates with obstructed pulmonary veins. The presence of TAPVC is an indication for operative repair. Operation should be performed on an emergent basis if pulmonary venous obstruction is significant and metabolic acidosis begins to develop. If there is no pulmonary venous obstruction and the infant is hemodynamically well compensated, the operation can be performed electively, but little is gained by delaying more than 1 or 2 weeks after diagnosis.

Surgical correction of TAPVC requires anastomosis of the common pulmonary venous channel to the left atrium, obliteration of the anomalous venous connection, and closure of the interatrial communication. Deep hypothermia and a short period of circulatory arrest are usually employed to optimize visualization and facilitate accurate performance of a widely patent anastomosis in neonates and small infants. Postoperative management is focused on avoiding episodes of pulmonary hypertension, which can acutely overload the right ventricle and result in sudden decompensation and death. Pulmonary artery pressure is monitored with a pulmonary artery catheter, and the infants are deeply anesthetized with fentanyl and pancuronium for a minimum of 48 hours after surgery.

Currently, operative mortality is less than 1% in patients over 1 year of age and between 5% and 10% in infants younger than 1 year. The most significant postoperative complication is residual or recurrent pulmonary venous obstruction, which has been noted in 5% to 10% of survivors. The long-term follow-up of patients surviving without postoperative pulmonary venous obstruction shows functional Class I status without late morbidity or mortality.

When some but not all the pulmonary veins connect anomalously, partial anomalous pulmonary venous connection (PAPVC) exists. The most common form of PAPVC involves connection of the right upper and middle lobe veins to the superior vena cava and is associated with a sinus venosus atrial septal defect. Surgical repair requires a pericardial patch that baffles the anomalous pulmonary venous return over to the left atrium.

Pulmonary vein stenosis is a rare anomaly characterized by localized narrowing of the pulmonary veins at or near their junctions with the left atrium. Patients with this condition usually present in infancy with unevenly distributed pulmonary venous congestion and failure to thrive. Prognosis is poor with or without surgery.

Cor triatriatum is a rare congenital anomaly in which a diaphragm or membrane within the left atrium obstructs pulmonary venous return. Diagnosis is made with two-dimensional echocardiography, and surgical excision of the membrane restores normal physiology and long-term survival.

VI

Ventricular Septal Defect

Henry L. Walters III, M.D., Albert D. Pacifico, M.D., and James K. Kirklin, M.D.

DEFINITION AND MORPHOLOGY. A ventricular septal defect (VSD) is a hole in the interventricular septum (IVS) and is, in its isolated form, the most commonly recognized congenital heart defect. While VSDs are most commonly single, they also may be multiple. These defects vary widely in size and location and may be associated with a variety of associated minor and major cardiac anomalies, including pa-

---

See the corresponding chapter or part in the *Textbook of Surgery,* 15th edition, pp. 2005–2018, for a more detailed discussion of this topic, including a comprehensive list of references.

tent ductus arteriosus (PDA), aortic insufficiency, pulmonary stenosis, and coarctation of the aorta.

VSDs can be grouped according to the rims (or boundaries) of the defect as well as the region of the morphologic right ventricle into which the defect opens. Variations in the boundaries and locations of VSDs produce three general classes of defects: perimembranous, muscular, and doubly committed/juxta-arterial.

Perimembranous lesions occupy the area of the membranous portion of the interventricular septum adjacent to the antero-septal commissure of the tricuspid valve. They can extend from the perimembranous region into the inlet portion of the right ventricle (also widely known as *atrioventricular canal defect*), into the outlet portion, or into both regions. These defects are accurately described as being perimembranous with inlet, outlet, or inlet plus outlet extension, respectively. The conduction tissue in all these perimembranous lesions runs along the posteroinferior rim of the defect.

Lesions with an exclusively muscular rim are called *muscular defects.* When considering a muscular defect that does not extend into the perimembranous region of the interventricular septum, the course of the conduction tissue remains as it is in the normal heart. When the muscular defect opens into the right ventricle directly below the septal leaflet of the tricuspid valve *(inlet muscular defect),* the conduction tissue runs along its anterosuperior margin. When a purely muscular defect opens into the right ventricular outlet *(outlet muscular defect),* the conduction tissue runs posteroinferiorly to the VSD but is protected by the muscular rim that forms the posterior edge of the defect. Muscular defects that open into the apical-trabecular region of the right ventricle *(apical-trabecular muscular defects)* can be either single or multiple and are usually far removed from the main axis of the conduction tissue. A multitude of these apical-trabecular muscular defects produces what is called a *Swiss cheese septum.*

Doubly committed/juxta-arterial defects are described as being doubly committed because they open beneath both the aortic and pulmonary valves. They are juxta-arterial because their superior border is formed by fibrous tissue between the leaflets of the aortic and pulmonary valves (and *not* by muscle). In most of these defects there is a muscular posteroinferior rim that protects the conduction tissue. These defects can be associated with prolapse of the leaflets of the aortic valve, causing progressive aortic insufficiency, although this also can occur with perimembranous defects.

PATHOPHYSIOLOGY. The size of VSDs can vary considerably. A large VSD is approximately the size of the aortic valve orifice or larger and causes systemic right ventricular systolic pressure. Small VSDs have insufficient size to raise right ventricular systolic pressure, and the ratio of pulmonary to systemic flow ($Q_p:Q_s$) does not increase above 1.75. Moderate-sized VSDs are *restrictive* but have sufficient size to raise the right ventricular systolic pressure to approximately half the left ventricular systolic pressure and may cause a $Q_p:Q_s$ of 2 to 3.5. The direction and size of the shunt in patients with VSDs depend on the size of the defect, the differences in pressure between the ventricles during systole and diastole, and the differences in compliance between the two ventricles.

NATURAL HISTORY. Many patients with VSDs have small defects and few or no symptoms, since the left-to-right shunt is small. Pulmonary hypertension with pulmonary vascular disease does not tend to develop in this group of patients. Infants born with large VSDs have moderate elevation of pulmonary vascular resistance owing to persistence of the medial thickening of the small pulmonary arteries present in the normal fetus. As the pulmonary vessels mature in the first few weeks of life, pulmonary resistance declines. The magnitude of the left-to-right shunt across the defect increases, and symptoms develop. Such infants may die of severe congestive heart failure during this period. If they survive and the hemodynamic state stabilizes, low cardiac output and breathlessness can cause severe failure to thrive. If surgical repair is not undertaken, death may occur from the sequelae of congestive heart failure, usually within the first year of life. In a small number of infants with large VSDs who survive the neonatal period, severe pulmonary vascular disease and a significant increase in pulmonary vascular resistance begin to develop by the age of 6 to 12 months. When, as a result of the hypertensive pulmonary vascular disease, the shunting becomes dominantly right to left across the defect, the patients become cyanotic and can be considered to have Eisenmenger's complex. Operation is then contraindicated. Spontaneous closure or narrowing of VSDs, even large ones, has been estimated to occur in more than 80% of infants. The probability of eventual spontaneous closure is inversely related to the age at which the patient is observed.

CLINICAL PRESENTATION. Infants with large VSDs usually do not have symptoms until they reach the age of 6 weeks to 3 months. Tachypnea, poor feeding, growth failure, recurrent respiratory infections, exercise intolerance, and severe cardiac failure may then develop. On palpation, a thrill is present in the third to fifth left intercostal spaces as well as a loud systolic murmur. The second heart sound at the base is usually loud and may be split. A mid-diastolic murmur may be heard at the apex, indicating a large flow across the mitral valve.

DIAGNOSIS. The chest roentgenogram of patients with large VSDs, mild elevation of pulmonary vascular resistance, and large left-to-right shunts demonstrates large pulmonary arteries, both centrally and peripherally. The right and left ventricles are enlarged, as is the left atrium. The diagnosis is usually established by two-dimensional echocardiography. Cardiac catheterization confirms the diagnosis and detects secondary or multiple defects. In addition, the pulmonary and systemic arterial pressures and flows are measured, and the pulmonary vascular resistance is calculated.

INDICATIONS FOR OPERATION. At any age, the presence of pulmonary vascular disease so severe that the pulmonary vascular resistance is greater than 10 to 12 units per sq. m. is considered a contraindication to operation. If the pulmonary vascular resistance is 8 to 10 units per sq. m., operation is generally advised, realizing that an unsatisfactory long-term result due to progressive pulmonary vascular disease may occur. The presence of severe pulmonary hypertension is not a contraindication to operation if the resistance is less than 10 units per sq. m.

Prompt intracardiac repair is indicated in infants with large defects, large shunts, and pulmonary hypertension who present with severe and intractable left ventricular failure, recurrent pulmonary infections, severe growth failure, or evidence of rapidly increasing pulmonary vascular resistance. An inverse relationship exists between the probability of eventual spontaneous closure of a VSD and the age at which the patient is observed. This is highly relevant to clinical decisions concerning individual patients. For example, a significant number of patients have moderate-sized VSDs associated only with modest elevations of pulmonary artery pressure, moderate cardiomegaly and pulmonary plethora, a $Q_p:Q_s$ up to 3, and few, if any, symptoms. These patients can be observed to approximately 4 years of age, expecting spontaneous reduction in size or actual closure of the defect. If the defect is closing gradually during this interval, operation can be deferred. If there is no change in the defect, operation is advised before the patient reaches school age. Small VSDs not associated with symptoms, cardiomegaly, pulmonary plethora, elevated pulmonary artery pressure, or a $Q_p:Q_s$ greater than 1.5 to 1.8 can be observed safely. When the patient reaches 10 to 12 years of age, the likelihood of spontaneous closure is remote, and the choice of surgical intervention versus observation is controversial. When aortic valvular incompetence develops in a child with a VSD, prompt closure of the defect should be undertaken to prevent further prolapse of the aortic cusps and to prevent progression of this aortic valve pathology.

SURGICAL TREATMENT. The right atrial approach is preferred for most perimembranous, inlet muscular, and some apical-trabecular muscular, outlet muscular, and doubly committed/juxta-arterial defects. The right ventricular approach provides consistently good exposure for outlet muscular and doubly committed/juxta-arterial defects. A longitudinal anterior right ventriculotomy with or without extension around the apex is useful for many apical-trabecular muscular defects that may not be well exposed through the right atrium. In general, the right atrial approach is preferred because it avoids an incision in the right ventricle. After exposure of the VSD, the lesion is always repaired with a patch. The location of the specialized conduction tissue and its positional relationship to the VSD must be understood clearly in order to avoid creating atrioventricular dissociation by inappropriate placement of the sutures. The rare Swiss cheese septum may require a left ventricular approach and may require placement of a patch over the majority of the interventricular septum.

When aortic valve incompetence coexists with a VSD, the severity of the incompetence should be assessed fully preoperatively. If the incompetence is mild, only closure of the VSD is indicated. If the aortic incompetence is moderate or severe, plication of the aortic leaflets should be performed through an aortotomy before closure of the VSD.

Neonates with a large VSD and coexisting severe coarctation of the aorta initially are stabilized with an infusion of PGE_1 to maintain ductal patency and peripheral perfusion. The authors prefer to initially repair the coarctation through a left thoracotomy. The use of concomitant pulmonary artery banding is controversial. Some employ it selectively when the defect is large or when multiple VSDs are present. Others prefer to observe the patient after isolated coarctation repair. Repair of the VSD is then performed during the same hospitalization if the patient develops intractable congestive heart failure; otherwise, the patient is followed conservatively. If the VSD fails to close over time, the usual indications for VSD repair, as discussed previously, apply. Pulmonary artery banding is used infrequently but continues to have a place in the management of some infants with multiple cardiac anomalies and in some infants with severe heart failure from multiple (Swiss cheese type) VSDs.

RESULTS OF SURGICAL REPAIR. Closure of VSDs can be accomplished safely in most centers properly prepared for this type of procedure. Hospital mortality and complications are directly related to the preoperative condition of the patient and to the conduct of the operative procedure. Hospital mortality now approaches 0%. Major associated lesions, particularly when present in symptomatic infants with large VSDs, do have an incremental risk effect on hospital mortality.

Postoperative progression of pulmonary vascular disease is uncommon when the VSD is repaired before the age of 2 years. Nearly all patients with large VSDs and mild elevation of pulmonary vascular resistance have an excellent prognosis. Improved physical development is a prominent feature of the late postoperative course after repair of large VSDs in infants. There is an impressive increase in weight and usually complete relief of symptoms. Premature late death occurs rarely when pulmonary vascular resistance is low preoperatively. These deaths presumably follow arrhythmias, either ventricular fibrillation or the sudden late development of heart block. Severe pulmonary hypertension postoperatively can increase with time and cause premature late death. However, some patients with pulmonary hypertension and elevated pulmonary vascular resistance late postoperatively have neither progression nor regression of their disease.

VII

Tetralogy of Fallot

Ross M. Ungerleider, M.D.

Tetralogy of Fallot (TOF) is one of the most common congenital heart malformations and can be present in 3 to 6 infants per 10,000 births. The anomaly was described originally by Fallot in 1888 and was felt to consist of (1) pulmonary stenosis, (2) an intraventricular communication (VSD), (3) dextroposition of the aorta, and (4) hypertrophy of the right ventricle. In 1944, Alfred Blalock performed a subclavian artery–to–pulmonary artery anastomosis, and the creation of this "shunt," which provided increased pulmonary blood flow for a severely cyanotic 4.5-kg. child, has been considered by many to be the beginning of modern congenital heart surgery. For many years surgical treatment of tetralogy of Fallot consisted of two stages, with aortopulmonary shunts being placed for symptomatic infants followed by complete repair using cardiopulmonary bypass at a later age. Now, in 1996, most pediatric heart surgeons offer elective complete one-stage repair for infants with tetralogy of Fallot within the first year of life.

ANATOMY

As is true for most congenital heart lesions, there is wide variability in the anatomic spectrum of TOF. This can encompass the size of the right ventricle, the size and distribution of the pulmonary arteries, the location of the pulmonary stenosis, as well as additional sources of pulmonary blood flow. The most common variability involves the degree of pulmonary stenosis and the size of the pulmonary arteries. Patients with high-grade obstruction of the right ventricular infundibulum or pulmonary valve present with cyanosis immediately after birth as the ductus arteriosus begins to close. Patients with less severe pulmonary outflow obstruction may receive enough antegrade pulmonary flow from the right ventricle to appear only mildly cyanotic in infancy. Likewise, patients with hypoplastic pulmonary arteries present with more obstruction to pulmonary blood flow and increased cyanosis at an earlier age. Occasionally, one of the pulmonary arteries may be absent. TOF also encompasses the spectrum of defects with atresia of the main pulmonary artery, and in these patients there is complete obstruction between the right ventricle and pulmonary arteries such that all right ventricular blood flow exits the heart through the aorta by way of the VSD.

See the corresponding chapter or part in the *Textbook of Surgery*, 15th edition, pp. 2018–2033, for a more detailed discussion of this topic, including a comprehensive list of references.

Some patients with TOF (5%) also may have abnormalities to the coronary arteries, with the most frequent anomaly being origin of the left anterior descending coronary artery from the right coronary artery such that it crosses the right ventricular outflow tract just below the pulmonary valve annulus. A right aortic arch (25% of patients) or a retroesophageal subclavian artery (5% to 10%) also may be found. The degree of the pulmonary blood flow depends on the size of the pulmonary arteries and the degree of right ventricular outflow tract obstruction. Furthermore, additional sources of pulmonary blood flow (a ductus arteriosus or bronchial collaterals) also can influence the amount of pulmonary blood flow present in each individual patient. The predominant physiology is right-to-left shunting across the ventricular septal defect. This shunt flow is increased by a fall in systemic vascular resistance, causing further diminishment of pulmonary blood flow and increased cyanosis ("tet spell"). Pulmonary blood flow in these patients can be enhanced by increasing systemic vascular resistance (either by the patient, if they are old enough, by squatting or by the physician by giving pharmacologic agents such as ephedrine).

NATURAL HISTORY AND DIAGNOSIS

Natural history studies demonstrate a 30% mortality by age 6 months that increases to 50% by 2 years. Only 20% of patients can be expected to reach 10 years of age, and not more than 5% to 10% live to reach 21. The greatest risk that these patients face is of paradoxical emboli, cerebral or pulmonary thrombosis, or subacute bacterial endocarditis. Older patients may appear smaller than expected for age and usually have cyanosis to some degree. Almost all patients present with a systolic ejection murmur, and the second heart sound is usually single and rarely increased in intensity. Pulmonary hypertension is distinctly unusual in this patient population. In early infancy, the chest film may appear normal. The pulmonary vascular markings may be somewhat decreased depending on the amount of pulmonary blood flow across the patent ductus arteriosus as well as the natural right ventricular outflow tract. With time, a classic boot-shaped heart (*coeur en sabot*) may develop and is the recognized hallmark of tetralogy of Fallot. The chest x-ray also may show evidence of a right aortic arch, and this finding in the presence of cyanosis is very suggestive of TOF.

Recent advances in two-dimensional echocardiography and color-flow Doppler have elevated the diagnostic capabilities of this technology, and almost all babies with tetralogy of Fallot can be diagnosed with this procedure. Classically, these images will demonstrate a large perimembranous ventricular septal defect with an overriding aorta and bidirectional shunting across the VSD. The pulmonary outflow tract will appear narrowed or even atretic. Angiography with cardiac catheterization is usually not necessary for diagnosis but is helpful to demonstrate the pulmonary artery anatomy and any additional sources of pulmonary blood flow in selected patients. Typical findings at catheterization include equal RV and LV pressures (due to the unrestrictive VSD) and mild to moderate systemic arterial desaturation from right to left shunting.

SURGICAL CORRECTION

As suggested by the natural history of this lesion, most patients will require surgical intervention. Current trends are to provide surgical correction as soon as possible (usually electively within the first year of life) and generally by the time the patient has reached the age of 2 years. The urgency with which surgery is performed is affected by numerous variables, which include the symptoms at presentation, age at presentation, and associated lesions. The use of prostaglandins (PGE_1) to stabilize patients with diminished pulmonary blood flow has greatly influenced the emergent care of these patients. Prostaglandins reopen the ductus arteriosus and help to maintain its patency, thus providing pulmonary blood flow to these critically ill infants. This enables transport of these infants to institutions with tertiary facilities so that appropriate action can be taken. Prior to the recognition of the value of prostaglandins in these patients, infants were transported with critical cyanosis and marginal pulmonary blood flow and often reached the referral institution in a condition that placed them far beyond salvage.

Surgical management for these patients can be varied and ranges from total correction of the entire defect in early infancy to palliation in infancy followed by total correction at a later time. Total operative correction during infancy is preferred in most instances and is accomplished with the utilization of cardiopulmonary bypass. It includes patch closure of the ventricular septal defect and enlargement of the right ventricular outflow tract to provide unobstructed flow into the pulmonary bed. This occasionally requires placement of a patch from the right ventricle across the pulmonary valve annulus extending out the main pulmonary artery to the bifurcation of the right and left branches. Some surgeons prefer placement of a shunt as an initial procedure for patients with TOF, since this often can be done without the use of cardiopulmonary bypass and in their experience enables staged correction at a later date with results similar to early total correction. The only problem with this strategy is that the mortality that occurs with palliation or with waiting for corrective surgery, along with the distortion of anatomy created by palliation, may actually cause morbidity and mortality that is significantly higher than that achieved by groups who attain appropriate results with early complete repair. Surgeons who favor shunts choose between the Blalock-Taussig shunt (subclavian artery to pulmonary artery), the modified Blalock-Taussig shunt (a prosthetic tube—usually Gore-Tex—placed between the subclavian artery and pulmonary artery), and a central shunt (a prosthetic tube placed between the aorta and the pulmonary artery). Each of these shunts provides for an increase in pulmonary blood flow and alleviates the cyanosis while enabling deferment of total surgical correction until a later date. Tetralogy of Fallot is now being corrected with an ever-diminishing mortality. Overall, survival with operative repair should be greater than 95% when the repair is done primarily or after a single systemic-to-pulmonary artery shunt. Improved techniques of myocardial protection with hypothermia, cold cardioplegia, or even total circulatory arrest are enabling more precise anatomic repairs in younger infants with excellent results. Early postoperative risks include the creation of heart block, which should occur in less than 1% of patients of all ages, and residual ventricular septal defects, which should occur in less than 4% of patients.

PULMONARY STENOSIS WITH INTACT VENTRICULAR SEPTUM

Stenosis of a pulmonary valve with an intact ventricular septum can range from a highly favorable to a highly lethal lesion. The most important prognostic factor is the size of the right ventricular chamber and tricuspid valve leading into it. Patients who present at an older age often are in a more favorable category with respect to long-term outcome. This is not necessarily true if a patient with a hypoplastic right ventricle presents at a later age because pulmonary blood flow has been adequately maintained through a patent ductus arteriosus during the interim period. Patients with severe hypoplasia of the right ventricle may never be candidates for a biventricular repair and may instead need to be staged toward a Fontan-type operation. In a Fontan operation, the systemic venous return is diverted directly into the pulmonary bed. This utilizes the single adequate ventricle as the systemic pumping chamber.

These patients are usually managed with the placement of a systemic-to-pulmonary artery shunt at the time of initial presentation in infancy. This enables the pulmonary artery to grow so that conversion to Fontan physiology can be accomplished by the time the patient reaches the age of 5 years old. Twenty per cent of these patients also may have severe coronary artery anomalies resulting in coronary ischemia with myocardial infarction. These patients, especially if they need to be staged toward a Fontan operation, may be more suitable candidates for cardiac transplantation. Those patients with right ventricles that approach a more normal size may be treated adequately with enlargement of the pulmonary outflow tract alone, and the long-term outcome in this group can be quite satisfying.

VIII

Double Outlet Right Ventricle
Albert D. Pacifico, M.D., and Henry L. Walters III, M.D.

DEFINITION AND MORPHOLOGY. Double outlet right ventricle (DORV) is a congenital cardiac anomaly in which both the aorta and the pulmonary arteries arise wholly or in large part from the right ventricle. A ventricular septal defect (VSD) represents the only outlet from the morphologic left ventricle. A DORV is present when more than 50% of the aorta and pulmonary artery arise from the morphologic right ventricle. An exception to this rule is found in defects that also have severe obstruction of the right ventricular outflow tract, which are categorized as tetralogy of Fallot until the aorta arises more than 90% from the right ventricular cavity. When more than 90% of the aorta arises from the right ventricular cavity, these lesions are then called DORV with pulmonary stenosis. A VSD is almost uniformly present but may vary in size and in its relationship to the great vessels. The VSD may thus be categorized as subaortic (50%), subpulmonary (Taussig-Bing malformation, 30%), doubly committed (to both great vessels, 10%), or noncommitted (10%). DORV exists with or without valvular and/or subvalvular pulmonary stenosis. The hemodynamics, clinical course, and specific type of operation employed depend on the size of the VSD, its relationship to either great artery, the relationship of the great arteries to each other, the presence or absence of pulmonary stenosis, and the presence or absence of major associated anomalies.

PATHOPHYSIOLOGY AND CLINICAL COURSE. Patients with large subaortic, doubly committed, or noncommitted VSDs without pulmonary stenosis present with congestive heart failure due to excessive pulmonary blood flow. Their presentation is indistinguishable from that of patients with an isolated and large VSD. In contrast, patients with a subpulmonary VSD and no pulmonary stenosis have a course more similar to that of patients with transposition of the great arteries with VSD, with cyanosis being present usually from birth. These patients tend to develop early congestive heart failure or severe pulmonary vascular disease and usually are symptomatic within the first few months of life. Pulmonary stenosis is usually present in hearts with subaortic VSDs and usually absent in those with subpulmonary defects. Patients with pulmonary stenosis exhibit varying degrees of cyanosis due to restricted pulmonary blood flow, and their clinical course often resembles that of patients with tetralogy of Fallot.

DIAGNOSIS. High-quality angiocardiograms, combined

See the corresponding chapter or part in the *Textbook of Surgery,* 15th edition, pp. 2033–2039, for a more detailed discussion of this topic, including a comprehensive list of references.

with two-dimensional echocardiography, provide knowledge of the great artery relationships, size and location of the VSD, functional and anatomic status of each atrioventricular valve, and the presence and severity or absence of pulmonary stenosis.

SURGICAL METHODS, TIMING, AND RESULTS. The goals of corrective surgery are to relieve pulmonary stenosis, to provide separate and unobstructed outflow pathways from each ventricle to the correct great vessel, and to separate the pulmonary and systemic circulation.

The repair for patients with subaortic or doubly committed VSDs without pulmonary stenosis consists of connecting the left ventricle to the aorta with an intracardiac tunnel. As a group these patients tend to develop pulmonary vascular disease within the first few years of life; therefore, these conditions should be repaired by 6 months of age or sooner if poorly controlled heart failure is present. In the current era the risk of death early after repair of these lesions approaches 0%, and the actuarial 15-year survival including hospital death is 96%.

In patients with subaortic or doubly committed VSDs with coexisting pulmonary stenosis, the techniques of repair are similar to those described for repair of TOF, except the VSD is closed with the tunnel technique rather than with a straight patch. If it is thought that a totally intracardiac repair can be performed, primary repair is generally advised in symptomatic patients or at 6 to 12 months of age, whichever comes first. The use of palliative systemic-to-pulmonary artery shunts should be minimized but may be required in patients with severe pulmonary artery hypoplasia or in patients in whom an extracardiac conduit may be required for the repair. The functional status of survivors of repair of DORV with subaortic or doubly committed VSDs and pulmonary stenosis is excellent.

Repair of DORV with subpulmonary VSD (Taussig-Bing malformation) is complex, and many approaches have been proposed. The most attractive surgical option is a totally intraventricular repair described by Kawashima. This procedure can best be accomplished when the great arteries are in a more or less side-by-side relationship, with the aorta to the right of the pulmonary artery. The infundibular septum must first be resected generously to provide an unobstructed pathway from the VSD to the aorta. The VSD, and hence the left ventricle, is then connected directly to the aorta by an intraventricular tunnel that runs posterior to the pulmonary artery. Kawashima's most recent report documents 10 patients in whom there were no early or late deaths, and reoperation was required in only 1 patient for residual pulmonary stenosis. The most common approach to the repair of the Taussig-Bing malformation is the arterial switch procedure combined with tunnel repair of the VSD to the pulmonary artery. In this technique, tunneling of the VSD to the adjacent pulmonary artery creates transposition of the great arteries with an intact interventricular septum. The arterial switch procedure then re-establishes ventriculoarterial concordance. In a recent series, the hospital mortality was 14.3%, and there were no late deaths at the time of follow-up. Patients with the Taussig-Bing malformation in the absence of pulmonary stenosis tend to develop severe congestive heart failure or pulmonary vascular disease early in life. This poor natural history mandates operation within the first 3 months of life.

When pulmonary stenosis is present in patients with the Taussig-Bing malformation, repair is accomplished most commonly by constructing a tunnel that connects the VSD with the origin of the aorta (and includes the origin of the pulmonary artery), closing the pulmonary artery, and using a valved extracardiac conduit to restore continuity between the right ventricle and the pulmonary artery. The *réparation à l'étage ventriculaire* repair (REV) consists of aggressive resection of the infundibular septum, tunneling of the VSD (and hence the left ventricle) to the aorta, and closure of the pulmonary artery orifice. Right ventricular-to-pulmonary artery continuity is established by connecting the main pulmonary artery directly to a vertical incision in the right ventricular outflow tract rather than using an extracardiac conduit. There is no general consensus as to the best timing for surgical repair of patients with the Taussig-Bing malformation and pulmonary stenosis. An initial systemic-to-pulmonary artery shunt may be advisable in symptomatic patients in whom eventual repair will include the placement of an extracardiac conduit. This will allow the placement of an initially larger conduit at 2 to 3 years of age and possibly reduce the future number of obligatory conduit replacements.

Repair of hearts with DORV and noncommitted VSD can be accomplished by constructing an intraventricular tunnel (or Dacron patch partition) connecting the VSD (which usually must be enlarged anterosuperiorly) with the aorta, closing the pulmonary artery, and placing a valved extracardiac conduit from the right ventricle to the pulmonary artery. Alternatively, when appropriate anatomic and hemodynamic criteria exist, repair can be accomplished by a modification of the operation described by Fontan. Repair of this complex malformation generally has been associated with a higher hospital mortality. Patients with DORV and noncommitted VSD without pulmonary stenosis should have pulmonary artery banding in the first 6 months of life to control heart failure and to prevent the development of advanced pulmonary vascular disease. When pulmonary stenosis is present, an initial systemic-to-pulmonary artery shunt is performed to relieve cyanosis in patients less than approximately 2 years of age. Definitive repair in this subset of patients (valved extracardiac conduit or a modification of the Fontan procedure) should be delayed until approximately 2 to 3 years of age.

IX

Tricuspid Atresia
Erle H. Austin III, M.D.

Tricuspid atresia represents 1.4% of congenital heart malformations and is the third most common cyanotic heart defect. It is characterized by an absent connection between the right atrium and the right ventricle, which causes an obligatory right-to-left shunt at the atrial level. Blood achieves access to the lungs through a ventricular septal defect if the great arteries are normally related (Type I, 70%) or directly from the left ventricle if they are transposed (Type II, 30%). Presentation, natural history, and management of patients with tricuspid atresia depend on anatomic and physiologic factors that control pulmonary blood flow. In most cases some degree of pulmonary stenosis (Type IB and IIB) exists, restricting pulmonary blood flow and accentuating the degree of cyanosis. If pulmonary atresia exists (Type IA and IIA), the only flow to the lungs is through a patent ductus arteriosus. Less frequently there is no obstruction to pulmonary blood flow (Type IC and IIC), and pulmonary blood flow may become excessive. The volume overload of the left ventricle in these patients results in significant congestive heart failure. When these patients also have transposition of the great arteries (Type IIC), some obstruction of flow to the systemic circulation (subaortic stenosis, coarctation of the aorta) may coexist, worsening the congestive heart failure and diminishing systemic perfusion. Without surgery, prognosis is best in patients with equal flow to the systemic and pulmonary circulations. Patients with too little pulmonary blood flow die of hypoxia within the first weeks of life, whereas those with too much pulmonary blood flow die of congestive heart failure within the first months of life.

Clinical presentation is consistent with the degree of pulmonary blood flow. Patients with tricuspid atresia and pulmonary atresia or significant pulmonary stenosis demonstrate marked cyanosis, while patients with tricuspid atresia and unobstructed pulmonary blood flow show only mild cyanosis but exhibit symptoms of congestive heart failure. Definitive diagnosis is made with two-dimensional echocardiography.

The goal of initial management is to adjust pulmonary blood flow to provide adequate tissue oxygenation without volume overloading the left ventricle. This approach is designed to best prepare the patient for the performance of a Fontan procedure between 2 and 4 years of age. In newborn infants with severe cyanosis (oxygen saturations less than 70%), pulmonary blood flow is augmented by the perfor-

See the corresponding chapter or part in the *Textbook of Surgery*, 15th edition, pp. 2039–2044, for a more detailed discussion of this topic, including a comprehensive list of references.

mance of a modified Blalock-Taussig shunt, which consists of placing a 4- or 5-mm. polytetrafluoroethylene tube graft from the left subclavian artery to the left pulmonary artery. Infants with congestive heart failure from excessive pulmonary blood flow undergo banding of the main pulmonary artery to diminish flow and prevent the development of irreversible pulmonary vascular disease. Infants presenting after 3 months of age with either too much or too little pulmonary blood flow are well served by anastomosing the divided superior vena cava end to side into the right pulmonary artery and closing the main pulmonary artery and any other major sources of pulmonary blood flow. This bidirectional superior cavopulmonary (Glenn) anastomosis provides satisfactory pulmonary blood flow without volume overloading the left ventricle. Unfortunately, the Glenn anastomosis cannot be performed safely in the neonatal period because of the high pulmonary vascular resistance at that time.

The best long-term treatment for tricuspid atresia is the Fontan procedure, which separates the pulmonary and systemic circulations and directs all the systemic venous return to the lungs. The Fontan operation is best performed between 2 and 4 years of age, when pulmonary vascular resistance is low and myocardial function is still good. Patients must be selected carefully, being certain that pulmonary vascular resistance is less than 4 Woods units and left ventricular enddiastolic pressure is less than 15 mm. Hg. Left ventricular ejection fraction should be at least 30%. Other risk factors, such as mitral valve insufficiency and pulmonary artery distortion, must be considered and corrected at the time of the Fontan procedure or combined with a preliminary bidirectional superior cavopulmonary anastomosis.

The currently favored technique of Fontan correction involves creating a tunnel within the right atrium from the inferior vena cava to the superior vena cava, dividing the superior vena cava, and anastomosing both ends end to side into the right pulmonary artery, thereby producing a total cavopulmonary anastomosis. This technique minimizes energy loss from turbulent flow, decreases the amount of atrial tissue exposed to high atrial pressures, and results in fewer atrial dysrhythmias in the long term.

Operative mortality for the Fontan procedure is now between 5% and 10%. Over 85% of patients are in good to excellent condition after recovering from surgery, but with time this percentage slowly decreases. Actuarial survival indicates a minimal attrition for the first 5 to 10 years, followed by an increasing rate of death from arrhythmias and sudden unexplained mortality. Despite these imperfect results, the Fontan procedure has provided significant improvements in exercise capacity, quality, and quantity of life for many patients born with tricuspid atresia.

X

Hypoplastic Left Heart Syndrome
Erle H. Austin III, M.D.

Hypoplastic left heart syndrome is characterized by an inadequately developed left ventricle and ascending aorta. It includes a spectrum of anomalies, ranging from aortic and mitral atresia with complete absence of the left ventricle to severe aortic stenosis with a left ventricle too small to sustain the systemic circulation. Hypoplastic left heart syndrome is the most common cardiac defect causing death of the newborn infant. It occurs in 0.15 per 1000 live births at a frequency similar to that of transposition of the great arteries and tetralogy of Fallot. Without intervention, this lesion is uniformly fatal, with over 90% of infants dying before 1 month of age.

The absence of a functional left ventricle places the burden of the circulation on the right ventricle, which is required to supply blood to the lungs via the branch pulmonary arteries and to the body via a patent ductus arteriosus. *In utero* this circulation is well tolerated, permitting survival to full term with a normal birth weight in the majority of infants. These children usually appear completely normal at birth, but within 24 to 48 hours of life they become tachypneic and mildly cyanotic. As the ductus arteriosus begins to close, delivery of blood to the systemic and coronary circulations is compromised, and the major portion of the right ventricular output is diverted to the lungs and recirculated back to the overwhelmed single right ventricle. If prostaglandin E_1 is not administered, systemic perfusion worsens, resulting in oliguria, metabolic acidosis, and eventual death.

Newborn infants that present with tachypnea, cyanosis, and marginal peripheral perfusion should be assumed to have hypoplastic left heart syndrome and started on prostaglandin E_1 immediately. Definitive diagnosis can then be made with two-dimensional echocardiography. Cardiac catheterization is usually not required.

In addition to ensuring ductal patency with prostaglandin E_1, initial management is directed at achieving a balanced delivery of blood flow to the systemic and pulmonary circulations. Assuming the ductus arteriosus is patent, distribution of flow is determined by the relative vascular resistances of the two circulations. The normal postnatal decrease in pulmonary vascular resistance causes a natural tendency for pulmonary blood flow to exceed system blood flow. To avoid a further decrease in pulmonary vascular resistance, supplemental oxygen is strictly avoided. Evidence that pulmonary and systemic blood flow are balanced ($Q_p/Q_s \approx 1$) includes a

---

See the corresponding chapter or part in the *Textbook of Surgery*, 15th edition, pp. 2045–2052, for a more detailed discussion of this topic, including a comprehensive list of references.

peripheral oxygen saturation of 75% to 80%, and arterial blood gases demonstrating a P_{O_2} of 40 mm. Hg, a P_{CO_2} of 40 mm. Hg, and a pH of 7.40. Patients presenting with balanced circulations can be treated expectantly. However, those with arterial saturations exceeding 85% and metabolic acidosis from inadequate systemic perfusion often require tracheal intubation, neuromuscular blockade, and mechanical ventilation. In these cases, the P_{CO_2} is adjusted to 40 to 45 mm. Hg by controlling the minute ventilation and adding CO_2 to the inspired gas mixture. Positive end-expiratory pressure (PEEP) also may be applied to selectively increase pulmonary vascular resistance and redirect a greater proportion of the cardiac output toward the systemic circulation.

Once patients are stabilized, further management may include staged surgical reconstruction, cardiac transplantation, or compassionate care (no treatment). The first stage of surgical reconstruction, the Norwood procedure, entails creation of an unobstructed pathway from the right ventricle to the aortic arch, insertion of a small shunt between the systemic arterial and pulmonary arterial circulations, and excision of the interatrial septum to ensure unimpeded pulmonary venous return and adequate mixing in the right atrium. A second stage is performed between 3 and 9 months of age and consists of changing the systemic arterial shunt to a systemic venous shunt by anastomosing the divided superior vena cava end to side into the proximal right pulmonary artery (a bidirectional Glenn shunt). This operation diminishes the volume load on the single right ventricle. Between 18 months and 3 years of age, a fenestrated Fontan procedure is performed. With this procedure, virtually all the systemic venous return is directed to the pulmonary circulation.

Staged reconstruction can be applied to most patients with satisfactory right ventricular function without a prolonged and uncertain wait for definitive treatment. The expense and side effects of immunosuppression are also avoided. On the other hand, operative mortality for this approach has been high. Some early reports have described hospital mortalities exceeding 50% for the first stage. More recent reports, however, indicate that the initial stage can be performed at a risk as low as 15%, with a 5% risk for the other two stages. Long-term outlook for these patients is unknown at this time.

Cardiac transplantation requires stabilization of these ill infants until an appropriate donor is identified. Implantation of the donor heart often requires reconstruction of the aortic arch with a generous portion of the donor's own aorta. Immunosuppression is provided with cyclosporine, azathioprine, and prednisone, with an attempt to wean the patient off steroids within the first posttransplant year. Cardiac transplantation can be performed in these infants with an operative mortality of 10% to 15%. Unfortunately, 25% of patients die before a donor heart becomes available. Short- and intermediate-term survival and functional capacity have been excellent in infants who have survived heart transplantation. However, the long-term outcome for these patients is also unknown.

XI

Truncus Arteriosus
Richard A. Hopkins, M.D., and Robert B. Wallace, M.D.

ANATOMY AND CLASSIFICATION. Truncus arteriosus is a rare congenital cardiac malformation characterized by a single arterial vessel arising from the heart, receiving blood from both ventricles, and supplying blood to the aorta, lungs, and coronary arteries. Truncus arteriosus is due to a lack of partitioning of the embryonic conus during the first few weeks of fetal development and is usually associated with a ventricular septal defect. Collett and Edwards classified truncus arteriosus into four types based on the origin of the pulmonary arteries. In Type I, a single arterial trunk gives rise to the aorta and main pulmonary artery. In Type II, the right and left pulmonary arteries arise immediately adjacent to one another from the dorsal wall of the truncus. In Type III, the right and left pulmonary arteries arise from either side of the truncus. In Type IV, the proximal pulmonary arteries are absent, and pulmonary blood flow is by way of bronchial arteries.

HEMODYNAMICS. All the blood from both the left and the right ventricles is ejected into the truncus arteriosus. As with isolated ventricular septal defect, the pulmonary vascular bed in truncus arteriosus is exposed to high flow at systemic pressure, a condition that, untreated, may produce progressive pulmonary vascular obstructive disease.

PROGNOSIS, SYMPTOMS, AND DIAGNOSIS. Most patients with persistent truncus arteriosus die in early infancy from congestive heart failure. Death for those who survive the first 2 years of life is generally related to pulmonary vascular obstructive disease.

Physical examination usually reveals a systolic thrill and murmur over the left third and fourth intercostal spaces parasternally. When truncal valve incompetence is present, a diastolic murmur follows the second heart sound. Chest roentgenography shows cardiomegaly with biventricular enlargement. The peripheral pulmonary vasculature is increased unless there is advanced pulmonary vasculature obstructive disease. The electrocardiogram is nonspecific.

Heart catheterization and angiocardiographic studies are indicated in all older patients suspected of having truncus arteriosus. Neonates may have anatomy defined adequately by echocardiography alone.

TREATMENT. Definitive treatment for truncus arteriosus is complete repair. Ideally, operation should be performed in the first 3 months of life, preferably in the first 30 days of life. Operation at this age protects against the development of

See the corresponding chapter or part in the *Textbook of Surgery*, 15th edition, pp. 2052–2057, for a more detailed discussion of this topic, including a comprehensive list of references.

pulmonary vascular obstructive disease. Although conduit re-replacement is required when operation is performed in early infancy, it has been shown that this can be accomplished at a low risk.

Complete Surgical Repair. The operation is performed through a median sternotomy with utilization of total cardio-pulmonary bypass and deep hypothermia, either with total circulatory arrest or low flow. Myocardial protection is pro-vided by cold cardioplegic arrest during aortic cross-clamping. The pulmonary arteries usually can be excised from the trun-cus as a single segment. The incision in the right ventricle is made high in the ventricle in the planned direction of the conduit. If truncal regurgitation is severe, valve replacement must be considered. A patch is used to close the ventricular septal defect. An appropriate-sized valved Dacron or homo-graft conduit is cut to proper length and used to establish continuity between the right ventricle and the pulmonary ar-teries.

RESULTS. Recent experiences from institutions in which elective repair in infancy has been performed indicate that this can be accomplished at an acceptable mortality. Ebert reported an 11% hospital mortality in 100 consecutive patients operated on under 6 months of age. Eighty-six patients were alive at 16 months to 8 years postoperatively, and 55 of the survivors required conduit replacement (accomplished with-out mortality). Bove and colleagues have reported neonatal repairs in 11 patients with a 9% mortality. Hanley and the Boston group have reported 100% survival in neonatal truncus repair when there are no concomitant coronary artery anoma-lies, truncal valve regurgitation, or interrupted aortic arch anatomy. Early complete repair with a homograft is currently the procedure of choice.

XII

Transposition of the Great Arteries
Thomas L. Spray, M.D.

Complete transposition of the great arteries is a congenital cardiac defect in which there is anatomic reversal of the rela-tionship with the great arteries: The aorta arises entirely or largely from the right ventricle, and the pulmonary artery arises entirely or largely from the left ventricle (ventriculoar-terial discordant connection). Because the resulting abnormal-

---

See the corresponding chapter or part in the *Textbook of Surgery*, 15th edition, pp. 2057–2070, for a more detailed discussion of this topic, including a comprehensive list of references.

ity is of separate pulmonary and systemic circulations existing in parallel instead of in series, the lesion is incompatible with life without surgical intervention. Transposition is associated with an intact ventricular septum in 50% of patients, a ventricular septal defect in an additional 25%, and a ventricular septal defect and left ventricular outflow obstruction in 25%. Common associated anomalies include coarctation of the aorta and patent ductus arteriosus.

PATHOPHYSIOLOGY

D-Transposition of the great arteries is a relatively common form of congenital heart disease accounting for 9% of infants with congenital heart disease and representing a frequency of 0.206 per 1000 live births. A distinct male predominance is noted. Untreated, 90% of children with D-TGA and an intact septum will die by 1 year of age. Because the pulmonary and systemic circulations exist in parallel instead of in series in D-TGA, mixing of the circulations at the atrial, ventricular, or great vessel level is mandatory for survival.

CLINICAL MANIFESTATIONS

The most common clinical finding in the infant with TGA is cyanosis (arterial Po_2 of 25 to 40 mm. Hg), which varies depending on the degree of mixing or the presence of associated anomalies. Congestive heart failure may be a predominant clinical finding in children with large ventricular septal defect or patent ductus arteriosus. Examination typically reveals an overactive precordium with a soft systolic murmur and a single and loud second heart sound due to the proximity of the aorta to the anterior chest wall. The electrocardiogram may be normal at birth but over time shows signs of increasing right ventricular biventricular hypertrophy. Chest x-ray findings include an egg-shaped cardiac configuration, narrow superior mediastinum, and increased pulmonary markings with cardiomegaly, although the chest x-ray may be normal at birth and show progressive cardiomegaly and pulmonary markings with age.

MANAGEMENT

Echocardiography has now generally supplanted cardiac catheterization in the majority of patients with D-TGA, and catheterization is often indicated only for children who have inadequate shunting and require balloon atrial septostomy or if intra- or extracardiac abnormalities require clarification. Since the majority of coronary arterial variations can be addressed successfully at surgical correction, identification of the origins of the coronary arteries by echocardiography is usually sufficient to permit operation without catheterization. Initiation of prostaglandin E_1 to maintain ductal patency, volume infusion to improve the degree of interatrial shunting, and

Rashkind atrial septostomy may stabilize patients while awaiting operative intervention.

SURGICAL CORRECTION

Satisfactory correction of D-TGA results in rerouting of systemic venous blood to the pulmonary circulation and pulmonary venous blood into the systemic arterial circulation at either the atrial, ventricular, or great arterial level. The earliest repairs of D-TGA involved rerouting the systemic and pulmonary venous returns at the atrial level (Senning and Mustard repairs), resulting in an adequate physiologic repair but not an anatomic repair, since the morphologic right ventricle continues to be the systemic ventricle. Both ventricular (Rastelli) and great artery (arterial switch or Jatene) repairs provide more anatomic corrections, using the morphologic left ventricle as the systemic ventricle.

The Senning and Mustard atrial diversion repairs for D-TGA were associated with excellent results, although late development of atrial arrhythmias and gradual ventricular dysfunction in a small portion of patients has led to abandonment of these techniques in the majority of cardiac centers.

The first successful use of an arterial reconstruction in D-TGA was by Jatene in 1975. The principles of successful anatomic correction involved dividing the aorta and pulmonary artery and excising the origins of the coronary arteries with a button of aortic wall, repositioning the coronary arteries to the posterior great vessel (pulmonary artery) and repositioning the pulmonary bifurcation to the anterior great vessel. The defects in the aorta from which the coronary arteries have been excised are reconstructed with additional tissue, and then the posterior great vessel is anastomosed to the distal aorta.

The arterial switch procedure was utilized initially in infants with ventricular septal defect and TGA who had maintenance of systemic ventricular pressures in the pulmonary ventricle and therefore had an adequately prepared left ventricle for use as a systemic ventricle. Improvement in these operations in infants has permitted the application of the arterial switch routinely in infants with TGA and an intact septum or TGA and ventricular septal defect, and the arterial switch is now the procedure of choice. Successful application of the arterial switch technique to infants with an intact septum results from the fact that elevated pulmonary vascular resistance is present at birth and the left ventricle is therefore at relatively high pressure and able to adequately support the systemic circulation after the operation. In addition, improvements in the techniques of coronary transfer, myocardial protection, and neonatal vessel reconstruction have resulted, with improved survival statistics in the arterial switch procedure that now rival the results with the atrial baffle operations.

Infants with significant left ventricular outflow tract obstruction represent a small proportion of children with D-TGA. Since left ventricular outflow tract obstruction is often dynamic, primary arterial switch may still be performed in many of these infants. When significant fixed obstruction is present in the left ventricular outflow tract, repair is by the Rastelli operation, where pulmonary venous blood is directed by a patch through the VSD across to the anterior aorta and a valved conduit is placed from the right ventricle to the distal pulmonary arteries. By relocating the pulmonary bifurcation anterior to the aorta, it is possible in some cases to avoid the requirement of a valved conduit from the anterior ventricle to the pulmonary artery (the REV procedure of Lecompte).

OPERATIVE RESULTS

The results with the arterial repair for transposition of the great arteries have been excellent, with survival of 93% to 95% of infants undergoing primary repair. Left ventricular size, mass, functional status, and contractility appear to be normal at intermediate-term follow-up, with no evidence of late deterioration. In addition, atrial and ventricular arrhythmias after the arterial switch operation are unusual, with a 96% incidence of sinus rhythm following the procedure. These results have confirmed the superiority of the anatomic arterial switch over atrial repairs.

XIII

Congenital Aortic Stenosis
Erle H. Austin III, M.D.

Congenital aortic stenosis represents 5% to 10% of congenital heart defects. Obstruction to left ventricular outflow occurs most commonly at the level of the valve (70% to 80%) but also may occur above or below it.

In patients with isolated valvular stenosis, the valve leaflets are thickened, with varying degrees of fusion at the commissures. Most commonly the right and left coronary cusps are completely fused, forming a bicuspid valve. The degree of fusion at the remaining two commissures dictates the amount of obstruction. In patients presenting as neonates, the valvular deformity may be such that only one commissure is identifiable. The next most common form of congenital aortic stenosis occurs below the valve (10% to 20%). Fixed subaortic stenosis occurs most often as a fibrous membrane that encircles the outflow tract several millimeters below the aortic valve. In severe cases, the subaortic ring can consist of a long, narrow tunnel of fibromuscular tissue. Another unrelated and less

See the corresponding chapter or part in the *Textbook of Surgery,* 15th edition, pp. 2070–2082, for a more detailed discussion of this topic, including a comprehensive list of references.

common form of subaortic stenosis is called *hypertrophic ob-structive cardiomyopathy*. This hereditary disease of cardiac muscle results in muscular hypertrophy of the interventricular septum, creating a dynamic obstruction of the left ventricular outflow tract. The least common form of congenital aortic stenosis is supravalvular. In the discrete form the aortic root is narrowed at the top of the valve commissures, creating an hourglass appearance. In the rarer diffuse form, the wall of the ascending aorta is thickened for a variable distance, caus-ing severe luminal narrowing that may extend into the aortic arch and its branches.

Regardless of the level of obstruction, aortic stenosis causes systolic left ventricular hypertension and a compensatory con-centric increase in left ventricular mass. Systolic function may be preserved by this hypertrophy, but left ventricular compli-ance is decreased, and higher end-diastolic pressures are re-quired to achieve adequate ventricular filling. When the hy-pertrophy is severe, the combination of high systolic wall tension and increased myocardial mass may cause subendo-cardial ischemia. Symptoms of congestive heart failure de-velop as left ventricular end-diastolic pressure rises. Symp-toms of angina or syncope begin to occur during exertion when myocardial oxygen demands are increased. The degree of hypertrophy correlates with the severity of stenosis, which is graded on the basis of the pressure gradient measured across the obstruction. For mild stenoses, the systolic outflow gradient is less than 50 mm. Hg. In moderate stenoses, the gradient is between 50 and 75 mm. Hg. Any gradient greater than 75 mm. Hg represents severe stenosis.

Valvular aortic stenosis has a bimodal form of presentation. When it presents in the neonate, the infant is commonly in severe congestive heart failure. Rapid circulatory deterioration often results in the death of these infants if the stenosis is not expeditiously relieved. When valvular aortic stenosis presents in the older child, it is often discovered as an asymptomatic systolic ejection murmur on a routine physical examination. The natural history in these patients is much less ominous than that of the neonate.

Surgical relief of valvular aortic stenosis is indicated in all newborns presenting with congestive heart failure and in older children with gradients that exceed 75 mm. Hg. The preferred operative approach includes cardiopulmonary by-pass and direct exposure of the aortic valve. The fused com-missures are opened to within 1 mm. of the aortic wall. Currently, the mortality for this procedure is between 10% and 15% in neonates and less than 1% in older children.

Replacement of the aortic valve with a prosthetic device is rarely necessary at initial operation in children with aortic stenosis. When aortic valve replacement becomes necessary in a small child, enlargement of the aortic valve annulus may be required. Mechanical valve prostheses have been preferred in children because of the limited durability of xenograft valves in the young age group. Recently, however, children and young adults have been well served by the pulmonary auto-graft technique, which transplants the patient's own pulmo-nary valve to the aortic position, replacing the pulmonary valve with a pulmonary allograft. Durability of the autograft exceeds other tissue valves and lifelong anticoagulation is not required.

In addition to left ventricular hypertension, fixed subaortic stenosis may result in damage to the aortic valve leaflets. For this reason, surgical treatment is indicated when the systolic gradient exceeds 40 mm. Hg. Resection of the fibrous membrane is performed through an aortotomy with retraction of the aortic valve leaflets. A concomitant transaortic septal myectomy is usually performed to decrease the risk of recurrent subaortic stenosis. Operative mortality for resection of the subaortic membrane with or without septal myectomy is between 1% and 3%. When tunnel subaortic stenosis exists, adequate relief of left ventricular outflow tract obstruction may require opening the right ventricle and incising the interventricular septum.

Muscular subaortic stenosis (hypertrophic obstructive cardiomyopathy) is primarily managed medically with beta blockers and calcium-channel blockers. Symptomatic patients failing medical therapy are candidates for transaortic septal myectomy. Plication of the anterior leaflet of the mitral valve may further relieve the outflow obstruction. Hospital mortality is between 1% and 5%.

Supravalvular aortic stenosis should be repaired when symptoms occur or when the systolic gradient exceeds 50 mm. Hg. Repair of the discrete form requires excision of the intimal shelf and insertion of a patch to enlarge the aortic root at the level of the narrowing. The most anatomic reconstruction results when all three sinuses of Valsalva are enlarged. However, satisfactory relief of obstruction has been achieved with enlargement of only one or two sinuses. Mortality for surgical repair approaches 1%. When diffuse supravalvular aortic stenosis involves the aortic arch, the patch is extended into the arch and head vessels using a brief period of total circulatory arrest after core cooling on cardiopulmonary bypass to a temperature of 18° C.

XIV

The Coronary Circulation
D. Duane Davis, Jr., M.D.,
and David C. Sabiston, Jr., M.D.

Atherosclerotic coronary artery disease remains the leading cause of death in the United States, accounting for over

See the corresponding chapter or part in the *Textbook of Surgery*, 15th edition, pp. 2082–2094, for a more detailed discussion of this topic, including a comprehensive list of references.

500,000 deaths annually. Although the incidence and case mortality rates have declined since the 1960s, the prevalence, mortality, and economic cost of coronary artery disease continue to escalate due to the growth and the aging of the population.

ANATOMY

The right and left main coronary arteries are the first branches of the aorta arising from the anterior and posterior sinuses of Valsalva, respectively. The left main coronary bifurcates into the left anterior descending (LAD) artery and the left circumflex artery. The LAD artery proceeds distally over the interventricular septum, extending around the apex into the posterior interventricular groove. Branches of the LAD artery include septal perforators, which course along the right ventricular (RV) side of the anterior septum; diagonal branches, which course obliquely across the left ventricular (LV) free wall; and right ventricular free wall branches. The left circumflex artery diverges from the left main artery at a 90-degree angle and continues in the left atrioventricular groove. Branches to the LV from the circumflex artery, termed *marginal arteries,* course over the lateral and inferior surface of the heart. The right coronary artery (RCA) courses anteriorly in the right atrioventricular groove. At the acute margin of the heart where the vessel turns posteriorly toward the crux of the heart, the acute marginal branch artery arises and courses toward the apex of the heart. At the crux of the heart the RCA usually (90%) gives rise to the branch artery to the atrioventricular (AV) node before bifurcating into the posterior descending artery (PDA) and posterolateral artery.

Dominance of the coronary artery system is defined by which system gives rise to the posterior descending artery. The PDA arises solely from the RCA in 75% of patients (right dominance), solely from the left circumflex artery in 10% (left dominance), and in 15% of patients, the RCA and left circumflex artery are in continuity (codominance). The PDA courses in the posterior interventricular groove providing branches to the RV, LV, and perforating branches to the septum. The sinoatrial (SA) node is supplied by a proximal branch of RCA in 55% of patients and from a branch of the left main or circumflex artery in 45% of patients. The AV node artery arises from the PDA. The His bundle and proximal bundle branches are supplied by the AV node artery. The distal bundle branches and Purkinje system are supplied by septal perforators off the LAD artery.

The venous drainage of the heart is via superficial and deep circuits. The superficial veins conduct most of the venous blood and accompany the respective coronary arteries draining into the coronary sinus or the anterior cardiac vein, which drain into the right atrium. The deep veins communicate with both the atrial and ventricular cavities via thesbian veins and sinusoidal channels.

NORMAL PHYSIOLOGY

Coronary blood flow removes the by-products of metabolism and provides oxygen and metabolic substrate to generate chemical energy that is converted into mechanical energy. Normal coronary blood flow is between 0.6 and 0.9 ml. per gm. of myocardium per minute. Myocardial oxygen consumption is normally 0.8 to 0.15 ml. oxygen per gm. myocardium per minute. Because the heart relies on aerobic metabolism to generate its energy requirements, the measurement of oxygen consumption provides an accurate measure of myocardial energy use. The major determinants of myocardial oxygen consumption are the development of systolic wall tension, heart rate, and contractility. Because the myocardium already extracts the majority of available oxygen, an increase in myocardial oxygen consumption requires an increase in myocardial perfusion. Coronary perfusion can be increased three- to six-fold over basal conditions. Regulation of coronary blood flow occurs predominantly in precapillary sphincters, although epicardial conductance vessels and the transmural resistance vessels are capable of vasoregulation. The coronary circulation maintains relatively constant coronary flow when coronary perfusion pressure is in the range of 60 to 130 mm. Hg. The majority of LV perfusion occurs during diastole due to the transmission of compressive forces on the intramural coronary vessels by the development of wall tension during systole. Because wall tension development is less in the RV, systolic flow is proportionally greater in the RV as compared with the LV. Paralleling the differences in wall tension development between the subendocardium and subepicardium, the ratio of blood flow is 1.25. This requires that the subendocardial vasculature is relatively vasodilated, which implies a limited vasodilator reserve and more susceptibility to ischemia.

Coronary vascular resistance is altered by a number of neurogenic, metabolic, and hormonal factors. Although coupling of coronary blood flow to myocardial oxygen consumption has been well demonstrated, the mechanisms have not been elucidated completely. The endothelium is important in regulating coagulation and coronary resistance. The endothelium produces a number of vasoactive substances that are predominantly vasodilators; in addition, it transduces responses to a number of neurohumoral agents. Prostacyclin (PGI_2) and endothelial-derived relaxing factor (EDRF), a nitric oxide analog, appear to be the most important vasodilators released by the endothelium. EDRF is released in response to acetylcholine, bradykinin, histamine, serotonin, and ADP. The vasodilatory and anticoagulant activities of the intact endothelium are in direct opposition to those of activated platelets. Importantly, in processes that injure the endothelium, such as atherosclerosis and hypercholesterolemia, paradoxical vasoconstriction and procoagulant activity occur.

PATHOLOGIC ANATOMY

Coronary atherosclerosis is a progressive process that results as a response to injury. The anatomic distribution of atherosclerotic lesions is not uniform throughout the coronary vasculature. The lesions occur most frequently in the proximal large coronary arteries, usually in association with branching vessels. In patients undergoing coronary arteriography, involvement of the LAD artery is most common, followed by the RCA and the circumflex arteries. Approximately 5% to 10% have involvement of the left main artery. The majority of patients have more than one vessel involved. Approximately 40% have three vessels involved, 30% have two vessels involved, and 25% have single-vessel disease. Importantly, 80% to 90% of patients have disease amenable to surgical bypass.

Fissuring of atherosclerotic plaques occurs, particularly those located eccentrically. By accumulating blood within the fissure or by clot formation, a rapid increase in plaque volume can occur. These complicated plaques are associated with acute transmural myocardial infarction when the plaque causes coronary occlusion and unstable angina when subtotal obstruction occurs.

ISCHEMIC PATHOPHYSIOLOGY

Impairment to blood flow may be secondary to fixed obstructive lesions or due to vasospasm. Stenosis of the arterial lumen greater than 75% of the cross-sectional area, which corresponds to a 50% reduction in vessel diameter, causes a critical resistance that effectively limits flow. Although flow may be adequate during steady-state conditions, increases in myocardial oxygen consumption or decreases in perfusion pressure causes ischemia. Maximally vasodilated vessels distal to a critical stenosis are unable to further augment flow. Subendocardial tissue is particularly susceptible to ischemia.

Ischemic myocardium rapidly ceases to contract. It also fails to relax normally and is less compliant. Restoration of blood flow does not immediately restore systolic or diastolic function to baseline. The delay before returning to normal function is referred to as *stunning*. The duration of stunning is proportional to the duration and severity of ischemia.

Myocardial cell death may occur as early as 20 minutes after the onset of ischemia. Cell death occurs as a wavefront phenomenon. Subendocardial cell death occurs earliest, usually within 60 minutes following total cessation of flow, and extends across the myocardial cell wall to the subepicardium after 4 to 6 hours. This emphasizes the importance of early restoration of myocardial blood flow to salvage myocardial tissue. Although the presence of adequate collaterals limits the size of a myocardial infarction, unlike other arterial beds, the human heart has a marginal ability to develop collaterals.

CLINICAL PRESENTATION

The most common presentation of coronary artery disease is angina pectoris. Anginal chest pain is usually located retrosternally and is often described as pressure, tightness, or as Heberden noted in his initial description in 1759, a sense of strangling. Pain may radiate or be located in the arms, particularly the ulnar aspect of the left arm, the neck and jaw, and the epigastrium. Nausea, vomiting, and diaphoresis may be associated with angina. Anginal equivalents such as dyspnea, palpitations, and breathlessness may occur. A small percentage of patients never have symptoms associated with myocardial ischemia. These patients are more likely to have diabetes mellitus and hypertension.

Anginal episodes are classically associated with increased physical activity, emotional stress, following eating, or with cold exposure. The typical anginal episode lasts between 10 seconds and 30 minutes. Pain lasting longer than 30 minutes is characteristic of unstable angina or myocardial infarction. In patients who have fixed coronary artery stenoses, angina may occur with a surprisingly reproducible amount of activity. A circadian rhythm exists: Anginal threshold is lower and infarct incidence is higher in the morning. The severity of angina is graded by the activity required to induce symptoms. *Unstable angina* is defined as angina occurring at rest, new-onset Class IV angina, postinfarction angina, or crescendo angina, the progression in New York Heart Association (NYHA) classification over a short time. Postinfarction angina and rest angina are associated with the presence of complicated atherosclerotic plaques and with greater cardiac morbidity. Higher NYHA classification correlates with increasing severity of anatomic disease, as well as with an increased risk of myocardial infarction and cardiac death.

In patients with an acute myocardial infarction (AMI), the symptoms of chest pain are usually greater in severity and duration, generally persisting longer than 30 minutes. Symptoms of LV failure such as dyspnea and breathlessness may be predominant, particularly in elderly patients with AMI. The amount of myocardium affects the clinical presentation: 15% is associated with a decrease in LV ejection fraction and elevated ventricular filling pressures; 25% is associated with overt symptoms of congestive heart failure; and more than 40% is associated with cardiogenic shock.

In patients with coronary artery disease, the physical examination is often unremarkable. Evidence of impaired LV compliance may be manifest by the presence a third heart sound and rales. Although the resting electrocardiogram (ECG) is often normal, particularly during anginal episodes or stress testing, inverted T waves and alterations in the ST segments may be present. Persistent ST-segment elevation or depression and the development of Q waves are indicative of an AMI. Exercise testing using ECG, echocardiography, and nuclear cardiography is useful in assessing the functional significance in a patient with coronary artery disease. Although stress testing may be used as a screening technique for the presence of coronary artery disease (CAD), false-negative and false-positive responses occur. Importantly, exercise testing provides useful information regarding prognosis. Patients with early positive studies are likely to have severe coronary artery disease and are more likely to suffer AMI and cardiac death. Particularly, the LV ejection fraction measured during exercise is a powerful predictor of survival.

Cardiac catheterization and coronary arteriography are required to diagnose the presence and anatomic severity of CAD. The relative amount of myocardium at risk and the degree of ventricular impairment present can be assessed, allowing determination of prognosis and optimal therapy. In addition, the anatomic road map is crucial before embarking on revascularization using catheter techniques or bypass grafting.

MANAGEMENT

Optimal management of patients with CAD requires an assessment of the patient's relative risk for an adverse myocardial event, such as AMI and death, as well as the severity of the patient's symptoms. The natural history of patients with CAD is such that with increasing amounts of myocardium at risk for ischemia, survival is decreased. Obstructions occurring proximally as compared with distally, involving the LAD artery as compared with the RCA, and involving the left main or three-vessel disease as compared with two-vessel or single-vessel disease are associated with impaired survival. Additional risk is imparted by an increase in the severity of symptoms, impaired LV function, and ischemia that is inducible by low levels of exercise.

Differences in survival based on treatment modality have been demonstrated in certain groups of patients with CAD. A significant survival advantage in patients treated with coronary artery bypass grafting (CABG) has been demonstrated in a number of randomized clinical trials in the following patient groups: patients with more than 75% stenosis of the left main artery; patients with three-vessel or two-vessel disease with proximal LAD artery involvement, and in association with one of the following—moderate to severe anginal symptoms (NYHA Class III–IV), impaired LV ejection fraction (LVEF < 50%), or easily inducible ischemia with exercise. CABG is recommended as therapy in these patients, although some may be amenable to treatment with PTCA. In randomized trials comparing revascularization with PTCA or CABG, there was no survival advantage at 3 years of follow-up, but there were fewer repeat interventions in those treated with CABG. In the BARI trial, there were no differences in survival or myocardial infarction between *nondiabetic* patients treated with CABG or PTCA. In *diabetic* patients, there was a significant survival advantage and fewer myocardial infarctions in those treated with CABG. In a study comparing long-term survival benefits based on different treatments of CAD, those patients with greater severity of disease benefited more from CABG. Patients with three-vessel and two-vessel disease with 95% or greater proximal LAD artery stenosis benefited from bypass surgery compared with angioplasty. All patients with single-vessel disease, except those with 95% or greater proximal LAD artery stenosis, benefited from angioplasty as compared with bypass surgery. Patients with two-vessel disease without severe proximal LAD artery involvement or those with isolated severe proximal LAD artery disease were treated equally well with CABG or PTCA. CABG is indicated in patients with anginal symptoms refractory to medical management, particularly when the anatomy is not appropriate for PTCA.

Patients who are assessed to have low risk for coronary events are managed medically. The primary agents that have been effective in either reducing the frequency of anginal episodes or preventing AMI or cardiac death include nitrates, beta blockers, calcium-channel blockers, and aspirin. Modification of known risk factors associated with CAD should be initiated, including cessation of tobacco use, control of hypertension, reduction of serum lipids, and, when appropriate, weight reduction. Successful diminution of these risk factors has been shown to decrease the incidence of AMI, lead to regression of atherosclerosis, and in patients having undergone CABG, improve graft patency.

Patients with unstable angina initially should be managed medically. Because of the strong association of complicated plaques with the development of unstable angina, heparin and aspirin are effective agents. Early coronary arteriography is indicated in patients who continue to have angina. Approximately 80% of patients will have multivessel or left main occlusive disease. The incidence of adverse myocardial events is increased over the initial months following presentation, particularly in patients with multivessel disease, rest pain, complex lesion morphology, intracoronary thrombi, ischemia demonstrated during Holter monitoring, or those who are elderly. In patients with persistent angina, institution of an intra-aortic balloon pump (IABP) is efficacious. Revascularization using PTCA or CABG is frequently indicated, although the risk of a periprocedural myocardial infarction or mortality is approximately twice that of elective procedures.

Herrick, in 1912, initially made the observation that AMI was associated with thrombosis of the coronary artery, with subsequent studies demonstrating that 90% of transmural infarcts are associated with a totally occluded infarct-related vessel. Recent clinical evidence has reinforced the importance of obtaining myocardial reperfusion as early as possible. Thrombolytics have been shown to decrease mortality, decrease infarct size, and preserve ventricular function. The benefit is greatest when they are given early after onset of pain. Less benefit is achieved when they are given greater than 6 hours after the onset of pain. Importantly, the adjuvant use of heparin and aspirin has limited reocclusion and reinfarction rates. Patients who do not achieve reperfusion with a thrombolytic, have a contraindication to thrombolytic therapy, or have recurrent ischemia benefit from reperfusion using PTCA. Unfortunately, less than 25% of patients with AMI receive thrombolytic therapy due to delays in presentation after the onset of pain and delays in diagnosis. Patients at a high risk for subsequent cardiac events should undergo cardiac catheterization. Patients with multivessel disease in which the proximal LAD artery is involved have a survival benefit with revascularization.

Mechanical complications of AMI occur due to tearing of myocardial tissue. Such complications include rupture of the ventricular free wall, ventricular septal defect, and rupture of a papillary muscle with severe mitral regurgitation. Echocardiography can establish the diagnosis. These complications occur less frequently in patients treated with thrombolytics and more frequently in those taking corticosteroids and NSAIDs and the elderly. The mortality in patients treated medically with these complications exceeds 90%.

Rupture of the ventricular free wall causes hemopericardium and resulting tamponade. This accounts for 10% of hospital deaths due to AMI. Pericardiocentesis can confirm the diagnosis and provide temporary hemodynamic relief. Urgent surgical therapy with ventricular reconstruction can lead to survival.

Postinfarction VSD is manifest by the new onset of a harsh holosystolic murmur, often associated with a thrill. Hemodynamic compromise with ventricular failure occurs early. In addition to color-flow echocardiography, right-sided heart catheterization demonstrating an oxygen saturation stepup at the level of the right ventricle can establish the diagnosis. Except in moribund patients, correction by patch closure of the VSD and bypass grafting should be undertaken. Rarely, the patient may be stable, and the operation can be delayed, allowing the infarct tissue to heal. Better results are obtained in these patients, with survival approaching 90%. In the majority of patients, urgent operation is required. Use of an IABP provides a degree of hemodynamic support. Survival following surgical correction is approximately 50% to 75%.

Rupture of the papillary muscle leads to severe mitral regurgitation and rapid development of pulmonary edema and hypotension. A holosystolic murmur is usually present. Echocardiography is diagnostic. Unlike postinfarction VSD, papillary muscle rupture is often associated with a limited infarction size. Frequently, limited circumflex or RCA disease is present. IABP use provides hemodynamic support. Early operative therapy with mitral valve repair, when possible, or mitral valve replacement in conjunction with bypass grafting is indicated. Survival is reported as approximately 50% to 70%.

SURGICAL PROCEDURE

Although a number of indirect procedures were devised to treat CAD in the first half of this century, the first effective and direct approach was the coronary endarterectomy performed initially in 1956 by Bailey and subsequently modified by Longmire. However, endarterectomy is applicable to a minority of patients, and the long-term patency rates are poor. The first coronary artery bypass was performed by Sabiston in 1962 using a reversed saphenous vein. Although this patient succumbed to a perioperative cerebrovascular accident (CVA), later clinical success, particularly by Favalaro and associates at the Cleveland Clinic in the 1960s, demonstrated the clinical efficacy of CABG.

Coronary artery bypass grafting is usually performed using a median sternotomy to expose the mediastinum, heart, and great vessels. Conduits used to bypass the coronary artery obstruction are most commonly the internal mammary artery, harvested off the chest wall as a tissue pedicle, and the saphenous vein. The saphenous vein is reversed in direction, with the distal vein anastomosed to the ascending aorta and the proximal vein anastomosed to the coronary artery distal to the obstruction. The proximal end of the internal mammary artery is left in continuity with the subclavian artery, and the distal end is anastomosed to the coronary artery, usually the LAD artery. These anastomoses are performed routinely while the patient is on cardiopulmonary bypass. The coronary artery anastomoses are done after the ascending aorta is occluded and after the heart is arrested by delivery of a cardioplegia solution. Although different techniques exist for myocardial protection during the period when blood flow is interrupted, the majority of centers use cold cardioplegia and topical hypothermia on the heart. By cooling the heart to less than $10°$ C and inducing diastolic arrest, myocardial energy expenditure is reduced 100-fold. This approach provides a motionless heart and a dry field. All coronary arteries with greater than 60% stenosis and which are larger than 1.5 mm. in diameter are bypassed. Emphasis is placed on complete revascularization. Following completion of the bypass grafts, assurance of hemostasis around the anastomoses, and placement of temporary epicardial pacing wires, the patient is weaned from cardiopulmonary bypass. The mediastinum and opened pleural spaces are drained with large-bore chest tubes.

RESULTS

Mortality is approximately 3% in large series of patients undergoing CABG. Mortality is significantly increased by advanced age, incomplete revascularization, reoperative CABG, preoperative hemodynamic instability, unstable angina, female sex, and impaired ventricular function as measured by LV ejection fraction, particularly in those patients with mitral regurgitation or symptoms of congestive heart failure. In patients without significant risk factors, mortality approaches 1%. Long-term survival at 5, 10, and 15 years is approximately 90%, 75%, and 65%, respectively. Long-term survival is adversely affected by low ejection fraction, particularly as measured during exercise, advanced age, diabetes mellitus, and not using the internal mammary artery for grafting.

Early after CABG, rates of relief of anginal symptoms and freedom from myocardial infarction are excellent, approximately 85% and 95% at 5 years, respectively. After 5 years, recurrence of angina and myocardial infarction rates increase, reflecting progression of atherosclerosis in the coronary vasculature and occlusive disease in bypass grafts, particularly those using the saphenous vein. The 1-year patency rate of bypass grafts using the internal mammary artery and the saphenous vein is 95% and 90%. Graft patency at 10 years remains good using the internal mammary artery, 85% to 90%. The patency rate of grafts using the saphenous vein begins to decrease after 4 years and is only 50% to 60% after 10 years.

Since many venous grafts and a lesser number of internal

mammary artery grafts become stenotic or occluded, severe isolated coronary lesions may be amenable to endarterectomy. Endarterectomy for isolated left main coronary artery stenosis has been reported to be the preferred procedure under these circumstances, since the long-term results have been quite favorable. For example, a patient with a severe left main lesion (95%) and unstable angina who was operated on emergently in 1964 using this technique is alive 32 years later without return of symptoms of myocardial ischemia.

CABG significantly improves both myocardial function and patient performance. Exercise tolerance is markedly improved in patients after CABG and remains better than in patients treated medically as long as 10 years following operation. Regional wall function and exercise ejection fraction are both improved within 2 weeks following operation. Similar improvements in diastolic function as measured by ventricular compliance occur following CABG.

SURGICAL MANAGEMENT OF FAILED ANGIOPLASTY

Peter Van Trigt III, M.D.

As percutaneous transluminal coronary angioplasty (PTCA) has gained increasing popularity as a primary treatment for coronary atherosclerotic heart disease (with more than 400,000 PTCA procedures performed in 1995), surgeons have encountered a concomitant rise in the need for emergency surgical myocardial revascularization for acute coronary angioplasty failure. Emergency coronary artery bypass grafting for acute myocardial ischemia secondary to vessel dissection, thrombosis, or spasm (recoil) has significant morbidity and definite mortality. Currently, a PTCA failure rate of 4% to 5% is reported by most centers performing a large number of coronary angioplasties, and these patients require expeditious surgical revascularization. Rapid surgical revascularization with careful management of the patient during the period of vessel closure for minimization of ischemia is required for optimizing the clinical outcome of these compromised patients.

Percutaneous transluminal coronary angioplasty utilizes intracoronary balloon inflation to approximately 4 atmospheres of pressure for production of localized trauma to the coronary artery wall; the intended result is atheroma fracture and arterial expansion that produce an increase in luminal area. Unfortunately, balloon inflation or guidewire and catheter manipulation can cause more extensive arterial wall damage, with medial dissection and creation of an occlusive intimal flap. Thrombosis or spasm also may occur at the dilation site. In the absence of a well-developed collateral circulation, acute coronary occlusion produces severe myocardial ischemia and

---

See the corresponding chapter or part in the *Textbook of Surgery,* 15th edition, pp. 2095–2100, for a more detailed discussion of this topic, including a comprehensive list of references.

evolving myocardial infarction. The intracoronary reperfusion catheter has been used clinically to sustain coronary flow beyond an occlusion following failed angioplasty and can reverse myocardial ischemia and allow stabilization of the patient during transport to the operating room. Re-establishment of coronary flow through the reperfusion catheter before operation can have a direct influence on reducing the extent of myocardial infarction, which occurs in 30% to 40% of angioplasty failures despite successful later surgical revascularization. Reversal of acute ischemia also provides time to harvest the internal mammary artery for use in surgical revascularization as the optimal bypass conduit. The intra-aortic balloon pump also has been used to stabilize patients following failed PTCA, especially in those patients demonstrating persistent ischemia. Diastolic augmentation from the intra-aortic balloon pump does not greatly alter blood flow through the occluded vessel but can assist in maintaining viability of marginal myocardium supplied by collateral vessels at the border of the infarct zone. It should be emphasized that rapid transport of the patient to the operating room and placement on cardiopulmonary bypass are the *major objectives* during the period of vessel closure, since this has been shown to be the only effective means of reducing a significant perioperative myocardial infarction rate.

Most recent series of emergent coronary surgical revascularization following angioplasty failure cite an operative mortality of approximately 5%, with a perioperative infarction incidence of approximately 30%. If active ischemia is present on the preoperative electrocardiogram following failed PTCA, the postoperative myocardial infarction rate approaches 50% despite successful surgical revascularization. This is the result of a necessary period for transportation of the patient from the catheterization laboratory to the operating room, placement of the patient on cardiopulmonary bypass, and establishment of surgical revascularization. The predictors of operative mortality in patients undergoing emergency coronary artery bypass grafting for failed PTCA include cardiogenic shock, age greater than 70 years, previous coronary artery bypass surgery, and the presence of multiple-vessel disease. Some series report improved surgical outcome in this group of emergency CABG patients with the use of warm blood (substrate enhanced) cardioplegia. A 10-year experience reviewing emergency CABG after failed PTCA at Emory reported an overall surgical mortality of 3.1% with an incidence of perioperative myocardial infarction of 18%. However, when the most recent 3-year cohort of patients was examined, the mortality was higher (7.1%). This increased mortality reflected the increased incidence of factors associated with poor outcome after CABG in current patients undergoing PTCA (older age, multivessel disease, decreased LV ejection fraction, prior CABG, and diabetes).

Management of the patient who has sustained a failed coronary angioplasty and required emergent coronary artery bypass grafting requires careful attention to strategies for minimizing myocardial ischemia incurred following vessel closure and before surgical revascularization can be accomplished.

Of paramount importance is rapid surgical revascularization, which requires cardiac anesthesia and cardiac surgery well coordinated with the cardiac catheterization laboratory. Current experience has shown that operative mortality can be reduced to a low level (although not equivalent to elective surgical coronary mortality). However, the in-hospital morbidity remains quite high, especially perioperative myocardial infarction of approximately 30%. Attempts to reduce this rate of perioperative infarction must involve intervention techniques for restoration of perfusion to the ischemic region preoperatively.

REOPERATIVE CORONARY SURGERY

Stanley A. Gall, Jr., M.D.

The greater number of patients undergoing coronary artery bypass grafting (CABG), the greater number of patients surviving longer after CABG, and the technical and technological advances reducing the risk of reoperative coronary surgery have increased the importance of reoperative CABG. Reoperation will be accomplished following primary CABG in a cumulative 3% to 3.4% of patients after 5 years and 5.5% to 11% after 10 years. The annual risk of requiring reoperation increases markedly after 5 to 7 years, from 1.1% to 3.2% and 3.9% at 5, 10, and 12 years, respectively. The majority of patients (82%) present with both vein graft stenosis and progression of native vessel disease. Factors that increase the risk of requiring reoperation, by multivariate analysis, include the absence of an internal mammary artery (IMA) graft, younger age, incomplete revascularization, congestive heart failure, and Class III or IV angina. When all cardiac events are considered as end points, diabetes mellitus, severe angina, systolic hypertension, and diminished ejection fraction are predisposing risk factors for reoperation. Younger patients have an increased risk of interventions but maintain a superior survival. Although the risk of damaging an intact IMA is 3% to 5%, the benefits of a functioning IMA are so great that the presence of this graft does not pose a risk factor for reoperative morbidity or mortality. In higher-risk patients, percutaneous angioplasty may temporize symptomatic stenoses in native coronary vessels, in the IMA, and in saphenous vein grafts (SVGs). Angioplasty of SVG stenoses has an initial success rate of 85% to 95%, with complications such as distal coronary atheroembolism, perforation, myocardial infarction, rupture of the graft, or death occurring in 4% to 7% of patients. Restenosis occurs in 50% to 60% of lesions in the body of saphenous vein grafts within 6 months but in only 8% to 14% of IMA anastomoses and 26% of SVG anastomoses.

See the corresponding chapter or part in the *Textbook of Surgery*, 15th edition, pp. 2100–2106, for a more detailed discussion of this topic, including a comprehensive list of references.

Strong indications for reoperation include the acute complications of vessel dissection or perforation at catheterization or angioplasty, left main equivalent anatomy, unstable angina, or postinfarction angina. Those who are unable to control symptoms medically, have congestive heart failure, have a positive exercise tolerance test after myocardial infarction, or have silent ischemia with a large proportion of myocardium at risk also should be considered for reoperation. If stenosis is present distal to the IMA and disease in other vein grafts has progressed or a large portion of myocardium is at risk, reoperation is recommended. Patients with stenosed SVGs to the LAD coronary artery, even with stable Class I or II angina, have a significantly improved survival with reoperation as compared with medical management. Contraindications to reoperation include evolving myocardial infarction, cardiogenic shock, concurrent sepsis, and poor medical condition. Emergent revascularization can be accomplished technically but has poor immediate- and longer-term results, including a higher mortality and earlier return of anginal symptoms. Unstable patients must achieve physiologic stability and normalize or stabilize end-organ dysfunction through the use of maximal medical treatment, including the use of intra-aortic balloon counterpulsation, prior to reoperation. Although harvesting bilateral internal mammary arteries does not consistently subject the patient to an increased risk of mediastinal infection or sternal dehiscence, this risk is magnified in the elderly, female, and diabetic populations. The sequential use of the contralateral IMA in successive coronary procedures does not predispose to sternal healing complications.

Technical factors that increase the difficulty of reoperative CABG, in comparison with primary CABG, include more advanced native vessel disease, a longer time to initiate cardiopulmonary bypass, a longer cross-clamp time, a longer cross-clamp time per graft, and an increased blood loss. The risk factors, by multivariate analysis, for heightened morbidity and mortality following reoperative CABG include advanced age, diminished ventricular function, absence of an IMA graft, and diabetes mellitus. Additional risk factors include female sex, emergency procedure, and an interval between operations of greater than 10 years. Repeat median sternotomy is the most common incision for reoperation. Patients with limited grafting requirements may undergo a left or right thoracotomy to approach the heart. When the left anterior descending coronary artery distribution or both the right and left coronary distributions require bypass grafting, then a repeat sternotomy is required. Recent sternotomy, adhesion of the right ventricle or the internal mammary artery to the sternum, ascending aortic aneurysm, right ventricular hypertrophy, multiple prior sternal entries, or a history of mediastinitis increases the risk of injury during repeat sternotomy. High-risk patients may require exposure of the femoral vessels, cannulation of the femoral vessels, or even initiation of cardiopulmonary bypass via the femoral vessels prior to sternotomy. The oscillating saw is used to divide the anterior sternal table over the entire length of the sternum and then to carefully divide the posterior table, taking care not to injure underlying structures. The structures most often damaged are the right ventricle, the aorta, the right atrium, the innominate vein, saphenous vein grafts, and prior IMA grafts.

The conduct of a reoperative coronary procedure has been modified as the frequency of this operation has increased. The evolution of the technique to the current state, whereby minimal dissection is performed prior to cardiopulmonary bypass and cardioplegic arrest and retrograde cardioplegia supplements antegrade delivery, is believed to be responsible for the stable or improving outcome results despite a progressively higher-risk population of reoperative candidates. Bypass anastomoses are performed in a similar manner as in primary CABG. Pericarditis from primary CABG and more diffuse coronary disease may preclude identification of optimal vessels for grafting. Patent saphenous vein grafts are at risk for injury during repeat sternotomy, may be a source of embolism, and are at risk for later stenosis or thrombosis if not electively replaced. In patients in whom an SVG to the LAD artery was replaced by the IMA, 16% to 19% developed a hypoperfusion syndrome in the anterior circulation diagnosed by the presence of anterior ischemia, sudden hypotension, elevated filling pressures, diminished contractility, and ventricular dysrhythmias. The lowest mortality and myocardial infarction rates occurred when the stenotic SVG was left in place and an IMA anastomosis to the distal LAD was constructed.

The mortality of a reoperative coronary procedure exceeds that of primary CABG by two- to fivefold. Mortality after primary CABG is most often the result of noncardiac endorgan failure. Mortality after reoperation occurs almost exclusively as a result of cardiac causes (78% to 82%). Morbid events also follow reoperative CABG more frequently than primary CABG; these include a greater volume of shed mediastinal blood, a higher rate of intra-aortic balloon counterpulsation, a higher risk of requiring reoperation for mediastinal bleeding or tamponade, and higher myocardial infarction and pulmonary complication rates. Aprotinin has a demonstrated benefit in reducing chest tube output, total donor exposures, and total transfusion requirements after reoperative coronary surgery. Myocardial infarction is twice as prevalent in reoperations (2.1% to 6.9%) as in primary coronary procedures and may result from inadequate myocardial protection during aortic cross-clamp, atheroembolism, or incomplete revascularization. While long-term survival may approach that of primary CABG, return of angina occurs sooner and more frequently after reoperative coronary bypass surgery. Survival rates of 66% to 90% at 5 years and 35% to 88% at 10 years are significantly enhanced by the construction of an IMA to LAD artery anastomosis and good preoperative ventricular function. Factors adversely affecting 10-year survival include advanced age (>65), more severe anginal symptoms, left main occlusion, poor left ventricular function, both native vessel disease and graft failure, and the absence of an IMA graft. Return of angina occurs at a rate of 47% for the first year after reoperation, much greater than the 20% rate for primary CABG. Anginal symptoms thereafter recur at an annual rate similar to primary CABG (2.8% versus 2.7%). Control of hypercholesterolemia and hypertension may ameliorate the effects of these disease processes and decrease the risk of subsequent graft failure.

RADIONUCLIDE EVALUATION OF CORONARY ARTERY DISEASE

Robert H. Jones, M.D.

MEASUREMENT OF CARDIAC FUNCTION

The two radionuclide techniques that can be used to measure left ventricular function noninvasively in patients are initial-transit radionuclide angiocardiography and gated equilibrium ventriculography. Data are acquired for the gated equilibrium technique during 100 to 300 heartbeats after an intravenously injected blood pool tracer reaches equilibrium. Counts are synchronized to the cardiac cycle by the electrocardiogram and compressed into a single averaged heartbeat to permit assessment of wall motion on dynamic images and calculation of left ventricular ejection fraction from left ventricular count changes.

Initial-transit radionuclide angiocardiography uses a high-sensitivity gamma camera to dynamically record a single transit of a discrete tracer bolus through the heart. Assessment of the left ventricular function requires data from less than 10 heartbeats. The short imaging time makes initial-transit radionuclide angiocardiography especially useful for obtaining hemodynamic measurements during the stress of exercise.

MYOCARDIAL PERFUSION AND METABOLISM

Radionuclides that have a high extraction during initial myocardial transit can be used to assess regional blood flow. Thallium-201 is a potassium analog used extensively to assess the distribution of regional myocardial blood flow. Newer technetium-99m–labeled agents with superior imaging characteristics are increasingly replacing thallium-201 in clinical use. These tracers, injected during the peak of exercise stress and imaged soon thereafter, depict the distribution of myocardial blood flow during exercise. Perfusion defects on exercise images correspond to myocardium beyond a stenosis that fails to augment blood flow normally during exercise. During the initial few hours after injection, thallium-201 gradually redistributes in myocardium proportional to tissue potassium content. Therefore, redistribution images are influenced more by

See the corresponding chapter or part in the *Textbook of Surgery*, 15th edition, pp. 2106–2111, for a more detailed discussion of this topic, including a comprehensive list of references.

myocardial mass than by differences in regional myocardial blood flow. Ischemic myocardial regions typically show defects during exercise that normalize on redistribution images. In contrast, regions of prior myocardial infarction and scar cause defects on exercise images that persist on redistribution images. The three-dimensional distribution of gamma-emitting tracers, such as thallium-201, is commonly quantitated using single photon emission computed tomography (SPECT). Technetium-99m–labeled perfusion agents that provide better images and comparable biologic information are increasingly used in place of thallium-201 for cardiac perfusion imaging.

APPLICATION OF RADIONUCLIDE TECHNIQUES IN PATIENTS WITH CORONARY ARTERY DISEASE

Radionuclide techniques are most useful for risk stratification of patients with known or suspected coronary artery disease. Global and regional function and perfusion abnormalities are highly sensitive indicators of myocardial ischemia, which usually appear at a lower ischemia threshold than evokes chest pain or electrocardiographic change. Radionuclide techniques measuring ventricular function and myocardial perfusion reflect similar biologic processes because of the close link between myocardial integrity and blood flow.

The three variables on thallium-201 studies that relate most closely to the risk of death from coronary artery disease are the number of reversible thallium defects, the magnitude of initial reversible defect, and the maximal heart rate achieved during exercise. The variable on radionuclide angiocardiography that relates most to subsequent cardiac death or myocardial infarction is the exercise ejection fraction. A lesser amount of prognostic information is contributed by the exercise increase in heart rate and the resting end-diastolic volume. Measurement of the magnitude of myocardial ischemia by these radionuclide tests provides prognostic information not available from cardiac catheterization or routine clinical assessment. The accuracy of physiologic assessment obtained simply and at a relatively low cost makes radionuclide measurements ideally suited for initial evaluation of patients with coronary artery disease. Patients recognized by radionuclide testing to have a high risk of subsequent cardiac event should undergo cardiac catheterization and evaluation for possible interventional therapy.

Patients with good anatomic results after interventional therapy commonly normalize cardiac function and myocardial perfusion during exercise. The amount of improvement in individual patients objectively documents the effectiveness of interventional therapy and relates to subsequent freedom from untoward cardiac events. Radionuclide studies are also useful to evaluate the magnitude of recurrent ischemia in patients who subsequently become symptomatic to identify those who might benefit from repeat interventional procedures.

VENTRICULAR ANEURYSM

William A. Gay, Jr., M.D.

Although true aneurysms of the left ventricle may be caused by trauma or congenital cardiac malformations, the majority follow acute transmural myocardial infarction. The typical ventricular aneurysm has been described as "a thinned-out transmural scar that has completely lost its trabecular pattern." It is estimated that approximately 10% of patients sustaining an acute transmural myocardial infarction develop a left ventricular aneurysm. However, it is likely that this incidence will decrease with recent advances in the care of patients with acute infarcts, including careful hemodynamic control and aggressive reperfusional efforts.

Although the relationship between coronary occlusion and aneurysm formation has been well established, until recently it was poorly understood why some infarctions produced aneurysms and others did not. Recent studies indicated that the absence of significant collateral circulation in the distribution of the left anterior descending coronary artery is a major determining factor in the formation of ventricular aneurysm following anterior infarction.

Whereas some patients with ventricular aneurysm may be asymptomatic, most have some combination of dyspnea, angina, and palpitations. Peripheral arterial embolization from mural thrombi within the aneurysm is rare. Those patients whose aneurysms produce symptoms should be considered candidates for surgical resection. Although ventricular aneurysm may be diagnosed accurately by use of noninvasive means, ventriculography and selective coronary arteriography should be done in all patients being considered for operation. Visualization of the coronary arteries allows bypass of all significant occlusive lesions at the time of aneurysmectomy.

Aneurysmectomy is performed via a midline sternotomy incision with use of cardiopulmonary bypass. Ideally, all non-contractile areas of the ventricle are resected or excluded, and the ventricle is reconstructed geometrically to maximize its functional capacity. Early operative mortality is 5% to 10%, with 80% of survivors living 4 years later; in contrast, nearly 90% 5-year mortality occurs among patients whose aneurysms were not resected. Factors that increase operative risk include advanced age (more than 65 years), left main coronary artery disease, renal failure, and New York Heart Association (NYHA) Class IV status. Long-term survival is negatively affected by poor left ventricular function (EF < 20%) and/or the presence of left main coronary disease. Survivors of operation experience symptomatic improvement, but until recently, there has been little objective evidence of improved cardiac performance. With the use of multiple-gated acquisition scans (MUGA), intraoperative transesophageal echocardiography

See the corresponding chapter or part in the *Textbook of Surgery*, 15th edition, pp. 2111–2114, for a more detailed discussion of this topic, including a comprehensive list of references.

(TEE), and magnetic resonance imaging (MRI), improvements in ejection fraction and lessening of valvular regurgitation can be documented.

KAWASAKI'S DISEASE

Thomas A. D'Amico, M.D.

Kawasaki's disease, a vasculitic disorder of undetermined etiology, is the leading cause of acquired heart disease in children in the United States. Aspects of this disease yet to be explained include etiology, selectivity for children, and ability to progress to severe stages in view of its usually benign and self-limited nature. Initial therapy for Kawasaki's disease is directed toward reducing coronary artery and myocardial inflammation. Therapy in the later stages of the disease is designed to prevent coronary thrombosis by inhibiting platelet aggregation. Specific therapy for Kawasaki's disease awaits the discovery of the etiologic agent.

CLINICAL MANIFESTATIONS. The diagnosis of Kawasaki's disease is secured by the presence of five of the six major criteria. The principal presenting symptom is fever, which usually has an abrupt onset, is generally high and spiking, and does not respond to antibiotics. The appearance of fever is often accompanied by the presence of congested conjunctivae, bilateral and sterile. After the appearance of conjunctivitis, several changes in the lips and oral cavity occur. By the third day of illness, a polymorphous macular erythematous rash appears. The rash begins with reddening of the palms and soles; individual lesions may coalesce as the rash progresses proximally to spread over the trunk. In approximately 50% of patients, nonpurulent cervical lymphadenopathy develops.

Cardiovascular manifestations are prominent in the acute phase of the illness and the leading cause of morbidity and mortality. Examination of the heart may reveal tachycardia, distant heart sounds, or a gallop, suggestive of myocarditis or congestive failure; a holosystolic murmur signifies mitral valve insufficiency. Leukocytosis is invariably present and often is accompanied by a leftward shift in the differential. Anemia and thrombocytosis may be present. The electrocardiogram is abnormal in 70% of patients. Echocardiograms are positive in 45% of patients, providing early objective evidence of cardiovascular dysfunction.

NATURAL HISTORY. The pathologic basis of Kawasaki's disease is the progression of a nonspecific vasculitis that involves the microvasculature of the aorta and its major branches, manifested by endarteritis of the vasa vasorum of the coronary, brachiocephalic, celiac, renal, and iliofemoral systems. As the inflammatory process of the intima and ad-

---

See the corresponding chapter or part in the *Textbook of Surgery*, 15th edition, pp. 2114–2118, for a more detailed discussion of this topic, including a comprehensive list of references.

ventitia progresses, aneurysms form in these vessels and lead to stenosis, thromboembolism, ischemia, rupture, or healing. A spectrum of cardiovascular manifestations may occur, but they are usually self-limited; cardiac fatalities occur in less than 1% of patients. Myocarditis is present in as many as 50% of patients. Mitral regurgitation occurs in only 5% of patients; however, in patients with coronary aneurysms, the incidence is 25%. Myocardial infarction, a rare complication of Kawasaki's disease, may occur after diffuse ischemia or a thromboembolic event.

The most serious complication of Kawasaki's disease is the formation of coronary artery aneurysms, which has an incidence of 10% to 40%. Coronary artery aneurysms are responsible for at least 85% of the mortality associated with Kawasaki's disease. Most patients are found to have multiple aneurysms, but only aneurysms that reach 4 mm. in diameter are considered clinically significant. Patients with giant coronary aneurysms (greater than 8 mm.) have the worst prognosis, and this group constitutes nearly all the late deaths from Kawasaki's disease.

MANAGEMENT. After the diagnosis of Kawasaki's disease is secured, patients are treated with intravenous gamma globulin (2 gm. per kg.) and high-dose aspirin (100 mg. per kg. per day), which is continued until defervescence. Thereafter, they are maintained on low-dose aspirin (3 to 5 mg. per kg. per day) for 8 weeks. In children who develop aneurysms, low-dose aspirin therapy may be continued indefinitely.

Patients with no coronary changes on echocardiography at any stage of the illness require no pharmacologic therapy after the acute phase of the illness resolves. Patients with single coronary aneurysms (small to medium) are maintained on low-dose aspirin until the abnormalities resolve. Patients with multiple coronary aneurysms or with one or more giant coronary aneurysms are maintained on low-dose aspirin indefinitely. Coronary arteriography is performed if other studies suggest the presence of coronary stenoses.

Advanced cardiovascular complications require surgical intervention. The internal mammary artery (IMA) has been demonstrated to be the graft of choice for myocardial revascularization for children with Kawasaki's disease. A retrospective multicenter study analyzing the long-term outcome of myocardial revascularization in patients with Kawasaki's disease was completed recently. Actuarial analysis demonstrated a significantly higher survival at 90 months after operation in the IMA group than in the saphenous vein graft (SVG) group, and the actuarial patency rate was significantly higher for the arterial grafts than for the vein grafts.

XV

Ebstein's Anomaly
Theodore C. Koutlas, M.D.

Ebstein's anomaly is an uncommon cardiac defect that accounts for less than 1% of congenital heart disease. The malformation, described in 1866 by Wilhelm Ebstein, is characterized by the downward displacement of the septal and posterior leaflets of the tricuspid valve into the right ventricle. The anterior leaflet is attached normally to the annulus but is large and redundant. The abnormal tricuspid valve divides the right ventricle into two parts. The area between the tricuspid annulus and the displaced valve is referred to as the *atrialized ventricle*, while the trabecular and outlet portions below the valve make up the *functional ventricle*. The atrialized ventricle is thin and fibrotic and may even be aneurysmal. Atrial septal defects are present in most patients, and other less frequent abnormalities include pulmonary atresia, ventricular septal defects, and atrioventricular canal defects. Ebstein's anomaly of the left atrioventricular valve is common with corrected transposition of the great arteries but is exceedingly rare alone. Wolff-Parkinson-White syndrome is seen in 10% to 18% of patients, with accessory pathways localized to the right ventricular free wall or the posterior septum.

The tricuspid valve in Ebstein's anomaly is usually regurgitant but uncommonly may be stenotic or even imperforate. The atrialized ventricle impedes forward flow of blood into the pulmonary circulation, and the redundant anterior leaflet contributes to the functional obstruction of the right ventricle. Impaired filling of the functional right ventricle creates systemic venous hypertension and right-to-left shunting across the atrial septal defect, resulting in cyanosis. The right atrium and atrialized ventricle subsequently dilate massively, and this worsens the tricuspid regurgitation.

Variability in the morphology of Ebstein's anomaly leads to a broad spectrum of clinical manifestations. Almost half the patients present before 1 month of age, usually with cyanosis or heart failure. Infants diagnosed with Ebstein's anomaly have a poor prognosis, and their mortality approaches 50%. The remainder of patients present early in childhood or adolescence, although diagnosis in adult life is not uncommon. Symptoms usually consist of fatigue, dyspnea, palpitations, or cyanosis, although occasionally asymptomatic patients are found on routine chest x-ray or electrocardiogram. Arrythmias are seen in 25% to 40% of patients. Exercise tolerance is markedly abnormal, and without intervention, patients develop progressive heart failure or suffer sudden death.

See the corresponding chapter or part in the *Textbook of Surgery*, 15th edition, pp. 2118–2124, for a more detailed discussion of this topic, including a comprehensive list of references.

Physical examination findings include split first and second heart sounds, a systolic murmur along the left sternal border, and jugular venous distention with prominent v waves. The electrocardiogram (ECG) is always abnormal; right-axis deviation, right bundle-branch block, and right atrial hypertrophy are common findings. Chest radiography demonstrates a narrow vascular pedicle with a globular heart due to right atrial enlargement. Echocardiography is the primary diagnostic tool for Ebstein's anomaly, allowing precise determination of valve morphology, ventricular size and function, and associated cardiac defects. Cardiac catheterization is reserved for patients with complex malformations or previous shunts.

The surgical treatment of Ebstein's anomaly must be individualized due to the wide variability of the defect. Indications for surgery include functional Class III or IV symptoms, significant cyanosis, massive cardiomegaly, right ventricular (RV) outflow tract obstruction, or evidence of ventricular pre-excitation. Neonatal Ebstein's malformation may be difficult to treat due to the high pulmonary vascular resistance after birth. Prostaglandin (PGE_1) infusion and extracorporeal membrane oxygenation have been used successfully to palliate neonates with severe forms of Ebstein's anomaly. A technique described to repair neonatal Ebstein's anomaly combines oversewing of the tricuspid valve, atrial septectomy, and placement of a systemic-pulmonary shunt. These patients later undergo a modified Fontan procedure. In older children and adults, tricuspid valve repair is the procedure of choice. One successful repair combines plication of the atrialized ventricle, posterior tricuspid annuloplasty, closure of the atrial septal defect, and excision of the redundant atrium. Operative mortality was 7.3%, with the majority of the patients having trivial or mild tricuspid regurgitation. Only 3% of patients subsequently required tricuspid valve replacement. Christaan Barnard performed the first successful tricuspid valve replacement for Ebstein's anomaly in 1962. When tricuspid valve replacement is required, bioprosthetic valves are recommended because of their excellent durability in the tricuspid position and low incidence of thromboembolic complications. The operative mortality rate for tricuspid valve replacement has been reported as 5.8% to 20%. Patients with Wolff-Parkinson-White syndrome should undergo accessory pathway ablation during their surgical repair. Long-term results of the surgical treatment of Ebstein's anomaly are excellent, and over 90% of patients are functional Class I or II. Improvements in exercise tolerance, oxygen saturation, and symptomatic arrhythmias also have been reported after surgical repair of Ebstein's anomaly.

XVI

Congenital Lesions of the Coronary Circulation

James E. Lowe, M.D., James D. St. Louis, M.D., and David C. Sabiston, Jr., M.D.

CORONARY ARTERY FISTULAS

Coronary artery fistulas represent the most common of the congenital coronary malformations. They are characterized by normal origin of the involved coronary artery from the aorta with a fistulous communication with the atria or ventricles or with the pulmonary artery, coronary sinus, or superior vena cava.

CLINICAL MANIFESTATION. It is commonly believed that most patients with coronary artery fistulas are asymptomatic. However, 55% are symptomatic at the time of presentation. Because the underlying pathophysiology is essentially that of a left-to-right cardiac shunt, it follows that the most common manifestation is congestive heart failure. Angina pectoris is another common symptom of the defect. It is secondary to a steal of coronary arterial flow through the fistulous communication and subacute bacterial endocarditis. The major clinical finding secondary to a coronary artery fistula is a continuous murmur over the site of the abnormal communication. This murmur may closely resemble that of a patent ductus arteriosus.

The right coronary artery is involved most often in the development of a congenital coronary artery fistula (56%) and most often communicates with a chamber of the right side of the heart. The fistula usually involves the right ventricle (39%), followed closely in incidence by drainage into the right atrium (33%), including the coronary sinus and superior vena cava, or the pulmonary artery (20%). Left coronary artery fistulas are less common but usually drain into the right ventricle or right atrium. Rarely, coronary artery fistulas may drain into the left atrium or left ventricle.

EVALUATION. The successful surgical management of patients with congenital coronary artery fistulas depends on a thorough preoperative evaluation that precisely defines the anatomy and pathophysiology of the anomaly. In patients with a large fistula, injection of contrast medium into the aortic root may clearly delineate the lesion. In patients with a smaller fistulous communication from both coronary arteries, selective coronary arteriography is preferable and may be essential to establish the diagnosis.

See the corresponding chapter or part in the *Textbook of Surgery,* 15th edition, pp. 2124–2135, for a more detailed discussion of this topic, including a comprehensive list of references.

SURGICAL MANAGEMENT. Patients with a single communication that is easily dissected can be surgically corrected without cardiopulmonary bypass for suture obliteration. However, in patients with multiple communications or large, tortuous draining channels, the fistula is best obliterated by opening the recipient cardiac chamber with the patient on bypass in order to completely close all fistulous tracts.

RESULTS. Thirty-eight patients with congenital coronary fistulas have been evaluated at the Duke University Medical Center, and 31 of these patients have had operative repair. The mean time of follow-up for these 31 patients has been 10 years.

There were no operative deaths, and all patients are well and do not have evidence of recurrent fistula formation, although one patient with a complex fistula of the circumflex coronary artery to the right ventricle has a small residual shunt.

CONGENITAL ORIGIN OF THE LEFT CORONARY ARTERY FROM THE PULMONARY ARTERY

Anomalous origin of the left coronary artery from the pulmonary artery is an unusual but important cause of congestive heart failure, mitral insufficiency, and left ventricular infarction in infants and children. Without surgical intervention, it has been estimated that 95% of patients with the left coronary artery originating from the pulmonary artery die within the first years of life.

CLINICAL MANIFESTATIONS. The vast majority of patients (90% or more) with anomalous origin of the left coronary artery from the pulmonary artery develop symptoms during infancy. The infant usually appears normal at birth, since the pulmonary artery pressure at this age is elevated and allows perfusion of the left coronary from the pulmonary artery for a brief period of time. Symptoms may be present at birth, especially if there are associated cardiac defects. Symptoms are most likely to occur during the first several months of life as left ventricular ischemia becomes more pronounced. The chief symptoms are intimately associated with the onset of heart failure and include dyspnea and tachycardia.

On physical examination the characteristic findings include a rapid respiratory rate, tachycardia, and cardiac enlargement. A murmur is not usually present early in life, and congenital origin of the left coronary artery from the pulmonary artery is one of the few malformations that in infancy can cause congestive heart failure *without* a murmur. The liver is characteristically enlarged, and the spleen is palpable in a smaller number of patients. Occasionally, patients first present with signs of cardiovascular collapse and shock similar to those manifested by adults with sudden coronary artery occlusion.

EVALUATION. Characteristic electrocardiographic changes can establish the diagnosis. The first description of myocardial ischemia on the electrocardiogram of an infant with this condition was made in 1933 by Bland and associates. Based on

the work, congenital origin of the left coronary artery from
the pulmonary artery also has been referred to as *Bland-White-
Garland syndrome*. On angiography, the right side of the heart
is usually normal. The pulmonary vasculature may show subpectoral engorgement and enlargement. The most striking
feature is enlargement of the left atrium and left ventricle.
The wall of the left ventricle may be quite thin, especially
on its anterolateral aspect near the apex. A true ventricular
aneurysm with paradoxical pulsations may be present, and
mitral insufficiency is quite common.

Contrast medium in the aorta demonstrates a single right
coronary artery, although selective coronary arteriography is
more reliable for precise demonstration of this feature. Right
ventricular and pulmonary artery pressures may be elevated.
It is usually possible to demonstrate left-to-right shunting at
the pulmonary artery level by contrast. Although the oxygen
saturation may at times show a significant increase from the
right ventricle to the pulmonary artery, this is not always
present, even when it can be demonstrated that the left coronary arises from the pulmonary artery.

SURGICAL MANAGEMENT. Simple ligation at the site of
origin from the pulmonary artery is useful in the very young
when the left coronary artery is quite small. Ligation at its
origin is effective if enough collaterals from the right coronary
exist to supply the left coronary system. Ligation prevents the
steal of right coronary collateral flow into the low-pressure
pulmonary system. If collateral flow from the right coronary
artery is inadequate, or if the patient is an older infant, the
initial repair can be designed to reconstruct a two-coronary-
artery system. This is best accomplished by either ligation and
saphenous vein bypass grafting or ligation and left or right
subclavian artery–left coronary artery anastomosis. In
younger children and infants, the latter form of therapy has
technical advantages, because in this group the subclavian
artery is usually larger than the autologous saphenous vein.
Direct implantation of the anomalous left coronary artery into
the root of the aorta is a method of establishing a two-coro-
nary-vessel circulation by recreating the normal anatomy. In
addition, a two-coronary-artery system also can be created by
intrapulmonary conduits from the left coronary ostium to the
aorta. Segments of saphenous vein, free subclavian arterial
grafts, flaps of pulmonary artery, pericardial tubes, and prosthetic conduits have all been used successfully, but their long-
term patency rates are unknown. Because of the 95% to 100%
mortality in those treated nonoperatively, surgical therapy is
always indicated following diagnosis.

ORIGIN OF THE RIGHT CORONARY
ARTERY FROM THE PULMONARY ARTERY

St. John Brooks in 1886 originally described this rare malformation in two cadavers. Both lesions occurred in adults, neither of whom had evidence of heart disease. Brooks noted
dilated collaterals from the left coronary artery feeding the
right coronary artery and correctly postulated, based on this

observation, that flow in the right coronary artery might actually be retrograde into the pulmonary artery.

CLINICAL MANIFESTATIONS. The clinical manifestations of this condition are usually minimal or absent. In 17 collected cases the abnormal artery was discovered in individuals whose age ranged from 17 to 90 years. The malformation was thought to have been associated with death in only 2 cases. Even though origin of the right coronary artery from the pulmonary artery is a rare anomaly with a benign natural history in most patients, it can lead occasionally to myocardial ischemia, infarction, congestive heart failure, and myocardial fibrosis. Because it can be corrected safely when diagnosed, operative correction may be indicated.

EVALUATION. In the rare patient with this condition who comes to medical attention, the diagnosis is established by aortography and selective coronary arteriography. The left coronary artery is found to be dilated, and large intercoronary collaterals supply the right coronary artery. Flow in the right coronary artery is retrograde, emptying into the pulmonary artery. Contrasting with patients who have the more frequently occurring malformation of origin or the left coronary artery from the pulmonary artery, there are usually no electrocardiographic or radiographic abnormalities.

SURGICAL MANAGEMENT AND RESULTS. At operation, a narrow rim of tissue from the pulmonary artery is removed with the origin of the right coronary artery and reimplanted into the ascending aorta. This is the ideal form of surgical management and has been performed with no operative or late mortality. Other alternatives include simple ligation at the site of anomalous origin with or without saphenous vein bypass grafting.

ORIGIN OF BOTH CORONARY ARTERIES FROM THE PULMONARY ARTERY

Twenty-five infants in whom both coronary arteries, the left and the right, arose from the pulmonary artery have been reported. The malformation has been diagnosed by cardiac catheterization, and surgical repair has been successful.

ANEURYSMS OF THE CORONARY ARTERIES

Congenital aneurysms of the coronary arteries are most often asymptomatic until complications occur. Complications include thrombosis or embolization with subsequent myocardial ischemia or infarction or actual rupture of the aneurysm. Surgical management of a coronary artery aneurysm is indicated if the aneurysm is symptomatic, especially if there is evidence of emboli arising from the aneurysm with production of myocardial ischemia in the distal coronary bed.

XVII

Acquired Disorders of the Aortic Valve and Subaortic Valve

David A. Fullerton, M.D., and Alden H. Harken, M.D.

AORTIC STENOSIS

PATHOLOGY. Acquired aortic stenosis usually results from calcification of the valve leaflets following rheumatic fever or from degeneration of the valve. Congenitally bicuspid aortic valves become stenotic in the sixth to eighth decades, when they calcify.

PATHOPHYSIOLOGY. Progressive narrowing of the aortic valve leads to pressure overload of the left ventricle. The ventricle hypertrophies, decreasing its compliance and requiring a higher left ventricular end-diastolic pressure (LVEDP) to generate the same volume of cardiac output. The ventricle is therefore very dependent on the atrial kick; loss of the atrial kick, as with atrial fibrillation, leads to acute hemodynamic decompensation. The aortic valve area is determined by the Gorlin formula. The Gorlin formula may be simplified to

$$\text{area (sq. cm.)} = \frac{}{\text{cardiac output (ml. per min.)}/\sqrt{\text{gradient (mm. Hg)}}}.$$

DIAGNOSIS AND MANAGEMENT. A harsh systolic murmur is best heard over the base of the heart and radiates to the carotids. The pulse uptake is slow. Echocardiography estimates the gradient (Δ) across the valve by $\Delta = 4(\text{velocity}^2)$. Patients become symptomatic once the valve area is less than 1 sq. cm. Survival is limited once symptoms of angina, syncope, or heart failure are present; aortic valve replacement is indicated. Operative risk is 2% to 8% and determined by left ventricular function and other comorbid factors.

AORTIC INSUFFICIENCY

PATHOLOGY. Aortic insufficiency usually results from rheumatic fever, annuloaortic ectasia, endocarditis, Marfan's syndrome, or aortic dissection.

PATHOPHYSIOLOGY. The valve leaks during diastole, creating a widened pulse pressure and volume overload of the left ventricle. The left ventricle dilates, increasing wall stress and oxygen demand, and ultimately fails.

DIAGNOSIS AND MANAGEMENT. The pulse pressure is wide and creates a waterhammer (Corrigan's) pulse. There

---

See the corresponding chapter or part in the *Textbook of Surgery*, 15th edition, pp. 2135–2143, for a more detailed discussion of this topic, including a comprehensive list of references.

is a diastolic murmur heard over the base of the heart. A diastolic rumble (Austin-Flint) may be heard. The diagnosis is confirmed by echocardiography. Patients may remain asymptomatic for many years or be managed with afterload reduction and diuretics. Ten-year survival exceeds 70%. But once the ventricle begins to dilate, irreversible left ventricular failure is imminent and survival limited. Aortic valve replacement should be performed before end-systolic dimension exceeds 55 mm. or end-systolic volume exceeds 90 ml. per sq. m.

HYPERTROPHIC OBSTRUCTIVE CARDIOMYOPATHY

PATHOLOGIC ANATOMY AND PATHOPHYSIOLOGY. There is asymmetric hypertrophy of the interventricular septum, most pronounced in its basilar portion. Left ventricular output into the aorta is obstructed by this mound of muscle, hypercontractility of the left ventricular muscle, and the anterior leaflet of the mitral valve as it is drawn into the left ventricular outflow tract.

DIAGNOSIS AND MANAGEMENT. A harsh crescendo-decrescendo systolic murmur is present, exaggerated by Valsalva maneuver and decreased by squatting. Echocardiogram is diagnostic. Mortality is 6% per year for adults, usually from sudden death. Medical therapy is with beta blockade and/or calcium antagonists. Surgery (resection of the septum or mitral valve replacement) is indicated for a gradient greater than 50 mm. Hg in patients refractory to medical therapy.

XVIII

Mitral and Tricuspid Valve Disease
Donald D. Glower, M.D.

NORMAL ANATOMY AND PHYSIOLOGY

The normal mitral valve consists of two leaflets (anterior and posterior) that attach to the ventricular wall and the anterolateral and posteromedial papillary muscles via fibrous chordae tendineae. The tricuspid valve is composed of three leaflets—anterior, posterior, and septal. Recent evidence has demonstrated that the mitral valve apparatus does contribute to left ventricular function by maintaining continuity between the papillary muscles and the mitral valve annulus via the chordae.

See the corresponding chapter or part in the *Textbook of Surgery,* 15th edition, pp. 2143–2156, for a more detailed discussion of this topic, including a comprehensive list of references.

MITRAL STENOSIS

PATHOPHYSIOLOGY AND DIAGNOSIS. The most common causes of mitral stenosis are rheumatic fever and calcific degeneration. The leaflets and chordae are generally thickened, fused, and calcified. Long-standing mitral stenosis may produce atrial fibrillation and pulmonary hypertension. Symptoms of mitral stenosis may include exertional dyspnea, orthopnea, and hemoptysis. On examination, patients may have peripheral edema, hepatojugular reflux, and sternal heave. Cardiac auscultation may reveal an accentuated pulmonary component of the second heart sound, an opening snap shortly after the second heart sound, and a mid-diastolic rumbling murmur.

Chest radiograph may demonstrate left atrial enlargement, cephalization of pulmonary blood flow, Kerley B-lines, or pulmonary edema. Two-dimensional echocardiography can demonstrate leaflet immobility and thickening of the leaflets and subvalvular apparatus. At cardiac catheterization, a diastolic pressure gradient (ΔP) across the mitral valve of 10 mm. Hg or a mitral orifice area of 1 sq. cm. per sq. m. indicates significant stenosis. Area is calculated as $F/(38/\sqrt{\Delta P})$, where F is average diastolic mitral flow (ml. per sec.).

TREATMENT AND RESULTS. Medical treatment of mitral stenosis includes endocarditis prophylaxis, diuretics, maintenance of sinus rhythm, and control of heart rate in atrial fibrillation. Indications for percutaneous or operative treatment are calculated mitral valve area of less than 1 sq. cm. per sq. m. with Class III or Class IV symptoms or onset of atrial fibrillation. Percutaneous balloon valvotomy is the procedure of choice for patients with mobile mitral valve leaflets, minimal calcification, less than 2+ regurgitation, no atrial thrombus, and minimal subvalvular scarring. Surgical closed commissurotomy, open commissurotomy, or mitral valve replacement is indicated for patients who are not candidates for balloon valvotomy. Operative mortality varies from 1% to 10% depending on the operation performed, age, and other comorbidity. Ten-year survival after open commissurotomy or mitral valve replacement is 80% or 60%, respectively.

MITRAL REGURGITATION

PATHOPHYSIOLOGY AND DIAGNOSIS. Etiologies for mitral regurgitation include rheumatic fever, mitral valve prolapse, endocarditis, calcific degeneration, myocardial infarction or ischemia, and hypertrophic obstructive cardiomyopathy. Mitral regurgitation generally is caused by annular dilatation, prolapse of the leaflet edges, or restriction of the leaflet edge motion. Chronic mitral regurgitation may produce atrial fibrillation and right ventricular failure. Patients may die from biventricular heart failure and pulmonary edema. Symptoms of mitral regurgitation include exertional dyspnea, orthopnea, peripheral edema, and angina. On examination, jugular venous distention, irregular pulse, and a holosystolic murmur radiating to the axilla may all be present. Chest radiograph may demonstrate left atrial and left ventricular enlargement, Kerley B-lines, and pulmonary edema. Echocardiography may quantify the severity of regurgitation while visualizing ruptured chordae, vegetations, leaflet thickening or prolapse, and valvular calcification. Left- and right-sided heart catheterization can assess right ventricular pressures, degree of regurgitation, and left ventricular function and volume.

TREATMENT AND RESULTS. Medical treatment for mitral regurgitation includes endocarditis prophylaxis, diuretics, vasodilators, and control of heart rate in atrial fibrillation. Operation is indicated for moderate or severe regurgitation with Class III or Class IV symptoms, onset of atrial fibrillation, or impairment of left ventricular function. Mitral valve repair may be appropriate for patients without significant fibrosis or calcification of the leaflets or subvalvular apparatus; otherwise, mitral valve replacement is the procedure of choice. Operative mortality is 2% to 5% for mitral valve repair and 4% to 10% for replacement. Left ventricular function may be better preserved after mitral valve repair or replacement with preservation of papillary-annular continuity. Survival after mitral valve repair or replacement is roughly 60% at 10 years.

TRICUSPID VALVE DISEASE

PATHOPHYSIOLOGY AND DIAGNOSIS. Tricuspid stenosis may result from rheumatic fever or carcinoid. Tricuspid regurgitation may result from rheumatic fever, endocarditis, or functional dilatation of the tricuspid annulus. Both tricuspid stenosis and regurgitation produce right atrial hypertension, pedal edema, ascites, and hepatic congestion. Examination may reveal jugular venous distention, hepatic enlargement, ascites, pedal edema, or hepatojugular reflux. Tricuspid regurgitation produces a holosystolic murmur augmented by inspiration, and tricuspid stenosis produces an opening snap and end-diastolic rumble also augmented by inspiration. Chest radiograph typically shows right atrial or right ventricular enlargement. Echocardiography may visualize leaflet thickening along with quantification of diastolic tricuspid gradient or degree of tricuspid regurgitation. Right-sided heart catheterization can directly assess the tricuspid valve diastolic gradient, which is significant at 5 mm. Hg or more.

TREATMENT AND RESULTS. Medical management of tricuspid valve disease includes endocarditis prophylaxis, diuretics, and regulation of atrial fibrillation. Indications for operation include moderate tricuspid stenosis or regurgitation concurrent with other valvular disease requiring operation or severe stenosis or regurgitation that is symptomatic or associated with onset of atrial fibrillation. Available procedures include tricuspid valve repair for functional regurgitation, tricuspid valve replacement, or rarely, tricuspid valvectomy for patients with isolated tricuspid endocarditis and recent intravenous drug abuse. Operative mortality varies from 5% to 20% depending on concurrent operations and ventricular function. Survival and freedom from reoperation after tricuspid valve repair or replacement are generally 50% at 10 years.

OPERATIVE TECHNIQUE

Tricuspid or mitral valve operations are generally performed through a median sternotomy, although right anterolateral thoracotomy may be useful in certain patients with previous median sternotomy. Open commissurotomy is appropriate for mitral stenosis with good leaflet mobility, minimal valvular calcification or fibrosis, and less than 2 + regurgitation. The left atrium is opened, any left atrial thrombus is removed, the mitral commissures are opened with sharp and blunt dissection, and fused chordae are mobilized.

Mitral valve repair is most commonly performed as described by Carpentier for valves with annular dilatation, leaflet prolapse, or chordal rupture. Redundant or flail posterior leaflet tissue is resected, elongated chordae are shortened, and a prosthetic ring annuloplasty is performed.

Mitral valve replacement is indicated for severely fibrosed or calcified valves. The left atrium is opened, thrombus removed, and the prosthetic valve inserted. The posterior, and possibly the anterior, leaflet should be preserved if possible to minimize postoperative left ventricular dysfunction.

Tricuspid valve operation is performed most commonly during reperfusion on cardiopulmonary bypass after a mitral valve procedure. The right atrium is opened and inspected. Annular dilatation is treated with ring annuloplasty, bicuspidization annuloplasty, or DeVega annuloplasty. Organic valvular disease generally requires insertion of a valve prosthesis.

VALVE SELECTION

Biological valves have advantages of low rates of thromboembolism and generally not needing anticoagulation, with the disadvantage of lesser durability. Choice of mechanical versus biological prostheses should be based on patient ability to comply with anticoagulation, likelihood of hemorrhagic complications, expected patient longevity, and valve position. Bioprostheses may be most appropriate in elderly patients in normal sinus rhythm, young women desiring pregnancy, and most patients requiring tricuspid valve replacement. Mechanical mitral valves are most appropriate for young patients and patients in chronic atrial fibrillation.

POSTOPERATIVE CARE

Patients with mechanical prostheses or with chronic atrial fibrillation should be maintained on chronic anticoagulation with an INR of 2.5 to 3.5 with or without additional low-dose aspirin. Patients in normal sinus rhythm undergoing valve repair or replacement with a biological prosthesis generally may be managed with postoperative aspirin alone.

XIX

Surgical Treatment of Cardiac Arrhythmias

James L. Cox, M.D.

The contemporary therapy of cardiac arrhythmias, including antiarrhythmic drugs, catheter ablation, and surgery, is capable of curing essentially all supraventricular and ventricular tachyarrhythmias. Although the indications for surgical intervention have narrowed during the past 5 years, surgery remains an important therapeutic modality for the treatment of cardiac arrhythmias, especially for the most common of all arrhythmias, atrial fibrillation.

ATRIAL FIBRILLATION

Atrial fibrillation is present in 0.4% to 2.0% of the general population and in approximately 10% of the population over the age of 60 years, making it the most common of all sustained cardiac arrhythmias. Although atrial fibrillation is frequently considered to be an innocuous arrhythmia, it is associated with significant morbidity and mortality because of its three detrimental sequelae: (1) an irregularly irregular heartbeat, which causes patient discomfort and anxiety, (2) loss of synchronous atrioventricular contraction, which compromises cardiac hemodynamics and results in varying levels of congestive heart failure, and (3) stasis of blood flow in the left atrium, which increases the patient's vulnerability to thromboembolism.

Until recently, elective His bundle ablation, either by open-heart surgery or by endocardial catheter techniques, was the only effective means of treating atrial fibrillation nonpharmacologically. However, since these procedures do not actually ablate atrial fibrillation, they control only the ventricular rate and rhythm during atrial fibrillation. Unfortunately, His bundle ablation does not protect the patient from the other detrimental effects of atrial fibrillation, that is, loss of the atrial "kick" and the increased vulnerability to thromboembolism.

In 1991, we described the first surgical procedure designed specifically to cure atrial fibrillation, the so-called maze procedure. The maze procedure is now considered to be the surgical treatment of choice for medically refractory atrial fibrillation.

See the corresponding chapter or part in the *Textbook of Surgery*, 15th edition, pp. 2156–2170, for a more detailed discussion of this topic, including a comprehensive list of references.

Anatomic-Electrophysiologic Basis

During the past few years, epicardial template electrodes on the atria has been employed, both experimentally and clinically. The results of the studies documented complete re-entrant loops in some instances and partial loops in others and demonstrated that the re-entrant wavefronts could move through the septum around the pulmonary veins, inferior vena cava, or superior vena cava. The importance of these experimental and clinical studies lies in the fact that they have documented unequivocally that atrial flutter and atrial fibrillation are due to intra-atrial re-entry as first suggested by Moe and that the concept of multifocal automaticity is not operative in the genesis or perpetuation of atrial fibrillation in humans.

Surgical Indications and Contraindications

The major indication for surgery is intolerance of the arrhythmia. Major symptoms in the group with paroxysmal (intermittent) atrial fibrillation include dyspnea on exertion, easy fatigability, lethargy, malaise, and a general sense of impending doom during the periods of atrial flutter/fibrillation. All patients who are considered for surgery must have failed the maximum amount of tolerable drug therapy preoperatively. In addition, approximately one-fourth of the patients in the series had experienced at least one episode of cerebral thromboembolism that resulted in significant temporary or permanent neurologic deficit. Contraindications to the maze procedure include the presence of significant left ventricular dysfunction, not attributable to the arrhythmia itself, and concomitant cardiac or noncardiac disease that constitutes an excessive surgical risk.

Preoperative Electrophysiology Evaluation

A preoperative endocardial catheter electrophysiology study is performed routinely in all patients with atrial flutter and in patients with paroxysmal atrial fibrillation. The primary purpose of the preoperative study is to document the function of the sinoatrial (SA) node, particularly in the atrial fibrillation patients, and to determine both SA node function and the site of the re-entrant circuit in patients with atrial flutter. Preoperative electrophysiology studies are not performed in patients with chronic atrial fibrillation because the SA node cannot be evaluated without electrical cardioversion, which we believe would introduce too great a risk of thromboembolism.

Surgical Results

Between September 25, 1987 and June 25, 1994, 32 patients had the maze I procedure, 15 had the maze II procedure, and 76 had the maze III procedure for the treatment of atrial flutter and/or atrial fibrillation. Once the atrium healed from surgery (3 months), the recurrent arrhythmia rate has been less than 10% overall and 0% in patients having the maze III procedure. Thus 90% of patients were cured of atrial fibrillation by the surgery alone, and 9% of patients were cured with a combination of surgery and postoperative medicine, an overall postoperative cure rate of 99%. In the patients who had the maze III procedure, 75% returned to a normal sinus rhythm postoperatively, and 25% required a permanent atrial pacemaker for sick sinus syndrome. The maze procedure itself resulted in injury of the sinus node in only 2 patients in the entire series.

WOLFF-PARKINSON-WHITE SYNDROME

The introduction of endocardial catheter techniques utilizing radiofrequency energy has had its most dramatic impact on the treatment of supraventricular arrhythmias due to the Wolff-Parkinson-White (WPW) syndrome. Nevertheless, occasional patients still present for surgery, thus requiring cardiac surgeons to maintain an understanding of the anatomy, physiology, and surgical techniques related to this abnormality. The WPW syndrome is characterized by the presence of an abnormal muscular connection between the atrium and ventricle ("accessory atrioventricular connection" or "accessory pathway") that is capable of conducting electrical activity. Since these patients also have a normal His bundle that connects the atria to the ventricles electrically, they have two routes by which an electrical impulse may travel between the atria and ventricles. For tachycardia to occur, antegrade (from the atrium to the ventricle) conduction across the accessory pathway must first be blocked.

Indications for Surgery

The major contemporary indication for surgical intervention in the WPW syndrome is failure of radiofrequency catheter ablation (RFCA). The dramatic change from surgical therapy to catheter ablative therapy can be appreciated by noting that during the past 45 months, we have operated on only 15 patients for the WPW syndrome, all of whom had failed multiple attempts at RFCA of the accessory pathway(s). Only a third of these patients were completely free of some type of associated anomaly capable of making RFCA either more difficult or totally impossible to accomplish successfully. The other patients had various anatomic abnormalities or variations in normal anatomy, including an anomalous coronary sinus, Ebstein's anomaly, cardiac hypertrophy, mitral regurgitation, coronary artery disease, catheter perforation of the right ventricle, or a small heart due to age. This surgical experience with failed RFCA suggests that if one cannot ablate an accessory pathway in a reasonable period of time, it is highly probable that some type of anatomic abnormality exists that precludes one from doing so. Thus electrophysiologists should exercise common sense in knowing when to terminate their attempts at RFCA, since too much local radiofrequency trauma and injury can render a patient surgically incurable.

Preoperative Electrophysiologic Evaluation

Patients who are now subjected to surgery for the WPW syndrome have first undergone an endocardial catheter electrophysiologic study in association with their failed attempt at RFCA. The most important information for the surgeon to know prior to surgery is the location of the accessory pathway, the technique and number of ablative attempts employed by the electrophysiologist during the attempted RFCA, and the associated (if any) anatomic abnormalities to be encountered during surgery.

Intraoperative Electrophysiologic Mapping

Computerized mapping systems have obviated the need to use cardiopulmonary bypass for the intraoperative mapping of patients with the WPW syndrome. Antegrade and retrograde computerized mapping techniques are capable of detecting not only free wall pathways but also anterior septal and posterior septal accessory pathways. Accessory atrioventricular connections may be located anywhere around the anulus fibrosis of the heart except between the right and left fibrous trigones. However, from a surgical standpoint, their locations are classified, in decreasing order of frequency, as (1) left free wall, (2) posterior septal, (3) right free wall, and (4) anterior septal. Two surgical approaches are commonly employed to divide accessory atrioventricular connections. The endocardial technique is designed to divide the ventricular end of the accessory pathway, and the epicardial technique is directed toward division of the atrial end of the pathway. The results with both approaches are excellent, with virtual assurance of surgical cure of the abnormality.

PAROXYSMAL SUPRAVENTRICULAR TACHYCARDIA (PSVT)

PSVT is a clinical condition in which supraventricular tachycardia occurs suddenly in a patient who otherwise has a normal electrocardiogram (ECG). There are two abnormalities that account for essentially all PSVT: a concealed accessory atrioventricular connection and AV node re-entry.

Concealed Accessory Pathway

Accessory atrioventricular connections may be manifest or concealed. If an accessory pathway is capable of conducting in the antegrade (atrial-to-ventricular) direction, thereby causing a delta wave on the standard ECG, it is said to be *manifest*; that is, its presence is apparent electrocardiographically. Some patients harbor accessory atrioventricular connections that are capable of conducting in the retrograde direction only. Since antegrade conduction across the accessory pathway does not occur, the ventricles are activated only through the normal AV node–His bundle complex, and the standard ECG is normal. Therefore, such accessory pathways are said to be *concealed.* The surgical technique employed to divide concealed accessory pathways is the same as for patients with the classic WPW syndrome.

AV NODE RE-ENTRY TACHYCARDIA

AV node re-entry tachycardia is caused by a re-entrant circuit that is confined to the AV node or to the perinodal tissues of the lower atrial septum. The anatomic-electrophysiologic basis for this re-entrant circuit is the presence of two functional conduction pathways, one slow and one fast, through the AV node, the so-called dual AV node conduction pathways. During supraventricular tachycardia, antegrade conduction proceeds through the slow pathway and retrograde conduction through the fast pathway due to proximal antegrade block in the fast pathway. This results in nearly simultaneous activation of the ventricles and atria.

Surgical Indications and Contraindications

The surgical techniques designed to cure AV node re-entry tachycardia enjoyed excellent results. There were no operative deaths in any of the three major series reported. Following the perinodal cryosurgical procedure, smooth AV node conduction curves through the remaining single conduction pathway were demonstrated in all patients in our series, and none of the patients had inducible AV node re-entry tachycardia postoperatively. Presently, however, radiofrequency catheter techniques have replaced surgery as the procedure of choice for AV node re-entry tachycardia.

AUTOMATIC ATRIAL TACHYCARDIAS

Automatic atrial tachycardia is caused by an automatic focus of arrhythmogenic tissue lying outside the region of the normal anatomic SA node. Histologic examination of the atrial tissue excised at the site of origin of automatic atrial tachycardias has not revealed a specific finding common to all patients. Automatic atrial tachycardias frequently occur in pediatric patients, in whom the tachycardia may be asymptomatic or may present with vomiting and epigastric pain. Adult patients more commonly present with palpitations, presyncope, syncope, or symptoms of congestive heart failure. In patients with automatic atrial tachycardia, the standard ECG demonstrates a P-wave morphologic pattern that is different from that seen in sinus rhythm, suggesting the presence of an ectopic focus remote from the sinus node. Of the 125 patients with automatic atrial tachycardia reported to date, the location of the automatic focus was specified in 89 patients. Sixty-one (68%) were located in the right atrial free wall, 5 (6%) within the atrial septum, and the remaining 23 (26%) within the left atrium. If the site of origin of an automatic atrial tachycardia can be localized precisely by intraoperative mapping, the arrhythmogenic focus may be either excised or cryoablated. Automatic foci located in the free wall of the left atrium or in either of the atrial appendages are ideal for excision or cryoblation. Automatic atrial tachycardias arising near the orifices of the pulmonary veins are best treated either by pulmonary vein isolation or by left atrial isolation. Electrophysiology-guided operative procedures have been performed in 63 of the 125 patients available for review. Fifty-six (89%) have been completely cured without the need for permanent pacemaker implantation or postoperative antiarrhythmic therapy.

ARRHYTHMOGENIC RIGHT VENTRICULAR DYSPLASIA

Fontaine and associates described a previously unrecognized form of cardiomyopathy localized to the right ventricle which they termed *arrhythmogenic right ventricular dysplasia*. This syndrome is a congenital cardiomyopathy characterized by transmural infiltration of adipose tissue resulting in weakness and aneurysmal bulging of the infundibulum, apex, and/or posterior basilar region of the right ventricle. The syndrome is characterized clinically by intractable ventricular tachycardia originating from one or all of the three pathologic areas of the right ventricle. Our current approach to such patients employs a transmural encircling ventriculotomy that effectively isolates the arrhythmogenic myocardium from the remainder of the heart.

LONG Q-T SYNDROME

Ventricular tachycardia that occurs in association with the long Q-T syndrome is frequently of a distinct type called *torsades de pointes*. This term is derived from the appearance of the ventricular tachycardia on a standard ECG, on which the polarity of the tachycardia is inconstant. One of the most frequent causes of *torsades de pointes* is the administration of medications that prolong ventricular repolarization, particularly quinidine. The surgical treatment of recurrent ventricular tachycardia associated with long Q-T syndrome has centered around efforts to modify cardiac innervation. Left stellate ganglion resection has been reported to abolish symptoms in many patients with the long Q-T syndrome. However, our experience and that of others has been characterized by early success and late failure.

ISCHEMIC VENTRICULAR TACHYCARDIA

Anatomic-Electrophysiologic Basis

The arrhythmogenic regions of most re-entrant ischemic ventricular tachycardias are located in the endocardium and subendocardium, especially at the periphery of myocardial infarcts or ventricular aneurysms. Electrical activity is thought to be identifiable as part of the re-entrant tachycardia circuit if it precedes the onset of ventricular depolarization evident on the surface ECG and is required for the initiation and perpetuation of the tachycardia. The site of origin of the tachycardia is felt to be the area exhibiting the earliest presystolic electrical activity in the latter half of diastole and represents the region of myocardium that must be identified and removed at the time of surgery in order to prevent the arrhythmias.

Preoperative Electrophysiologic Evaluation

All patients who are to undergo surgical therapy for ventricular tachyarrhythmias should first undergo an endocardial catheter electrophysiology study. The objectives of the preoperative study are (1) confirmation that the arrhythmia is ventricular rather than supraventricular in origin, (2) demonstration that the ventricular arrhythmia can be induced and terminated by programmed electrical stimulation techniques (i.e., that it is a re-entrant arrhythmia), and (3) localization of the region of origin of the ventricular tachycardia by "catheter mapping" when possible. In addition to the preoperative electrophysiology study, patients with ventricular tachyarrhythmias routinely undergo cardiac catheterization and coronary angiography prior to surgical intervention.

Intraoperative Electrophysiologic Mapping

In patients undergoing surgery for ventricular tachyarrhythmias, the first step intraoperatively is to perform detailed electrophysiologic mapping procedures to guide the specific surgical technique to be employed.

Surgical Technique

MAP-GUIDED SURGERY. First, localize the site(s) of origin of the ventricular tachycardia. Then, with the heart in the normothermic beating state, preferably during ventricular tachycardia, the ventricle is opened through the infarct or aneurysm, and all the associated endocardial fibrosis is resected except that which extends onto the base of the papillary muscles. After resecting all visible endocardial fibrosis, endocardial cryolesions are applied to the site(s) of origin of the tachycardia as determined by the intraoperative mapping. The cryothermia is applied only after removal of the endocardial scar because, in our experience, approximately 10% of patients will still have inducible ventricular tachycardia intraoperatively after removal of all visible endocardial fibrosis. Once the extended endocardial resection and subsequent endocardial cryoablation have been completed, programmed electrical stimulation is applied in an attempt to reinduce the arrhythmia. If ventricular tachycardia is still inducible, it is again mapped and the remaining arrhythmogenic myocardium is cryoablated. If the arrhythmia is no longer inducible, the author feels confident that it has been permanently ablated. If other procedures are to be performed, such as coronary bypass grafting, they are then carried out under cardioplegic arrest.

REPAIR OF LEFT VENTRICULAR ANEURYSMS WITHOUT MAP GUIDANCE. During the past few years, two entirely new surgical techniques have been developed for the surgical resection and repair of left ventricular aneurysms. Both these techniques attempt to restore the normal contour of the left ventricle, eliminate the adverse effects of the septal component of the aneurysm, and realign the myofibrils of the left ventricular free wall to restore their optimal contractile function. The functional improvement of the left ventricle following either of these two procedures has been dramatic and remarkable when compared with the old technique of simply resecting the aneurysm and closing the ventricle. Of great interest is the unexpected observation that both these procedures appear to cure any ventricular tachyarrhythmias associated with the aneurysm. The surgical results include an operative mortality rate of 2% to 3% (comparable with that of ICDs), even in higher-risk patients, and a ventricular tachycardia cure rate of approximately 98%. Since these techniques are apparently capable of eliminating ventricular tachycardia and restoring cardiac function with operative mortality and recurrence rates comparable with those attained with ICDs, it is expected that the window of indications for the surgical treatment of ventricular tachycardia may again broaden.

XX

Cardiac Neoplasms

Norman A. Silverman, M.D.,
and David C. Sabiston, Jr., M.D.

Noninvasive imaging modalities have allowed cardiac tumors to evolve from pathologic curiosities to a surgically curable form of heart disease.

INCIDENCE AND CLINICAL PRESENTATION

Primary cardiac tumors are rare, having been found in 0.002% and 0.33% of autopsies. Eighty per cent of these tumors are benign, with myxoma being by far the most common. Primary malignancies are predominantly various forms of sarcoma. Cancer metastatic to the heart is, in contrast, increas-

---

See the corresponding chapter or part in the *Textbook of Surgery*, 15th edition, pp. 2170–2175, for a more detailed discussion of this topic, including a comprehensive list of references.

ingly common and is found in 10% to 20% of patients with known malignancy. Cardiac performance is compromised when an intracavitary tumor obstructs blood flow or prevents normal valvular function and when an intramural tumor infiltrates the ventricular myocardium. Systemic emboli are frequent with left atrial myxoma, but right-sided heart tumors also can embolize the pulmonary arteries. Particularly in the pediatric age group, these lesions cause recurrent dysrhythmias or injure the conduction system. Most intriguing are the systemic constitutional symptoms of fever, malaise, weight loss, polymyositis, and hepatic dysfunction associated with left atrial myxomas attributable to an autoimmune response.

DIAGNOSTIC MODALITIES

Echocardiography is the technique of choice in the initial evaluation of intracardiac tumors, providing real-time imaging of all cardiac chambers and more precise quantitation of tumor size and location. In selected patients, computed tomography (CT) is a valuable alternative for imaging the myocardial and intrapericardial extension of tumor not well visualized by ultrasonography. Magnetic resonance imaging (MRI) is a newer technique that also enables high-resolution tomography in three dimensions, but its cost precludes routine use. Invasive procedures risk tumor dislodgment and should be avoided.

BENIGN TUMORS

Myxomas constitute 50% of benign primary cardiac tumors. Seventy-five per cent originate in the left atrium, and 20% occur in the right atrium. Ventricular myxomas are rare. The majority of myxomas are solitary lesions unless associated with a familial syndrome characterized by multicentricity, skin lesions, and endocrine tumors. Myxomas rarely can undergo malignant degeneration. By obstructing the mitral orifice and embolizing, left atrial myxomas frequently masquerade as rheumatic mitral stenosis. When constitutional symptoms predominate, infective endocarditis, collagen-vascular disease, and occult malignancy or infection enter the differential diagnosis. Right atrial myxomas produce signs and symptoms of right-sided heart failure by obstructing vena caval return or the tricuspid valve orifice. Ventricular myxomas may induce syncope due to transient obstruction of the outflow tract.

Rhabdomyoma is a hamartoma and the most common cardiac tumor of childhood. These lesions are most often multicentric ventricular masses that cause recurrent tachyarrhythmias and have a poor prognosis. In contrast, the rare cardiac *fibromas* are well-circumscribed, solitary ventricular tumors of childhood that are more amenable to surgical cure. Tumors of fatty, blood vessel, and nerve cell or sheath origin also have been reported to arise from the heart. The diagnosis of primary cardiac tumor mandates prompt operative intervention. After complete tumor resection, the prognosis is excellent, with complete symptomatic relief and less than 1% recurrence.

PRIMARY MALIGNANT AND METASTATIC TUMORS

Primary malignancies are sarcomatous lesions usually originating from the right side of the heart. The characteristic clinical presentation is progressive, unrelenting congestive heart failure, cardiomegaly, chest pain, fever, hemopericardium, and arrhythmia. Unfortunately, the growth pattern of these lesions makes them unresectable, and irradiation and chemotherapy have been ineffective. Tumors that most frequently metastasize to the heart include lung and breast carcinoma as well as leukemia, lymphoma, and melanoma. Pericardial metastases cause tamponade or constriction. Myocardial metastases often cause rhythm disturbances or congestive heart failure. Surgical intervention is indicated to decompress symptomatic pericardial effusion.

XXI

Cardiac Pacemakers
James E. Lowe, M.D.

Artificial pacing has clearly prolonged and improved the lives of thousands of patients with symptomatic bradyarrhythmias. The recognition of this impact on patient care has steadily increased pacemaker implantations worldwide. In the United States, approximately 360 pacemakers are inserted annually per 1 million population, and this has been increasing at a rate of about 19 implants per million per year. Analysis of trends since 1975 indicates an increasing awareness of the benefits of pacing in patients with sinus node dysfunction. Implantation of a pacemaker for sinus node dysfunction accounted for 23% of primary implants in 1975 and 48% by 1989. Atrioventricular node and His-Purkinje conduction disturbances were indications for pacing in 45% of patients in 1989, drug-induced bradycardia in 4%, and tachyarrhythmias in 2%. Furthermore, there has been an increasing dependence on dual-chamber pacing in a number of clinical conditions as the multiple benefits of this pacing modality are demonstrated. It is estimated that over 30% of pacemakers implanted today are dual-chamber devices, and this percentage is anticipated to increase further in the next decade. In addition, the availability of various sensors to increase the pacemaker rate during periods of physiologic stress have improved exercise capabilities in patients receiving pacemakers. Single-chamber,

See the corresponding chapter or part in the *Textbook of Surgery*, 15th edition, pp. 2175–2198, for a more detailed discussion of this topic, including a comprehensive list of references.

rate-responsive devices now account for another third of all pacemakers implanted. As pacemaker technology continues to improve, new indications for pacemakers are identified, and the percentage of the elderly in the population increases, it is anticipated that the need for permanent pacemakers will continue to increase.

Although there is still some controversy regarding indications for permanent cardiac pacing as well as the type of pacing system chosen, most physicians would agree with the following guidelines.

INDICATIONS FOR PERMANENT PACING

Implantation of a permanent pacemaker commits the patient to a lifetime with an implantable device, with its associated costs, inconveniences, and potential complications. Therefore, the decision to implant a permanent pacemaker must consider both the benefits and the risks and complications associated with its use. Fortunately, pacemaker and lead technology and implantation techniques have been so greatly improved that the acute and long-term risks associated with permanent pacemakers are small. Nonetheless, the decision to implant a permanent pacemaker needs to be made with the aim of improving the patient's quality of life and longevity.

Because controversy exists about appropriate indications for implantation of a permanent pacemaker, guidelines have been written by a task force of the American College of Cardiology and American Heart Association (Committee of Pacemaker Implantation, 1991). Indications for permanent pacemaker implantation have been grouped in this report into three classifications:

Class I: Conditions for which there is general agreement that a permanent pacemaker should be implanted.

Class II: Conditions for which permanent pacemakers are frequently used but in which there may be a divergence of opinion with respect to the necessity of their implantation.

Class III: Conditions in which there is general agreement that permanent pacemaker implantation is not indicated.

Thus Class I and II indications are those in which the patient definitely or probably benefits from implantation of permanent pacemaker, whereas in Class III indications, there is no or minimal potential benefit to the patient.

Acquired Atrioventricular (AV) Block in Adults

Before permanent pacemakers were available, 50% of patients with complete heart block died within 1 year. The most common cause of acquired complete heart block is sclerodegenerative disease of the cardiac skeleton and AV conduction system. Other causes of complete heart block include ischemic heart disease, cardiomyopathic processes, Chagas' disease, and traumatic injury. Permanent pacemaker implantation is indicated in any patient with symptomatic complete, high-grade, or second-degree AV block. Symptoms include congestive heart failure, altered mental status, or other end-organ failure, particularly if it can be shown that temporary pacing improves the symptom. Permanent pacing is usually recommended for surgically induced complete heart block that persists more than 1 week after the operation. Symptomatic complete or high-grade AV block in the setting of atrial fibrillation or other atrial tachyarrhythmias is also an indication unless the AV block is due to digitalis or other drugs and these drugs are not necessary for the patient's management. In patients with second-degree AV block, symptoms should be shown to be related to the episodes of AV block. Patients with asymptomatic Mobitz Type II are frequently considered to benefit from permanent pacing, given the high risk for development of complete heart block in these patients. Patients with Wenckebach (Mobitz Type I) second-degree AV block shown to be due to block in or below the His bundle during electrophysiologic testing are also candidates for permanent pacing because their risk for developing complete heart block is similar to that of patients with classic Mobitz Type II second-degree AV block. Patients with Wenckebach second-degree AV block due to intra- or infra-Hisian Wenckebach conduction patterns usually have associated bundle-branch block. Wenckebach second-degree AV block with a narrow QRS complex is almost always due to AV nodal block, and three-fourths of the cases associated with bundle-branch block are also due to AV nodal block and thus are not indications for permanent pacemaker implantation.

AV Block after Myocardial Infarction

Unlike those for acquired AV block in other conditions, indications for permanent pacemaker implantation in the setting of recent myocardial infarction do not necessarily require the presence of symptoms. Patients with persistent complete or high-grade AV block after myocardial infarction, whether associated with symptoms or not, should be permanently paced given their poor prognosis. In addition, patients with transient complete heart block during acute myocardial infarction who have persistent bundle-branch block have been shown in some studies to have a high risk of late complete heart block and thus should be permanently paced. Because alternating bundle-branch blocks have high rates of progression to complete heart block, they also should be permanently paced, even if episodes of transient complete or high-grade AV block have not been documented.

Chronic Bifascicular and Trifascicular Block

Bifascicular and trifascicular blocks suggest extensive damage to the His bundle and bundle branches. Although the overall risk for progression to permanent or symptomatic complete heart block is low, certain patients with bi- and trifascicular blocks are at considerably higher risks. Patients with bi- or trifascicular block with intermittent complete heart block, high-grade AV block, or Mobitz Type II second-degree AV block represent such a high-risk group and should undergo permanent pacemaker implantation. Because syncope is the usual symptom associated with transient complete or high-grade AV block, patients with syncope and bi- or trifascicular block should undergo electrophysiologic testing to determine if infra-Hisian block can be induced by pacing, in which case a pacemaker should be implanted. It also has been suggested that even asymptomatic patients with a markedly prolonged infranodal conduction time (HV interval > 100 msec.) should undergo prophylactic permanent pacing, given their high risk for progression to complete heart block. Even in the absence of pacing-induced infra-Hisian block or a markedly prolonged HV interval, patients with syncope and bi- or trifascicular block in whom a cause for syncope cannot be identified with extensive testing should receive a permanent pacemaker, given the high probability that their syncope was secondary to a high-grade though transient conduction disturbance and their potential increased risk of death from a bradyarrhythmia. Although patients with bi- and trifascicular disease have a relatively high mortality rate, this is largely due to the underlying heart disease that caused the conduction disorder, not to the development of complete heart block. Thus routine implantation of pacemakers in asymptomatic patients with bi- and trifascicular block is not indicated.

Sinus Node Dysfunction

Patients with sinus node dysfunction may develop a number of arrhythmias, such as inappropriate sinus bradycardia, chronotropic incompetence, sinoatrial exit block, and sinus arrest. This group of rhythm disorders typically occurs in older patients with or without underlying heart disease and is collectively known as the *sick sinus syndrome*. In addition, many patients with sick sinus syndrome have associated atrial tachyarrhythmias, particularly atrial fibrillation. This association of atrial tachyarrhythmias in patients with the sick sinus syndrome is called the *tachycardia-bradycardia* (or *tachy-brady*) *syndrome*. Patients with symptomatic bradycardia not due to reversible causes are candidates for permanent pacing. In addition, patients with the tachycardia-bradycardia syndrome frequently require digitalis, other AV nodal blocking agents, or antiarrhythmic drugs to control atrial tachyarrhythmias, which cause an exaggerated suppression of sinus node function. If these drugs are not avoidable in this situation, then permanent pacing will be needed to protect against drug-induced bradycardia. Some patients with intermittent symptoms suggestive of bradycardia and documented bradycardias with rates less than 40 beats per minute but in whom the symptoms have not been documented to occur with bradycardia may be candidates for permanent pacing. However, a concerted effort should be made to confirm the presence of bradycardia with symptoms.

Neurovascular Syndromes

Several neurovascular syndromes cause exaggerated para-sympathetic tone with resultant sinus bradycardia, asystole, and transient high-grade AV block (cardioinhibitory effect). In addition, reflex withdrawal of sympathetic tone may further exacerbate the bradyarrhythmias and also cause profound vasodilation (vasodepressor effect), sometimes without significant bradyarrhythmias. The most common of these syndromes is the carotid sinus hypersensitivity syndrome, when it is associated with a significant cardioinhibitory response and syncope. In these patients, mild carotid sinus massage will cause significant asystole (> 3 sec.). Some individuals, however, may have a hypersensitive response to carotid sinus massage and remain asymptomatic. For this reason, it is useful to document significant bradyarrhythmia during a spontaneous episode of syncope or near-syncope in patients suspected of having carotid sinus hypersensitivity syndrome. However, in some patients with recurrent syncope, clear documentation of bradycardia during a spontaneous episode is not possible, although demonstration of a hypersensitive response to carotid massage suggests the diagnosis. The most common neurovascular syndrome is the neurally mediated syncope syndrome, which results from an exaggerated Bezold-Jarisch reflex induced when relative hypovolemia and increased sympathetic tone create left ventricular chamber obliteration during systole. Some patients may have palliation of symptoms with permanent pacing to alleviate the bradycardia component of the Bezold-Jarisch reflex if temporary pacing demonstrates improvement in symptoms during provocative tilt table testing.

Tachyarrhythmias

Permanent pacing can be useful in some cases of medically refractory supraventricular and ventricular tachycardia if pacing the atria or ventricles, respectively, at tolerated rates above the intrinsic heart rate prevents arrhythmia recurrence (overdrive suppression). However, a prolonged period of overdrive suppression using a temporary pacemaker should be tried before implanting a permanent pacemaker to demonstrate the efficacy of this approach. Patients with symptoms and *torsades de pointes* can be treated effectively with overdrive pacing if reversible causes are not found. Permanent pacemakers have been designed to detect and terminate with pacing both supraventricular and ventricular tachycardias. With the advent of highly effective catheter ablation techniques for treatment of paroxysmal supraventricular tachycardias, the use of pacemakers for overdrive suppression or termination of supraventricular tachycardias is rarely needed. Pacemakers that only pace terminate ventricular tachycardia can accelerate the tachycardia to a poorly tolerated ventricular tachycardia or fibrillation. These have been incorporated as part of implantable defibrillators to administer high-energy shocks if pacing causes degeneration of an initially hemodynamically stable arrhythmia.

Intractable Congestive Heart Failure and Cerebral or Renal Insufficiency Benefited by Temporary Pacing

Patients with refractory congestive heart failure and decreased perfusion causing cerebral or renal insufficiency may be improved occasionally by increasing heart rate with temporary pacing. If temporary pacing has proved to be effective under these conditions and long-term therapy is indicated, permanent pacing should be considered. Most of these patients require atrial contraction to improve cardiac output. Therefore, dual-chamber atrial synchronous pacing is usually indicated in this subgroup. Recent studies have suggested that AV sequential pacing with relatively short AV intervals may improve left ventricular function in patients with dilated cardiomyopathies without overt bradycardia, but further evaluation of this phenomenon is needed before this indication can be recommended. Patients with hypertrophic obstructive cardiomyopathy are also favorably influenced by ventricular pacing, presumably because of the asyneresis induced by pacing the ventricular apex that partially alleviates outflow tract obstruction.

THE IMPULSE GENERATOR

An implantable cardiac pacemaker consists of an impulse generator, lead wire, and electrode. The impulse generator contains a power source or battery, hybrid circuits, and a lead connector. All these components are kept in a hermetically sealed metal container. The size and weight of the impulse generator depend on the size of the battery and the number of electronic components. Impulse generators are usually kept in rectangular or oval packages with rounded edges and weigh between 20 and 50 gm.

PHYSIOLOGY OF PACING

Perhaps the most dramatic example of the advancement in pacemaker technology is the various ways in which the heart can be paced. The way in which an impulse generator functions is referred to as the *pacing mode*. An accurate description of pacing mode must convey not only the chamber of the heart that is being paced but also the chamber sensed by the pacemaker and the manner in which the pacemaker responds to sensed activity. Simple descriptive terms such as *ventricular-demand pacemaker* sufficed well for single-chamber devices but have become more awkward as the complexity of pacemakers increases. Devices that pace and sense both atrial and ventricular activity are now frequently implanted. To meet the need for a uniform method of describing pacemaker function, the Intersociety Commission for Heart Disease Resources (ICHD) recommended a five-letter code that succinctly and accurately describes various pacing modes.

The ICHD code uses the letters A and V for atrium and ventricle. The letter D stands for dual, indicating both chambers, or, when indicating a mode of response, more than one mode. The two traditional response modes to sensed activity, either inhibition or triggering, are indicated by I and T. When no function or response is possible, the letter O is used. In the three-letter code system, the first letter designates the chamber(s) paced, the second letter the chamber(s) sensed, and the third letter the mode of response of the pacemaker to sensed activity. Thus a pacemaker that paces only the ventricle senses ventricular activity when intrinsic beats are present and it responds to the sensed activity by inhibiting its output (the well-known ventricular-demand pacemaker) is designated VVI in the ICHD code. An asynchronous ventricular pacemaker that does not sense but that paces at a constant rate regardless of intrinsic cardiac rhythm would be designated VOO (the ventricle is paced, neither chamber is sensed, and there is therefore no response mode to sensed events). In the case of the standard AV sequential pacemaker, in which both the atrium and ventricle are paced but only ventricular activity is sensed, the designation is DVI.

XXII

The Use of Cardiovascular Pharmacologic Agents in Surgical Patients

Jeffrey H. Lawson, M.D., Ph.D.,
and Robert W. Anderson, M.D.

Recent advances in medical care have lead to changes in the population of patients who are referred for surgical treatment. Many patients are now older and have multiple medical problems, which often include cardiovascular disease. Optimal surgical care of these patients requires that the surgeon be knowledgeable about the basic principles of cardiovascular pharmacology. This chapter outlines basic aspects of cardiovascular pharmacology so that appropriate treatment plans for these patients can be formed.

The first aspect of patient care prior to any surgical procedure or use of cardiovascular drugs is an assessment of the

See the corresponding chapter or part in the *Textbook of Surgery*, 15th edition, pp. 2198–2209, for a more detailed discussion of this topic, including a comprehensive list of references.

patient's overall health and cardiovascular status. When a careful history and physical examination are placed into the context of the planned surgical procedure, an assessment of cardiovascular risk can be formulated. No further preoperative workup is required for low-risk patients who plan to undergo routine surgical procedures. As a patient's cardiovascular risk increases, judicial preoperative testing of the patient's cardiovascular health is indicated to specifically define and treat the cardiovascular defect prior to the surgical procedure. If a specific cardiovascular defect is identified prior to surgery, cardiovascular therapeutics can then be used in operative management of the surgical patient.

The categories of drugs that are commonly used in the management of cardiovascular diseases include (1) antihypertensives and diuretics, (2) agents for the management of congestive heart failure, (3) antianginal drugs, (4) inotropic drugs, (5) antiarrhythmics, and (6) anticoagulants.

ANTIHYPERTENSIVES AND DIURETICS

Hypertension is a common problem, and the number of patients being treated for this disorder has increased substantially during the past two decades. Antihypertensive drugs function by disrupting normal physiologic pathways that regulate vascular pressure. For this reason, these agents may be potentially dangerous in surgical patients, in whom the stress of disease and the use of general anesthetic agents may unmask potentially hazardous physiologic responses.

Diuretic agents, such as the thiazides and furosemide, are employed most commonly for the treatment of mild or moderate hypertension. These agents increase the urinary excretion of salt and water, which may lead to hypovolemia, tachycardia, and hypotension when anesthetics are administered that blunt the normal homeostatic response to decreasing blood pressure. In addition, hypokalemia may occur following the chronic administration of diuretics, which can lead to cardiac arrhythmias if total body potassium stores are not repleted.

Adrenergic inhibitors are drugs that inhibit specific actions of the sympathetic nervous system reflex arc. Peripherally acting agents such as reserpine and guanethidine may depress cardiac output and result in hypotension by blunting the normal sympathetic response to volume depletion and general anesthetic agents. This problem is not observed with centrally acting adrenergic inhibitors such as clonidine, which are much better tolerated during anesthetic administration. Because abrupt withdrawal of adrenergic inhibitors may lead to a rebound hypertensive crisis in the perioperative period, caution must be used if discontinuation of these drugs is required.

Beta blockers are well tolerated in surgical patients and offer a significant degree of protection from postoperative cardiac rhythm disturbances and rebound hypertension. It is usually safe to continue beta-blocker use during the perioperative period and to utilize specific beta agonists if hypotension or bradycardia develops. Abrupt withdrawal of beta blockers has been associated with acute myocardial infarction and should be avoided.

Alpha-receptor antagonists are rarely used in the management of uncomplicated hypertension. Patients taking agents such as prazosin, phenoxybenzamine, or phentolamine may develop a relative volume loss, which often requires preoperative fluid replacement. When possible, alpha-receptor antagonists should be discontinued prior to performing any elective surgical procedure unless specific indications exist, such as a pheochromocytoma, that require the continuation of these agents.

Vasodilators are rarely used in the management of chronic hypertension. Hydralazine, if given without a beta blocker, will commonly elicit reflex tachycardia, limiting its usefulness. Nitroprusside administered intravenously is the agent of choice for the treatment of hypertensive emergencies but should be used only under conditions of proper intraoperative or intensive care unit monitoring.

Angiotensin-converting enzyme inhibitors are useful in the treatment of hypertension in patients with elevated renin levels. These agents lower total peripheral vascular resistance and appear not to interfere with normal cardiovascular responses to anesthesia or volume shifts during the operative period. Because abrupt withdrawal of these agents may result in severe hypertension, these agents should be continued throughout the operative period, if possible.

Calcium antagonists selectively block the movement of calcium across the intracellular membranes. These agents have become widely used in the management of hypertension, cardiac arrhythmias, and angina. Nifedipine has strong peripheral vasodilatory effects and has become very popular in the treatment of uncomplicated hypertension. For minor surgical procedures, it is reasonable to continue most patients on their regular dose of calcium-channel blockers. For major noncardiac surgical procedures it is best to discontinue the agent prior to surgery and closely monitor the patient's hemodynamic status during the perioperative period. For patients who require aggressive calcium-channel blockade in the perioperative period, intravenous nicardipine is available. Due to its rapid onset and potent action, this agent is only recommended for use in the intensive care unit setting. In general, calcium antagonists are safe to use in the perioperative period, but one must pay close attention to the patient's hemodynamic and volume status when surgical patients are taking these agents.

AGENTS FOR THE MANAGEMENT OF CONGESTIVE HEART FAILURE

The management of congestive heart failure is best achieved by reduction in cardiac work through the use of vasodilators rather than stimulation of the failing heart with inotropic agents. Drugs that promote vasodilatation of the vascular smooth muscle improve the performance of the heart by decreasing peripheral vascular resistance. This causes a shift of the blood out of the central circulation to the peripheral venous capacitance beds, which decreases preload and end-diastolic volume in the heart. By enhancing stroke volume and ventricular emptying, the overall function of the failing heart improves.

When a surgical patient presents with evidence of congestive heart failure, a comprehensive evaluation of the patient's overall cardiac status is required. Optimal medical therapy, which includes the use of afterload-reducing agents and careful fluid management, should be instituted as soon as possible. Operative preparation also should include the judicious use of invasive intraoperative cardiovascular monitoring. With aggressive use of vasodilators and careful intraoperative fluid management, patients with congestive heart failure can undergo most surgical procedures safely; however, patients must be followed very carefully in the perioperative period for any evidence of cardiac dysfunction.

ANTIANGINAL DRUGS

Surgical patients with any history of ischemic heart disease must be evaluated thoroughly and managed optimally from a cardiac standpoint. Evaluation of the patient requires a careful history and physical examination, noninvasive cardiac testing, and if indicated, cardiac catheterization to identify clinically significant cardiac ischemia. Following a careful preoperative evaluation, the patient's medical therapy should be optimized to prevent a perioperative myocardial infarction. Furthermore, if severe coronary artery disease is identified, coronary artery revascularization should be considered prior to a large elective surgical procedure.

If the patient is managed medically, there are, in general, three classes of pharmacologic agents specifically used for the perioperative treatment of angina pectoris. These agents include nitrates, beta blockers, and calcium antagonists. Nitrates are the first-line agents for relief of anginal symptoms and present no particular risk to the patient at the time of the surgical procedure. If intraoperative nitrates are required, either the transdermal or intravenous nitrates are appropriate, depending on the magnitude of the operative procedure. Beta blockers are also useful to avoid myocardial stress associated with the operative procedure, particularly if the patient has been on a beta blocker preoperatively. Abrupt withdrawal of beta blockers should be avoided due to the possibility of induced cardiac arrhythmias or ischemic complications. Calcium antagonists are useful in patients with chronic obstructive pulmonary disease because these agents are not associated with side effects such as bronchospasm. Calcium antagonists, however, may produce profound hypovolemia following volume loss due to their powerful vasodilating effects on the peripheral vasculature. Therefore, these agents must be used with caution and appropriate intraoperative monitoring.

INOTROPIC DRUGS

Inotropic drugs play an important role in the management of heart failure patients with cardiovascular instability due to primary cardiac dysfunction or peripheral vascular disease. The most common agents used for inotropic stimulation include the digitalis compounds, the sympathomimetic amines, and the phosphodiesterase inhibitors. Digitalis compounds can be troublesome in surgical patients because of the toxic manifestations of these agents. Hypoxia and hypokalemia increase myocardial susceptibility to digitalis-induced ventricular arrhythmias. It is generally recommended to withhold digitalis compounds in the perioperative period and support the heart with safer inotropic agents. The sympathomimetic amines stimulate cardiac beta receptors, which augment the myocardial contractile system. Dopamine is the drug of choice for patients with myocardial failure who require inotropic support for hemodynamic stability. Dobutamine is a synthetic analog of dopamine with an inotropic effect on the heart and causes a mild peripheral vasodilatation. Dobutamine is useful in patients who have had long-standing myocardial failure in whom endogenous catecholamine levels are depressed as well as in patients with coronary artery disease undergoing general or cardiac surgical procedures. Phosphodiesterase inhibitors function by inhibiting intracellular phosphodiesterase type II, which leads to an increase in intracellular cyclic AMP. These compounds possess strong inotropic effects as well as causing arterial and venous dilatation. Amrinone and milrinone are both widely used and seem to be most effective in patients with low cardiac output and with mitral and aortic valve insufficiency. These agents are also useful in patients with severe congestive heart failure that is resistant to beta$_1$ stimulants.

ANTIARRHYTHMIC AGENTS

The surgical patient is predisposed to the development of cardiac arrhythmias because of the possible development of hypoxia, electrolyte abnormalities, cardiotoxicity of anesthetics, hemodynamic changes, anemia, and myocardial infarction. In surgical patients, initial therapy should always be directed toward the correction of any of these abnormalities. For cardiac arrhythmias that produce significant hemodynamic compromise, pharmacologic therapy should be initiated to control the nature of the rhythm disturbance.

Premature ventricular contractions are only significant if they occur more than 10 times a minute from a single focus, are multifocal, occur in couplets, or fall near the T wave. These ectopic beats may produce ventricular tachycardia or fibrillation and should be suppressed by the use of intravenous lidocaine. If lidocaine is ineffective, procainamide is a useful second-line agent.

Atrial dysrhythmias are common in the postoperative period. Initial therapy must always include the correction of any underlying electrolyte or metabolic abnormality. For atrial flutter and fibrillation, therapy should be directed toward slowing the ventricular response. Digoxin and atenolol are currently the drugs of choice for initial therapy. If patients are resistant to digoxin or atenolol or develop signs of hemodynamic compromise, cardioversion or the use of intravenous verapamil may be required to slow the ventricular response to the atrial dysrhythmias.

ANTICOAGULANTS

Most surgical patients with significant cardiac risk factors, cardiac dysrhythmias, or angina pectoris will be treated with anticoagulant therapy to decrease their risk for coronary artery thrombosis or cardiac embolism. The most common anticoagulant drugs used in cardiac patients are aspirin and Coumadin. Aspirin is widely used in patients with coronary artery disease due to its antiplatelet effects, while Coumadin is more commonly used in patients with atrial dysrhythmias, mechanical heart valves, or a history of deep venous thrombosis. For patients undergoing minor surgery, it is often safe to continue with aspirin therapy during the procedure, but only if proceeding with meticulous surgical hemostasis. When performing larger surgical procedures with patients on either aspirin or Coumadin, the risk of bleeding from the procedure must be weighed against the risk of thrombosis. If anticoagulation is required, then most patients should be converted to intravenous heparin therapy preoperatively. The surgical procedure can then be performed during a heparin window, where the level of anticoagulation can be easily titrated or reversed using protamine.

XXIII

Cardiopulmonary Bypass for Cardiac Surgery

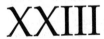

William L. Holman, M.D., David C. McGiffin, M.D., and James K. Kirklin, M.D.

PUMP OXYGENATOR APPARATUS FOR CARDIOPULMONARY BYPASS (CPB)

A *venous reservoir* stores excess volume and allows escape of air bubbles returning with venous blood. The *oxygenator* provides oxygen to the blood and eliminates carbon dioxide. Currently bubble oxygenators, membrane oxygenators, and microporous hollow-fiber oxygenators are available for clinical use. An efficient *heat exchanger* is necessary for control of the perfusate temperature to achieve systemic cooling and

---

See the corresponding chapter or part in the *Textbook of Surgery*, 15th edition, pp. 2209–2218, for a more detailed discussion of this topic, including a comprehensive list of references.

rewarming during CPB. The *arterial pump* is usually a roller pump.

PHYSIOLOGIC RESPONSE TO CARDIOPULMONARY BYPASS

Many complex physiologic changes occur when a patient is temporarily supported by means of an oxygenator system. Two main types of physiologic variables exist during CPB: *externally controlled variables,* which are controlled by the surgeon, anesthesiologist, and perfusionist, and *patient variables,* which are less easily regulated.

Externally Controlled Variables

The *perfusion flow rate* and *temperature of the perfusate* are variables controlled by the perfusionist under the direct guidance of the operating surgeon. We utilize some degree of hypothermia for nearly all cardiac operations, and we regard the decision as to perfusion temperature as one of the most important decisions to be made during CPB. Although no absolute criteria exist for safe flow rates at a given temperature, organ damage appears least likely to occur when the microvasculature is perfused at flows that maintain nearly normal tissue oxygen levels and maximal oxygen consumption. Experimental and clinical data indicate that normothermic perfusion flow rates of 1.7 L. per min. per sq. m. or greater are usually acceptable, but flow rates of 2.0 to 2.5 L. per min. per sq. m. provide a more secure margin of safety for organ perfusion.

During CPB the *systemic venous pressure* and *pulmonary venous pressure* (left atrial pressure) should be maintained near zero on total cardiopulmonary bypass, and the *hematocrit* of the patient-oxygenator system should be maintained between 20% and 30%. A low hematocrit during hypothermic perfusion theoretically provides optimal perfusion of the microcirculation by lowering blood viscosity; however, this advantage of hemodilution is balanced by an increase in extravascular extravasation of fluid as intravascular osmotic pressure decreases.

If the projected patient-oxygenator hematocrit is adequate, then an *asanguineous priming solution* is used. The *glucose concentration* of the priming solution is increased to provide an energy source and promote an osmotic diuresis. *Arterial oxygen levels* are maintained between 100 and 250 mm. Hg, while the *arterial carbon dioxide pressure* is maintained between 30 and 40 mm. Hg (measured at 37° C.).

Patient Variables

The body's physiologic response to CPB is extremely complex and only partially understood. The *systemic vascular resistance* falls abruptly with the onset of CPB. The patient's oxygen consumption and venous oxygen saturation are both partially controlled by the perfusion flow rate and the patient's temperature. It is generally assumed that the microcirculation is being effectively perfused if the mixed venous oxygen pressure during CPB is 30 to 40 mm. Hg. Extracellular fluid is increased after CPB. The magnitude of this increase is directly related to the duration of CPB and the degree of hemodilution.

DAMAGING EFFECTS OF CARDIOPULMONARY BYPASS

The vast majority of patients suffer no clinically apparent ill effects of CPB; however, an occasional patient develops sever multiorgan dysfunction despite an otherwise accurate cardiac repair. In its most severe form the *postperfusion syndrome* is characterized by a diffuse whole-body inflammatory reaction, with elements of increased capillary permeability, extravascular extravasation of plasma, increased interstitial fluid, leukocytosis, fever, peripheral vasoconstriction, breakdown of red blood cells, and a diffuse bleeding diathesis. Two risk factors for an adverse clinical response to CPB include *age* (very young and very old) and *duration of bypass* (sharply increased risk after 4 hours of CPB).

It is the *exposure to unphysiologic surfaces* that produces the greatest damage during CPB. The most critical surfaces are probably those of the oxygenating device. Exposure to the pump oxygenator promotes platelet aggregation, resulting in decreased platelet numbers and function after cardiopulmonary bypass. Platelet activation is probably mediated by fibrinogen adsorption to the surfaces of the oxygenator and tubing. Methods to attenuate postoperative bleeding by improving postbypass platelet function are being actively investigated.

The *humoral amplification system* is a complex system of plasma proteins that responds to a local stimulus with a self-perpetuating and expanding series of reactions. The components of the humoral amplification system include the *coagulation cascade*, the *fibrinolytic cascade*, the *kallikrein system*, and the *complement system*. We believe that the damaging effects of CPB are related in large degree to the humoral amplification system, which initiates a whole-body inflammatory response during CPB.

Complement activation is likely a key feature of CPB-induced inflammation and is important in neutrophil activation and degranulation during CPB. Studies have correlated cardiac, pulmonary, renal, and hematologic dysfunction after CPB, with higher levels of C3a after bypass, longer elapsed times of bypass, and younger age at operation.

CONDUCT OF CPB

After the patient is heparinized, cannulation of the venous and arterial circulations is achieved and CPB is initiated. After full CPB is established, the perfusion temperature may be decreased. The intracardiac portion of the operation is generally performed with the aorta cross-clamped and with cardioplegic-induced cardiac arrest. The precise perfusate temperature selected during cardioplegic arrest depends on the expected duration of the ischemic period as well as the anticipated needs for low perfusion rates or total circulatory arrest.

Approximately 5 minutes before removing the aortic cross-clamp, rewarming is initiated, and the flow rate is increased to 2.0 to 2.5 L. per min. per sq. m. The arterial line blood temperature should not exceed 39° C. to prevent heat damage to the blood elements. Air is evacuated from the cardiac chambers before the cross-clamp is removed. Suction is continued on the aortic needle vent until cardiopulmonary bypass is discontinued. When the cardiac action is vigorous, the venous line is partially occluded. This will elevate the left atrial pressure and promote effective cardiac action for debubbling the heart. Cardiopulmonary bypass is then gradually discontinued. Polyvinyl catheters are placed in the left and right atria to facilitate postoperative hemodynamic management, and atrial and ventricular temporary pacing wires are placed for postoperative pacing and arrhythmia management.

XXIV

Intra-Aortic Balloon Counterpulsation: Physiology, Indications, and Techniques

W. Randolph Chitwood, Jr., M.D.,
and Joseph R. Elbeery, M.D.

The intra-aortic balloon pump (IABP) is the circulatory assist device used most frequently. Balloon pumping results in concurrent diastolic coronary flow augmentation and systolic ventricular afterload reduction with mild preload reduction. These advantages often enable jeopardized myocardium to function more efficiently.

PHYSIOLOGIC EFFECTS OF INTRA-AORTIC BALLOON PUMPING

Intra-aortic balloon counterpulsation imparts multiple physiologic benefits on the impaired heart. Major determinants of myocardial oxygen consumption include pulse rate, transmural wall stress, and intrinsic contractile properties. The IABP

See the corresponding chapter or part in the *Textbook of Surgery*, 15th edition, pp. 2218–2228, for a more detailed discussion of this topic, including a comprehensive list of references.

has been shown to modify left ventricular ejection pressure by altering afterload. During periods of cardiac failure, increased ventricular dilatation and afterload result in augmented wall tension (stress). Maximal wall stress and oxygen requirements occur during isovolumic systole. Rapid collapse of the balloon reduces impedance to aortic flow by creating an instant "abyss" or void in aortic blood volume. The additive effects from this singular event usually decrease ventricular end-diastolic pressure and ischemia. Secondary benefits are decreased heart rate and diminished peripheral vascular resistance. In damaged hearts, most IABP benefits probably result from diastolic coronary flow augmentation. With ischemic myocardium, autoregulatory reserves generally are expended, with transmural flow becoming more pressure-dependent. Under these conditions, the IABP increases the diastolic driving pressure, reducing ventricular end-diastolic pressure concurrently and augmenting endocardial perfusion pressure significantly. Clinically, the diastolic pressure may be increased up to 90% by counterpulsation.

INDICATIONS FOR INTRA-AORTIC BALLOON PUMPING

The intra-aortic balloon pump is effective for treating *pharmacologically refractory angina* and enables angiography and angioplasty to be done more safely. At least 80% of patients obtain pain relief from balloon pumping. Survival in patients with medically refractory angina has been excellent using IABP support if followed by surgical revascularization. Although the benefits of intra-aortic balloon pumping during a myocardial infarction are controversial, coronary flow appears to be augmented effectively after successful thrombolysis or an emergent angioplasty.

Balloon pumping has been very helpful in weaning patients from cardiopulmonary bypass who have ventricular failure *following cardiotomy* (3% to 6%). These patients either had a severely damaged ventricle preoperatively and incurred additional ischemic injury or had good ventricular function and experienced profound intraoperative myocardial depression. Of patients requiring IABP insertion during cardiopulmonary bypass, 75% to 85% can be weaned effectively, and of these, 50% to 80% experience long-term survival. Specific guidelines have been established to aid in instituting balloon pumping following cardiac surgical operative procedures.

Following myocardial infarction, severe *acute mitral insufficiency,* and *acute ventricular septal defect,* or *intractable arrhythmias* may occur, and these patients often benefit from early IABP support. However, the salutary effects may be short-lived, and surgery should proceed rapidly. Most commonly, papillary muscle rupture or dysfunction results from an inferior myocardial infarction with resultant severe mitral insufficiency. The IABP decreases afterload and atrial shunting, augmenting left ventricular ejection. In approximately 60% of those with acute ventricular septal defects, rapid hemodynamic deterioration occurs. The combination of IABP support and early repair has decreased the operative mortality to as low as 30%. Long-term survival has been about 70%. IABP stabilization reduces left-to-right shunting, right ventricular failure, and pulmonary wedge pressure, effecting an increase in cardiac output and systemic pressure. Significant ventricular arrhythmias occur in 10% to 50% of patients following acute myocardial infarctions. Up to 55% may resolve following IABP institution. When ischemia is the etiology, placement of an IABP usually controls ventricular irritability. Ventricular aneurysms develop in up to 20% of patients following myocardial infarctions. Significant irritability may occur with acute aneurysms; however, only about 10% require surgical intervention to treat arrhythmias. Those having congestive failure or residual ischemia usually improve hemodynamically with the IABP.

For patients requiring emergent surgery because of a *failed angioplasty,* balloon counterpulsation provides optimal stabilization. This is especially important for complex angioplasty with multivessel coronary disease or markedly impaired ventricular function. Because of effective IABP stabilization, most patients can be revascularized emergently using the internal mammary artery instead of all vein grafts. More recently, the IABP has been used to support patients during complex three-vessel and left main coronary angioplasty.

The IABP is effective for treating end-stage cardiomyopathy patients while *awaiting cardiac transplantation,* and the importance of the method has increased with a declining donor heart supply. The IABP may provide sufficient afterload reduction to obviate the need for a more invasive left ventricular bridge or assist device.

CONTRAINDICATIONS TO BALLOON PUMPING

With severe *aortic insufficiency,* balloon pumping enhances valvular regurgitation. However, patients with minor degrees of insufficiency tolerate balloon pumping well. The presence of a thoracic or abdominal *aortic aneurysm* may be a relative contraindication. *Diffuse atherosclerosis* may preclude femoral artery insertion in 10% to 25% of patients. Newer guidewire methods as well as axillary artery and transthoracic introduction may now allow use in patients either with complicated aortoiliac disease or aneurysms.

INSERTION AND REMOVAL TECHNIQUES

The percutaneous method for IABP catheter insertion is used now for most patients. Currently, the smallest dual-lumen percutaneous catheter (70 cm. long) is No. 8.5 French (O.D.) and has a standard 40-ml. balloon. After obtaining pulsatile flow from a common femoral artery needle puncture, a guidewire is passed to above the iliac bifurcation. A vessel dilator and introducer sheath are passed sequentially, with the balloon catheter introduced over the wire until the tip is positioned just distal to the left subclavian artery. Sheathless insertion has helped reduce limb ischemia. Although required infrequently, femoral surgical insertion techniques may become necessary. These catheters either are inserted through a 10-mm. Dacron/PTFE graft, sewn to the femoral artery, or inserted directly into the artery with suture hemostasis. To allow patient mobility, balloon catheters can be inserted via the axillary artery and passed retrograde into the descending aorta. When aortoiliac disease precludes retrograde insertion during surgery, the transthoracic approach has been helpful. Extremity pulses, color, and temperature, as well as motor and sensory activity, should be assessed frequently. Although anticoagulation should be avoided immediately after surgery, in general patients should be heparinized while the IABP catheter is in place.

For balloon removal, heparin should be stopped 6 hours in advance, with a platelet count and coagulation factors determined. Surgical balloons may be removed in the intensive care unit under the appropriate sterile technique. Balloons must be evacuated completely prior to removal to reduce catheter size. Following withdrawal of percutaneous balloons, groin pressure should be applied constantly for 30 minutes, with the distal pulses monitored either by palpation or Doppler ultrasound. Transthoracic and axillary catheters usually require return to the operating room for removal.

COMPLICATIONS

Major complications of IABP usage include *limb ischemia* from primary thrombosis, emboli, or vascular dissection; intra-abdominal and intrathoracic *hemorrhage* from perforation and/or dissection; groin *hematomas; lymph drainage;* femoral artery *false aneurysms;* local *wound infections;* systemic *sepsis; renal failure* and *bowel infarction* from balloon malposition; *thrombocytopenia and hemolysis; device malfunction* in dependent patients; and *neurologic complications,* including paraplegia. Between 2% and 10% require vascular repair, including either patch angioplasty or femoral-femoral bypass grafting. The incidence of major IABP complications has been reported to be higher with percutaneous balloon catheters. In most situations, ischemic complications can be obviated by early removal, sheathless insertion, or partial withdrawal of the introducer sheath. The time period of counterpulsation, presence and degree of vascular disease, and female sex appear to be the most significant determinants of vascular complications. Although the total number of complications has remained stable over the last 10 years, the severity of complications and death rate have decreased significantly.

TIMING OF COUNTERPULSATION AND WEANING

Balloon inflation can be timed from either a peripheral or direct ventricular electrogram, radial arterial catheter, or the IABP central pressure channel. Since inflation delays (50 to 120 msec.) may occur using peripheral catheters, central aortic pressure seems preferable. Malpositioned sensing electrodes, radial artery spasm, arrhythmias, pacing, and electrocautery interference can cause timing problems. The IABP should inflate 40 msec. before the dicrotic notch (ascending T wave) and deflate during early isovolumic contraction (after P wave). Total deflation must occur before ejection (R wave). Significant decreases in aortic systolic and end-diastolic pressures usually occur. Early inflation results in premature aortic valve closure with reduced stroke volume, and late inflation causes inadequate diastolic pressure augmentation. Early deflation effects poor afterload reduction, and late deflation impedes systole with increased cardiac work.

Many surgeons prefer to wean the majority of inotropic medications before withdrawal of the IABP. Inotropic and vasopressor drugs should be minimal (i.e. dopamine < 5 μg. per kg. per min.) before establishing a 1:2 pumping ratio. The inflation ratio and remaining cardiotonic drugs then are weaned simultaneously.

Transport of Balloon Pump Patients

The development of mobile intensive care units and specially equipped helicopters has made transport of patients with balloon pumps in place safe and effective. In many centers, transport of balloon pump–dependent patients from another hospital is routine, since accurate in-transit monitoring has become standard for mobile ICU care.

XXV

The Artificial Heart
William S. Pierce, M.D.

The concept of replacement of the human heart by miniature artificial ventricles came about in the late 1950s. The first experimental work was performed by William Kolff, the developer of the artificial kidney. The first artificial hearts to work successfully in experimental animals were pneumatically powered hearts with separate left and right ventricles. Each ventricle employs a valved diaphragm or sack-type pump and a pneumatic air port that leads outside the chest to a valved air compressor. Cardiac outputs of 8 L. per min. of air can be realized, and inlet and outlet pressures can be maintained within the physiologic range. Artificial heart implantation is performed in much the same manner that a heart transplant is performed.

In the early 1980s it became apparent that a significant

See the corresponding chapter or part in the *Textbook of Surgery,* 15th edition, pp. 2228–2232, for a more detailed discussion of this topic, including a comprehensive list of references.

number of patients who may be transplant candidates die before a suitable donor heart is identified. The concept of using the artificial heart as a "bridge" to heart transplantation was developed. Accordingly, to date, over 200 artificial hearts have been used as a bridge to transplantation. The most commonly used device has been the Jarvik-7 or Jarvik-70 artificial heart manufactured by Symbion, Inc. The Symbion artificial heart has been shown to adequately support the circulation, but complications, including thromboembolism and infection, have been frequent. Overall, approximately 40% of patients who underwent artificial heart implantation were subsequently discharged from hospital having had a successful heart transplantation. In 1989, Symbion, Inc., closed. During the past several years, the remnants of the Symbion Company were reconstituted into CardioWest Technologies, Inc. Thirty-five pneumatic artificial hearts of the CardioWest design have now been implanted in patients with improved results. However, most surgeons favor the use of left or biventricular support as a bridging technique for heart transplantation.

In 1983, Dr. William DeVries, then of the University of Utah, believed that the Jarvik artificial heart was suitable for "permanent" heart replacement. A pneumatic artificial heart was implanted in Dr. Barney Clark, whose heart disease and medical condition did not allow cardiac transplantation. While Dr. Clark only lived 112 days with the artificial heart, the device functioned satisfactorily and allowed him to be ambulatory for a period of time. While Dr. DeVries implanted pneumatic hearts in several other patients as permanent devices, problems of thromboembolism, infection associated with the percutaneous drive lines, and the requirement for a bulky power unit have relegated the use of the pneumatic artificial heart for permanent heart substitution to historical considerations only.

About one decade ago, development of an artificial heart that was powered by an implanted electric motor was begun. This motor can actuate a pusher plate–type blood pump or can pressurize a hydraulic fluid which, by hydraulic valve orientation, will alternately pump the left and right ventricles. Much of the information developed for blood pump design and control systems for the pneumatic artificial hearts has been applicable to the electric devices. The implanted artificial heart has, in addition to the implanted energy converter, an electronic control system, a small implanted battery that will allow the device to run from 30 to 45 minutes without any type of external energy, and in most designs a small compliance chamber (a gas-filled chamber that minimizes pressure changes in the gas surrounding the pumping chambers). High-frequency electrical energy is transmitted across the chest by inductive coupling (the transformer principle). Accordingly, a battery-energized flat coil (the primary coil) is positioned over a secondary coil that is positioned just beneath the skin. Energy transmission by inductive coupling has eliminated the need for any percutaneous tubes or wires. With this system, animals have survived over a year (electric motor pusher plate system) and for 3 to 4 months (hydraulic system).

At the present time, three groups in the United States are performing extensive mock circulatory loop and animal testing of these hearts. At the current rate of development, it appears that by the year 2000, Food and Drug Administration (FDA) approval will have been obtained for these devices to permit initial clinical evaluation.

INDEX

Note: Page numbers followed by the letter t refer to tables.